DIAGNOSTIC IMAGING OF INFANTS AND CHILDREN

Volume II

Cranium and Brain

Spine

Extracranial Head and Neck

DIAGNOSTIC IMAGING OF INFANTS AND CHILDREN

DIAGNOSTIC IMAGING OF INFANTS AND CHILDREN

Volume II

Cranium and Brain

Spine

Extracranial Head and Neck

Robert J. Starshak, MD
Robert G. Wells, MD
John R. Sty, MD
David C. Gregg, MD
Children's Hospital of Wisconsin
Milwaukee, Wisconsin

AN ASPEN PUBLICATION®
Aspen Publishers, Inc.
Gaithersburg, Maryland
1992

Library of Congress Cataloging-in-Publication Data
(Revised for vol. 2)

Diagnostic imaging of infants and children.

Includes bibliographical references and indexes.
Context: v. 1. Genitourinary system, gastrointestinal system, liver, pancreas, and spleen—v. 2.
Cranium and brain, spine, extracranial head and neck.
1. Pediatric diagnostic imaging. I. Sty, John R.
[DNLM: 1. Diagnostic Imaging—in infancy & childhood.
WN 200 D5363]
RJ51.D5D53 1991
618.92' 00754
91-18267
ISBN: 0-8342-0257-3 (v. 2)

The authors have made every effort to ensure the accuracy of the information herein, particularly with regard
to drug selection and dose. However, appropriate information sources should be consulted, especially for new
or unfamiliar drugs or procedures. It is the responsibility of every practitioner to evaluate the appropriateness
of a particular opinion in the context of actual clinical situations and with due consideration to new
developments. Authors, editors, and the publisher cannot be held responsible for any typographical or other
errors found in this book.

Editorial Services: Jane Coyle Garwood

Library of Congress Catalog Card Number: 91-18267
ISBN: 0-8342-0257-3

Printed in the United States of America

1 2 3 4 5

Table of Contents

Preface

Radiologists and clinicians involved in the care of neonates, children, and adolescents are frequently faced with the dilemma of determining the most accurate, least invasive, and most compassionate diagnostic approach that can document a specific disease or establish a useful differential diagnosis. A variety of factors are involved in this process. Continual changes in imaging technology and the rapidly expanding wealth of information in the medical literature challenge the ability of physicians to remain current on the clinical, diagnostic, therapeutic, and scientific aspects of pediatric diseases. This burgeoning knowledge base is at least in part responsible for the ever-increasing tendency to fragment clinical and radiologic practice into smaller and smaller subspecialities. The medical literature also has become fragmented so that medical professionals must turn to an increasing number of sources to stay abreast of pertinent information in their own fields and in related fields.

The appropriate selection, performance, and interpretation of diagnostic imaging procedures in pediatrics require not only a thorough knowledge of the principles of imaging procedures but also an understanding of pertinent clinical factors. This correlation is particularly important in pediatrics because the types of diseases and the manifestations of specific diseases may change greatly according to a patient's age. Because of this, the correlation of data from imaging studies with clinical findings is mandatory for the appropriate practice of pediatric radiology.

In addition, a basic understanding of the capabilities and limitations of the expanding armamentarium of imaging modalities is essential for clinicians involved in the care of children. Technical considerations and the health status of the child must be weighed by both radiologists and clinicians in selecting an approach to evaluate diseases in different age groups. In many cases dissimilar imaging modalities can be used to provide similar diagnostic information. The expertise of individual radiologists with specific imaging modalities and the availability of imaging equipment at individual institutions will influence the selection of imaging techniques.

We developed this text to present concisely the pertinent clinical features and imaging characteristics of pediatric diseases. Findings from the use of standard radiographs, sonography, computed tomography, magnetic resonance imaging, and nuclear medicine imaging are described for every disease addressed. The interrelationships among the various imaging modalities and clinical findings are stressed. Where appropriate, the embryology, pathology, and physiology of disease processes are also reviewed.

Diagnostic Imaging of Infants and Children is divided into three volumes, each of which contains three chapters arranged according to organ system. Volume I addresses the genitourinary tract; the gastrointestinal tract; and the liver, pancreas, and spleen. Volume II deals with the cranium and brain; the spine; and the extracranial head and neck. Volume III focuses on the cardiovascular system; the chest; and the musculoskeletal system. Within each chapter, diseases are grouped according to major etiologic categories: developmental, infectious, inflammatory, traumatic, neoplastic, vascular, and metabolic. Representative illustrations of imaging findings are included wherever appropriate.

The information in this text was accumulated from our collective personal experience and from current information in the medical literature. Virtually all important pediatric diseases whose management involves diagnostic imaging studies are included. While this information will be most useful for pediatric radiologists, this text is also intended to be a valuable resource for general radiologists, radiologists in training, and clinicians involved in the care of children.

Acknowledgments

We wish to extend our sincere thanks to all who aided us in the preparation of this work. Thanks go to Gary Colpaert and the entire technical staff of the Department of Radiology of Children's Hospital of Wisconsin for their valuable assistance in producing the images used. Special thanks are extended to Molly Youngkin and Jean Jolliffe of the Todd Wehr Library of the Medical College of Wisconsin for their valuable assistance in verifying the references. Beth Gregg also provided valuable assistance in verifying the references. The illustrations were produced by the Department of Audiovisual Services of Children's Hospital of Wisconsin. Our thanks go to Dean Van Hoogen and his staff, Walter Earhart, Arnold (Ted) Heyel, Debi Mortl, Jeff Surges, and Betty Terry for the consistently excellent quality of the figures. Several line drawings were produced by Edith Wells, to whom we express our thanks. The editorial and publishing expertise of Aspen Publishers, Inc., especially that of Jack Bruggeman, Jane Coyle Garwood, and Deborah B. Leser, is clearly evident on every page of this text. Our undying gratitude is extended to Shirley Laszewski, who typed the many drafts of the manuscript of this text. Without her expertise and assistance, it would not exist.

Chapter 1

The Cranium and Its Contents

CONGENITAL ANOMALIES AND MALFORMATIONS

Congenital Lesions of the Skull

Development of the Skull

Development of the skeletal system begins during gestation week 3. Mesenchyma derived from the mesoderm forms fibroblasts, chondroblasts, and osteoblasts. The flat surface bones of the calvaria ossify directly from mesenchymal tissue (membranous ossification) to form the cranial vault; this portion of the skull is termed the membranocranium. The smaller bones of the base of the skull and the inferior portion of the occipital bone change from mesenchyma to cartilage before ossification begins (enchondral ossification); these bones make up the chondrocranium. The membranocranium (calvaria) and the chondrocranium encase the brain and together make up the neurocranium. The viscerocranium comprises the remaining bones of the skull and face. These are partly derived from neural crest cells in the cephalic region of the growing embryo. The base of the skull, including the foramen magnum, develops in a relatively complex process of enchondral ossification from numerous centers and is therefore more prone to developmental defects than the membranocranium.

In the fetus and infant, the membranous (flat) bones of the skull are joined together by connective tissue at the sagittal, coronal, lambdoidal, metopic, and squamosal sutures. The anterior fontanelle is the intersection of the metopic, coronal, and sagittal sutures. The anterior fontanelle normally closes between 6 and 20 months of age. The posterior fontanelle is the junction of the lambdoidal and sagittal sutures. It closes by the age of 3 months.

Numerous developmental variations can occur in the skull, the majority of which are of no clinical significance. Wormian bones are accessory bones that occur in the sutures, especially in the lambdoidal suture. Most often these are a normal variation, but multiple wormian bones can be identified in a number of developmental disorders (Table 1-1).

Lacunar Skull

Lacunar skull (craniolacuna or lückenschädel) is characterized by defective ossification of the cranial vault. Only the membranous portions of the calvaria are involved. This abnormality occurs in newborn infants who have spina bifida or other major structural anomalies of the central nervous system. Lacunar skull is a developmental anomaly; it does not reflect elevated intracranial pressure. This abnormality generally resolves within the first 6 months of life.

Lacunar skull is demonstrated on radiographs and bone window computed tomography (CT) as poor mineralization of the membranous calvaria with a soap-bubble pattern of rarefaction. The findings are usually most pronounced in the parietal and frontal squamosa, with lesser involvement of the occipital squamosa being seen. The enchondral portion of the skull is normal (Fig. 1-1).

Sinus Pericranii

Sinus pericranii is a rare vascular anomaly in which there is an abnormally large communication between the intracranial and extracranial venous circulations. This results in an extra-

Table 1-1 Conditions Associated with Multiple Wormian Bones

Normal variant
Cleidocranial dysplasia
Hypophosphatasia
Hypothyroidism
Menkes (kinky-hair) syndrome
Pyknodysostosis
Osteogenesis imperfecta

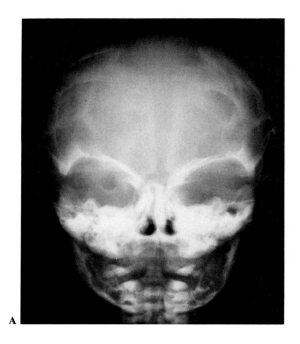

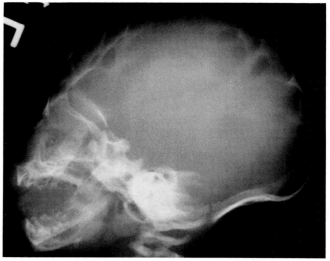

B

Fig. 1-1 Lacunar skull. **(A)** Anteroposterior (AP) and **(B)** lateral skull radiographs demonstrate poor mineralization of the membranous calvaria in the parietal and frontal regions. The typical soap-bubble pattern of lacunar skull (craniolacunia) is present. This infant had a lumbar myelomeningocele.

cranial mass of dilated vascular structures. The mass is soft and easily compressible. Variation in size is observed with the changes in venous pressure that occur with crying, with the Valsalva maneuver, or with the patient assuming a head-down position.

The etiology of sinus pericranii is unknown in most cases. A developmental etiology is most common. Secondary post-traumatic forms have also been reported. Sinus pericranii is most often identified in children and young adults. There is a 2:1 male predominance.

Sinus pericranii is demonstrated radiographically as an oval radiolucency in the calvaria. The lesion is most often located in the frontal or parietal regions. Bilateral lesions may occur; radiographically, these may mimic parietal foramina.

A definitive diagnosis of sinus pericranii is provided by angiography, magnetic resonance imaging (MRI), or CT. The lesion is of slightly higher attenuation than brain on unenhanced CT and enhances in concert with the intracranial venous structures after intravenous contrast material administration. Nonenhancing areas due to thrombus may be present. Bone window images show that the vascular structure passes through an osseous defect that has well-defined margins.

Spin-echo T_1-weighted MRI of sinus pericranii usually shows a mixed signal character with signal voids due to rapidly flowing blood and areas of moderate signal intensity due to stagnant blood or clot. Slow-flowing blood produces high signal intensity on T_2-weighted images. The lesion demonstrates marked enhancement with paramagnetic contrast material. One or more areas of communication between the extracranial mass and the intracranial venous structures are usually demonstrable on MRI.[1,2]

Parietal Foramina

Parietal foramina are ossification defects in the parietal squamosa. They vary in size from a few millimeters to several centimeters. The defects are symmetric and are located on either side of the sagittal suture (Fig. 1-2). If sufficiently large, they may be palpable. Parietal foramina are transmitted as an autosomal dominant trait. They are of no clinical significance.

Craniosynostosis

Craniosynostosis is the result of premature fusion of one or numerous cranial sutures. Both primary and secondary forms of craniosynostosis occur. The exact etiology of primary craniosynostosis is unknown but may be related to an abnormality of the mesenchymal layer of the ossification centers in the calvaria. The process of premature sutural closure usually begins in utero. A primary pathologic bony defect restricts normal bone growth and causes a variable degree of deformity of the skull and face. This may in turn limit brain growth and cause secondary neurologic deficits.

Most cases of craniosynostosis are sporadic and occur without associated anomalies. The incidence has been reported to be approximately 5 in 10,000 live births. There is a 3:1 male

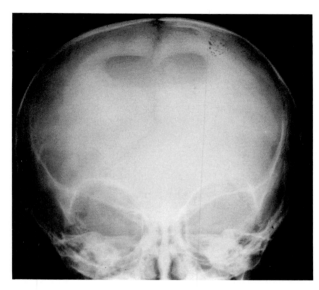

Fig. 1-2 Frontal skull radiograph demonstrating bilateral parietal foramina. The symmetric ossification defects are located on each side of the sagittal suture and have smooth, well-defined margins.

predominance. Approximately 2% to 8% of cases of isolated craniosynostosis are familial.

Secondary forms of craniosynostosis may be produced by intracranial pathology. Normal development of the skull depends on adequate brain growth. Deficient brain growth, such as occurs in microcephaly or after surgical shunting of severe hydrocephalus, may result in secondary premature closure of cranial sutures. Craniosynostosis may also occur in association with hematologic disorders that cause bone marrow hyperplasia, endogenous or exogenous hyperthyroidism, and abnormalities of calcium and phosphorus metabolism such as rickets, hypercalcemia, and hypophosphatasia.

Craniosynostosis is also associated with various genetic and sporadic craniofacial syndromes. These include Crouzon disease and Apert, Saethre-Chotzen, Carpenter, and Pfeiffer syndromes. These have extracranial manifestations such as syndactyly, polydactyly, dysmorphic facial appearance, midfacial hypoplasia, a beaklike nose, and proptosis. Common to all these syndromes is bilateral coronal and basal skull synostosis.

Normal growth of the skull occurs perpendicular to each of the sutures. If one suture is fused before birth or early during infancy, compensatory growth occurs parallel to the fused suture or across the nonunited sutures. This results in an abnormal head shape that is characteristic of the specific suture involved. More complex abnormalities of head shape and size occur if multiple sutures are closed. The most severe of these is the cloverleaf skull malformation (kleeblattschädel).

Craniosynostosis is classified according to the suture that is involved. Sagittal synostosis refers to premature fusion of the sagittal suture. It is the most common form of craniosynostosis, accounting for approximately 60% of all cases. The great majority of these patients are boys. The defect may be inherited. Sagittal synostosis results in elongation of the calvaria and a decrease in the transverse diameter of the skull; this is termed scaphocephaly. The abnormal head shape is usually recognizable at birth. There is a palpable ridge over the closed sagittal suture. These patients are neurologically normal. Sagittal craniosynostosis should not be confused with the elongation of the calvaria that commonly occurs in premature infants as a result of positional molding.

Radiographically, sagittal craniosynostosis is demonstrated as marked elongation of the skull in the anteroposterior dimension. The sagittal suture is sclerotic (Fig. 1-3). A midline ridge of bone is frequently identifiable on tangential views.

Coronal synostosis represents approximately 20% of cases of craniosynostosis. This type is more common in girls. If both

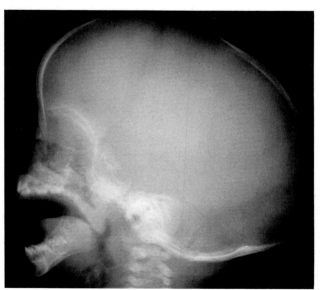

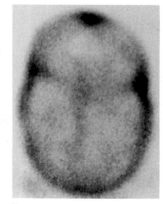

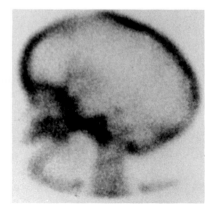

Fig. 1-3 Sagittal craniosynostosis. (**A**) Lateral radiograph demonstrates elongation of the skull. The sagittal suture is sclerotic, indicating sagittal craniosynostosis. The coronal and lambdoidal sutures are normal in appearance. (**B**) Vertex and (**C**) lateral images from bone scintigraphy demonstrate prominent activity in the region of the sagittal suture, indicating that sutural closure is occurring. There is less prominent uptake in the normal coronal and lambdoidal sutures.

A   B   C

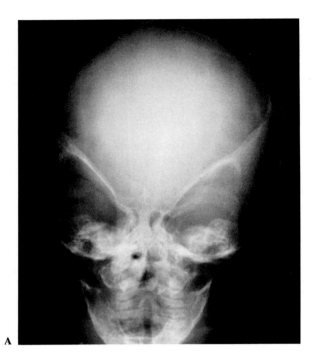

A

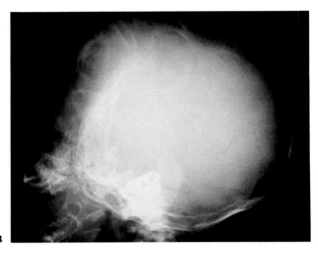

B

Fig. 1-4 Coronal craniosynostosis. **(A)** Frontal and **(B)** lateral radiographs show sclerosis of both coronal sutures and undergrowth of the frontal bones. The anterior cranial fossa is shallow and foreshortened, and the lambda is elevated. The skull is brachycephalic. The frontal view shows the typical elliptic appearance of the orbits that is due to bilateral coronal synostosis.

coronal sutures close, the skull is short in the anteroposterior dimension and is widened in its transverse diameter (brachycephaly). The occiput and forehead are flattened. The anterior fontanelle is displaced anteriorly. Ridges may be palpable over the prematurely closed coronal sutures.

Radiographically, the anterior cranial fossa appears shallow and foreshortened in cases of bilateral coronal synostosis. The anterior fontanelle is displaced anteriorly, and the lambda is higher than usual. The upper-outer margins of the orbits have an elliptical appearance on frontal views. The coronal sutures appear sclerotic (Fig. 1-4).[3]

Premature closure of multiple cranial sutures results in the cloverleaf skull malformation. This is demonstrated radiographically as sclerosis and fusion of the coronal, lambdoidal, and sagittal sutures. Excessive growth occurs in the squamosal regions. The cranium becomes markedly misshapen. The orbits are shallow, causing severe exophthalmos (Fig. 1-5).

Plagiocephaly

Plagiocephaly describes an asymmetric skull. This deformity is nonspecific and can be produced by a number of types of synostosis. Unilateral closure of a coronal suture, a lambdoid suture, or both will result in an asymmetric skull. With unilateral coronal synostosis the orbit is elliptic (harlequin eye appearance), and the anterior fontanelle is displaced toward the side of the closed suture (Fig. 1-6). With unilateral lambdoid synostosis, the ipsilateral ear is displaced anteriorly. The contralateral frontal bone is larger than the ipsilateral frontal bone, and the occipital bones manifest similar but contralateral asymmetry. This causes the shape of the cranium to be skewed, resembling a parallelogram.

Trigonocephaly

Trigonocephaly is the result of premature closure of the metopic suture. This results in a pointed forehead and a prominent ridge in the midline. There is relative hypotelorism. The forehead is narrow, and the anterior skull appears triangular when viewed from above. Some patients with trigonocephaly have related abnormalities such as cleft palate, orbital coloboma, anomalies of the urinary tract, and holoprosencephaly.

Oxycephaly

Oxycephaly is the result of premature closure of both the coronal and the sagittal sutures. The skull is excessively high and narrow, producing a tower shape. Oxycephaly may cause increased intracranial pressure and can have significant neurologic sequelae. Some patients also have choanal atresia. The internal auditory canals are frequently narrowed, causing auditory and vestibular disturbances.[4]

Craniotubular Bone Modeling Disorders

Significant abnormalities of the skull occur with various skeletal dysplasias (Table 1-2). In general, these disorders are

Table 1-2 Craniotubular Bone Modeling Disorders

Craniometaphyseal dysplasia
Craniodiaphyseal dysplasia
Osteopetrosis
Sclerosteosis (osteopetrosis with syndactyly)
Generalized cortical hyperostosis

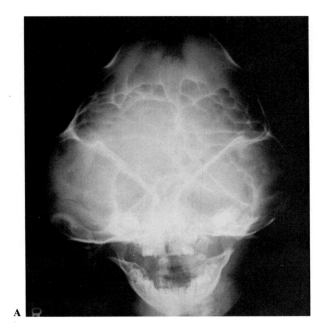

A

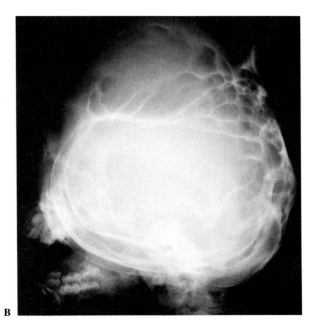

B

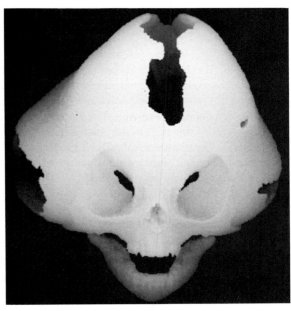

C

Fig. 1-5 Cloverleaf skull. (**A**) Frontal and (**B**) lateral radiographs show severe deformity of the skull. The temporal squamosa bulge laterally and anteriorly, and the parietal bones bulge superiorly. The coronal, lambdoidal, and most of the sagittal sutures are fused. There are prominent internal ridges throughout the majority of the calvaria. (**C**) Three-dimensional CT re-formation (anterior view) shows the severe calvarial deformity of cloverleaf skull. There is marked bulging and thinning of the temporal squamosa. The orbits are markedly shallow.

the result of a disequilibrium between the processes of bone formation and bone resorption, leading to defective modeling and remodeling of bone.[5] In the presence of severe hyperostosis, especially of the skull base, neurologic symptoms often occur; these include cranial nerve deficits, brainstem compression, and elevated intracranial pressure.[6]

Craniometaphyseal Dysplasia. Craniometaphyseal dysplasia is a rare hereditary condition with features that overlap with those of metaphyseal dysplasia. Clinically, these patients are taller than average for their age. The tubular bones are palpably enlarged. If the calvaria is extensively involved, encroachment on neural structures may cause diminution of visual acuity, progressive deafness, and cranial nerve palsies.

Radiographically, children with craniometaphyseal dysplasia demonstrate flaring and lack of tubulation of the long bones. The cortex in the area of flaring is relatively thin, but elsewhere the cortex is of normal thickness. The cranium is markedly involved, with the changes being most dramatic at the skull base. There is diffuse, marked thickening of the bones that leads to progressive compression of the neural foramina. The calvaria is diffusely thickened, although the portions of the neurocranium composed of enchondral bone are more severely affected than the membranous portions (Fig. 1-7).[7–9]

Osteopetrosis. Osteopetrosis is a rare disease of defective bone resorption that results in generalized bone sclerosis and fragility. The basic defect is failure of absorption of the primary spongiosa during the process of enchondral ossification, probably resulting from impaired lysosomal function of osteoclasts and monocytes, their precursor cells. There is bone formation by osteoblasts but without the dynamic remodeling and resorption of bone by osteoclasts. This results in bone sclerosis and thickening and obliteration of the medullary spaces.[10]

There are two forms of osteopetrosis. One is transmitted as an autosomal recessive trait and the other as an autosomal dominant trait. The autosomal recessive (infantile or congenital) type presents with signs of constriction of cranial

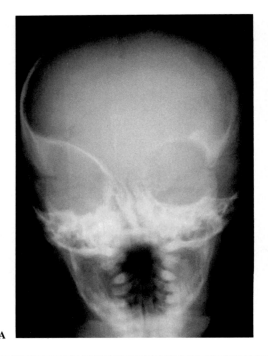

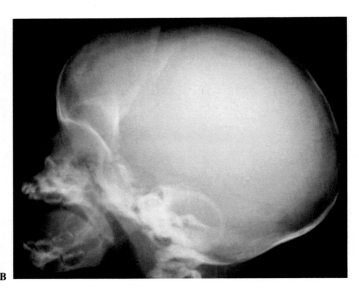

Fig. 1-6 Coronal craniosynostosis. **(A)** Frontal and **(B)** lateral radiographs showing sclerosis of the right coronal suture. The frontal view shows the typical harlequin eye appearance of the right orbit, which is due to unilateral coronal synostosis.

neural foramina, pathologic fractures, and compromised bone marrow function with anemia, thrombocytopenia, hepatosplenomegaly, and increased susceptibility to infection. Infants with autosomal recessive osteopetrosis often have optic atrophy. The overgrowth of bone may also compromise the carotid canals and the jugular foramina.[11] The autosomal

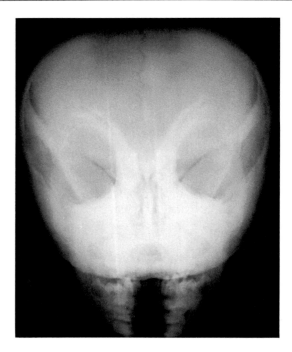

Fig. 1-7 Craniometaphyseal dysplasia. Frontal radiograph demonstrates severe thickening of the skull base and less marked thickening of the calvaria. There is marked narrowing of the orbital fissures.

dominant (tarda) type usually presents later in life than the recessive variety. These patients mainly have pathologic fractures and defective dentition.

Radiographically, osteopetrosis is demonstrated as a diffuse increase in the density of the skeleton. The cortices of the long bones are thickened, frequently to the point where the marrow space disappears. Persistence of calcified cartilage in the marrow space causes a unique bone-within-bone appearance. The lack of osteoclastic activity results in undertubulation of the bones. The metaphyseal ends may become clublike. Cranial involvement is demonstrated as amorphous thickening and sclerosis of the skull base. This results in narrowing of the neural foramina. The membranous calvaria is not involved.[12]

Achondroplasia. Achondroplasia is a bone dysplasia that consists of short stature, dysmorphic features, congenital skeletal abnormalities, and neurologic impairment. It is the most common skeletal dysplasia, occurring in 1 in 25,000 live births. Achondroplasia entails abnormal enchondral ossification. In the skull, only the base of the skull, which forms from enchondral ossification, is directly involved. There is a compensatory increase in the growth of the membranous bones of the cranial vault. Clinically, patients with achondroplasia have short stature, a prominent bulging forehead, macrocephaly, and a trident hand. The condition is transmitted as an autosomal dominant trait, although approximately 80% of cases are new mutations.

Radiographs in cases of achondroplasia show a constricted appearance of the base of the skull. The foramen magnum and the jugular foramina are extremely small. The shortness of the skull base may lead to compression of the basal cisternae, reduction in the volume of the posterior fossa, and compression of the medulla at the foramen magnum (Fig. 1-8). Many

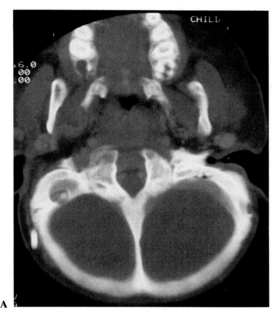
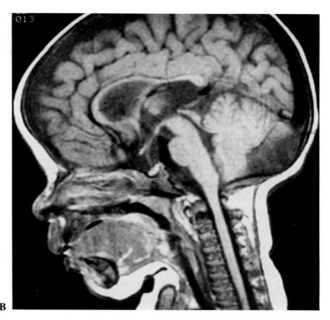

Fig. 1-8 Achondroplasia. (**A**) CT scan demonstrates marked narrowing of the foramen magnum. (**B**) Sagittal MR scan shows marked narrowing of the subarachnoid space at the level of the foramen magnum. There is also elevation of the base of the occipital bone, resulting in a small posterior fossa and causing an impression on the inferior aspect of the cerebellum.

patients with achondroplasia develop hydrocephalus. The exact cause of hydrocephalus in these cases is unknown, although many mechanisms have been postulated. These include aqueductal stenosis, osseous compression of the fourth ventricle or medullary foramina, and elevated intracranial venous pressure due to bilateral jugular vein compression.[13]

Congenital Malformations of the Brain and Meninges

Development of the Central Nervous System

The pathogenesis of malformations of the central nervous system is incompletely understood. The development of the central nervous system is complex; the process is of long duration, extending from the early formation of the neural tube in the second week of fetal life to the fully formed brain and spinal cord in the perinatal period and beyond. Therefore, a disorder of central nervous system organogenesis can lead to a wide variety of cerebral malformations. The great majority of morphologic anomalies are due to a developmental alteration that initially becomes manifest during the 8 weeks of the embryonic stage of development. In general, the earlier the disorder occurs, the more severe the malformation will be. The normal development of the central nervous system can be classified into four stages: neurulation, ventriculocisternal development, cell proliferation, and neuronal migration. Malformations may result from developmental alterations during any of these stages.

Primary Inductive Process (Neurulation). The primary inductive process (neurulation) begins in embryonic week 2, when mesoderm induces the overlying ectoderm to form the neural plate. During week 3, the mesoderm induces the neural plate to form the forebrain and the foregut entoderm to form the face. The lateral margins of the neural plate form the neural tube by fusion dorsally, beginning in the primitive cervical region. Failure of dorsal neural tube fusion results in dysraphisms such as anencephaly, cephalomeningocele, meningocele, Arnold-Chiari malformation with spinal rachischisis, and other conditions.

During week 4, the prosencephalic, metencephalic, and rhombencephalic vesicles develop from the anterior end of the neural tube. During week 5, the telencephalon and diencephalon develop from the line of dorsal fusion of the prosencephalon. The telencephalon expands laterally to form the cerebral hemispheres. Failure of the mesoderm to interact with the entoderm and ectoderm prevents bilateral expansion of the telencephalon and normal formation of the diencephalon. This may result in holoprosencephaly and midline facial anomalies such as cyclopia.

During week 6, the commissural plate is formed medially from the telencephalon as a primitive form of the corpus callosum. Disturbances in formation of the commissural plate produce the various forms of dysgenesis of the corpus callosum.

Ventriculocisternal Development (Diverticulation). During week 7 of embryonic development, the choroid plexus appears and begins to secrete cerebrospinal fluid into the primitive ventricular system. During week 8, the caudal end of the fourth ventricle perforates, and cerebral spinal fluid penetrates the primitive leptomeninges (meninx primitiva) to form the subarachnoid space. Disturbances in the development of the subarachnoid space may lead to arachnoid cysts or communicating hydrocephalus. Alterations during this stage also produce hydrocephalus with Arnold-Chiari malformation and hydrocephalus due to aqueductal stenosis.

Cell Proliferation. During weeks 3 through 6 of embryonic development, undifferentiated cells in the primitive ependymal zone that borders the embryonic ventricular system proliferate to become neuroblasts. Disturbances in this process of cell proliferation may result in cerebellar hypoplasia or Dandy-Walker malformation. The phakomatoses are due to abnormal proliferation of cell populations during this stage. Proliferation of perineural fibroblasts occurs with neurofibromatosis, proliferation of astrocytes occurs with tuberous sclerosis, and proliferation of endothelial cells occurs with Sturge-Weber syndrome.

Neuronal Migration. Neuroblasts migrate laterally from the periventricular region to form the mantle zone, which is a primitive form of the basal ganglia. Neurons send out processes to form the cell-poor marginal zone, which is a primitive form of hemispheric white matter. During week 7, neuroblasts make a second migration across the marginal zone to form the cortical plate, which is a primitive form of cortical gray matter. Symmetric failure of cell migration produces hydranencephaly and schizencephaly. Asymmetric migration results in porencephaly. Failure of neuroblasts to reach their final location produces heterotopy of gray matter. During week 20, the cortical plate thickens to form primary sulci. Disturbances in the formation of the sulci produce lissencephaly, pachygyria, and polymicrogyria. Secondary sulci normally develop between weeks 24 and 40, and tertiary sulci develop from weeks 36 to 60.

The cellular maturation of the central nervous system consists of neuronal and glial cell multiplication and maturation in germinal centers with subsequent migration to remote areas. This process culminates in the columnar organization in the mature cortex, complex synaptic organization, programmed cellular death, and myelination. The number of neurons at birth is approximately 100 billion, and there is little increase in that number after birth. The rate of neuron production during fetal development is estimated to be approximately 250,000 per minute. At birth, the brain contains approximately 1 trillion glial cells.

In the developing brain, cells migrate outward from a periventricular location in the germinal matrix to four basic embryonic zones in the cortical plate. These zones are as follows, from deep to superficial: ventricular, containing the proliferating cells that become neurons; subventricular, containing cells that give rise to neurons and macroglia; intermediate, which is the afferent axon region; and marginal, which is the outermost layer. The cortical plate forms the mature six-layered cerebral cortex between the intermediate and marginal zones.

The process of transformation of the cortical plate into neocortex involves several developmental stages. In fetal week 7, neuroblasts migrate superficially to establish the cortical plate. The plate thickens, condenses, and separates from the intermediate zone. The intermediate zone contains numerous fibers. There are two periods of cell migration. The first extends through fetal week 11, and the second is completed by week 13. The arrangement of neurons in the cortical plate is columnar or vertical. This cellular arrangement in the neocortex is predetermined by centrifugal migration of cells. Immature neurons are guided to a location in the distant cortex by radially oriented glial fibers. On reaching the level of the cortical plate, the neurons become aligned in a single vertical column with an inside-out pattern. Each neuron that follows a given radial guide will settle external to its predecessor. Eventually, the radially elongated glial cells disappear, probably becoming transformed into astrocytes.

Myelination. The process of myelination begins at about gestation month 5 with the myelination of the cranial nerves. It progresses in an orderly fashion. The process of myelination nears completion at about 2 years of age, although some myelination continues until early adulthood. Because myelin contains considerable amounts of lipid, the process of myelination alters the MR appearance of the brain, especially during the first 2 years of life.

At birth, some myelination can be seen in portions of the brainstem, the cerebellum, the posterior limbs of the internal capsule, the optic radiations, the centrum semiovale, and the parietal subcortical white matter. These areas of myelination are seen as areas of high signal on T_1-weighted images and of decreased signal on T_2-weighted images. They are best seen on T_1-weighted sequences.

Another factor that plays a role in the changing MR appearance of the brain in young children is the changing water content of gray and white matter. In the neonatal period, there is only minimal myelination. The white matter has an increased water content relative to the gray matter. Because of this, the signal intensity of the white matter on T_1-weighted images is less than, and on T_2-weighted images is greater than, that of the adjacent gray matter. Nonmyelinated areas of white matter are hypointense on T_1-weighted images and are hyperintense on T_2-weighted images. This MR appearance persists until approximately 6 months of age, with subtle differences progressing with brain maturation.

After approximately 6 months of age, the gray matter and nonmyelinated white matter become essentially isointense because the water content of these tissues is similar. Those areas that become myelinated show high signal on T_1-weighted images and low signal on T_2-weighted images.

After 1 year of age, the process of myelination has progressed to the point that it has significant influence on the MR appearance of the developing brain. By 2 years of age, 90% of the white matter tracts have become myelinated. At this point, the child's brain for all practical purposes resembles the adult brain. The signal intensity of white matter is greater than that of gray matter on T_1-weighted images and is less than that of gray matter on T_2-weighted images. Imaging protocols that use long repetition times (3000 msec or longer) and long echo times (120 msec or longer) will further increase the difference in signal intensities of gray and white matter. These sequences are especially valuable in assessing brain myelination in children younger than 2 years of age.[14,15]

Anencephaly and Exencephaly

Anencephaly is a severe congenital malformation in which both cerebral hemispheres are absent. Anencephaly is the most common neural tube defect. Its reported incidence is 1 in 1000 births. There is extensive cranioschisis. Most infants with anencephaly are stillborn; those born alive usually die shortly after birth.

There is a striking geographic variation in the prevalence rates of anencephaly. The highest prevalence is in Great Britain and Ireland, and the lowest is in Asia, Africa, and South America. Anencephaly is aproximately six times more common in whites than in African-Americans, and girls are affected more often than boys (4:1).

Anencephaly is the result of failure of closure of the anterior neural tube. This occurs between gestation days 21 and 26. The embryonic defect resulting in anencephaly probably occurs before closure of the anterior neuropore on day 26.

The cranial vault in infants with anencephaly is defective over the vertex, exposing a soft angiomatous mass of neural tissue (area cerebrovasculosa) covered by a thin membrane that is contiguous with the skin. The cranial vault defect may extend caudally to the cervical region. In some cases, the entire neural tube is open; this is termed craniorachischisis.

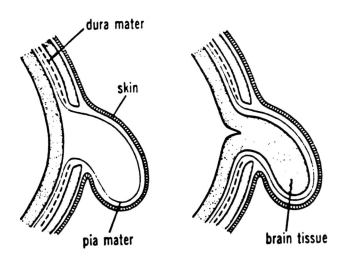

Fig. 1-9 Schematic drawing of the two major types of cephalocele. Protrusion of meninges and cerebrospinal fluid through a defect in the cranium and dura matter is termed a meningocele. If there is brain tissue included in the herniated structures, the lesion is termed an encephalocele. *Source:* Adapted from *Medical Embryology* (p 275) by J Langman, with permission of Williams & Wilkins Co, © 1963.

The eyes are usually protuberant because of inadequate formation of the bony orbits.

Anencephaly can be diagnosed on prenatal sonography beginning early in the second trimester. The diagnosis can be made as early as week 12. The sonographic diagnosis of anencephaly is highly reliable, with accuracy rates being 100% in experienced hands.[16] Absence of the cranial vault and brain cephalad to the level of the orbits is a constant and diagnostic feature in anencephaly. The base of the skull is nearly always present. A variable amount of soft tissue, representing the angiomatous stroma, can be seen protruding through the cranial defect. The anencephalic fetus has a typical froglike appearance and usually has a short neck.

Polyhydramnios frequently accompanies anencephaly. The exact etiology of this complication is unclear. Several hypotheses have been proposed, including fetal failure to swallow because of brainstem dysfunction, excessive micturition, and failure of reabsorption of cerebrospinal fluid.[17] A frequent accompanying phenomenon is increased fetal activity. The cause for this is unknown, although irritation of the meninges and neural tissue has been proposed as a mechanism.

Anencephaly must be differentiated from exencephaly. In exencephaly there is complete or partial absence of the calvaria and complete but abnormal development of the brain tissue. The enchondral portion of the skull base forms normally. Exencephaly is much less common than anencephaly.[18]

The pathogenesis of exencephaly is unknown, but evidence suggests that it represents an embryologic precursor to anencephaly. The absence of the calvaria can lead to brain destruction by exposing the developing brain to amniotic fluid and repeated episodes of trauma.

Exencephaly can be detected on prenatal sonography. The sonographic findings include absence of the cranial vault with exposure of dysplastic-appearing cerebral tissue to the amniotic fluid. The brain parenchyma appears relatively normal in volume but is heterogeneous and disorganized in its echo texture.

Cephalocele

Cephalocele is a congenital malformation that consists of a defect in the cranium and dura mater, through which intracranial structures can herniate. If the herniation consists only of leptomeninges filled with cerebrospinal fluid, this is termed a cranial meningocele. If the sac contains leptomeninges and brain tissue, the lesion is termed an encephalocele (Fig. 1-9). A defect in the calvaria that lacks a prolapse of brain or meninges is termed cranium bifidum occultum.

Cephaloceles occur in about 1 in every 4000 to 5000 live births. The overall prevalence shows little or none of the geographic variation that occurs with spina bifida and other malformations of the central nervous system. Cephaloceles are much less common than spina bifida cystica.

Although most cases of cephalocele are sporadic, there is an increased incidence of this anomaly in families with spina bifida and other malformations of the central nervous system. There is also an increased incidence of cephaloceles in the HARD ± E syndrome that associates *h*ydrocephalus, *a*gyria, *r*etinal *d*ysplasia, and (in about 50% of the cases) *e*ncephalocele.[19]

There are also geographic differences in the prevalence of different types of cephalocele, suggesting the influence of racial and perhaps environmental factors. Occipital cephaloceles are more common in Europe and the United States, whereas frontal locations are more common in southeast Asia and the Soviet Union. Approximately 75% of occipital encephaloceles occur in girls. Anterior encephaloceles are more common in boys.

The exact etiology of cephalocele is unknown. The variety of locations and nature of the many types of cephaloceles suggest that different pathologic mechanisms must occur. A defect in the primary inductive process of neurulation may explain the coexistence of anterior encephaloceles and cerebral and craniofacial malformations such as the various forms of prosencephaly, anomalies of the corpus callosum, anomalies of the visual and olfactory structures, and midline facial clefts. The coincidence of these lesions suggests an alteration at an early stage of gestation (28 to 35 days). It is at this time that the notochord, the neural tube, and the surrounding mesoderm form the cranial base and the facial structures.

A defect in the primary inductive process may also explain the association of posterior cephaloceles with cerebral malformations such as dysgenesis of the corpus callosum, dorsal cysts, callosal lipoma, and porencephaly. The coincidence of these lesions suggests that the cephalocele may interfere with the induction and formation of the membranous cranial roof, which occurs somewhat later in gestation (38 to 45 days).

Focal isolated cranial defects with cephalocele may arise at a still later stage of embryogenesis. Ossification of the chondrocranium begins with the coalescence of the multiple ossification centers, which occurs on about gestation day 35 and continues until after birth. Failure of these ossification centers to unite properly will result in a persistent defect between two enchondral ossification centers. This mechanism may explain certain basal cephaloceles.

Occipital Cephalocele. The occipital bone is formed by both enchondral and membranous ossification. Mesodermal cells proliferate and fuse around the notochord to form that portion of the skull that is termed the basiocciput. Exoccipital bones develop posterior to the basiocciput from parachordal mesoderm. They undergo ossification at about day 60 to form the lateral margins of the foramen magnum. The caudal boundary of the foramen magnum is formed by the supraoccipital bone. The interparietal bone, which lies above the supraoccipital bone, is the only portion of the occipital bone that undergoes membranous ossification. The supraoccipital bone is separated from the interparietal bone by the mendosal suture, which closes at approximately 3 months of age.

The occipital region is the most common location of cephaloceles in infants in North America and Europe. They

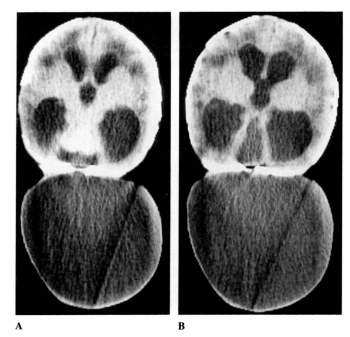

A   B

Fig. 1-10 Cephalocele. (**A**) Axial CT scan demonstrates a large occipital meningocele projecting through a small midline defect in the occipital bone. There is no herniated brain tissue. (**B**) Next higher image shows hydrocephalus and communication of the meningocele with a cystic area between the leaves of the tentorium. This is a combined infratentorial and supratentorial cephalocele.

can be entirely infratentorial, entirely supratentorial, or combined infratentorial and supratentorial. Meningoceles and cephaloceles occur with approximately equal frequency in the occipital region. The size of the cephalocele is variable, ranging from a few millimeters to a defect that contains a large portion of the brain. Small cephaloceles are usually covered by normal-appearing scalp. Larger cephaloceles are covered by a thin, translucent membrane that is contiguous with the scalp. The size of the defect in the cranium is best demonstrated on CT. The nature of the contents of a cephalocele may be suggested on CT but is best evaluated with MRI.

Approximately 50% of infratentorial occipital cephaloceles are associated with Chiari III malformation. In these cases, the defect is located in the supraoccipital bone, either at or a short distance from the foramen magnum. The cerebellum (particularly the cerebellar vermis) is displaced caudally, but herniation of cerebellar tissue through the defect in the occipital bone is minimal. The medulla and pons become oriented vertically, and the fourth ventricle is compressed and stretched caudally. Hydrocephalus is common with Chiari III malformation.

In those cases in which an occipital cephalocele is both infratentorial and supratentorial, any herniated brain tissue is nearly always supratentorial brain. Hypoplasia or abnormal implantation of the tentorium permits passage of herniated tissue into the posterior cranial fossa defect. The brainstem and cerebellum are displaced anteriorly and compressed. Hydrocephalus is common (Figs. 1-10 and 1-11).

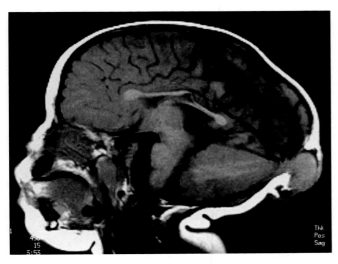

Fig. 1-11 Cephalocele. Sagittal T_1-weighted MR scan shows a defect in the superior aspect of the occipital bone. There is herniation of leptomeninges and cerebellar tissue through the defect. The medulla and pons have a vertical orientation, and there is deformity of the posterior aspect of the cerebellum. Also note thinning and dysplasia of the corpus callosum. This is a combined infratentorial and supratentorial occipital cephalocele.

In supratentorial occipital cephaloceles, brain herniation and hydrocephalus each occur in approximately 50% of cases (Fig. 1-12). There is a better prognosis with supratentorial than infratentorial cephalocele.

Frontoethmoidal Cephalocele. The membranous roof of the cranium is formed by about gestation day 38 to 40. The first two ossification centers of the frontal bone develop in the region of the future superciliary arches at gestation day 50 to 60. Membranous ossification begins in these two centers and spreads dorsally over the pars frontalis and into the pars orbitalis in the direction of the ethmoid and sphenoid bones. The two ossification centers of the frontal bone meet in the midline at the metopic suture.

The anterior wall of the nasal capsule lies posterior to the nasal and frontal bones. During gestation week 8, the nasal capsule is composed of cartilage that is divided by a median cartilaginous septum. The lateral walls of the capsule later undergo ossification to form the lateral masses of the ethmoid and the inferior concha bones. The anterior two-thirds of the midline nasal septum remains cartilaginous; the posterior one-third becomes ossified to form the perpendicular plate of the ethmoid bone and the crista galli.[20]

On the basis of the location of the bony defect, four types of frontoethmoidal cephalocele are recognized: nasofrontal, nasoethmoidal, naso-orbital, and interfrontal. The relative frequency of these different types has not been accurately determined. It is clear, however, that frontoethmoidal cephaloceles as a group are relatively rare in Europe and North America and more common in southeast Asia.

With nasofrontal cephalocele, a round or ovoid bony defect occurs in the bregma between two deformed orbits. The intra-

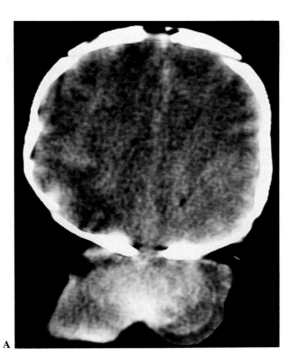

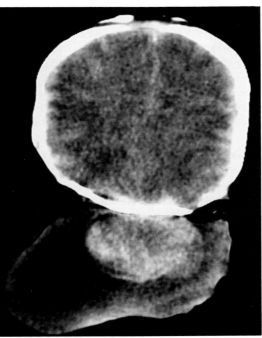

Fig. 1-12 Supratentorial occipital cephalocele. The herniation consists of leptomeninges, cerebrospinal fluid, and dysplastic brain. There is a small midline defect in the upper aspect of the occipital bone.

cranial orifice of the defect projects above the ethmoid bones and the crista galli (which is often bifid). Patients with nasofrontal cephaloceles have hypertelorism and a clinically identifiable mass at the glabella or at the base of the nose. These cephaloceles vary from a small mass measuring less

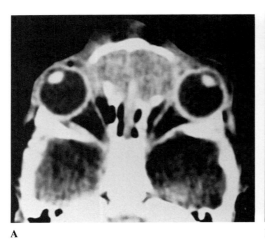
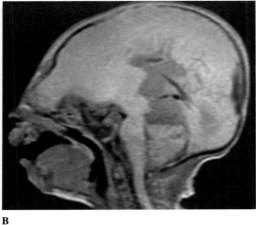
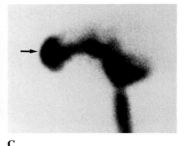

A   B   C

Fig. 1-13 Nasoethmoidal cephalocele. (**A**) Axial CT scan demonstrates inferior protrusion of the frontal lobes through a defect in the cribriform plate associated with fairly marked hypertelorism. The laminae papyraceae are deficient, and the brain tissue protrudes into the medial aspects of the orbits. (**B**) Sagittal proton-density MR scan clearly demonstrates the herniation of brain tissue through the bony defect into the nasal fossa. There is agenesis of the corpus callosum. (**C**) Lateral image from a radionuclide cisternogram shows communication between the cephalocele (arrow) and the subarachnoid space.

---

than 1 cm to a large sac containing the anterior part of the frontal lobes. Small nasofrontal cephaloceles may contain only meninges. Associated cerebral malformations, especially dysgenesis of the corpus callosum, are common.

With nasoethmoidal cephalocele, the herniated sac protrudes through a defect in the cribriform plate of the ethmoid bone into the nasal fossa. The defect may be unilateral or bilateral, median or paramedian. The most frequent presenting complaint in these cases is nasal obstruction. Physical examination reveals an intranasal mass that may be mistaken for a nasal polyp. Facial and cerebral malformations such as median facial clefts, hypertelorism, and dysgenesis of the corpus callosum are less common with nasoethmoidal cephaloceles than with other cephaloceles (Fig. 1-13).

With naso-orbital cephalocele, the bony defect is located between the ethmoid bone and the frontal process of the maxilla. Therefore, the cephalocele passes through the cribriform plate, the ethmoid sinus, and the lamina papyracea to enter the medial part of the orbit. Naso-orbital cephaloceles are extremely rare. On physical examination, there is a compressible, slightly pulsatile mass in the medial aspect of the orbit that causes lateral deviation of the globe and exophthalmos. Contiguity of the orbital mass with the intracranial structures can be demonstrated on CT or MRI.

Interfrontal cephaloceles usually occur in the inferior portion of the metopic suture but rarely can involve the entire length of the suture. The cranial defect is often quite large, and the anterior tips of the frontal lobes or the anterior halves of the cerebral hemispheres may protrude extracranially. Brain herniation may be asymmetric. The prognosis is poor because of compression of the herniated brain by a constricting ring that is formed by the frontal bone defect and because of the high incidence of associated cerebral malformations, especially the HARD associations. Interfrontal cephaloceles are rare.

Sphenoidal Cephalocele. The sphenoid bone develops at the anterior end of the notochord. It has four major components: the basisphenoid, which arises from prechordal mesoderm; the presphenoid, which is situated anterior and inferior to the basisphenoid; the orbitosphenoid, which gives rise to the planum sphenoidale and the lesser wings; and the alisphenoid, which gives rise to the greater wings of the sphenoid bone. Chondrification of the body of the sphenoid begins at about gestation day 40. The craniopharyngeal canal passes through the basisphenoid; it normally closes at about gestation day 50. Ossification centers first appear in the body of the sphenoid bone at gestation days 70 to 80. There are numerous ossification centers for each component.

Sphenoidal cephaloceles are extremely rare. The predominant clinical feature of a sphenoidal cephalocele is obstruction of the nasopharynx. This leads to breathing difficulties and may cause alteration of the cry. The cephalocele may be identifiable as a palpable, pulsatile mass that is covered by intact nasopharyngeal mucosa. The mass may increase in size with crying or jugular venous compression. Spontaneous fistulization and meningitis are rare.

Facial malformations of variable severity occur in all cases of sphenoidal cephalocele. Hypertelorism is universal. Other facial malformations may include labial fissures, palatine fissures, and median nasal fissures. Optic malformations are also common. They include coloboma or hypoplasia of the eye and orbit, bilateral optic nerve hypoplasia, hypoplasia of the chiasm, and retinal defects. Endocrine dysfunction occurs frequently and consists of deficits of somatotropin, gonadotropins, and antidiuretic hormone. The most frequent associated cerebral malformation is dysgenesis of the corpus callosum.

Skull radiographs in cases of sphenoidal cephalocele show absence of the center of the floor of the sella turcica. There is a pharyngeal mass of soft tissue density that is attached to the anterior surface of the body of the sphenoid bone. The dorsum sellae is normal.

Sphenoidal cephaloceles always contain the inferior portion of the third ventricle and the pituitary gland. This is best detected on MRI, especially in the sagittal plane. MRI will also demonstrate the pharyngeal component of the cephalocele, which usually abuts the posterior border of the nasal septum (Fig. 1-14).

Chiari Malformations

Chiari malformations are divided into three distinct types. Chiari I malformation describes caudal extension of the cerebellar tonsils below the foramen magnum. The intracranial structures are normal. Many cases of Chiari I malformation are asymptomatic. Symptoms are most likely to arise when the tonsils extend more than 1 cm below the foramen magnum. Symptoms of Chiari I malformation are often related to syringohydromyelia, which is present in 20% to 25% of patients with this anomaly. The inferior herniation of the cerebellar tonsils through the foramen magnum is best demonstrated on sagittal MRI.

There are clinical and etiologic subgroups of Chiari I malformation. Some cases of inferior tonsillar herniation appear to be due to intrauterine hydrocephalus. After birth, the tonsils have a pointed configuration and lie in an abnormal caudal position. Patients in this subgroup of Chiari I malformation usually present in infancy with hydrocephalus. A second subtype of Chiari I malformation is associated with cranial cer-

vical dysgenesis. Osseous abnormalities in these children include occipitalization of the atlas, Klippel-Feil anomaly, or other types of abnormalities of C-1, C-2, and the occiput. The tonsils are often somewhat large. Syringohydromyelia may be present. These children may exhibit cranial nerve dysfunction or anesthesia of the extremities. A third subtype of Chiari I malformation encompasses cases with acquired deformities of the foramen magnum, such as basilar invagination. The clinical manifestations may include cranial nerve dysfunction or symptoms related to syringohydromyelia.

The Chiari II (Arnold-Chiari) malformation is a complex malformation involving the hindbrain, spine, and various mesodermal structures. Supratentorial anomalies of variable severity are associated with this condition. The presence of Chiari II malformation is heralded at birth by the identification of a myelomeningocele. Symptoms of the Chiari II malformation itself are usually related to hydrocephalus and may become apparent several weeks or months after birth. Focal neurologic signs, such as cranial nerve palsies and pseudobulbar, pyramidal, or cerebellar signs, may appear later in childhood or adolescence. The pathologic features of Chiari II malformation are best demonstrated on MRI. Many of the important findings can also be appreciated on CT or, in infants, sonography.[21]

The hindbrain findings in Chiari II malformation are best understood as resulting from a small posterior fossa and a low tentorial attachment. Because the posterior fossa is diminutive, the cerebellum is indented superiorly by the tentorium and inferiorly by the foramen magnum. The pons is stretched and elongated inferiorly and narrowed in its anteroposterior

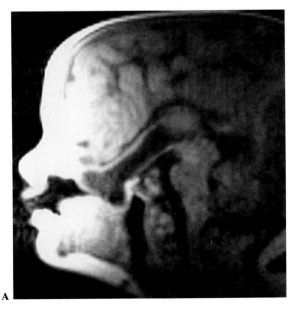
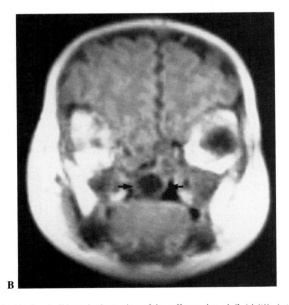

A   B

Fig. 1-14 Sphenoidal cephalocele. **(A)** Sagittal T₁-weighted MR scan shows a large defect in the skull base in the region of the sella turcica. A fluid-filled structure that is contiguous with the third ventricle projects inferiorly into the nasopharynx. There is agenesis of the corpus callosum. **(B)** Coronal T₁-weighted MR image shows slight inferior extension of the frontal lobes through the defect, especially on the right. The fluid component lies somewhat inferiorly (arrows). There is marked hypertelorism.

dimension. The medulla and cervical spinal cord are also stretched inferiorly. The medulla extends below the foramen magnum. The dentate ligaments that attach to the lateral aspect of the spinal cord allow for a variable amount of caudal displacement of the cord. These ligaments, however, eventually arrest further displacement of the cord. If the medulla extends more inferior than the dentate ligaments will allow the spinal cord to move, a characteristic cervicomedullary kink is formed. Patients in whom the cervicomedullary kink lies at C-4 or below are likely to be symptomatic, showing brainstem dysfunction. This is present in approximately 70% of patients with Chiari II malformation (Fig. 1-15).[22]

The cerebellum in Chiari II malformation extends anterolaterally into the cerebellopontine angles and partially encompasses the brainstem. The fourth ventricle is low in position and has an abnormal vertical orientation. The anteroposterior diameter of the fourth ventricle is narrowed. Occasionally, a portion of the fourth ventricle may form a cyst or diverticulum posterior to the medulla and caudal to the vermis. The vermis is usually displaced into the cervical spinal canal (Fig. 1-16). The portion of the cerebellum that is displaced below the foramen magnum tends to degenerate.

The mesencephalic tectum in Chiari II malformation has a beaked appearance on axial and sagittal images as a result of fusion of the superior and inferior colliculi. There may also be compression by the termporal horns when there is significant hydrocephalus. The tectum is stretched posteriorly and inferiorly. Axial CT images often demonstrate posterior con-

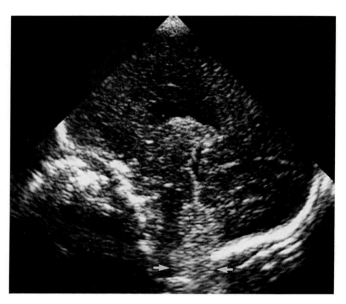

Fig. 1-16 Chiari II malformation. Midline sagittal cranial sonogram demonstrating caudal descent of the vermis through the foramen magnum (arrows). The fourth ventricle is also elongated and is displaced inferiorly by the Chiari II malformation. The corpus callosum is absent.

cavity of the petrous bones (in about 70% of cases), which is due to pressure effects of the cerebellum on the small posterior fossa (Fig. 1-17). This scalloping of the petrous bones is more difficult to appreciate on MR images. The internal auditory canals may be foreshortened. The foramen magnum is enlarged in about 70% of cases of Chiari II malformation. Bone window CT images may also show lacunar skull in these infants during the first several months of life.

The supratentorial abnormalities that occur with Chiari II malformation are best evaluated on MRI (Fig. 1-18). Abnormalities of the corpus callosum are seen in more than 85% of patients. The most common anomalies are hypoplasia or absence of the splenium and absence of the rostrum. Enlargement of the caudate nuclei is frequently seen, as is enlargement of the massa intermedia (Fig. 1-19). The falx cerebri is usually fenestrated, resulting in interdigitation of the gyri across the interhemispheric fissure. The gyral pattern as seen on sagittal MRI is often abnormal in the medial aspects of the occipital lobes, having the appearance of multiple small gyri. This is distinct from true polymicrogyria because the cortex is of normal thickness.[23]

Hydrocephalus of variable severity occurs in virtually all cases of Chiari II malformation. This is due to aqueductal stenosis in about 50% of cases. Obstruction to cerebrospinal fluid flow may also be produced by tonsillar and brainstem herniation at the foramen magnum. Ventricular dilatation is often most marked in the posterior aspect of the lateral ventricles (ie, colpocephaly).

The Chiari III malformation is a Chiari II malformation associated with a low occipital or a high cervical cephalocele. This anomaly is extremely rare.

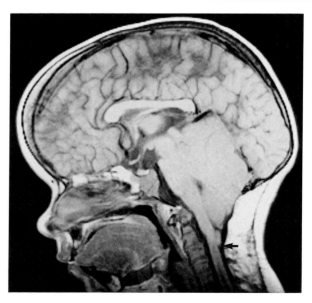

Fig. 1-15 Chiari II malformation. Sagittal T$_1$-weighted MR scan of a young child who had prior repair of a myelomeningocele shows caudal descent of the hindbrain. The medulla lies in the upper cervical region. The vermis and cerebellar tonsils are herniated through the foramen magnum. There is a kink at the cervicomedullary junction (arrow). The cerebellum is indented superiorly by the tentorium. There is enlargement of the massa intermedia and fusion of the colliculi. Note also hydromyelia in the upper cervical cord.

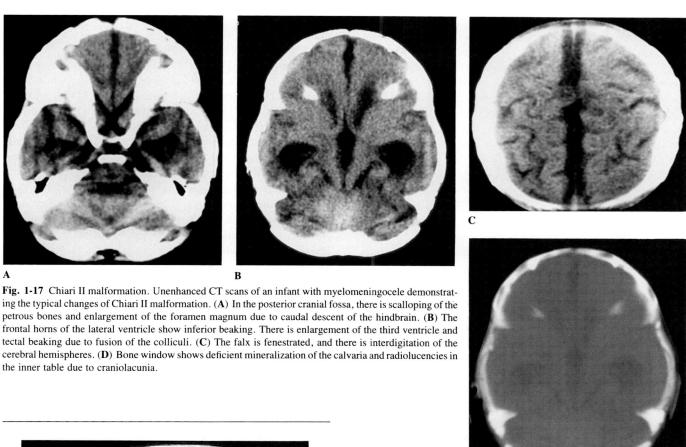

A   B

C

D

Fig. 1-17 Chiari II malformation. Unenhanced CT scans of an infant with myelomeningocele demonstrating the typical changes of Chiari II malformation. (**A**) In the posterior cranial fossa, there is scalloping of the petrous bones and enlargement of the foramen magnum due to caudal descent of the hindbrain. (**B**) The frontal horns of the lateral ventricle show inferior beaking. There is enlargement of the third ventricle and tectal beaking due to fusion of the colliculi. (**C**) The falx is fenestrated, and there is interdigitation of the cerebral hemispheres. (**D**) Bone window shows deficient mineralization of the calvaria and radiolucencies in the inner table due to craniolacunia.

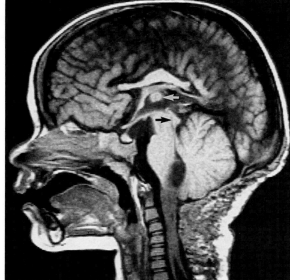

A

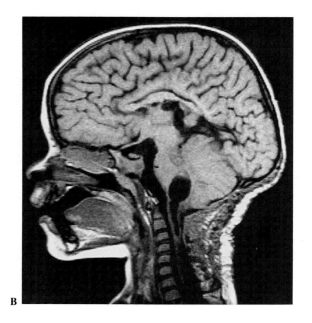

B

Fig. 1-18 Chiari II malformation. (**A**) Sagittal and (**B**) parasagittal T_1-weighted MR scans of a child with repaired myelomeningocele show moderate dysplasia of the corpus callosum. The genu and rostrum are hypoplastic, and the corpus callosum has an abnormal appearance, resembling a Napoleon hat. In addition, there is enlargement of the massa intermedia (white arrow in **A**) and beaking of the tectum due to fusion of the colliculi (black arrow in **A**). Syringobulbia is seen in the pons and upper medulla, and there is syringomyelia in the upper cervical cord. Note also that the gyri are small, especially in the occipital lobes. The cortex is of normal thickness.

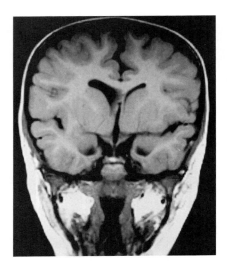

Fig. 1-19 Chiari II malformation. Coronal T_1-weighted MR image of a child with repaired myelomeningocele showing inferior beaking of the frontal horns of the lateral ventricles. Note also enlargement of the heads of the caudate nuclei.

Holoprosencephaly

Holoprosencephaly is a congenital anomaly in which there is lack of normal lateral cleavage into distinct cerebral hemispheres as well as a failure of transverse cleavage into a diencephalon and telencephalon. The underlying mechanism is thought to be defective development of the notochordal plate, resulting in lack of normal lateral migration of the telencephalic and optic vesicles. There is failure of division of the forebrain (prosencephalon) between weeks 5 and 6 of embryogenesis. This results in a complex facial and craniocerebral anomaly of variable severity.[24]

Holoprosencephaly may be isolated or may occur in association with any of several syndromes, most commonly trisomy 13 and trisomy 18. Facial dysmorphism, such as hypotelorism and midline facial clefts, often occurs in the more severe forms of holoprosencephaly.

Three subcategories of holoprosencephaly are recognized: alobar, semilobar, and lobar. As with many other classification systems, however, the divisions represent somewhat arbitrary indicators of the severity of the anomaly rather than distinct or clear categories. The three forms of holoprosencephaly represent a continuum. In all forms of holoprosencephaly, the septum pellucidum and the olfactory bulb are absent, and the sylvian fissures are poorly developed. The posterior fossa structures are usually normal. The intracranial pathology is usually best demonstrated on MRI or CT, although sonography may be useful in young infants and for prenatal detection.[25]

The incidence of holoprosencephaly is between 1 in 5,000 and 1 in 16,000 live births. Because many cases of holoprosencephaly undergo spontaneous abortion, the true incidence may be as high as 1 in 250 pregnancies.[26] Holoprosencephaly accounts for approximately 50% or more of all cases of ventricular dilatation detected prenatally.[27]

Alobar holoprosencephaly is the most severe form of this anomaly. The third ventricle is absent, and the thalami are fused. There is no interhemispheric fissure, and the falx cerebri is absent or markedly hypoplastic. The cerebrum is composed of a thin rim of tissue, which is usually most prominent

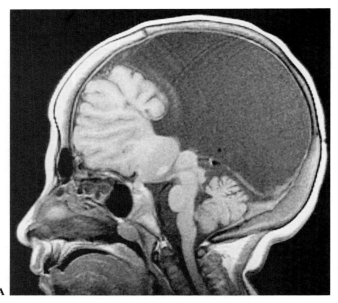
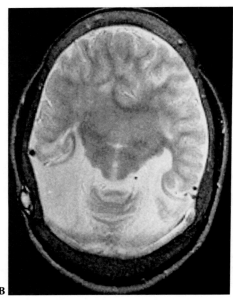

Fig. 1-20 Alobar type of holoprosencephaly. (**A**) Sagittal T_1-weighted and (**B**) axial T_2-weighted MR scans show absence of most of the hemispheres aside from the frontal lobes. The frontal lobes are fused, and the falx and interhemispheric fissure are absent. The more posterior aspect of the cranium contains a large cyst that is contiguous with the fused ventricles. There is also fusion of the thalami, and the third ventricle is absent. The brainstem is normal, but the cerebellum is slightly small.

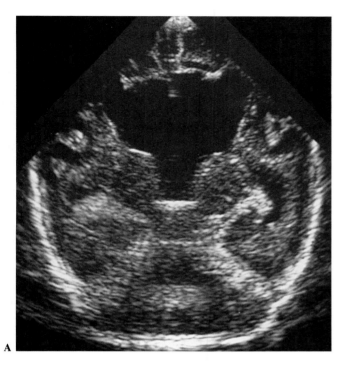

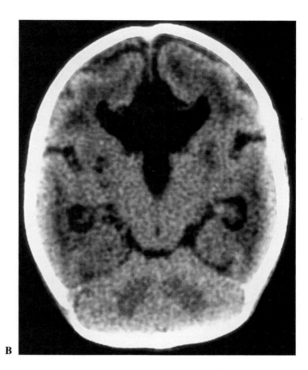

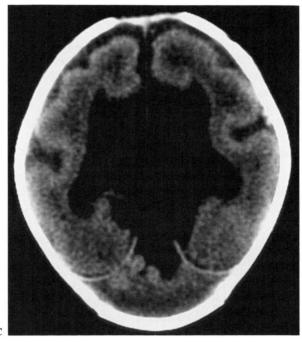

Fig. 1-21 Semilobar type of holoprosencephaly. (**A**) Coronal sonogram shows fusion of the large lateral ventricles and absence of the septum pellucidum. A rudimentary third ventricle is shown to communicate freely with the common lateral ventricles. The corpus callosum is absent. (**B** and **C**) Unenhanced axial CT scans also demonstrate the fused lateral ventricles. There is partial formation of the falx cerebri. The brain surface is abnormally smooth as a result of pachygyria.

in the frontal and occipital regions. Most of the intracranial space is occupied by a crescent-shaped single ventricle that is continuous with a large dorsal cyst (Fig. 1-20).

Many infants with alobar holoprosencephaly are stillborn or die in infancy. Physical examination usually identifies severe midline facial anomalies and hypotelorism resulting from absence or hypoplasia of the premaxillary portion of the face. A severe form results in cyclopia. Imaging of the facial structures demonstrates cleft palate, microphthalmia or anophthalmia, trigonocephaly, micrognathia, and absence of the nasal septum. Skull radiographs show a small anterior fossa, high superior arching of the orbits, and severe hypotelorism.

The dysmorphic features of the brain that occur in the semilobar type of holoprosencephaly are less severe than those in the alobar type. There is more cerebral tissue, and there is rudimentary formation of the frontal and occipital horns. The interhemispheric fissure is often partially formed posteriorly. The falx is usually present posteriorly but may not lie in the midline. The thalamic nuclei are partially separated by a small third ventricle. There are rudimentary temporal horns, although formation of the hippocampal gyrus is generally incomplete. As with all forms of holoprosencephaly, the septum pellucidum is absent, and the lateral ventricles are fused. The corpus callosum is absent in both the alobar and semilobar

forms, although a spleniumlike structure may be seen with semilobar holoprosencephaly (Fig. 1-21). Mild facial anomalies (cleft lip or cleft palate) may be seen. In most cases, the face is normal.[28]

In the lobar form of holoprosencephaly, the brain anomalies are relatively mild. The interhemispheric fissure and falx cerebri are at least partially formed. The anterior falx is usually dysplastic. The septum pellucidum is absent. The hippocampal formations are nearly normal, and the temporal horns and

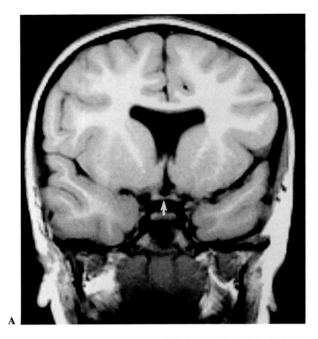
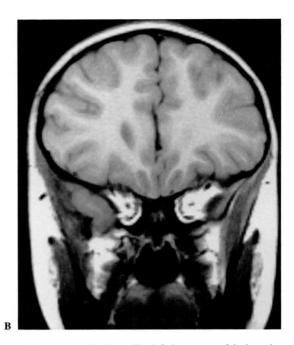

Fig. 1-22 Septo-optic dysplasia. (**A** and **B**) Coronal T$_1$-weighted MR images show absence of the septum pellucidum. The inferior aspects of the lateral ventricles are beaked. The optic chiasm (arrow in **A**) and optic nerves are hypoplastic. The falx cerebri is present.

third ventricles are better defined than in the alobar and semi-lobar forms. The ventricles are moderately dilated. The sylvian fissures are absent or small, and the frontal lobes may be hypoplastic. The corpus callosum may or may not be present. Lobar holoprosencephaly is distinguished from septo-optic dysplasia by identification of a normal falx cerebri in the latter.

Septo-optic Dysplasia

Septo-optic dysplasia is a rare congenital anomaly of the anterior midline structures of the brain. The pathologic features include hypoplasia of the optic nerves, optic chiasm, and hypothalamic infundibulum and hypoplasia or absence of the septum pellucidum. The clinical presentation of septo-optic dysplasia is quite variable. The visual symptoms may include wandering nystagmus, diminished visual acuity, or blindness, but some patients have normal or nearly normal vision. Hypotelorism is identified infrequently. Hypothalamic-pituitary dysfunction occurs in about two-thirds of cases, usually presenting as growth retardation due to deficient secretion of growth hormone and thyroid-stimulating hormone. Diabetes insipidus and precocious puberty may occur. In occasional cases, there is panhypopituitarism. Ophthalmologic examination demonstrates hypoplasia of one or both optic discs.

The features of septo-optic dysplasia may be demonstrated on CT or MRI, although the latter technique is optimal. Both coronal and axial images are helpful. There is hypoplasia or complete absence of the septum pellucidum, resulting in a boxlike configuration of the frontal horns (ie, the anteromedial aspects of the frontal horns are squared off on both axial and coronal images). On coronal images, there is beaking of the

floors of the frontal horns of the lateral ventricles (Fig. 1-22). Some degree of enlargement of the lateral ventricles is common. The optic nerves and canals are hypoplastic. Hypoplasia of the optic chiasm and hypothalamus sometimes results in bulbous dilatation of the anterior recess of the third ventricle and a large suprasellar cistern. Occasionally, hypoplasia of the hemispheric white matter causes mild ventricular enlargement. Schizencephaly accompanies septo-optic dysplasia in up to 50% of cases.[29,30]

In addition to the group of anomalies that make up septo-optic dysplasia, congenital absence of the septum pellucidum may also occur as an isolated abnormality. These patients may be clinically normal or have mental retardation or seizures. As described previously, the septum pellucidum is absent in the various forms of holoprosencephaly. There is a syndrome in which there is aplasia or severe hypoplasia of the septum pellucidum and porencephaly (often joining the sylvian fissures to the lateral ventricles), gray matter heterotopias (usually adjacent to the porencephaly and in the callosocaudal angle), and areas of microgyria.[31] The septum is hypoplastic or absent in some cases of Chiari II malformation. Acquired defects of the septum pellucidum may occur as a result of severe hydrocephalus.

Dysgenesis of the Corpus Callosum

The corpus callosum is divided into four sections: the rostrum, genu, body, and splenium. Dysgenesis of the corpus callosum can be complete or partial. When there is incomplete development of the corpus callosum, the dorsal portion is always affected. With a partially formed corpus callosum, the genu is virtually always present, the body may be absent, and the splenium and rostrum are frequently absent. This is because the normal temporal sequence of formation of the corpus callosum proceeds from genu to body to splenium to rostrum. These observations help differentiate true dysgenesis of the corpus callosum from secondary destruction; a small or absent genu or body in the presence of an intact splenium or rostrum may be produced by a destructive process but should not occur as a true developmental malformation.

Anomalies of the corpus callosum are frequently associated with other midline brain malformations. These include Dandy-Walker malformation, interhemispheric arachnoid cyst, heterotopic gray matter, cerebellar hypoplasia, cephalocele, and midline facial anomalies. Dysgenesis of the corpus callosum is common in children with Chiari II malformation. Associated anomalies, when present, often account for the major symptomatology in cases of dysgenesis of the corpus callosum. Isolated dysgenesis of the corpus callosum may be asymptomatic. Mild or moderate mental retardation occurs in some cases. Neurologic evaluation reveals visual and motor abnormalities that may be subtle.

In normal cerebral development, the fibers that form the corpus callosum cause an inversion of the cingulate gyrus and formation of the cingulate sulcus superior to the gyrus. With agenesis of the corpus callosum, the cingulate gyri remain everted, and the cingulate sulci do not form. Persistent eversion of the cingulate gyri results in extension of the medial hemispheric sulci into the third ventricle; this finding is one of the characteristic features of absence of the corpus callosum.

With absence of the corpus callosum, axonal fibers from the cerebral hemispheres fail to cross the midline. These fibers instead reach the medial hemispheric wall and turn to course parallel to the interhemispheric fissure. There, axonal fibers make up the longitudinal callosal bundles of Probst. The bundles of Probst lie lateral to the cingulate gyrus and medial to the lateral ventricles; the inferior margins merge with the fornices. The bundles of Probst invaginate the medial borders of the lateral ventricles. This results in a crescent shape of the lateral ventricles that is more noticeable in the rostral segments. The foramina of Monro tend to be enlarged. Because of the absence of the corpus callosum, the third ventricle is somewhat widened and extends superiorly into the interhemispheric fissure to form an interhemispheric cerebral collection of cerebrospinal fluid, which is generally called the interhemispheric cyst. This fluid collection usually is due to an upward extension of the third ventricle. The cyst may or may not communicate with the third ventricle, however.

The corpus callosum is in large part responsible for the shape of the lateral ventricles, especially posteriorly. The caudate heads and the lentiform nuclei keep the sizes of the frontal horns relatively normal, even with complete absence of the corpus callosum. Posteriorly, however, only loose white matter surrounds the ventricles when the callosal splenium is absent. With absence of the splenium, the ventricles enlarge superiorly and posteriorly into the underdeveloped white matter. This results in dilatation of the

trigones, occipital horns, and posterior horns of the lateral ventricles. This appearance is termed colpocephaly. The bodies of the lateral ventricles have a linear, parallel orientation when the callosal body is absent.

Dysgenesis of the corpus callosum is best evaluated on sagittal MRI. The diagnosis can also be established on CT and sonography. The imaging findings on axial images include characteristic lateral convexity of the frontal horns, parallel separated lateral ventricles, colpocephaly, upward extension of the third ventricle between the lateral ventricles, and communication of the third ventricle with the interhemispheric fissure anteriorly (Fig. 1-23). The anterior commissure is always present. Coronal images demonstrate persistent eversion of the cingulate gyri with the medial hemispheric sulcus extending to the third ventricle, crescent-shaped lateral ventricles due to impression on the medial wall of the ventricles by the bundles of Probst, and incomplete inversion of the hippocampal formation in the medial temporal lobes. If there is a partial absence, it is usually of the dorsal segment. Consequently, a dysgenetic corpus callosum may include the genu, the genu and a segment of the body, the genu and the entire body, or the genu, body, and splenium without the rostrum. Slight thinning of the posterior portion of the body of the corpus callosum is a common normal variation that should not be mistaken for dysgenesis.[32–35]

Lipoma of the Corpus Callosum

As with other intracranial lipomas, lipoma of the corpus callosum is a congenital malformation. It is thought to be due to abnormal persistence and maldifferentiation of the meninx primitiva (the mesenchymal anlage of the meninges). Callosal lipomas are almost always associated with anomalies of the corpus callosum. Cephalocele and cutaneous lipomas are frequently associated. Lipoma of the corpus callosum accounts for approximately 30% of all intracranial fatty lesions.

Skull radiographs in cases of lipoma of the corpus callosum are often normal, but occasionally they demonstrate midline calcifications with or without associated fat-density lucencies. CT shows a mass with the negative attenuation values of fat immediately above the lateral ventricles. Components of the lesion may extend inferiorly between the ventricles or anteriorly into the interhemispheric fissure. Calcification is frequently identified along the margins of the lesion. The character of the calcification is variable, but most frequently it is curvilinear and extends around the periphery; occasionally there is nodular calcification in the center of the lipoma. When the lipoma is associated with facial dysraphism, CT is important in defining the bony craniofacial anomalies.[36]

As with CT, MRI is highly accurate for the detection and characterization of corpus callosal lipoma. T_1-weighted MR scans show a hyperintense midline mass superior and posterior to the corpus. The mass may also involve the area of the lamina terminalis or fornix. The pericallosal vessels frequently course through the lipoma. Occasionally, a portion of the lipoma can be seen extending into the choroidal fissure of the lateral ventricles (Fig. 1-24).[37,38]

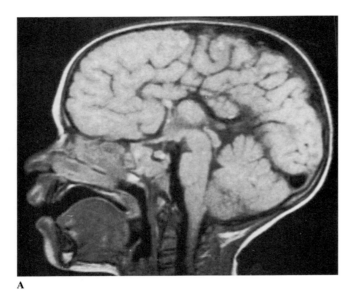

A

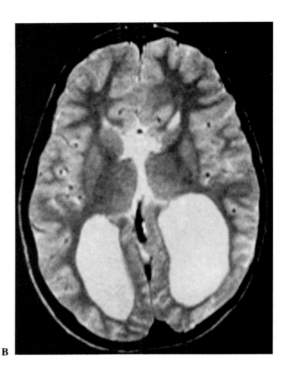

B

Fig. 1-23 Dysgenesis of the corpus callosum. (**A**) Sagittal T_1-weighted MR scan shows complete absence of the corpus callosum. The gyri are oriented in a radial configuration. The posterior fossa structures are normal. (**B** and **C**) Axial T_2-weighted images show colpocephaly and a separated and parallel configuration of the bodies of the lateral ventricles.

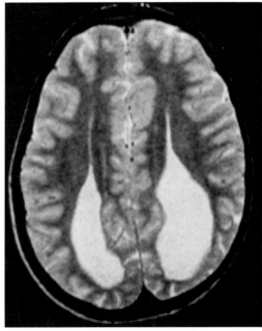

C

Congenital Lesions of the Pituitary Gland

The pituitary gland develops from two embryologically distinct sources. The anterior lobe arises from the epithelium of the craniopharyngeal duct (pouch of Rathke). This is a midline structure that extends from the roof of the oral cavity. Normally, the craniopharyngeal duct undergoes complete involution, leaving the anterior lobe of the pituitary gland as an isolated island of epithelial tissue in the intracranial cavity. The posterior lobe of the pituitary is composed of neural tissue that originates as an inferior extension of the hypothalamus. The posterior lobe remains connected to the hypothalamus by the pituitary stalk.

Pituitary hypoplasia is thought to result from interference with the normal migration of the embryologic precursors of the pituitary gland. Patients may or may not show evidence of pituitary hormone deficiency. CT and MRI show a small but otherwise normal-appearing pituitary gland. On MRI, the anterior and posterior lobes of the pituitary gland are easily differentiated on T_1-weighted sagittal images because the posterior lobe is hyperintense with respect to the anterior lobe as a result of intercellular lipid material. In young infants, both lobes of the pituitary are hyperintense on T_1-weighted images.

Idiopathic growth hormone deficiency is a disorder that is not clearly understood. There is an association with growth hormone deficiency and septo-optic dysplasia. In children with growth hormone deficiency, skull radiographs may show a small sella turcica. In many cases, however, the sella turcica is of normal size.

MR findings in patients with idiopathic growth hormone deficiency fall into two groups. Those patients who have multiple hormone deficiencies, including growth hormone deficiency, have an ectopic neurohypophysis approximately

90% of the time. This presents as a small, high-signal area on T_1-weighted images near the median eminence of the hypothalamus. In addition, these patients have absence of the infundibulum of the pituitary gland and absence of the normal high signal from the posterior pituitary gland. Among patients with isolated growth hormone deficiency, an ectopic neurohypophysis is found in only 10%. The anterior pituitary dysfunction in those patients who have an ectopic neurohypophysis is thought to be related to absence of the infundibulum, which carries the normal portal venous system of the pituitary gland.[39,40]

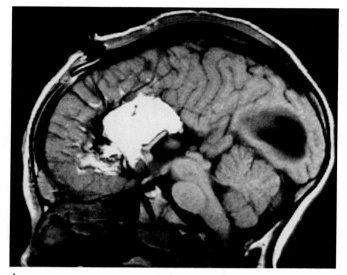

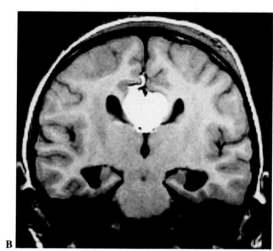

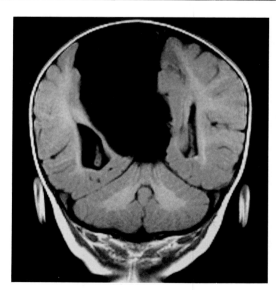

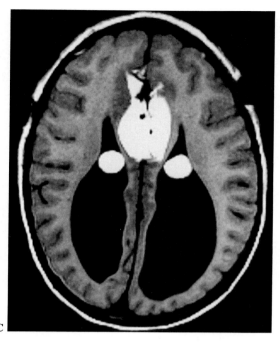

Fig. 1-24 Lipoma of the corpus callosum. (**A**) Sagittal, (**B**) coronal, and (**C**) axial T_1-weighted MR scans show agenesis of the corpus callosum and a hyperintense midline fatty mass. Vascular flow voids course through the mass. Portions of the lipoma extend into the lateral ventricles. Ancillary findings of agenesis of the corpus callosum, such as colpocephaly and radial arrangement of the paramedian gyri, are also demonstrated.

Arachnoid Cyst

Arachnoid cysts are congenital lesions in the arachnoid membrane that develop because of cerebrospinal fluid secretion. True arachnoid cysts differ from leptomeningeal cysts caused by trauma or inflammation in that the latter are loculations of cerebrospinal fluid surrounded by arachnoid scarring. True arachnoid cysts are intra-arachnoid in location. Congenital arachnoid cysts expand by the accumulation of cerebrospinal fluid that is actively secreted by cells in the wall of the lesion. Subarachnoid cysts are similar lesions that are lined by arachnoid externally and by pia and internal arachnoid velum internally. CT and MRI demonstrate arachnoid and subarachnoid cysts as sharply circumscribed, unilocular, homogeneous masses that have the imaging characteristics of cerebrospinal fluid.[41]

The sylvian fissures are the most common locations for arachnoid cysts, accounting for about half the lesions. The suprasellar, quadrigeminal plate, cerebellopontine angle, and posterior infratentorial midline cisternae each account for approximately 10%. Other less common locations include the intrahemispheric fissures, pericerebral subarachnoid spaces, and midline infratentorial region (Fig. 1-25). Hydrocephalus is present in 40% to 50% of patients with arachnoid cysts and may be of either communicating or noncommunicating varieties.

Suprasellar arachnoid cysts can extend inferiorly into the sella turcica, laterally into the middle cranial fossae, or posteriorly into the interpeduncular cisterna. With posterior

Fig. 1-25 Interhemispheric arachnoid cyst. Coronal MR scan demonstrating a large arachnoid cyst of the right side of the interhemispheric fissure. The hemispheres are widely separated at this site. The cyst does not communicate with the ventricular system.

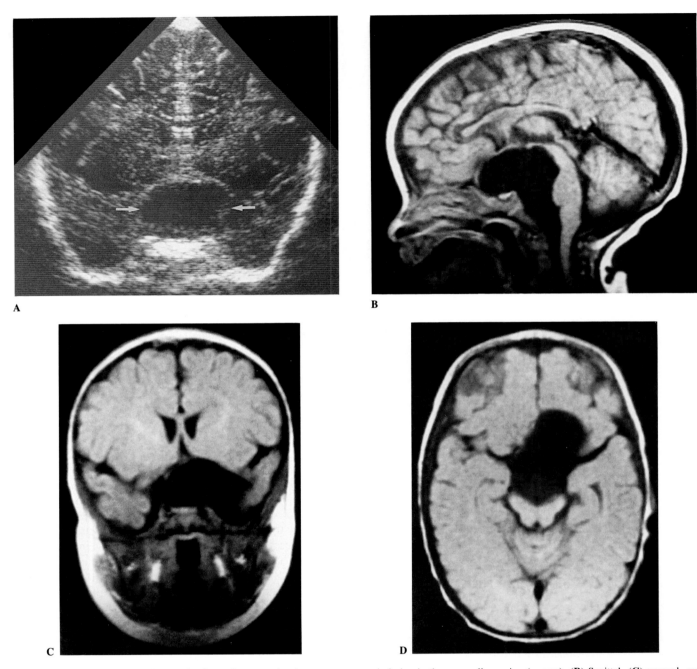

Fig. 1-26 Suprasellar arachnoid cyst. (**A**) Coronal sonography demonstrates a cystic lesion in the suprasellar region (arrows). (**B**) Sagittal, (**C**) coronal, and (**D**) axial T_1-weighted MR images more clearly define the anatomy of this suprasellar arachnoid cyst. There is extension into the left middle and anterior cranial fossae as well as into the interpeduncular cisterna. The brainstem is displaced posteriorly, and the cerebral peduncles are spread. The optic chiasm and tracts are displaced superiorly. The third ventricle is compressed. The aqueduct is patent; hydrocephalus has not developed.

expansion, the third ventricle is displaced in a cephalad direction. If the cyst is large the foramina of Monro may be obstructed, resulting in hydrocephalus. The posterior extent of the cyst may displace the pineal gland inferiorly and obstruct the aqueduct, also producing hydrocephalus. The optic chiasm, optic tracts, and intracranial portions of the optic nerves may be stretched and displaced by the cyst. The diagnosis is best established by MRI, with midline sagittal images

showing the cyst to displace the floor of the third ventricle cephalad. Extension into the middle cranial fossae is best viewed on coronal images (Fig. 1-26).[42]

The appearance of arachnoid cysts of the middle cranial fossa is somewhat variable, largely depending on the size of the lesion. Approximately 10% to 20% are small and biconvex, showing little mass effect and no bone erosion. Approximately half the middle cranial fossa cysts are of mod-

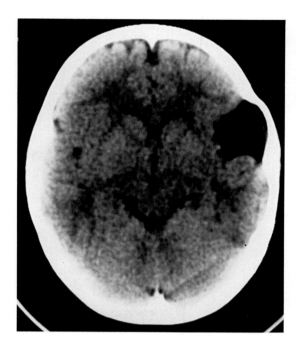

Fig. 1-27 Sylvian fissure arachnoid cyst. Axial CT scan showing a well-defined arachnoid cyst in the anterior aspect of the left sylvian fissure. Chronic mass effect has caused expansion and thinning of the adjacent portion of the calvaria. The margins of the left temporal lobe are effaced.

erate size. They often occupy the anterior and middle aspects of the temporal fossa and displace the tip of the temporal horn posteriorly, superiorly, and medially. Those located in the sylvian fissure cause separation and effacement of the fissure. Those located along the floor of the middle cranial fossa cause superior displacement of the temporal lobe. The calvaria adjacent to the lesion may be expanded (Fig. 1-27). Approximately 30% of middle cranial fossa arachnoid cysts are large enough to occupy virtually the entire fossa. These lesions cause marked mass effect with compression of brain and midline shift.[43]

Approximately 25% of arachnoid cysts arise in the posterior fossa. These cysts are usually large at presentation. The epicenter of the lesion may be anywhere in the posterior fossa. The cerebellopontine angle cisternae and inferior midline regions are the most common locations. Other sites include the quadrigeminal plate cisterna, the prepontine cisterna, and the lateral retrocerebellar region. Midline posterior fossa arachnoid cysts must be differentiated from the Dandy-Walker malformation. The distinction can frequently be made clinically. Patients with arachnoid cysts usually present with signs of cerebellar dysfunction that are due to compression by the cysts, whereas patients with the Dandy-Walker malformation present with signs of either hydrocephalus or developmental delay.

Diagnostic imaging shows sharply defined walls of the posterior fossa arachnoid cyst. Although it may be compressed and displaced, the cerebellar vermis is intact (Fig. 1-28). The cyst can be separated from the vallecula and fourth ventricle in

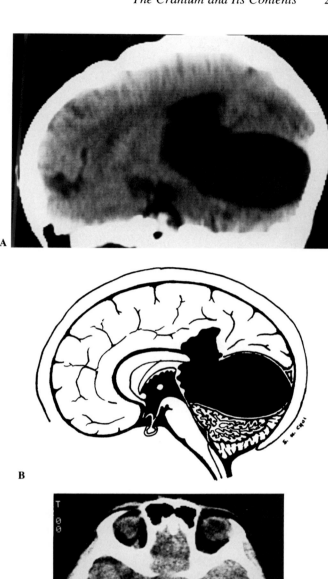

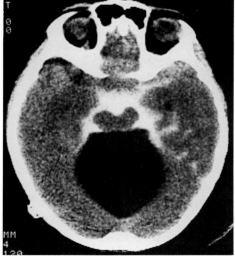

Fig. 1-28 Collicular arachnoid cyst. (**A**) Sagittal reformatted CT scan shows a large arachnoid cyst in the superior aspect of the posterior fossa. The cerebellum is displaced inferiorly. A portion of the cyst extends superiorly through the incisura of the tentorium. (**B**) Schematic representation of the cyst shows its relationships to adjacent structures. Most of the cyst lies inferior to the tentorium. The cerebellar vermis is intact and markedly compressed. (**C**) CT cisternography shows contrast material in the subarachnoid spaces. The posterior fossa cyst does not accumulate contrast material because of the lack of free communication with the subarachnoid space. The epicenter of this cyst is in the quadrigeminal or collicular plate cisterna.

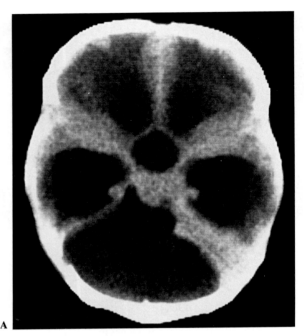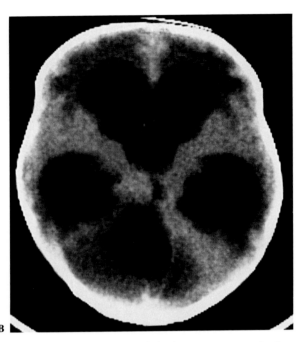

Fig. 1-29 Lateral retrocerebellar arachnoid cyst. (**A** and **B**) Unenhanced axial CT scans of a newborn with macrocephaly demonstrate a posterior fossa fluid collection that causes marked compression of the cerebellum. The straight sinus is displaced somewhat to the left. Because of the large size of the cyst, the aqueduct has become obstructed, causing hydrocephalus. There is transependymal migration of cerebrospinal fluid in the frontal and temporal regions.

all imaging planes, whereas the Dandy-Walker malformation is demonstrated as an extension of the fourth ventricle in conjunction with aplasia of the cerebellar vermis. Retrocerebellar arachnoid cysts must be differentiated from the normal variation of a prominent cisterna magna.[44–46]

Retrocerebellar arachnoid cysts are usually quite large. They may lie either in the midline or in a lateral location (Fig. 1-29). The key feature in differentiating a retrocerebellar arachnoid cyst from an enlarged cisterna magna is communication of the cisterna magna with the remainder of the cerebrospinal fluid spaces. This may be demonstrated on cisternography.

Posterior Fossa Cystic Malformations

Cystic developmental anomalies of the posterior fossa include Dandy-Walker malformation, Dandy-Walker variant, megacisterna magna, and arachnoid cyst. The Dandy-Walker malformation is a complex developmental anomaly that includes a high tentorium, dysgenesis or agenesis of the cerebellar vermis, and cystic dilatation of the fourth ventricle, which occupies most of the posterior fossa. The overall size of the posterior fossa is enlarged. The Dandy-Walker variant consists of dysgenesis of the cerebellar vermis and cystic dilatation of the fourth ventricle without significant enlargement of the posterior fossa. Megacisterna magna refers to enlargement of the posterior fossa because of a prominent cisterna magna; the cerebellar vermis and fourth ventricle are intact (Fig. 1-30). Posterior fossa arachnoid cyst is a distinct entity that has been discussed previously.[47–49]

Dandy-Walker malformation, Dandy-Walker variant, and megacisterna magna are thought to represent components of a spectrum of posterior fossa cystic malformations that result from insults to the development of the fourth ventricle and cerebellum. This spectrum of anomalies is sometimes termed the Dandy-Walker complex. It is proposed that megacisterna magna results from an insult primarily to the developing fourth ventricle. The Dandy-Walker variant is produced by an insult primarily to the developing cerebellar hemispheres, and the Dandy-Walker malformation results from an extensive insult that involves both the cerebellum and the fourth ventricle.[49]

One or more associated central nervous system or systemic anomalies are present in most patients with Dandy-Walker malformation. The most common associated abnormality is hydrocephalus. Hydrocephalus is unusual at birth but develops in up to 75% of these infants by 3 months of age. Hydromyelia of the spinal cord may occur. Dysgenesis of the corpus callosum occurs in about 25% of patients with Dandy-Walker malformation. This can be either complete agenesis or partial absence of the corpus callosum. About 5% of Dandy-Walker patients have polymicrogyria, heterotopic gray matter, or lissencephaly. There are unusual cases in which an occipital cephalocele occurs in association with Dandy-Walker malformation. Anomalies of other systems that are associated with Dandy-Walker malformation include polydactyly, cardiac defects, microphthalmos, microglossia, cleft palate, and facial hemangiomas.

The diagnosis of Dandy-Walker malformation and the related types of posterior fossa cystic malformations can be achieved with CT, MRI, or prenatal sonography. These stud-

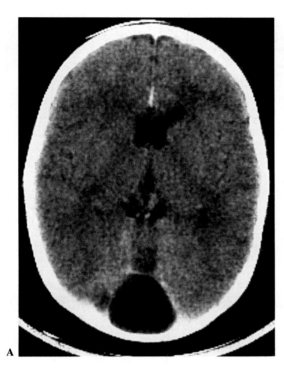

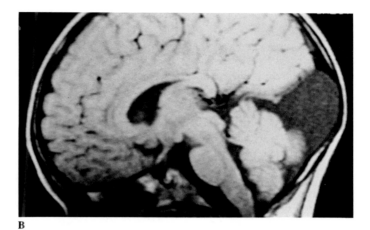

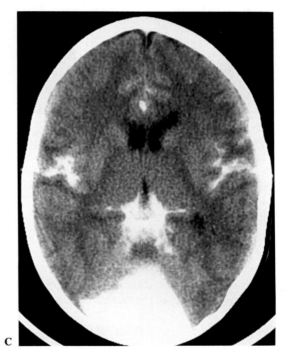

Fig. 1-30 Megacisterna magna. (**A**) Unenhanced axial CT scan shows a midline posterior fossa fluid collection. The cyst has attenuation characteristics identical to those of cerebrospinal fluid. (**B**) Sagittal T_1-weighted MR image shows the vermis of the cerebellum to be intact. The posterior fossa fluid collection lies posterior to the vermis. The straight sinus is somewhat elevated. (**C**) CT cisternography shows the megacisterna magna to communicate freely with the remainder of the subarachnoid space. The presence of a normal cerebellar vermis excludes Dandy-Walker malformation.

ies show hypoplasia or absence of the cerebellar vermis and hypoplasia of the cerebellar hemispheres. There is a large fluid-filled structure that occupies a large portion of the posterior fossa and widely communicates with the fourth ventricle. The posterior fossa may be enlarged, and the tentorium is elevated (Fig. 1-31).[49,50]

Congenital Destructive Brain Lesions

Hydranencephaly. Hydranencephaly is a condition in which most of the brain cortex and white matter are absent and replaced by cerebrospinal fluid. The fluid-filled hemispheres are lined peripherally by membranes that are composed of an outer layer of leptomeningeal tissue and an inner layer of remnants of cerebral cortex and white matter. The lateral ventricles are absent, and the cysts usually communicate with the third ventricle. Obstructive hydrocephalus of variable severity may be present as a result of obstruction of the aqueduct. The thalami are usually preserved, and the posterior fossa structures are relatively normal.[51]

Hydranencephaly is thought to be due to an event in utero that causes massive destruction and subsequent resorption of cerebral tissue. This condition probably represents a severe type of bilateral porencephaly. The precise mechanism of injury is unknown, and different factors may be involved in individual cases. Severe vascular occlusion, such as bilateral carotid artery occlusion, is probably responsible for most cases. Intrauterine infection may be involved in some instances. Toxoplasmosis and infection with cytomegalovirus have been shown to be involved in many cases of hydranencephaly. It is likely that a number of insults to the developing brain occurring at a time when the brain reacts by liquefactive necrosis can result in hydranencephaly.

Neonates with hydranencephaly may appear normal clinically. Neurologic findings develop within a few weeks after birth, however. Spasticity and myoclonic seizures are common. In some children hydrocephalus produces an enlarged head circumference, whereas lack of brain growth leads to microcephaly in others. Electroencephalography shows absent or markedly suppressed activity. Many affected children die during infancy.[52]

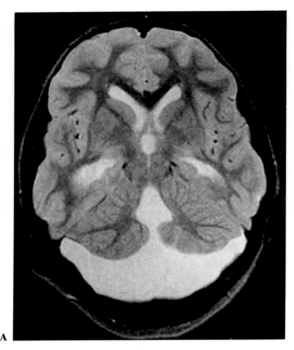

A

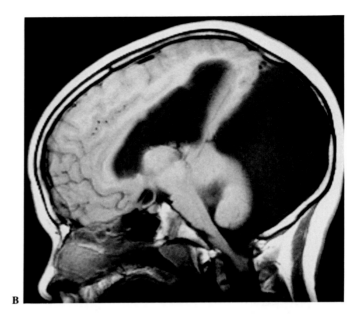

B

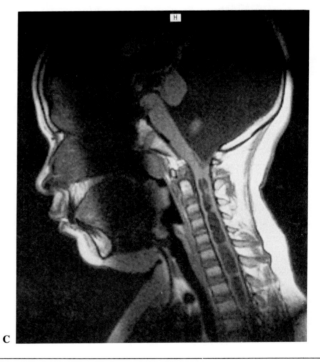

C

Fig. 1-31 Dandy-Walker malformation. **(A)** T$_2$-weighted axial and **(B)** T$_1$-weighted sagittal MR images show absence of the cerebellar vermis and hypoplasia of the cerebellar hemispheres. Note elevation of the tentorium and the torcula. The genu of the corpus callosum is present, but the body and splenium are absent. **(C)** Sagittal T$_1$-weighted MR image of the cervical spine shows extensive hydromyelia with internal ridges in the center of the cord.

The diagnosis of hydranencephaly can be established with sonography, CT, or MRI. Imaging reveals replacement of the cerebral hemispheres by cerebrospinal fluid, with a thin peripheral rim of tissue. The thalami are usually present. At times the inferior aspects of the frontal lobes and the inferomedial temporal lobes are preserved. The falx cerebri is usually present (Fig. 1-32). The cerebellum is normal in appearance, but the brainstem is often somewhat atrophic.

Hydranencephaly may be difficult to distinguish from severe hydrocephalus. In the latter, a definite rim or mantle of cerebral tissue should be visible surrounding the dilated ventricles; the membrane surrounding hydranencephaly is quite thin. The distinction is probably best achieved on MRI, although in the past angiography has been advocated. From a practical standpoint, both conditions are treated with diversionary shunting if there is macrocephaly. Hydranencephaly is differentiated from severe alobar holoprosencephaly in that, in the latter condition, the falx cerebri is absent, the thalami are fused, cerebral tissue inferior to the midline cyst is preserved, and a rudimentary third ventricle is usually identifiable.

Porencephaly. In the broad sense, the term *porencephaly* refers to an abnormal fluid-filled cavity in the brain. Various types of porencephaly may be recognized on the basis of presumed etiologic factors, morphology, and patient age. Encephaloclastic porencephaly refers to a smooth-walled, congenital cystic brain lesion that is not surrounded by signifi-

cant glial reaction; this type is thought to be due to localized brain destruction during the first half of gestation. Porencephaly resulting from insults later in fetal life or acquired after birth (by neonatal asphyxia, cerebrovascular accident, and the like) is more properly termed cystic encephalomalacia. This type is associated with significant glial reaction. Porencephaly may also be divided into communicating and noncommunicating types to reflect the presence or absence of connection with the ventricular system.[52]

Imaging studies demonstrate encephaloclastic porencephaly as a smooth-walled cavity, usually with wide communication with the ventricular system. On MRI, the cyst is

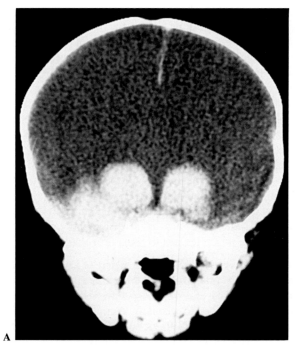
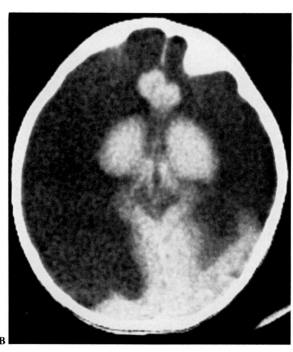

Fig. 1-32 Hydranencephaly. (**A**) Coronal and (**B**) axial CT scans of a 2-week-old infant show replacement of virtually all the cerebral hemispheres by cerebrospinal fluid. The thalami are present, and there are small residual areas of brain parenchyma in the right temporal lobe, the occipital lobes, and the paramedian aspect of the frontal lobes. The falx cerebri is present.

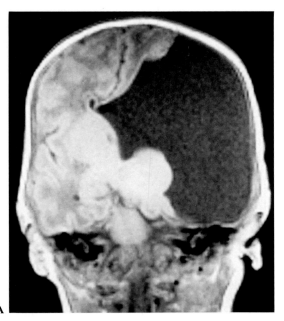
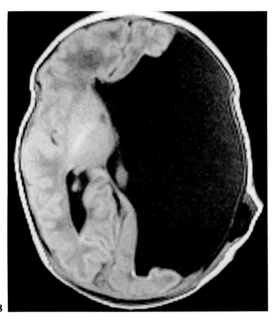

Fig. 1-33 Encephaloclastic porencephaly. (**A**) Coronal and (**B**) axial T_1-weighted MR scans demonstrate a large porencephalic cyst replacing a large portion of the left cerebral hemisphere. The left lateral ventricle and the interventricular septum are absent. The cyst communicates freely with the right lateral ventricle. There is minimal remaining left hemispheric parenchyma at the margins of the cyst.

isointense to cerebrospinal fluid on all imaging sequences (Fig. 1-33). With cystic encephalomalacia, the wall of the cyst is often irregular as a result of gliosis, and septations may be present. The cyst may or may not communicate with the ventricular system. The gliosis in the surrounding brain can often be demonstrated as areas of high signal intensity on T_2-weighted images. Glial septa in the cavity are best demonstrated on T_1-weighted sequences. Sonography is also quite sensitive for identifying the numerous glial septa that occur in cystic encephalomalacia.

Disorders of Neuronal Migration

Schizencephaly. Schizencephaly is a congenital anomaly in which a gray matter-lined cleft extends through the hemisphere from the lateral ventricle to the subarachnoid space. These clefts can be unilateral or bilateral. The most common location is in the region of the precentral and postcentral gyri. Cerebrospinal fluid is contained in the cleft. Microscopically, the gray matter that makes up the walls of the cleft shows the features of polymicrogyria. The cleft is lined by a pial-ependymal membrane. The clefts of schizencephaly can be fused or separated. In fused clefts the walls oppose each other, and the cerebrospinal fluid space in the cleft is largely obliterated. When the walls are separated, cerebrospinal fluid fills the resultant tract from the lateral ventricle to the convexity of the subarachnoid space. Schizencephaly is thought to be caused by an anomaly of neuronal migration.

The severity of symptoms in cases of schizencephaly roughly correlates with the size of the defect(s). A single fused cleft usually is associated with relatively mild symptoms, such as a seizure disorder or mild hemiparesis. Developmentally, this group of patients is usually normal. A unilateral separated cleft tends to result in mild to moderate developmental delay with some variation depending on the portion of the brain affected. Patients with bilateral clefts tend to have seizures and significant psychomotor retardation. These patients usually have severe motor anomalies and are frequently blind. The blindness is due at least in part to optic nerve hypoplasia, which occurs in one-third of patients with schizencephaly.

The diagnosis of schizencephaly can be established on CT or MRI, although the latter technique is the most specific. The anomaly is demonstrated as a cleft extending through the hemisphere. The cleft has irregular margins and is lined with gray matter. The gyral pattern of the cortex immediately adjacent to the cleft usually shows a structural abnormality such as polymicrogyria or pachygyria (Fig. 1-34). Gray matter heterotopias may be identified in the ventricle adjacent to the cleft. In almost all cases, there is a dimple along the wall of the lateral ventricle at the site of the cleft. This dimple is a helpful sign in establishing the diagnosis of schizencephaly, particularly in cases in which the segments are fused. In most cases of schizencephaly there are bilateral clefts, although they may not be symmetric. The septum pellucidum is absent in up to 90% of patients with schizencephaly (Fig. 1-35).[53–55]

Gray Matter Heterotopia. Gray matter heterotopia is a collection of normal nerve cells in an abnormal location. This anomaly is thought to be due to focally arrested neuronal migration. Gray matter heterotopia may be an isolated anomaly, but it often occurs in association with another structural brain anomaly such as schizencephaly, agenesis of the corpus callosum, or Chiari II malformation. These patients typically present with seizures. Other symptoms may be related to concomitant structural anomalies.

Because gray matter heterotopias are composed of normal nerve cells in abnormal locations, imaging studies show the lesions to have the characteristics of normal gray matter. Al-

though large heterotopias can be identified on CT, MRI is the most sensitive imaging technique for the evaluation of these lesions. MRI demonstrates a nodular region that is isointense to gray matter on all imaging sequences. The subependymal regions and the periventricular white matter are the most common locations. The size and number of lesions are quite variable. In severe cases, there are thick bands of heterotopic gray matter filling most of both cerebral hemispheres. As mentioned, agenesis of the corpus callosum is often associated with subependymal gray matter heterotopias.

Gray matter heterotopias can usually be readily distinguished from neoplasm by the MR features. Heterotopias are isointense to normal gray matter on all imaging sequences, including contrast-enhanced studies. There is no surrounding edema and little or no mass effect. Sequential examinations show the size of the lesions to remain unchanged.[56–58]

Lissencephaly and Pachygyria. There is a spectrum of neuronal migration anomalies in which there is deficient gyral formation. At one end of the spectrum is lissencephaly or agyria, which refers to virtually complete absence of gyri resulting in smooth hemispheric surfaces that lack primary fissures. At the other end of the spectrum is pachygyria, which refers to a decrease in number, broadening, and flattening of the gyri. In some cases, regions of agyria and pachygyria may be present in the same patient; this is sometimes termed incomplete lissencephaly. In these mixed forms, the agyria is most often localized to the parietal and occipital regions, and the pachygyria tends to occur in the frontal and temporal lobes.

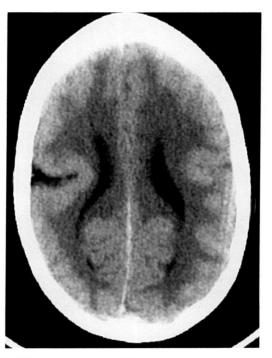

Fig. 1-34 CT scan demonstrating schizencephaly on the right with a cleft that is fused medially. The cleft is lined by a thick layer of gray matter. The gyral pattern in the right hemisphere adjacent to the cleft is abnormally smooth as a result of pachygyria. This is fused cleft schizencephaly.

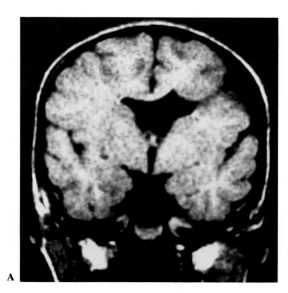

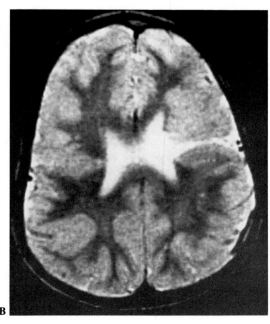

Fig. 1-35 Schizencephaly. (**A**) Coronal T$_1$-weighted and (**B**) axial T$_2$-weighted MR scans demonstrate complete cleft schizencephaly in the left hemisphere, resulting in communication between the pericerebral subarachnoid space and the left lateral ventricle. The cleft is lined by thickened gray matter. The septum pellucidum is absent.

Two major types of lissencephaly have been described. Classic, or type 1, lissencephaly is characterized by agyria (occasionally with some areas of pachygyria), deficient opercular development, colpocephaly, and a variable degree of hypoplasia of the corpus callosum. Miller-Dieker syndrome consists of type 1 lissencephaly associated with characteristic facial anomalies and postnatal growth deficiency. Small deletions of the short arm of chromosome 17 have been identified in many of these patients. Type 1 lissencephaly also occurs in Norman-Roberts syndrome.[60]

Type 2 lissencephaly refers to agyria or severe pachygyria in association with obstructive hydrocephalus and other severe malformations of the brain. Walker-Warburg syndrome refers to type 2 lissencephaly in association with hypoplasia of the cerebellar vermis, retinal dysplasia, and anterior chamber mesenchymal dysgenesis. When these features occur in association with congenital muscular dystrophy, the condition is termed cerebral oculomuscular syndrome. Minor facial anomalies, severe hypotonia, and a variable degree of mental retardation are additional features of type 2 lissencephaly.[61]

Lissencephaly and pachygyria can be demonstrated on CT, although the MR features are most distinctive. With type 1 lissencephaly, the surface of the cerebrum is smooth. Slight indentations in the regions of the expected sylvian fissures result in a figure-eight shape. The cortex is thickened, there is diminished white matter, and normal white-gray interdigitations are lacking. The ventricles are often slightly enlarged; enlargement is often most prominent in the posterior aspects of the lateral ventricles (ie, colpocephaly). The rostrum of the corpus callosum is often absent, and the splenium may be hypoplastic or absent (Fig. 1-36).

With type 2 lissencephaly, the lateral and third ventricles are enlarged, and obstructive hydrocephalus is typically present. The abnormal smooth surface of the brain is usually identifiable on MRI. On CT, however, the hydrocephalus may interfere with demonstration of the brain surface anatomy. The lack of normal white-gray interdigitation is usually visible. In many cases, a fairly well demarcated, smooth, low-attenuation line is visible midway between the cerebral surface and the ventricle. Other potential findings with type 2 lissencephaly include agenesis or hypoplasia of the corpus callosum, absence of the septum pellucidum, and hypoplasia of the cerebellar vermis (Fig. 1-37). Occasionally, true Dandy-Walker formation is present.

Imaging in cases of pachygyria demonstrates focal or diffuse areas of deficient gyral formation. There is a subnormal number of gyri in the affected region, and some degree of cortical thickening is identified. The sulci are decreased in number and are shallow (Fig. 1-38).[55]

Lissencephaly and pachygyria are thought to be caused by defective neuronal migration from the germinal matrix to the cortical surface. Normal gyral formation occurs during gestation weeks 26 through 28. Six cortical layers can normally be defined histologically. In patients with lissencephaly the cerebral cortex is thickened, and there are few layers. Along the inner margin of the cortex, there is a thick abnormal layer that contains a sparse population of large cells. Medial to this layer is a dense population of ectopic neurons that have presumably been prevented from migrating peripherally. In cases of pachygyria, the degree of cortical thickening is not as severe as with lissencephaly or agyria, and the expected six cortical layers can usually be identified. A medial layer of sparsely scattered large cells is present, but it is not as thick as with lissencephaly.[54,59]

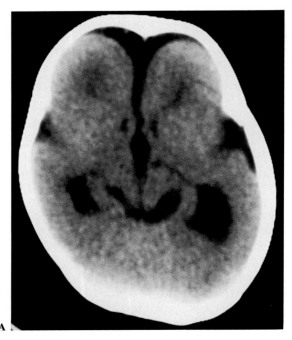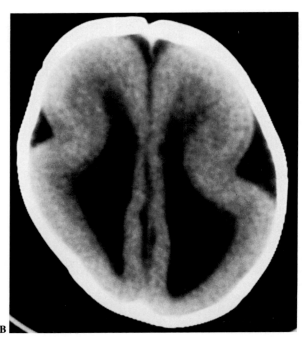

A   B

Fig. 1-36 Type 1 lissencephaly. (**A** and **B**) Axial CT scans demonstrate a smooth agyral cerebral cortex with lack of interdigitations of white matter. Indentations on the cortex in the region of the sylvian fissures produce the characteristic figure-eight shape on these axial images. The gray matter is thickened, and little white matter is visible. There is slight ventricular enlargement, particularly in the posterior aspects of the lateral ventricles. The corpus callosum is absent.

Polymicrogyria. Polymicrogyria is an anomaly of neuronal migration in which one or more portions of the cortex are thickened and contain multiple diminutive gyri. In this disorder, the neurons migrate sufficiently to reach the cortex but become distributed in an abnormal fashion, thereby forming multiple small gyri. The most common location is in the temporal and parietal lobes adjacent to the sylvian fissure. Polymicrogyria may occur in association with a number of other structural brain anomalies, such as unilateral megalencephaly and schizencephaly. Clinically, children with polymi-

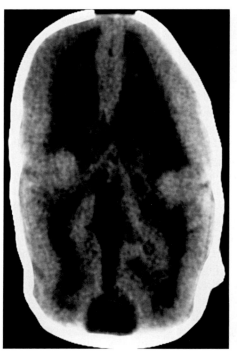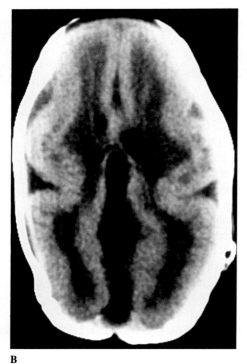

A   B

Fig. 1-37 Type 2 lissencephaly. (**A** and **B**) Axial CT scans in an infant shunted for hydrocephalus show an abnormal smooth appearance of the cerebrum. There is thickening of the gray matter and lack of normal interdigitations of white matter. The cerebellar vermis is hypoplastic.

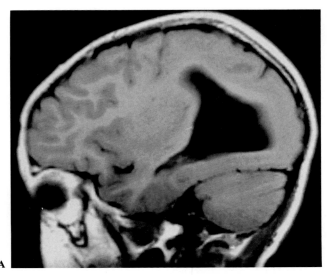

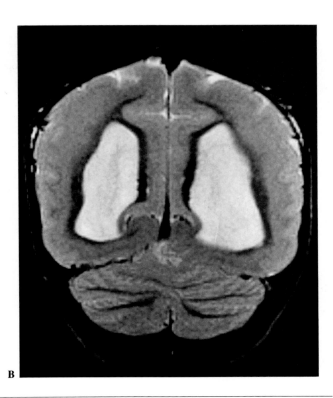

Fig. 1-38 Focal pachygyria. **(A)** Parasagittal T_1-weighted MR scan shows deficient gyral formation and cortical thickening in the parietal and occipital regions; there is more normal gyral formation in the frontal and temporal lobes. There is slight enlargement of the posterior aspect of the lateral ventricle. **(B)** Coronal T_2-weighted MR image shows marked deficiency in myelination and lack of white matter ramification in the involved portions of the hemispheres.

crogyria usually have some degree of developmental delay and seizures.

CT and MRI demonstrate polymicrogyria as a region of abnormally broad, thickened gyri. In general, the individual gyri are too small to be visualized, and the appearance mimics that of pachygyria. The identification of gliotic white matter adjacent to the abnormal cortex is helpful in confirming the diagnosis of polymicrogyria because this is not seen with pachygyria. The gliosis is demonstrated as abnormally decreased white matter attenuation on CT scans and high-signal abnormality on T_2-weighted MR images. Large superficial veins are sometimes identified adjacent to a region of polymicrogyria. This finding is most common when there is a large infolding of thickened cortex.

Unilateral Megalencephaly. Unilateral megalencephaly is a hamartomatous enlargement of all or part of one cerebral hemisphere. This anomaly is thought to be due to defective neuronal migration during the first trimester. The affected hemisphere contains regions of pachygyria, polymicrogyria, and gray matter heterotopias. There is gliosis in the white matter. The hemisphere is hypertrophied and dysplastic. Histologic evaluation demonstrates the presence of large, distorted neurons and glia. The anomaly may be focal, lobar, hemispheric, or (rarely) bilateral. These patients typically have severe seizure disturbances that begin in infancy. Hemiparesis, hemianopsia, and psychomotor delay occur to a variable degree.

CT and MRI in cases of unilateral megalencephaly show the involved hemisphere to be moderately to markedly enlarged.

There is pachygyria or agyria (or both) and a smooth cortical surface, shallow sulci, and cortical thickening. Gray matter heterotopias and gliosis occur in the white matter. The gliosis causes abnormal low attenuation in the white matter on CT scans and high signal intensity on T_2-weighted MR images. The border between the cortex and the subjacent white matter is indistinct or obliterated. On axial images, the frontal horn of the involved hemisphere tends to be straight and is directed anterolaterally (Fig. 1-39).[62,63]

HYDROCEPHALUS

Hydrocephalus is characterized by an abnormal balance of formation and absorption of cerebrospinal fluid. Because of this imbalance, excess cerebrospinal fluid in the central nervous system causes an increase in intracranial pressure. The degree and pattern of enlargement of the cerebrospinal fluid pathways and the amount of damage to central nervous system structures depend on both the degree and the etiology of the hydrocephalus. There is a fairly broad spectrum of clinical manifestations of hydrocephalus.

Mechanisms of Hydrocephalus

The rate of cerebrospinal fluid production in the brain is reasonably constant, and, with the exception of hydrocephalus

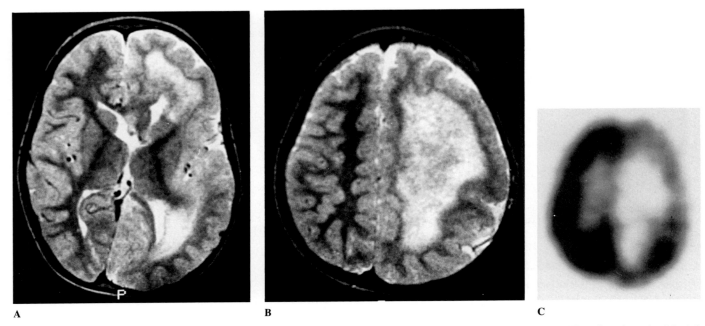

A   B   C

Fig. 1-39 Unilateral megalencephaly. (**A** and **B**) Axial T$_2$-weighted MR scans show enlargement of the left cerebral hemisphere. There is pachygyria of the left hemisphere with lesser involvement of the occipital lobe. There is marked abnormally high signal arising from the white matter of the abnormal hemisphere. The frontal horn of the left lateral ventricle has a straightened configuration. (**C**) Axial [^{123}I]iofetamine single-photon emission CT brain imaging shows deficient accumulation of tracer in the abnormal left hemisphere.

due to choroid plexus papillomas, overproduction of cerebrospinal fluid is not the cause of hydrocephalus in the great majority of cases. Hydrocephalus is almost invariably due to some mechanism that results in impaired resorption of cerebrospinal fluid. This can result from blockage of flow in the ventricular system, basal cisternae, or cerebral convexity. Diminished absorption may also result from abnormalities of the arachnoid villi.[64]

As intracranial pressure increases, cerebrospinal fluid may be absorbed through the arachnoid membrane or the stroma of the choroid plexus, or it may egress through the extracellular spaces of the cortical mantle. This latter phenomenon is termed transependymal cerebrospinal fluid flow (Fig. 1-40). As these new absorptive pathways develop, a new equilibrium is established between production and absorption of cerebrospinal fluid. This situation has been termed compensated hydrocephalus.

With transependymal flow of cerebrospinal fluid through the white matter, neuronal and astrocystic swelling develops in the gray matter, and atrophic changes occur in the nerve fibers of the cerebral hemispheres. The cilia that normally cover the ependymal surface of the ventricular system may disappear in hydrocephalic states. If the intraventricular pressure is great, and if there is marked ventriculomegaly, cerebral blood flow may be reduced. This is most prominent in the distribution of the anterior cerebral arteries. Compromised blood flow can lead to ischemic injury of the basal forebrain and medial cerebral hemispheres.

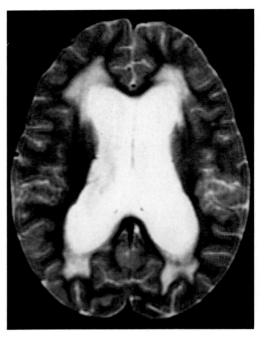

Fig. 1-40 Hydrocephalus. T$_2$-weighted axial MR scan showing moderate hydrocephalus. There is increased signal in the periventricular white matter as a result of transependymal cerebrospinal fluid flow. Note the predilection for involvement of the white matter in the frontal and occipital regions and relative sparing of the white matter adjacent to the bodies of the lateral ventricles.

Clinical Features of Hydrocephalus

Several factors influence the natural history of hydrocephalus. Among these are the age of the patient at the time of onset and the duration of the increased intracranial pressure. Also important are the rate of increase of pressure and the presence or absence of associated structural abnormalities. Before the age of 2 years, hydrocephalus is almost always accompanied by an enlargement of the head circumference. Chiari II malformation and aqueductal stenosis account for about 80% of cases of hydrocephalus in this age group. Other relatively common etiologies of hydrocephalus in infants include intrauterine infection, perinatal hemorrhage, and neonatal meningitis. Rare etiologies include midline tumors, choroid plexus papillomas, arachnoid cysts, and central arteriovenous malformations.

In infants with hydrocephalus, the head circumference increases at an abnormal rate, leading to macrocephaly. Clinically, the forehead is disproportionately large, and the skull is somewhat thin. The sutures are palpably spread, the anterior fontanelle bulges, and the scalp veins are visibly dilated. Potential ocular disturbances include paralysis of upward gaze (Parinaud syndrome), nystagmus, proptosis, and a diminished pupillary light reflux. Spasticity of the lower extremities is common.

Hydrocephalus first developing later in childhood is usually due to aqueductal stenosis or a posterior fossa tumor. The clinical features in these cases are determined by the severity of hydrocephalus and by the nature of the primary lesion, when present. In most patients, increased intracranial pressure results in early morning headaches that improve in the upright position. Vomiting, especially morning vomiting, is another frequent clinical sign of increased intracranial pressure. In many children, this leads to evaluation of the gastrointestinal tract before the fundamental lesion in the central nervous system is discovered.

Spastic and cerebellar signs predominate in the lower extremities. Papilledema and strabismus are identified in most patients at presentation. Endocrine abnormalities may be produced by compression of the hypothalamic-pituitary axis due to enlargement of the anterior recesses of the third ventricle. This can result in short stature, gigantism, menstrual irregularities, hypothyroidism, or diabetes insipidus.

Specific Types of Hydrocephalus

Hydrocephalus can be grouped into two major types. Hydrocephalus due to overproduction of cerebrospinal fluid is rare and is mainly due to choroid plexus papilloma. The great majority of cases of hydrocephalus are due to obstruction to normal cerebrospinal fluid flow or inadequate absorption. This category can be further divided into communicating hydrocephalus, in which there is an extraventricular obstruction to flow or diminished absorption, and noncommunicating hydrocephalus, which is caused by intraventricular obstruction, most often at the aqueduct of Sylvius.

Hydrocephalus Due to Excessive Cerebrospinal Fluid Formation

Papillomas of the choroid plexus account for 2% to 5% of childhood intracranial tumors. The clinical presentation occurs in infancy with signs of elevated intracranial pressure. The appearance of choroid plexus papillomas on CT and MRI is described later in this chapter. These tumors are most often located in the lateral ventricles near the trigone. The body of the lateral ventricle and the third ventricle are the next most common sites (Fig. 1-41). In contrast to the situation with adults, the fourth ventricle is an uncommon location of a choroid plexus papilloma in children.

Intraventricular Obstruction (Noncommunicating Hydrocephalus)

Intraventricular obstructive hydrocephalus, or noncommunicating hydrocephalus, can result from obstruction in any portion of the ventricular system, from the foramina of Monro to the foramina of Magendie and Luschka. The etiology of the obstruction may be congenital or acquired, and the obstruction may be intrinsic or extrinsic to the ventricular system (Table 1-3). A proper diagnosis of the specific etiology often requires correlation of the clinical history with the imaging findings. CT and, in young infants, sonography are well suited for detecting and characterizing obstructive hydrocephalus. In many cases, MRI provides additional information concerning the specific etiology. Because of the potential for even small neoplasms to cause obstructive hydrocephalus, MRI or contrast-enhanced CT should be performed in these cases.

Tumors. Tumors are among the more common lesions to cause ventricular obstruction at the level of the foramina of Monro. Midline lesions usually obstruct both foramina; unilateral or asymmetric tumors may cause unilateral obstruction, thereby trapping one or both of the lateral ventricles. Intraventricular tumors or cysts originating in the lateral or third ventricles can grow into the foramen of Monro. Examples of these lesions include intraventricular arachnoid cysts and colloid cysts of the third ventricle (Fig. 1-42). Suprasellar masses may displace the floor of the third ventricle superiorly and cause extrinsic obstruction of the foramina of Monro and third ventricle. In children with tuberous sclerosis, a subependymal nodule or giant cell astrocytoma can originate adjacent to the foramen of Monro and grow medially to obstruct the foramen.

Obstruction of the aqueduct of Sylvius by a tumor is a fairly common etiology of hydrocephalus in children beyond early infancy. Pineal tumors are a common cause of neoplastic obstruction at this level. These include germ cell tumors (germinoma, endodermal sinus tumor, and teratoma), pineocytoma, and pineoblastoma.[65] Varices of the vein of Galen may also present as a pineal region mass compressing the aqueduct.

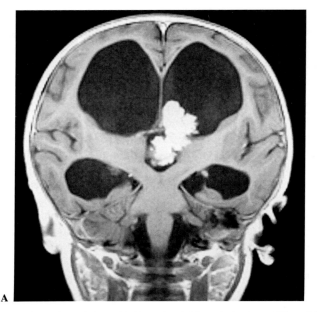

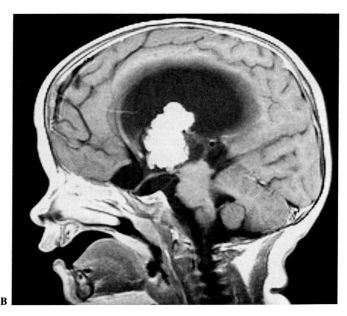

Fig. 1-41 Hydrocephalus. **(A)** Coronal and **(B)** sagittal enhanced T_1-weighted MR images show an intensely enhancing mass with frondlike borders in the third ventricle. The mass extends through the foramen of Monro into the left lateral ventricle. This is a choroid plexus papilloma that has resulted in hydrocephalus due to excessive formation of cerebrospinal fluid.

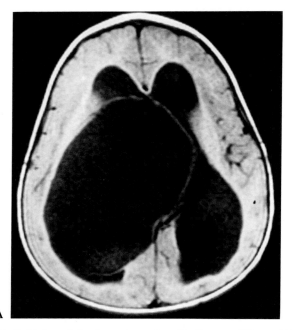

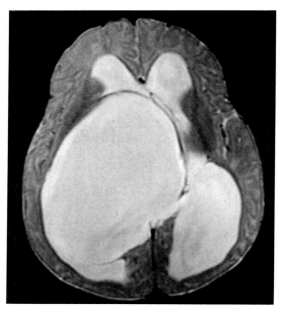

Fig. 1-42 Hydrocephalus due to obstruction of the foramen of Monro. **(A)** Axial T_1-weighted and **(B)** T_2-weighted MR images show a large intraventricular cyst in the right lateral ventricle that is associated with hydrocephalus. Intraventricular cysts most commonly arise from the choroid plexus, and the lateral ventricles are the most common location of these lesions.

Table 1-3 Causes of Noncommunicating Hydrocephalus

Intrinsic Causes	Extrinsic Causes
Congenital stenosis or atresia	Congenital mass (eg, arachnoid
Infection	cyst)
Hemorrhage	Neoplasm
Congenital intraventricular cyst	Vascular malformation
Intraventricular neoplasm	Cerebral edema

Gliomas of the tectum are uncommon tumors that, even when quite small, produce obstructive hydrocephalus by compression of the aqueduct (Fig. 1-43).

Tumors of the fourth ventricle and cerebellum can cause obstructive hydrocephalus. The most common posterior fossa tumor in children is medulloblastoma, which is followed in frequency by cerebellar astrocytoma and ependymoma. Posterior fossa tumors may cause hydrocephalus by invasion and

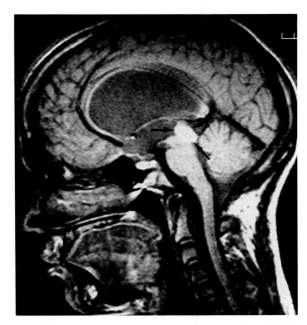

Fig. 1-43 Glioma of the tectum. Sagittal enhanced T$_1$-weighted MR image shows a small, intensely enhancing mass (arrows) in the tectum of the midbrain. The mass causes occlusion of the cerebral aqueduct and secondary hydrocephalus.

filling of the fourth ventricle or by extrinsic compression of the fourth ventricle or aqueduct. Hydrocephalus is not as common with intrinsic brainstem tumors.

Aqueductal Stenosis. Intrinsic aqueductal stenosis accounts for approximately 15% to 20% of cases of pediatric hydrocephalus. The incidence is about 1 in 1000 births. Most are developmental lesions, although acquired forms of aqueductal stenosis also occur, most often as a result of fibrillary gliosis related to prior hemorrhage or infection. A rare X-linked form of congenital aqueductal stenosis has also been described.[66] Obstruction of the aqueduct may be due to a membrane, focal or long-segment stenosis, or forking (replacement of the aqueduct by multiple narrow channels). Focal stenosis most often occurs either at the level of the superior colliculi or at the intercollicular sulcus.

Forking and stenosis of the aqueduct are frequently accompanied by fusion of the quadrigeminal bodies, fusion of the third nerve nuclei, and molding or beaking of the tectum. In some patients, the shape of the molded tectum is congruent with that of the medial aspects of the adjacent dilated temporal lobes.

The diagnosis of aqueductal stenosis can be established on CT or MRI, although the latter technique is somewhat more specific. Benign and neoplastic etiologies of aqueductal stenosis are best differentiated on MRI. The imaging features of intrinsic aqueductal stenosis include dilatation of the lateral and third ventricles and a normal-appearing fourth ventricle. With severe hydrocephalus, rupture of the septum pellucidum may occur. Stenosis of the proximal aqueduct, either at the level of the superior colliculus or at the entrance of the aqueduct immediately inferior to the posterior commissure, tends to produce severe hydrocephalus. Stenosis of the more distal portions of the aqueduct often causes minimal or moderate hydrocephalus. In these cases, there is dilatation of the proximal aqueduct and posterior displacement of the quadrigeminal plate (Fig. 1-44).[67]

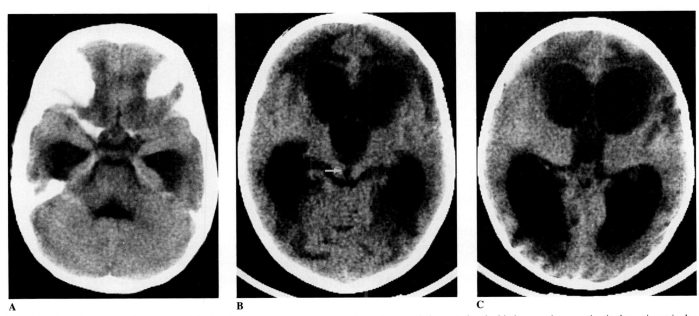

A   B   C

Fig. 1-44 Aqueductal stenosis. (**A**, **B**, and **C**) Axial CT scans demonstrating moderate hydrocephalus associated with decreased attenuation in the periventricular white matter resulting from transependymal cerebrospinal fluid flow. The fourth ventricle is normal in size. The superior aspect of the aqueduct is slightly dilated (arrow in **B**). The quadrigeminal plate is displaced posteriorly. These findings indicate hydrocephalus due to aqueductal stenosis. Contrast-enhanced images (not shown) revealed no evidence of an enhancing mass lesion.

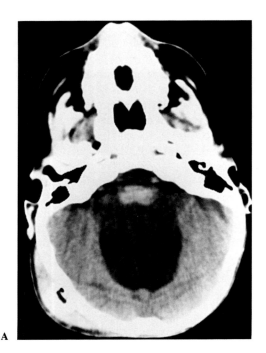

A

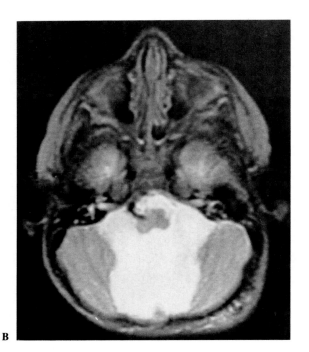

B

Fig. 1-45 Trapped fourth ventricle. **(A)** Axial CT scan of an infant shunted for obstructive hydrocephalus due to an intraventricular hemorrhage shows massive dilatation of the fourth ventricle, including dilatation of the lateral recesses. The brainstem is displaced anteriorly and is narrowed. **(B)** Axial T_2-weighted and **(C)** sagittal T_1-weighted MR images confirm massive dilatation of the fourth ventricle. There are posterior displacement and thinning of the cerebellar vermis. The brainstem is displaced anteriorly and is thinned. The sagittal image demonstrates the typical pear-shaped dilatation that occurs with trapped fourth ventricle.

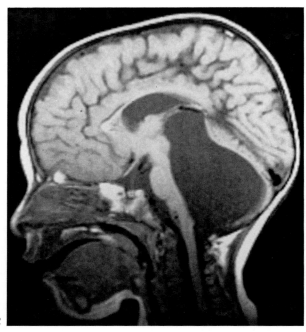

C

Outlet Obstruction of the Fourth Ventricle. Intraventricular obstructive hydrocephalus is occasionally due to an obstruction of the fourth ventricular foramina of Magendie and Luschka. The etiology of the obstruction may be developmental, mechanical, or postinflammatory. Imaging studies usually show dilatation of the entire ventricular system with disproportionate enlargement of the fourth ventricle.

Trapped Fourth Ventricle. Trapped, or isolated, fourth ventricle occurs when the aqueduct of Sylvius and the fourth ventricular outflow foramina are all obstructed. Continued cerebrospinal fluid production by the fourth ventricular choroid plexus leads to progressive cystic dilatation of this ventricle. This condition is usually due to mechanical or inflammatory abnormalities that cause stenosis or occlusion of the aqueduct and outlet foramina. It most commonly occurs in premature infants after intraventricular hemorrhage. Inflammatory changes associated with shunting or meningitis may also be responsible.

On imaging studies the isolated fourth ventricle appears as a large, round or pear-shaped, midline cystic structure in the posterior fossa (Fig. 1-45). The brainstem is displaced anteriorly, and the cerebellar vermis is displaced posteriorly. The lateral and third ventricles are dilated unless there is a functional ventriculoperitoneal shunt.[68]

Extraventricular Obstruction (Communicating Hydrocephalus)

Communicating hydrocephalus accounts for about 30% of childhood hydrocephalus. After passing through the outlet foramina of the fourth ventricle, cerebrospinal fluid normally enters the cisterna magna and basal cisternae and then flows into the cerebral and cerebellar subarachnoid spaces. Normal drainage can be impaired by meningeal thickening, adhesions in the subarachnoid spaces, or increased venous pressure in the arachnoid villi. The basal cisternae, the tentorial hiatus, the

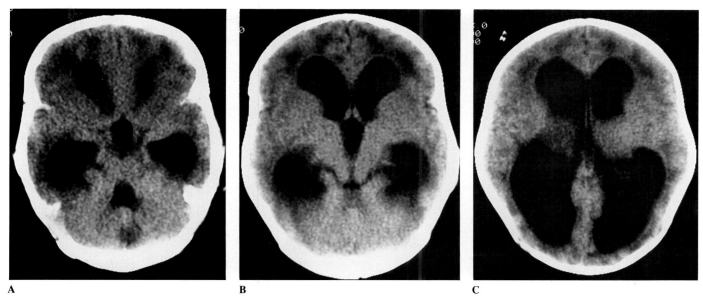

A   B   C

Fig. 1-46 Extraventricular obstructive hydrocephalus. (**A**, **B**, and **C**) Unenhanced CT scans of an infant recovering from *Hemophilus influenzae* type B meningitis show dilatation of the lateral, third, and fourth ventricles. There is transependymal flow of cerebrospinal fluid in the periventricular white matter.

spaces surrounding the cerebral hemispheres, and the arachnoid granulations represent potential sites of obstruction. Obstruction can occur as a sequela to bleeding, infection, or granulomatous meningitis (Fig. 1-46). Meningeal thickening and obstruction of the subarachnoid spaces may also be produced by cellular infiltration in cases of leukemia, lymphoma, and Langerhans cell histiocytosis. There are rare cases in which communicating hydrocephalus develops in children with obstruction of the superior vena cava, presumably as a result of interference with cerebrospinal fluid absorption by elevated venous pressures (Table 1-4).[69,70]

Meningitis. Meningitis results in a variable degree of alteration of cerebrospinal fluid flow dynamics, although clinically evident hydrocephalus is uncommon. During the acute phases of meningitis, thick, purulent fluid collects in the subarachnoid spaces and may impede cerebrospinal fluid flow. Inflammation of the arachnoid granulations also serves to block normal cerebrospinal fluid flow. These abnormalities usually resolve as the inflammatory process decreases during treatment. In the chronic phase of meningitis, fibrotic changes in the subarachnoid spaces may cause areas of permanent obstruction to normal cerebrospinal fluid flow; if these changes are extensive, hydrocephalus will result.

In current practice, significant hydrocephalus is uncommon in bacterial meningitis. The likelihood for the development of

Table 1-4 Causes of Communicating Hydrocephalus

Obliterative arachnoiditis (posthemorrhagic or inflammatory)
Leukemia/lymphoma
Langerhans cell histiocytosis
Venous obstruction
Subarachnoid tumor implants

hydrocephalus roughly correlates with the duration and severity of the infection (Fig. 1-47). In general, the longer the delay in therapy, the poorer the outcome. Different portions of the subarachnoid spaces may be more severely affected than others; bacterial meningitis tends to produce cerebral cortical arachnoiditis, and granulomatous diseases such as tuberculous meningitis more often cause obliteration of the cisternae.

Demonstration of mild ventricular dilatation on CT or MRI during the acute phase of meningitis does not necessarily portend permanent obstructive hydrocephalus. Follow-up studies after resolution of the infection are required to determine the ultimate prognosis. During acute meningitis, MR images enhanced with paramagnetic contrast material often show localized or diffuse meningeal enhancement; this finding is occasionally demonstrable on contrast-enhanced CT. Small subdural fluid collections are commonly seen in cases of meningitis.[71]

Meningeal Metastasis. Neoplastic processes that involve the subarachnoid spaces and meninges may produce extraventricular obstruction of cerebrospinal fluid flow. This may occur with cerebrospinal fluid tumor seeding, as in medulloblastoma and ependymoma, or with hematogenous neoplastic infiltration of the meninges, as in leukemia and lymphoma. In general, symptomatic hydrocephalus in these cases only occurs with extensive disease. CT and MRI show variable degrees of ventricular enlargement. MRI with paramagnetic contrast material shows thickening and abnormal enhancement of the meninges. There may be obliteration of some or all of the cisternae. With seeding of the cerebrospinal fluid, enhancing tumor nodules are usually visualized in the subarachnoid spaces. Similar findings may be appreciated on CT, although MRI is more sensitive for demonstrating meningeal abnormalities.

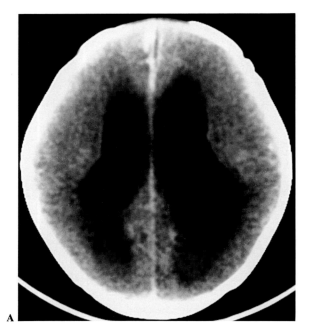 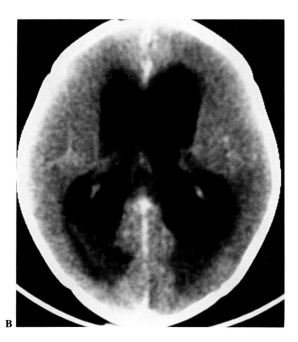

Fig. 1-47 Pyocephalus. (**A** and **B**) Contrast-enhanced CT scans in an infant with severe meningitis showing moderate hydrocephalus. There is layering of material in the dependent portions of the dilated lateral ventricles as a result of pyocephalus. The cerebral sulci are effaced. Abnormal meningeal enhancement is visible along the anterior interhemispheric fissure. The ependyma does not enhance abnormally.

Venous Obstruction. There are rare cases in which hydrocephalus is associated with venous outflow obstruction in the neck or head (Fig. 1-48). Presumably, elevation of the intracranial venous pressure interferes with normal cerebrospinal fluid absorption dynamics at the arachnoid villi. Infants and young children appear to be particularly prone to the development of hydrocephalus by this mechanism; patients older than 3 years of age who have venous outflow obstruction are more likely to develop pseudotumor cerebri. It is postulated that this age difference is related to the more pliable brain parenchyma and the ability of the calvaria to expand in infants, thereby allowing greater ventricular dilatation in response to pressure elevations. In older children and adults, the brain parenchyma is myelinated and less pliable, and sutural closure prevents calvarial expansion; therefore, intracranial venous hypertension causes pseudotumor cerebri without ventricular enlargement.

Hemorrhage

Hydrocephalus is a frequent complication of intraventricular hemorrhage in infants, especially premature infants. This is most often seen in infants who are born before gestation week 32. In the first few days after the hemorrhage, hydrocephalus may be produced by intraventricular or subarachnoid obstruction by clotted blood. Therefore, there is a combination of noncommunicating and communicating hydrocephalus. Hydrocephalus that occurs during this acute phase may persist or resolve spontaneously.[72]

A variable degree of scarring and fibrosis develops in the subarachnoid spaces within several days of the initial bleed.

This adhesive arachnoiditis tends to be most prominent in the region of the cisterna magna. With sufficient scarring and fibrosis of the subarachnoid spaces, subacute hydrocephalus may develop (Fig. 1-49). The development of subacute hydrocephalus after germinal matrix hemorrhage in a premature infant implies a poor functional prognosis.

Subarachnoid hemorrhage in full-term neonates is usually caused by birth trauma. The mechanisms by which hemorrhage causes hydrocephalus acutely and subacutely in these infants are similar to those in premature infants. There is a greater potential for spontaneous resolution of hydrocephalus in these infants.

Subdural hematoma is a potential cause of hydrocephalus in children of all ages. The hydrocephalus in these cases is usually of mild or moderate severity. Imaging studies show ventricular dilatation, subdural fluid, and slight dilatation of the subarachnoid space adjacent to the hematoma.

Hydrocephalus Associated with Congenital Anomalies

The Chiari II malformation is the single most common cause of hydrocephalus in children, accounting for approximately 40% of cases. The mechanism responsible for hydrocephalus in these children is incompletely understood; there is evidence that the connection between the spinal subarachnoid space and the subarachnoid space over the cerebral convexities is inadequate. The outlet foramina of the fourth ventricle in children with Chiari II malformation usually empty into the cervical spinal canal. In view of the limited capacity for cerebrospinal fluid absorption in the spinal canal, the poor commu-

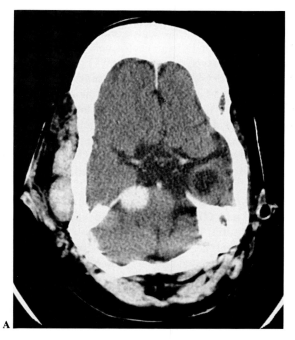

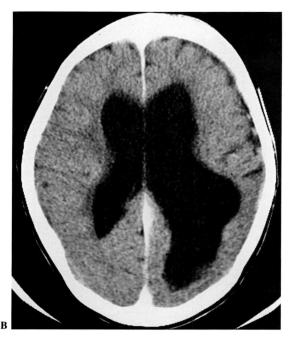

Fig. 1-48 Communicating hydrocephalus due to venous outlet obstruction. (**A**) Contrast-enhanced axial CT in the inferior aspect of the head demonstrates marked dilatation of the right sigmoid sinus. More inferior images showed dilatation of the ipsilateral jugular vein. This child had a large hemangiomatous and lymphangiomatous right neck mass that caused venous obstruction. (**B**) A more superior image shows moderate hydrocephalus.

nication with the subarachnoid spaces of the convexity presumably leads to hydrocephalus. In most cases, there does not appear to be significant obstruction in the ventricles or at the fourth ventricular foramina.[73]

Hydrocephalus occurs in approximately 75% of patients with Dandy-Walker malformation. It is usually not seen at birth, however. The etiology of hydrocephalus in most patients with Dandy-Walker malformation is unknown. It has been proposed that there is an increased susceptibility to subarachnoid hemorrhage from episodes of minor trauma. A large bleed or repeated small bleeds may impede absorption of cerebrospinal fluid and thereby result in communicating hydrocephalus. Less often, there is an anatomic obstruction at the level of the aqueduct.[74]

Benign Enlargement of the Subarachnoid Spaces

It is fairly common for imaging studies to demonstrate slightly enlarged subarachnoid spaces in the frontal and parietal regions in otherwise normal infants. This finding in an infant with normal ventricular size and no evidence of neurologic dysfunction should be considered a variation of normal (Fig. 1-50). A number of terms have been applied to this finding, such as benign extra-axial collections of infancy, external hydrocephalus, benign subdural effusions of infancy, and benign enlargement of the subarachnoid spaces. These infants often show evidence of macrocephaly or rapid increase in head circumference. The rate of head growth usually stabilizes

during the second year of life, and head circumference measurements eventually return to normal. Although not generally required, follow-up neuroimaging studies performed later in childhood show spontaneous disappearance of the prominent subarachnoid spaces.[75,76]

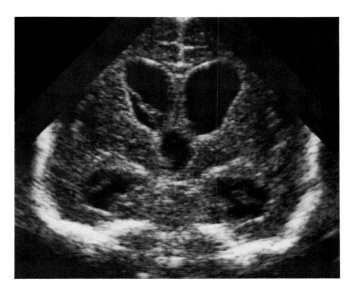

Fig. 1-49 Communicating hydrocephalus. Coronal sonography in a neonate 2 weeks after subependymal and intraventricular hemorrhage shows moderate hydrocephalus. There is a linear echogenic focus in the right lateral ventricle, representing a remnant of the prior hemorrhage. Communicating hydrocephalus in this infant is due to adhesive arachnoiditis related to perinatal germinal matrix hemorrhage.

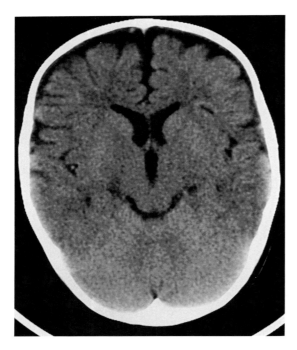

Fig. 1-50 Benign enlargement of the subarachnoid space. Axial CT scan in a 6-month-old infant with moderate macrocephaly shows slight prominence of the extra-axial cerebrospinal fluid spaces in the frontal regions. The cortical sulci are not compressed, and the ventricles are normal. This benign enlargement of the subarachnoid space is a common variation of normal in infants.

PHAKOMATOSES

The term *phakomatosis* describes a group of congenital malformations that predominantly affect ectodermal structures such as the skin, nervous system, and ocular structures. The major phakomatoses include neurofibromatosis, tuberous sclerosis, von Hippel–Lindau disease, Sturge-Weber syndrome, and ataxia-telangiectasia.

Neurofibromatosis

There are two major forms of neurofibromatosis. Neurofibromatosis type 1 (von Recklinghausen disease) accounts for at least 90% of all cases of neurofibromatosis. It is an autosomal dominant disease. An abnormality of the long arm of chromosome 17 near the centromere appears to be responsible for this disorder. Criteria developed by the National Institutes of Health indicate that the diagnosis of neurofibromatosis type 1 is based on the presence of two or more of the following: (1) six or more café au lait spots larger than 15 mm in postpubertal individuals or larger than 5 mm in young children; (2) one plexiform neurofibroma or two or more neurofibromas of any type; (3) an optic glioma; (4) abnormal axillary or inguinal skin pigmentation; (5) more than two pigmented hamartomas of the iris (Lisch nodules); (6) characteristic osseous manifestations, such as dysplasia of the sphenoid or

cortical thinning of the long bones; and (7) a diagnosis of neurofibromatosis in a first-degree relative.[77–79]

The most common primary central nervous system lesion in neurofibromatosis type 1 is optic pathway glioma. This tumor can involve one or both optic nerves. The presence of bilateral optic nerve gliomas is virtually pathognomonic of neurofibromatosis type 1. The tumor may extend into the chiasm and optic tracts; the disease may extend more posteriorly to involve the lateral geniculate bodies. At times, the lesion extends beyond the lateral geniculate bodies into the optic radiations. Most of these tumors are histologically low-grade gliomas.

Optic nerve lesions in children with neurofibromatosis can be evaluated with CT or MRI. Enlargement of the optic nerve is usually fusiform. The enlarged nerve may assume a tortuous or kinked appearance. The intracranial optic nerves, optic chiasm, optic tracts, and optic radiations are optimally evaluated on MRI. T_1-weighted or fat-suppression images demonstrate the degree of enlargement of the optic nerves, chiasm, or tracts. Tumor enhancement with intravenous paramagnetic agents is variable, ranging from minimal to marked. Extension into the optic radiations is shown as a high-signal abnormality on T_2-weighted images.

Hydrocephalus occurs in a small percentage of patients with neurofibromatosis type 1. This is most often due to obstruction at the level of the cerebral aqueduct. The obstruction may be due to intrinsic aqueductal stenosis or extrinsic compression by a glioma of the tectum or the tegmentum of the mesencephalon. Identification of the specific etiology is usually best achieved with MRI. With benign aqueductal stenosis, the proximal aqueduct is enlarged, and the tectum is thinned and displaced cephalad. Gliomas enlarge the tectum and completely obliterate the aqueduct. Gliomas demonstrate a variable degree of enhancement with intravenous contrast material on CT and with paramagnetic contrast material on MRI. In addition to the optic system and tectum, other common locations of gliomas in patients with neurofibromatosis type 1 are the brainstem and the cerebrum.

Dysplasias of the intracranial vessels may occur in neurofibromatosis type 1. Most often these are stenotic or occlusive lesions in the intracranial portions of the internal carotid arteries or the proximal portions of the middle or anterior cerebral arteries. There is also an increased incidence of vascular dysplasias in other regions of the body. Any child with neurofibromatosis type 1 who has seizures, mental retardation, paralysis, or severe headaches may have vascular dysplasia. Vascular dysplasia is difficult to identify on CT or MRI, although major vascular occlusions may be detectable. Angiography generally shows severe stenosis or occlusion of arteries in the region of the circle of Willis. A moyamoya type abnormality, with enlargement of the lenticulostriate arteries, is seen in approximately 65% of neurofibromatosis type 1 patients with cerebral vascular dysplasia.[80]

There is an increased incidence of cranial nerve neurilemmomas in neurofibromatosis type 1, although these lesions are still quite rare (Fig. 1-86). The optic nerve is the most frequently involved cranial nerve. Optic nerve neurilemmomas in these patients are rare, however, in comparison to the relatively common gliomas.

Intracranial complications may be produced by excessive growth of craniofacial plexiform neurofibromas. These lesions are benign, locally aggressive congenital tumors composed of Schwann cells, collagen, neurons, and an unorganized matrix. They may extend intracranially through foramina or along nerves. Intraorbital extension is common. On MRI and CT, a plexiform neurofibroma is demonstrated as a poorly defined, infiltrative, heterogeneous mass. These lesions tend to be of relatively low attenuation on CT and generally show minimal contrast enhancement. On MRI, the mass is hypointense to brain on T_1-weighted images and hyperintense to brain on T_2-weighted images. Heterogeneous enhancement occurs with paramagnetic contrast agents.

In some children with neurofibromatosis type 1, MRI demonstrates multiple areas of abnormally increased signal intensity in the brainstem, cerebrum, and cerebellum on T_2-weighted images. The pons and cerebellar white matter are the most common sites of involvement. These lesions are multiple, usually have no mass effect, and show no appreciable enhancement with paramagnetic contrast medium. They may be present in as many as 50% to 75% of patients with neurofibromatosis type 1. Because biopsy is usually not performed, the exact nature of these lesions is poorly understood; they are thought to represent foci of atypical glial cells, however (Fig. 1-51).[81]

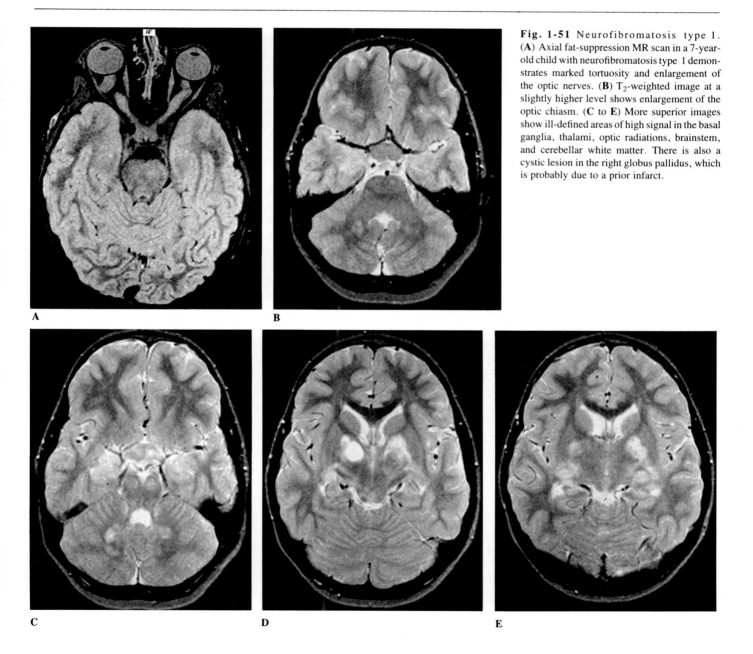

Fig. 1-51 Neurofibromatosis type 1. (**A**) Axial fat-suppression MR scan in a 7-year-old child with neurofibromatosis type 1 demonstrates marked tortuosity and enlargement of the optic nerves. (**B**) T_2-weighted image at a slightly higher level shows enlargement of the optic chiasm. (**C** to **E**) More superior images show ill-defined areas of high signal in the basal ganglia, thalami, optic radiations, brainstem, and cerebellar white matter. There is also a cystic lesion in the right globus pallidus, which is probably due to a prior infarct.

A   B

C   D   E

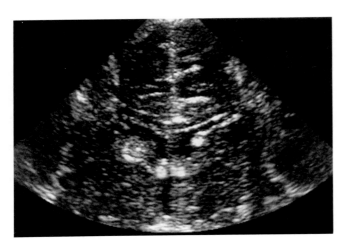

Fig. 1-52 Tuberous sclerosis. Coronal sonography in an infant being evaluated for seizures shows hyperechoic nodular lesions in the subependymal regions of the lateral ventricles. Note that some of these nodules are located immediately adjacent to the foramina of Monro. The more superior nodules could be confused sonographically with subependymal germinal matrix hemorrhage, although the region of the foramina of Monro would be an uncommon location for germinal matrix hemorrhage. These subependymal nodules of tuberous sclerosis are not yet calcified and, therefore, do not produce acoustic shadowing.

There is a form of neurofibromatosis distinct from neurofibromatosis type 1, in which bilateral acoustic neurinomas occur; this is termed neurofibromatosis type 2 or central neurofibromatosis. This type of neurofibromatosis is much less common than neurofibromatosis type 1. Neurofibromatosis type 2 is an autosomal dominant disorder that is associated with an abnormality of chromosome 22. In addition to bilateral acoustic neurinomas, meningiomas may also occur in this disorder. Fewer than half of the affected patients have café au lait spots. Lisch nodules are usually not identified. The diagnostic criteria for neurofibromatosis type 2 include bilateral cranial nerve VIII tumors or a first-degree relative with neurofibromatosis type 2 and the presence of either a unilateral cranial nerve VIII tumor or two of the following: neurofibroma, meningioma, glioma, schwannoma, or subcapsular lenticular opacity.

The imaging study of choice for the evaluation of neurofibromatosis type 2 is contrast-enhanced MRI. Because of the usual lack of obvious cutaneous and ocular manifestations, neurofibromatosis type 2 patients are usually not identified during childhood.[78]

Tuberous Sclerosis

Tuberous sclerosis (Bourneville disease) is a phakomatosis that involves multiple organ systems. There appears to be an autosomal dominant transmission with low penetrance. In many patients, the clinical manifestations represent a triad of mental retardation, adenoma sebaceum, and seizures. Adenoma sebaceum consists of a nodular, reddish-brown rash over the midface and nasolabial fold region. Histologically,

these lesions are angiofibromas. They may also occur on the trunk, gingiva, and periungual regions. Ash-leaf spots are hypopigmented lesions that are often identified on the trunk and extremities and are the cutaneous manifestation most often seen in young children. Other cutaneous manifestations include the shagreen patch and subungual fibroma.[82,83]

Myoclonic seizures occur by early childhood in most patients with tuberous sclerosis. The seizures often decrease in frequency with increasing age. Significant mental retardation occurs in 50% to 80% of patients. The severity of retardation is variable among patients.

The most common ocular abnormality in patients with tuberous sclerosis is a retinal hamartoma located near the optic disc. With the ophthalmoscope, this lesion is initially seen as a flat, semitransparent, whitish lesion that later develops a yellow, nodular appearance. These hamartomas are usually multiple and bilateral. When retinal hamartomas calcify, they sometimes can be identified on CT as tiny calcifications near the head of the optic nerve.

The most common intracranial abnormalities in tuberous sclerosis are subependymal hamartomas. These lesions are most often located along the ventricular surface of the body of the caudate nucleus. In severe cases, they may also be identified on the surfaces of the frontal or temporal horns or the third and fourth ventricles.

The subependymal hamartomas of tuberous sclerosis are demonstrated on neuroimaging studies as small, nodular lesions along the ventricular walls (Fig. 1-52). There is little or no change in size of the lesions on sequential scans. On CT, contrast enhancement is similar to that of normal brain. These lesions are often calcified, with the incidence of calcification increasing with age (Fig. 1-53). Calcification is rare during infancy.[84-86]

Subependymal hamartomas appear on MRI as nodules that protrude into the ventricular lumen. They are usually approximately isointense to white matter on all imaging sequences. They are best demonstrated on T_1-weighted images, where they contrast with the low signal intensity of cerebrospinal fluid. Enhancement with intravenous paramagnetic contrast material is usually identified (Fig. 1-54).

CT showing a large subependymal nodule that has prominent contrast enhancement suggests the presence of a giant cell astrocytoma (Fig. 1-55). Both hamartomas and giant cell astrocytomas enhance with paramagnetic contrast material on MRI, although the latter lesions tend to be larger and to enhance more intensely. Giant cell astrocytomas in children with tuberous sclerosis are usually located near the foramen of Monro. Sequential studies demonstrate gradual enlargement. The incidence of this lesion in tuberous sclerosis is about 5% to 10%. There is a histologic continuum between the subependymal hamartoma and the giant cell astrocytoma. These lesions protrude into the ventricle and are noninvasive. Obstructive hydrocephalus may occur if the lesion obstructs the foramen of Monro. At times, a giant cell astrocytoma may degenerate into a malignant tumor. This is suggested when imaging studies show evidence of invasiveness or particularly rapid enlargement.[87-89]

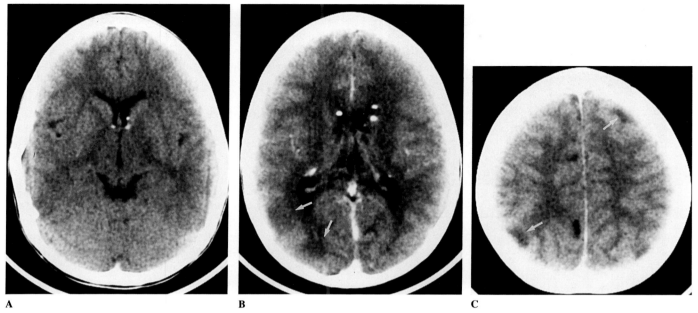

A   **B**   **C**

Fig. 1-53 Tuberous sclerosis. (**A**) Unenhanced axial CT scan shows three small calcified subependymal nodules along the inferior aspect of the lateral ventricles. (**B** and **C**) Contrast-enhanced CT scans show several more calcified subependymal nodules along the margins of the lateral ventricles. There are also ill-defined areas of abnormally low attenuation in the right posterior temporal and occipital lobes (arrows) and in the posterior aspect of the right parietal lobe (arrows). There is also a small area of abnormally low attenuation in the anterior aspect of the left frontal lobe (arrow). These low-attenuation lesions are cortical hamartomas of tuberous sclerosis.

Cortical hamartomas, or tubers, are common in tuberous sclerosis. These lesions are histologically distinct from subependymal hamartomas. They contain giant cells, areas of gliosis, and disorganized myelin sheaths. The number of cortical hamartomas is quite variable among patients, ranging from none to a few to a dozen or more. Malignant degeneration of these lesions is extremely rare.

In infants, a cortical hamartoma is demonstrated on CT as a low-attenuation lesion in an abnormally thickened cortical gyrus. With increasing age, these lesions tend to increase in

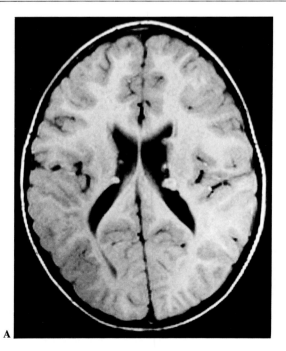
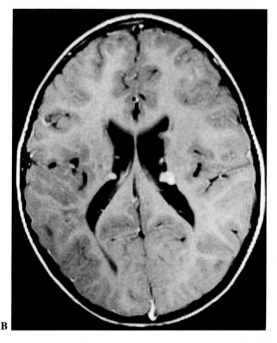

A   **B**

Fig. 1-54 Tuberous sclerosis. (**A**) T$_1$-weighted unenhanced and (**B**) enhanced MR images show multiple subependymal hamartomas along the walls of the lateral ventricles. Most of these hamartomas show moderate enhancement with paramagnetic contrast material. A more densely calcified hamartoma in the anterior aspect of the left lateral ventricle does not enhance. These small hamartomas show no evidence of invasion of the adjacent structures.

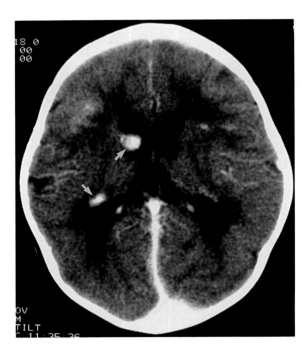

Fig. 1-55 Tuberous sclerosis. Contrast-enhanced CT scan shows two intensely enhancing, partially calcified, subependymal nodules in the right lateral ventricle (arrows). This degree of enhancement raises the possibility of degeneration into giant cell astrocytomas. Also visible are ill-defined areas of faint calcification in the white matter of both frontal lobes; these are foci of heterotopic cells.

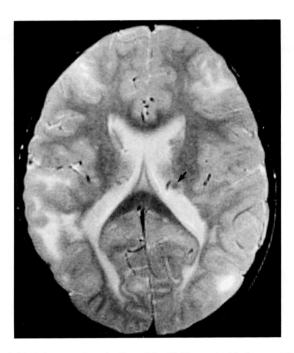

Fig. 1-56 Tuberous sclerosis. T_2-weighted MR scan in this 8-year-old child shows a high-signal abnormality involving several gyri in both cerebral hemispheres. The hyperintense abnormality involves both gray and white matter, although there is a peripheral rim of normal-appearing cortex adjacent to these lesions. The inner margins of the lesions are poorly defined. These areas of signal abnormality are due to cortical hamartomas. Also note a low-signal calcified subependymal hamartoma in the midportion of the body of the left lateral ventricle (arrow).

attenuation such that they become more difficult to distinguish from normal brain. Some cortical hamartomas calcify. The number of calcified lesions increases with age; at least one calcified cortical hamartoma can be identified in most patients by 10 years of age.

The MR appearance of cortical hamartomas in tuberous sclerosis also changes with age. During infancy, MRI demonstrates a focally enlarged gyrus that produces relatively low signal intensity on T_1-weighted images and high signal intensity on T_2-weighted images. The inner margins of the tubers are poorly defined. The peripheral margin tends to be fairly well defined, and there is often a thin rim of normal-appearing cortex overlying the lesion. In older children and adults, cortical hamartomas are often isointense to white matter on T_1-weighted images but remain hyperintense on T_2-weighted images (Fig. 1-56).

In addition to subependymal hamartomas and cortical hamartomas, foci of heterotopic cells are often present in the white matter of patients with tuberous sclerosis. These lesions consist of clusters of abnormal neurons in a matrix of gliosis and demyelination. Many of these lesions are too small to be identified on imaging studies. Those of sufficient size are identified on CT as well-defined, low-attenuation foci in the cerebral white matter. There is no appreciable enhancement with intravenous contrast material. Calcification of these lesions may occur and, when present, involves part or all of the nodule (Fig. 1-57). On MRI, these nodules are isointense or

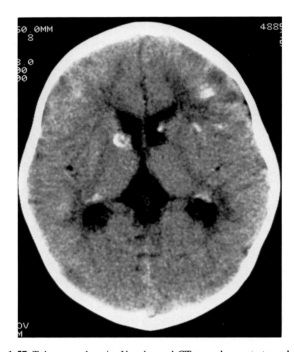

Fig. 1-57 Tuberous sclerosis. Unenhanced CT scan demonstrates calcified subependymal hamartomas in the walls of the lateral ventricles. There are ill-defined calcifications in the white matter of the left frontal and parietal lobes and an ill-defined surrounding low-attenuation abnormality. These are due to regions of heterotopic cells in association with tuberous sclerosis.

slightly hypointense to normal white matter on T_1-weighted images. They are demonstrated as well-demarcated regions of high signal intensity on T_2-weighted images. Calcifications of sufficient size produce signal voids on all imaging sequences.

Cerebellar lesions occur in about 10% of patients with tuberous sclerosis. The cerebellar lesions are histologically identical to the subependymal, cortical, and white matter lesions that occur in the cerebrum; the imaging features are also identical. Subependymal hamartomas are probably the least common of the cerebellar lesions seen in tuberous sclerosis.

Sturge-Weber Syndrome

Sturge-Weber syndrome (encephalotrigeminal angiomatosis) is a congenital disorder that is characterized by angiomatosis of the face, choroid of the eye, and leptomeninges. The facial lesion is often described as a port wine vascular nevus. This can involve any portion of the face and is present at birth. Aside from the facial and ocular findings, most children with Sturge-Weber syndrome are asymptomatic until they begin to have seizures. This occurs in 90% of patients within the first few years of life, often in infancy. The seizures usually become progressively refractory to therapy. Thirty percent of patients develop hemiparesis. Homonymous hemianopsia often accompanies the hemiparesis. Mental retardation of variable severity affects almost all patients.

The characteristic central nervous system manifestation of Sturge-Weber syndrome is meningeal angiomatosis. The angiomatosis is typically confined to the pia mater. The meningeal lesions consist of multiple small venous channels that are matted together on the brain surface. The arteries are also abnormal, although less so. With time, fibrotic changes often occur. The location of the meningeal angiomatosis correlates with the pattern of the facial nevus. Occipital angiomatosis is typically accompanied by facial lesions in the distribution of the ophthalmic division of cranial nerve V, parietal angiomatosis is associated with nevi in the maxillary division, and angiomatosis involving an entire hemisphere usually is accompanied by skin lesions in all three divisions of the trigeminal nerve. There are rare patients who have the cerebral angiomatosis but lack the cutaneous manifestations. The combination of facial and meningeal angiomatosis is believed to be due to persistent primordial sinusoidal vascular channels that are present from gestation weeks 4 through 8. Although unilateral in most cases, the pial and facial lesions can be bilateral.[90]

The most frequent CT finding in cases of Sturge-Weber syndrome is calcification in the cerebral cortex underlying the pial angiomatosis. The calcifications may occur throughout the cortex but are most common in the second and third cortical layers. The calcifications conform to the contours of the involved gyri. They are usually located in the temporoparietooccipital regions; frontal involvement is less common, and posterior fossa involvement is rare. Bilateral calcifications

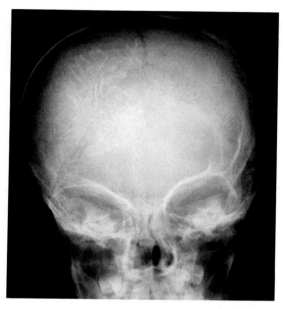

Fig. 1-58 Sturge-Weber syndrome. Anteroposterior skull radiograph showing intracranial calcifications on the right with a gyriform pattern. This is typical of Sturge-Weber syndrome.

occur in about 20% of cases. The gyral calcification produces low signal intensity on MRI. This finding is often best identified on T_2-weighted images. Dense gyral calcifications may also be demonstrated on skull radiographs in some cases (Fig. 1-58). The pial angiomatosis of Sturge-Weber syndrome may result in abnormal contrast enhancement on both CT and MRI. This enhancement characteristically has a gyriform pattern. On CT, this finding may be difficult to appreciate in older children when dense calcifications are present. On MRI, gyriform enhancement is usually appreciable in patients of all ages (Fig. 1-59).[91]

The ipsilateral choroid plexus is sometimes enlarged in patients with Sturge-Weber syndrome. This phenomenon is thought to be due to hyperplasia of the choroid plexus, although angiomatous malformations of the choroid plexus have been reported in some cases. CT shows enlargement and abnormal enhancement of the choroid plexus ipsilateral to the pial angiomatous malformation. On MRI, the choroid plexus is enlarged and hyperintense with respect to brain parenchyma on T_1-weighted images.

In many patients with Sturge-Weber syndrome, the ipsilateral cerebral hemisphere is decreased in size. The white matter in the atrophic hemisphere exhibits abnormally low attenuation on CT and slight prolongation of T_1- and T_2-relaxation times on MRI. The white matter changes are thought to be due to ischemia-induced gliosis.

Imaging studies may also show cranial asymmetry due to cerebral hemiatrophy. There is calvarial thickening ipsilateral to the atrophic hemisphere, and the ipsilateral mastoid air cells and paranasal sinuses are enlarged. Occasionally, the hemicranium ipsilateral to the angiomatosis is enlarged as a result of chronic or recurrent subdural hematomas.

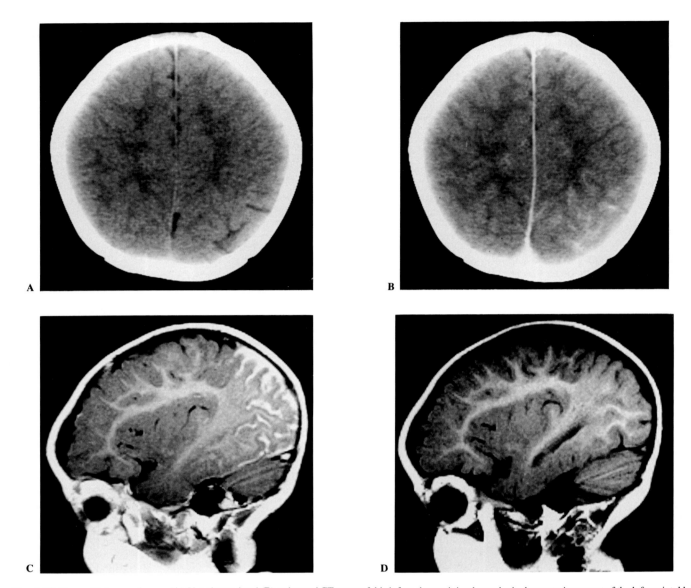

Fig. 1-59 Sturge-Weber syndrome. (**A**) Unenhanced and (**B**) enhanced CT scans of this infant show minimal atrophy in the posterior aspect of the left parietal lobe and abnormal enhancement along the sulci of these atrophic gyri. (**C**) Unenhanced and (**D**) enhanced parasagittal T_1-weighted MR scans also show slight atrophy of the gyri in the posterior parietal and occipital lobes on the left. There is intense pial enhancement in this region as a result of pial angiomatosis.

In some cases of Sturge-Weber syndrome, CT and MRI show enlarged veins in the subependymal and periventricular areas. The pial angiomatosis causes dysgenesis of and diminished outflow through the superficial venous system. Therefore, deep venous blood is shunted through the medullary veins into the deep venous system of the brain. With time, these vessels may enlarge to the degree that they become noticeable on imaging studies. Arteriovenous malformations also can occur in association with Sturge-Weber syndrome but are much less common than the simple enlargement of the deep venous system that is due to internal shunting.[92]

Significant ocular abnormalities occur in about 25% of patients with Sturge-Weber syndrome. The most important pathology is choroidal angiomatosis. This may lead to glaucoma or retinal detachment. Fetal glaucoma in these cases may progress to buphthalmos, which is demonstrated on imaging studies as enlargement and elongation of the globe. Rarely, contrast-enhanced MR images may demonstrate a retinal angioma.[93]

von Hippel–Lindau Disease

von Hippel–Lindau disease (central nervous system angiomatosis) is an autosomal dominant disorder with incomplete penetrance. This phakomatosis is characterized by retinal angiomas, cerebellar and spinal cord hemangioblastomas, renal cell carcinomas, pheochromocytomas, angiomas of the liver and kidney, and cysts of the pancreas, kidneys, liver, and epididymis. Criteria for diagnosis of von Hippel–Lindau disease include the presence of more than one central nervous system hemangioblastoma, or one central nervous system hemangioblastoma in conjunction with a visceral manifestation of the disease, or any manifestation of the disease in a patient with a known family history.

The manifestations of von Hippel–Lindau disease usually do not become clinically evident until adolescence or early adulthood. The most common presenting complaints are related to retinal involvement. Retinal hemangioblastomas lead to retinal inflammation, exudate, hemorrhage, and detachment. These changes cause progressive loss of visual acuity. Cerebellar signs are also common early manifestations of this disorder. Cerebellar hemangioblastoma may cause vertigo, nausea and vomiting, headache, and a number of more specific cerebellar signs, such as a positive Romberg sign.[94,95]

Cerebellar hemangioblastomas occur in at least 50% of patients with von Hippel–Lindau disease. Most often, there is a small tumor nodule in the wall of a large fluid-filled cyst in one hemisphere of the cerebellum. About 30% of these tumors are solid, however. CT usually shows a hemispheric cyst with a small enhancing mural nodule.[96] If the nodule is very small, it may not be visible. A solid hemangioblastoma is demonstrated as an ill-defined, enhancing hemispheric mass.

On MRI, a hemangioblastoma typically is slightly hypointense to brain on T_1-weighted images and hyperintense on T_2-weighted images.[97] The associated cyst shows the MR characteristics of fluid, although material in the cyst may slightly alter the appearance in comparison to cerebrospinal fluid. In those cases without a cyst, the margins of the lesion are usually poorly defined. Small tubular areas of flow void in the tumor nodule are sometimes visible; these are due to feeding and draining vessels. The tumor usually shows prominent enhancement with paramagnetic contrast material; this provides increased sensitivity for detection of small lesions. Angiog-

raphy demonstrates hemangioblastoma as a highly vascular neoplasm (Fig. 1-60).

NEOPLASMS

Brain tumors are the most common solid neoplasms in children and are second in frequency only to leukemia. There are approximately 1,000 to 1,500 new central nervous system neoplasms diagnosed in the United States every year. Fifteen percent to 20% of all primary brain tumors occur in pediatric patients. The estimated incidence in children younger than 15 years of age is 2.4 per 100,000.[98]

In the pediatric population as a whole, intracranial neoplasms occur with approximately equal frequency in supratentorial and posterior fossa locations. The incidence does, however, vary somewhat in different age groups of children. Supratentorial tumors are more common in infants and children up to 3 years of age, and infratentorial tumors predominate from 4 to 11 years of age. The incidence is approximately equal in children older than 11 years of age.

Neonatal brain tumors (those that present within the first 2 months of life) account for less than 2% of all pediatric brain tumors. The majority are supratentorial. The most common lesions are teratomas, primitive neuroectodermal tumors, astrocytomas, and choroid plexus papillomas.[99]

Potential presenting signs and symptoms in infants with an intracranial neoplasm include progressive macrocephaly, nausea and vomiting, and lethargy. Older children may experience headaches, nausea and vomiting, seizures, dizziness, visual impairment, and various focal neurologic signs such as cranial nerve palsy, ataxia, and hemiparesis. Hypothalamic or pituitary involvement may cause endocrine dysfunction such as diabetes insipidus, growth failure, or precocious puberty.

Central nervous system tumors are categorized by location and histologic type. The most widely used classification system is based on the World Health Organization nomenclature (Table 1-5).[100]

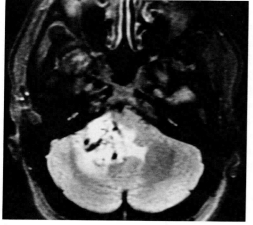

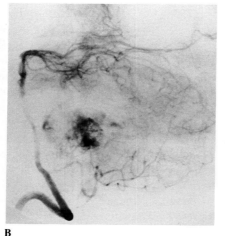

Fig. 1-60 Hemangioblastoma in von Hippel–Lindau disease. **(A)** T_2-weighted axial MR image shows a hyperintense mass in the right cerebellum with extension into the pons. There are tubular signal voids indicating large vessels in this tumor. There is surrounding edema in the cerebellum and brainstem. **(B)** Lateral vertebral angiogram shows intense tumor blush and neovascularity in this vascular neoplasm.

A   B

Table 1-5 Pathologic Classification of Pediatric Brain Tumors

Neuroepithelial tumors
  Glial tumors
    Astrocytic tumors
      Astrocytoma
      Anaplastic astrocytoma
      Subependymal giant cell astrocytoma
      Gigantocellular glioma
    Oligodendroglial tumors
      Oligodendroglioma
      Anaplastic oligodendroglioma
    Ependymal tumors
      Ependymoma
      Anaplastic ependymoma
      Myxopapillary ependymoma
    Choroid plexus tumors
      Choroid plexus papilloma
      Anaplastic choroid plexus carcinoma
    Mixed gliomas
    Glioblastomatous tumors
      Glioblastoma multiforme
      Giant cell glioblastoma
      Gliosarcoma
    Gliomatosis cerebri
  Neuronal tumors
    Gangliocytoma
    Anaplastic gangliocytoma
    Ganglioglioma
    Anaplastic ganglioglioma
  Primitive neuroepithelial tumors
    Primitive neuroectodermal tumor
    Medulloepithelioma
    Medulloblastoma
  Pineal cell tumors
    Pineoblastoma
    Pineocytoma
Tumors of the meninges and related tissues
  Meningiomas
    Meningioma
    Papillary meningioma
    Anaplastic meningioma
  Meningeal sarcomatous tumors
  Primary melanocytic tumors

Tumors of nerve sheath cells
  Neurilemmoma (neurinoma, schwannoma)
  Anaplastic neurilemmoma
  Neurofibroma
  Anaplastic neurofibroma (neurofibrosarcoma)

Primary malignant lymphomas

Tumors of blood vessel cells
  Hemangioblastoma
  Hemangiopericytoma
  Angiosarcoma

Germ cell tumors
  Germinoma
  Embryonal cell carcinoma
  Choriocarcinoma
  Endodermal sinus tumor
  Teratomatous tumors
    Mature teratoma
    Immature teratoma
    Teratocarcinoma
  Mixed germ cell tumor

Malformative tumors
  Lipoma
  Dermoid cyst
  Epidermoid cyst
  Craniopharyngioma
  Rathke cleft cyst
  Colloid cyst
  Enterogenous or bronchogenic cyst
  Granular cell sarcoma (choristoma)
  Hamartoma

Neuroendocrine tumors
  Anterior pituitary tumors
    Adenoma
    Pituitary carcinoma
  Paraganglioma

Posterior Fossa Neoplasms

Cerebellar Astrocytoma

Forty percent to 50% of all primary pediatric intracranial neoplasms are astrocytomas. Approximately 60% of astrocytomas in children occur in the posterior fossa; of these, about 65% arise in the cerebellum and 35% in the brainstem. Cerebellar astrocytoma accounts for about 12% of all brain neoplasms in children younger than 15 years of age.[101] It is the second most common neoplasm of the cerebellum in children, having an incidence slightly lower than that of medulloblastoma.[102,103]

A classification system for cerebellar astrocytomas has been developed on the basis of the histologic features. This classifi-

cation has important prognostic implications.[104] In this classification, the demonstration of microcysts, leptomeningeal deposits, Rosenthal fibers, and foci of oligodendroglial fibers indicates a glioma A variety. These patients have approximately a 95% 10-year survival rate after surgical resection. In contradistinction, the glioma B variety is characterized by pseudorosette formation, high cellularity, necrosis, mitoses, and calcifications. These patients have approximately a 30% 10-year survival postoperatively.

The usual age range of cerebellar astrocytoma extends from infancy to adolescence, and the mean age is approximately 7 years. Anaplastic varieties tend to occur in the 10- to 15-year age range. There may be a slight male predominance. The most common presenting signs are due to increased intracranial pressure, which may be of long duration. Specific cerebellar signs and symptoms vary depending on the location of the tumor. Midline lesions tend to cause truncal ataxia, whereas hemispheric tumors are often associated with appendicular dysmetria of the ipsilateral limbs. Other potential findings include torticollis or head tilt and motor abnormalities. Cranial nerve palsies are uncommon.

Astrocytomas may arise anywhere in the cerebellum. Most originate in the vermis; extension into the cerebellar hemispheres occurs in 25% to 30% of cases. Occasionally, a vermian astrocytoma will extend predominantly anteriorly into the fourth ventricle. Lesions limited to the cerebellar hemisphere account for about 15% of cases; these are more often cystic than midline astrocytomas.

Cerebellar astrocytomas are usually quite large at the time of presentation. These tumors can be predominantly cystic, solid, or solid with a necrotic center. The cystic lesions typically have a mural nodule, with the remainder of the cyst wall consisting of nonneoplastic compressed cerebellar tissue; this type accounts for about 50% of all cerebellar astrocytomas. They are almost always of the glioma-A type. About 40% to 45% of cerebellar astrocytomas are solid with a fluid-filled necrotic center. These are often of the glioma-B type. The necrotic portion sometimes has a multiloculated or polycystic appearance. Purely solid tumors are seen in less than 10% of cases. Cystic lesions without significant necrosis usually have a better prognosis than solid or necrotic lesions. Microscopic calcification is present in 20% to 25% of cerebellar astrocytomas, most commonly in the solid variety.[105–107]

Cerebellar astrocytomas are readily detected on CT or MRI. A large vermian or hemispheric mass, often having a predominantly cystic composition, is demonstrated. The attenuation of the solid component of the neoplasm is less than or equal to that of normal brain tissue on unenhanced CT. There is contrast enhancement of the solid component, although the pattern and intensity of enhancement vary somewhat among cases. A mixed enhancement pattern occurs in approximately 50% of cases.[108]

In those cases with a large cyst and a mural nodule, the cyst is usually round or oval, and the mural nodule may be round, oval, or even waferlike. The cyst is usually of slightly higher attenuation than clear cerebrospinal fluid, but shows no contrast enhancement. The nodule exhibits intense homogeneous contrast enhancement. The wall of the cyst may be of slightly higher attenuation on unenhanced CT but shows little or no contrast enhancement unless there is extension of the tumor along the cyst wall.

Solid cerebellar astrocytomas are usually oval, lobulated, and fairly well defined. Calcification is identified in a minority of cases. In those cases in which there is a cyst that is the result of necrosis of a solid astrocytoma, a well-defined mural nodule is absent. These cysts may be unilocular or multilocular. The cyst wall and the septations of the cyst enhance. The enhancement often extends into the cerebellum beyond the border of the cyst wall.

As with CT, the MR appearance of a cerebellar astrocytoma is somewhat variable. The solid components produce slightly lower signal than normal brain on T_1-weighted images and high signal intensity on T_2-weighted images. The signal characteristics of cystic components are determined by the contents. A cyst associated with an isolated mural nodule usually contains relatively clear fluid that has signal characteristics similar to those of cerebrospinal fluid (Fig. 1-61). Cysts due to necrosis may contain material that produces slightly higher signal than cerebrospinal fluid on T_1-weighted images. The cyst contents produce bright signal on T_2-weighted images. The tumor is also frequently surrounded by significant edema that can blur the margins of the lesion. In some cases, it is difficult to differentiate the solid and cystic components on unenhanced MR scans. Enhanced images obtained after injection of paramagnetic contrast material, however, typically show significant increase in solid tumor signal on T_1-weighted images. Edema in adjacent portions of the brain produces high signal on T_2-weighted images, but contrast enhancement does not occur (Fig. 1-62).[109]

Medulloblastoma

Medulloblastoma is the most common posterior fossa tumor of childhood, but it is only slightly more common than cerebellar astrocytoma. This tumor accounts for approximately 20% of pediatric intracranial neoplasms and 35% to 40% of posterior fossa neoplasms in childhood. Forty percent are identified during the first 5 years of life and 75% by the age of 10 years.[110,111]

Approximately 50% of patients with medulloblastoma have had symptoms for less than 1 month before diagnosis. This is in contradistinction to cerebellar astrocytoma, which usually has a long symptomatic course before diagnosis. The most common signs and symptoms in children with medulloblastoma are nausea, vomiting, headaches, progressive macrocephaly, and ataxia. The high incidence of vomiting may be related to effects on the area postrema; this is the emetic center of the brain and is adjacent to the inferior portion of the fourth ventricle. Progressive macrocephaly is a common presenting feature in infants. In older children, vomiting and ataxia are the most common symptoms. Head tilt is also a common clinical presentation of medulloblastoma. This may be due to either ophthalmoparesis or incipient cerebellar herniation. Head tilt may accompany or precede other clinical signs. It is frequently associated with neck stiffness. Potential motor symptoms in children with medulloblastoma include hypotonicity, decreased or absent reflexes, and ataxia that is usually truncal.

Medulloblastoma is a primitive neuroectodermal tumor that may show a variable degree of differentiation. These tumors may differentiate along ependymal, astroglial, or neuroblastic cell lines. About half of medulloblastomas are composed almost entirely of undifferentiated cells. Pathologically, medulloblastomas are soft and fleshy and are usually well demarcated. They are highly cellular. Hemorrhage, cyst formation, and calcification are uncommon.

About two-thirds of medulloblastomas in children arise in the vermis. The resulting midline mass causes lateral displace-

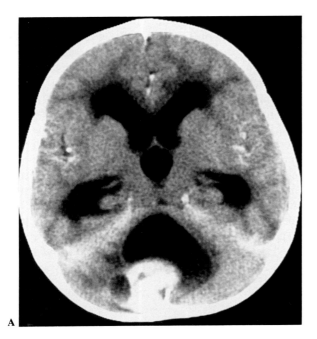

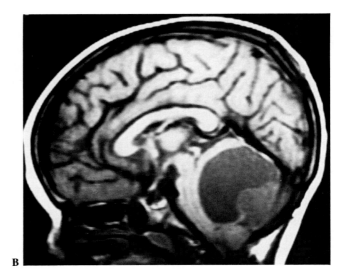

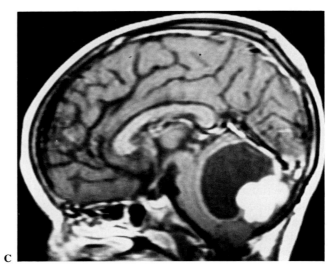

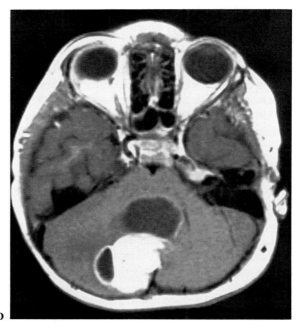

Fig. 1-61 Cystic cerebellar astrocytoma. **(A)** Contrast-enhanced CT scan shows a large, predominantly cystic mass in the midportion of the cerebellum. There is an intensely enhancing mural nodule posteriorly. The mass causes compression of the fourth ventricle and aqueduct, resulting in secondary obstructive hydrocephalus. **(B)** Sagittal T_1-weighted MR scan and **(C)** sagittal and **(D)** axial contrast-enhanced T_1-weighted MR scans show the cystic component of the lesion to have the signal characteristics of fluid. There is a thin, minimally enhancing rim surrounding most of the cystic component. The mural nodule shows intense enhancement with intravenous gadopentetate dimeglumine. The sagittal images clearly demonstrate the severe mass effect on the brainstem and confirm the epicenter of the lesion to be in the midportion of the cerebellum. The superior extent of the mass lies against the tentorium. This type of astrocytoma is associated with a favorable prognosis.

ment of the cerebellar tonsils. The anterior aspect displaces or invades the roof of the fourth ventricle and causes at least partial obstruction of the flow of cerebrospinal fluid. Invasion of the brainstem is seen in about one-third of patients. The posterior component of the mass often projects into the cisterna magna and may extend inferiorly to the region of the foramen magnum. Rarely, the mass may extend into the cerebellopontine angle cisternae.

Leptomeningeal invasion and subarachnoid dissemination are fairly common with medulloblastoma. Intracranially, subarachnoid metastases are often most prominent along the skull base and in the sylvian fissures. Intraventricular tumor nodules may occur but are uncommon. Drop metastases in the spinal subarachnoid space occur in about 40% of patients. The single most common site of drop metastases is the caudal sac. Nerve root involvement may occur. Tumor nodules sometimes attach to the surface of the cord and may secondarily invade the cord. Intramedullary spinal metastases due to central canal dissemination have been reported rarely. Systemic metastases are not common initially but may be identified if there is tumor recurrence. The usual areas of involvement include the

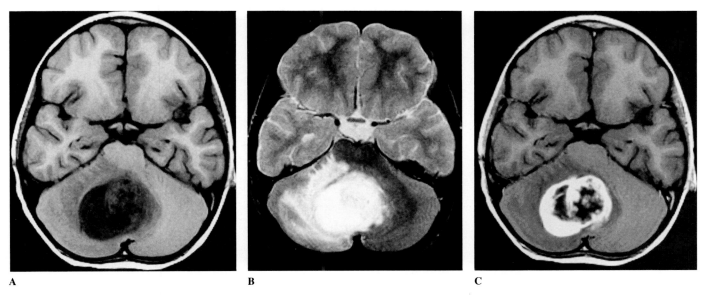

Fig. 1-62 Cerebellar astrocytoma. (**A**) T_1-weighted axial MR image shows a mass of low signal intensity in the middle and right portions of the cerebellum. The fluid components produce slightly higher signal than cerebrospinal fluid. (**B**) T_2-weighted image shows high-signal edema in the cerebellum adjacent to the mass, particularly in the right hemisphere. Both the solid and the cystic components of the tumor produce high signal intensity on this T_2-weighted image. There is vasogenic edema in the cerebellar white matter. (**C**) Contrast-enhanced T_1-weighted axial MR scan shows intense enhancement of the solid portions of the neoplasm. The necrotic changes in this cerebellar astrocytoma and the extensive surrounding edema indicate a less favorable prognosis than that associated with a predominantly cystic lesion that has a mural nodule.

skeletal system, lymph nodes, and lung. Metastatic spread to the peritoneal cavity by way of a diversionary shunt system placed to relieve hydrocephalus can occur, but this is uncommon.[112–115]

On CT, a typical medulloblastoma presents as a well-defined mass arising from the vermis with or without extension into the cerebellar hemisphere. Isolated involvement of the hemisphere in children is not common, in contradistinction to the situation in adult patients. In essentially all cases, the tumor is of higher attenuation than the surrounding cerebellar tissue on unenhanced CT. This is due to the highly cellular nature of these tumors. This finding is quite helpful in the differentiation of this lesion from cerebellar astrocytoma because astrocytomas are typically of slightly lower attenuation than normal brain on unenhanced CT.

Unenhanced CT often shows low-attenuation edema adjacent to a medulloblastoma. The edema is rarely extensive. Enhancement of the tumor varies from homogeneous to patchy. Twenty percent of medulloblastomas contain cystic or necrotic nonenhancing areas. Hemorrhage in the substance of the tumor is uncommon, however. Calcification is occasionally identified. Hydrocephalus is present in a high percentage of patients at the time of presentation. The fourth ventricle is compressed or invaded (Fig. 1-63). Metastatic lesions of sufficient size may be demonstrated as enhancing nodules in the subarachnoid spaces.

MRI provides the most accurate depiction of tumor morphology in cases of medulloblastoma. The mass is most often identified arising in the inferior aspect of the vermis. The signal characteristics of medulloblastomas vary somewhat among patients. Most often, the mass is hypointense to normal brain parenchyma on T_1-weighted images. The lesion is usually moderately hyperintense on T_2-weighted images, although this is not invariable. There is usually significant enhancement of the tumor with gadopentetate dimeglumine, like the enhancement patterns identified on CT (Fig. 1-63). In many cases, indistinctness of the cerebellar folia and fissures can be observed on midline sagittal MR images as a result of coating of the folia by cerebrospinal fluid metastases. Subarachnoid tumor nodules are best detected on enhanced images. The imaging evaluation for cerebrospinal fluid metastases should include evaluation of the ventricles, basal cisternae, and spinal canal. Drop metastases in the spinal canal can also be accurately detected on myelography or CT myelography.[116]

Ependymoma

Ependymoma accounts for slightly less than 10% of all primary central nervous system tumors in children and approximately 15% of all posterior fossa lesions. About 70% of intracranial ependymomas in pediatric patients are located below the tentorium. Two age peaks have been identified for this lesion, the first occurring between 1 and 5 years of age and the second in the third decade. About 60% of ependymomas occur in children younger than 5 years of age, and only 4% occur in patients older than 15 years of age. In many cases of posterior fossa ependymoma, there is a relatively insidious onset of symptoms. Obstructive hydrocephalus is common. Many patients have ataxia and other cerebellar signs.[117]

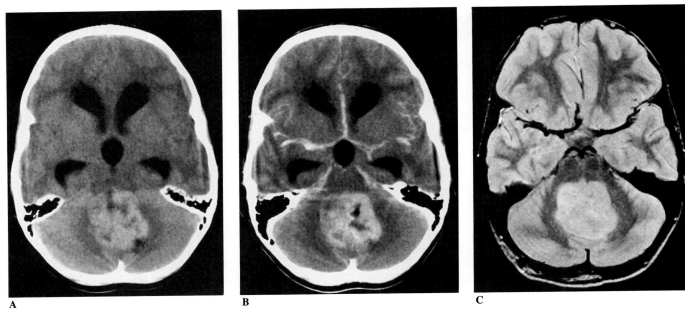

A   **B**   **C**

Fig. 1-63 Medulloblastoma. **(A)** Unenhanced CT scan shows a lobulated midline posterior fossa mass. The solid components of the tumor are of slightly higher attenuation than normal brain; this is a characteristic feature of medulloblastoma. The fourth ventricle is compressed, and obstructive hydrocephalus is present. There is minimal edema adjacent to the mass. **(B)** There is moderate, slightly heterogeneous enhancement of this medulloblastoma on contrast-enhanced CT. **(C)** Axial T_2-weighted MR image shows the midline medulloblastoma to have slightly higher signal than gray matter. There are scattered areas of higher signal indicating foci of necrosis. There is essentially no edema in the surrounding cerebellar white matter.

Posterior fossa ependymomas usually arise from ependymal cells in the lining of the fourth ventricle, most commonly in the floor. This tumor can also arise from extraventricular ependymal cell rests; the most common extraventricular site of origin in the posterior fossa is the cerebellopontine angle cisternae. Most ependymomas have a soft character that allows the neoplasm to extend through the local subarachnoid space and to insinuate around vessels and nerve roots. These lesions frequently extend through the outlet foramina of the fourth ventricle and infiltrate the surrounding cisternae. Approximately 10% to 15% of lesions arising in the region of the fourth ventricle extend to the cerebellopontine angle cisternae through the foramina of Luschka, and 60% to 70% extend through the foramen of Magendie into the cisterna magna. Inferior extension into the cervical spinal canal occurs in about 10% of cases. Ependymomas often penetrate the ventricular wall; frank invasion of the cerebellar parenchyma occurs in at least 30% of patients. Complete resection of ependymomas is often impossible, and local recurrences are common.[118,119]

Pathologically, most ependymomas are fairly well-defined, partially encapsulated tumors. Significant cystic areas are present in 10% to 15% of posterior fossa ependymomas. Calcifications are identified in at least 45%. There is a histologic spectrum of malignancy. In general, high-grade ependymomas are more common in the supratentorial region. In those cases with distant metastases, seeding of the cerebrospinal fluid is the usual mechanism; the risk for this complication is greatest with high-grade ependymomas of the posterior fossa.

The usual appearance of a posterior fossa ependymoma on CT is a midline mass that obliterates the fourth ventricle.

Extension through a foramen of Luschka into the cerebellopontine angle cisterna or through the foramen magnum into the cervical spinal canal is relatively characteristic of this tumor. On unenhanced images, the attenuation of most ependymomas is approximately equal to or slightly lower than that of normal cerebellum. There is usually low-attenuation edema adjacent to the mass. Calcifications are visible in nearly half of these tumors. The calcifications are usually punctate and distributed throughout most of the mass. Conglomerate calcifications are seen occasionally. Mild to moderate heterogeneous contrast enhancement is usually demonstrated. Small, nonenhancing cystic areas are present in a minority of cases.[120]

Ependymomas characteristically are heterogeneous on MRI. On T_1-weighted images, the tumor is usually slightly hypointense to normal brain parenchyma. Foci of marked hypointensity are sometimes present, representing cystic or necrotic changes. These foci produce high signal intensity on T_2-weighted images. At times, fluid-fluid levels may be identified in these regions. Solid portions of the tumor are hyperintense to brain on proton-density and T_2-weighted images. Calcifications or old hemorrhage results in areas of low signal intensity on both T_1- and T_2-weighted images (Fig. 1-64). The lesion shows intense, patchy enhancement after administration of paramagnetic contrast material. Peritumoral edema is hyperintense on T_2-weighted images and does not enhance on T_1-weighted contrast-enhanced images.[121]

The imaging features of ependymoma do not allow a definitive diagnosis because there is considerable overlap with the features of cerebellar astrocytoma and medulloblastoma. There are, however, several CT and MR findings that are suggestive of ependymoma. Ependymomas usually are iso-

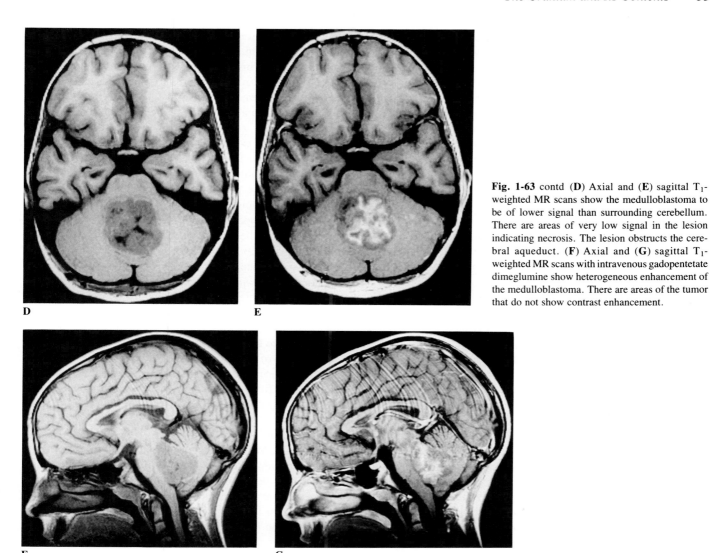

Fig. 1-63 contd **(D)** Axial and **(E)** sagittal T_1-weighted MR scans show the medulloblastoma to be of lower signal than surrounding cerebellum. There are areas of very low signal in the lesion indicating necrosis. The lesion obstructs the cerebral aqueduct. **(F)** Axial and **(G)** sagittal T_1-weighted MR scans with intravenous gadopentetate dimeglumine show heterogeneous enhancement of the medulloblastoma. There are areas of the tumor that do not show contrast enhancement.

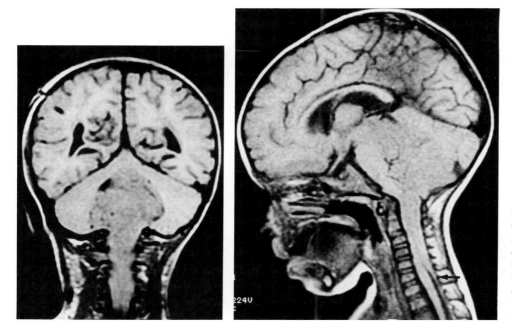

Fig. 1-64 Ependymoma. **(A)** Coronal and **(B)** sagittal T_1-weighted MR scans demonstrate a large, slightly hypointense, midline cerebellar tumor. The mass fills and expands the fourth ventricle and extends inferiorly through the foramen of Magendie into the cervical spinal canal (arrow in **B**). There are foci of low signal intensity in the mass, representing calcification.

dense or hypodense to normal brain on unenhanced CT, whereas medulloblastomas are typically hyperdense. Ependymoma has the highest rate of calcification of these three tumors, and the calcifications tend to be small and multifocal. Large cysts are uncommon in an ependymoma, although small cysts are often present. Probably the most specific finding is extension of the tumor through the foramen of Magendie into the cisterna magna and cervical spinal canal or extension through the foramen of Luschka into a cerebellopontine angle.

Brainstem Glioma

Intrinsic neoplasms of the brainstem represent 10% to 20% of all pediatric central nervous system tumors and account for approximately 20% to 25% of infratentorial brain tumors. The great majority of these are either fibrillary or pilocytic astrocytomas or glioblastomas; as a group, these are termed brainstem gliomas.[101,103] The peak incidence of brainstem glioma is between 3 and 9 years of age. About 80% of all brainstem tumors occur in patients younger than 20 years of age. Boys and girls are affected equally.

The classic clinical presentation of a brainstem tumor is the triad of long tract signs, cranial neuropathies, and ataxia. Ataxia is due to either damage of cerebellar crossing fibers in the pons or invasion of the cerebellum. Nystagmus is common. A number of oculomotor gaze disturbances may occur. Other potential findings include swallowing dysfunction, bulbar signs, and an absent gag reflex. Behavioral problems including somnolence, hyperactivity, and emotional lability are not uncommon. In general the prognosis is poor, with the 5-year survival rate being less than 20% in most series, although there are occasional long-term survivors.[122]

The pons is the most common site of origin of brainstem gliomas and is followed by the midbrain and medulla. These tumors are locally aggressive and infiltrative. Pontine gliomas frequently extend inferiorly into the medulla or posteriorly into the cerebellum. Superior extension from the midbrain results in thalamic involvement. Cyst formation, hemorrhage, or necrosis occurs in about one-quarter of brainstem gliomas; cysts may be seen in both low- and high-grade lesions, whereas necrosis and hemorrhage are more frequent in high-grade lesions.

Some degree of exophytic growth occurs in at least 50% of brainstem gliomas. Tumor may extend into the fourth ventricle or cerebellopontine angle cisterna. There may be extension anteriorly into the prepontine cisterna or posteriorly and inferiorly into the cisterna magna.

The usual CT appearance of a brainstem glioma is a focally expanded area of the brainstem. A well-defined mass is often not visible. The fourth ventricle is displaced posteriorly. Obstructive hydrocephalus is not as common as with other posterior fossa neoplasms. The tumor may extend into the cerebellar peduncles. On unenhanced CT images, tumor attenuation may be equal to or slightly lower than that of normal brainstem tissue. High-attenuation areas indicating hemorrhage are uncommon. Contrast enhancement is visible in at least 50% of these tumors, but the degree and character of contrast enhancement are extremely variable. Enhancement patterns range from none to intense and from homogeneous to heterogeneous or ringlike (Fig. 1-65). The pattern of contrast enhancement is not a reliable indicator of the histologic grade of the neoplasm.

As with CT, MRI demonstrates brainstem glioma as a focal area of expansion of the brainstem. MR images often provide a more accurate depiction of the extent of the lesion. As with other neoplasms, brainstem glioma is isointense or slightly hypointense to normal tissue on T_1-weighted images and hyperintense on T_2-weighted images (Fig. 1-66). Cystic areas or areas of hemorrhage are identified occasionally. The character of tumor enhancement with intravenous gadopentetate

A

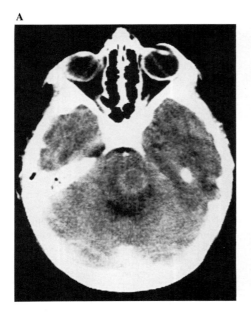

B

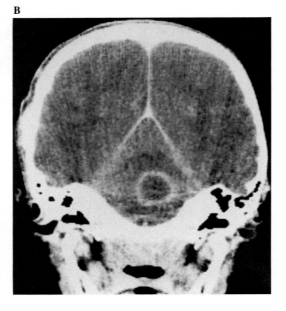

Fig. 1-65 Intrinsic brainstem glioma. (**A**) Axial and (**B**) coronal contrast-enhanced CT scans demonstrate enlargement of the pons and a ringlike area of enhancement. The margins of the lesion are poorly defined. These tumors are usually much more extensive than the pattern of contrast enhancement would suggest.

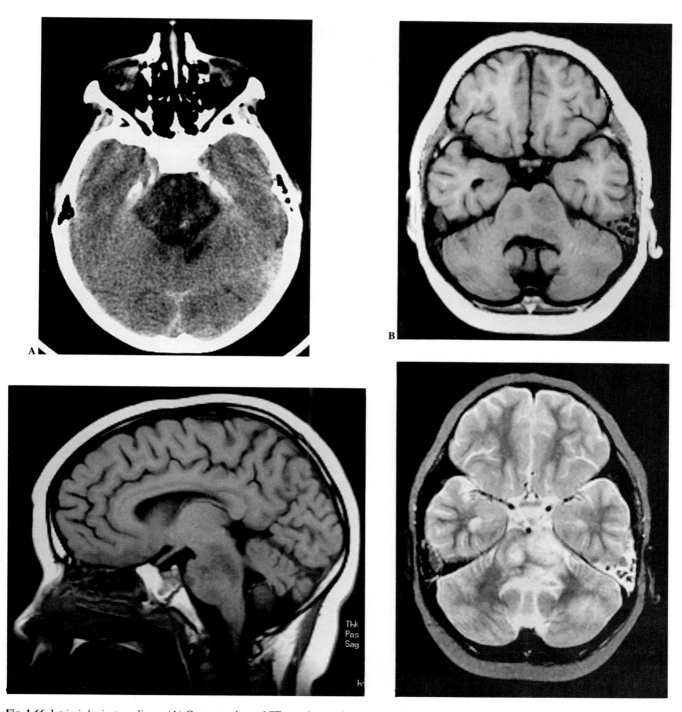

Fig. 1-66 Intrinsic brainstem glioma. (**A**) Contrast-enhanced CT scan shows enlargement and decreased attenuation of the upper portion of the brainstem. There are small, ill-defined areas of contrast enhancement. (**B**) T_1-weighted axial and (**C**) sagittal MR images show enlargement of the pons and midbrain with slightly heterogeneous decreased signal intensity. The anterior wall of the fourth ventricle is slightly compressed. (**D**) T_2-weighted MR image shows high signal intensity in the mass.

dimeglumine roughly parallels the findings described above for CT contrast enhancement.

Significant exophytic extension of a brainstem glioma may cause confusion as to the site of origin of the lesion (Fig. 1-67). In the great majority of cases of brainstem glioma, the fourth ventricle is narrowed, stretched, and dis-placed posteriorly. The lateral aspects of the fourth ventricle may be flattened if there is extension of the tumor into the cerebellar peduncle. Exophytic extension of tumor into the cisterna magna may cause paradoxic anterior displacement of the fourth ventricle, and the appearance on axial images may mimic that of a cerebellar tumor. MRI provides a more accu-

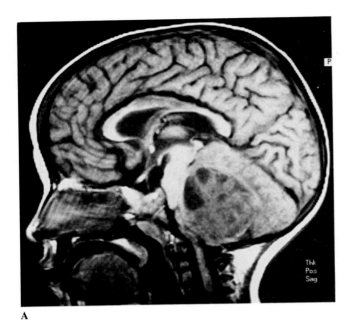

A

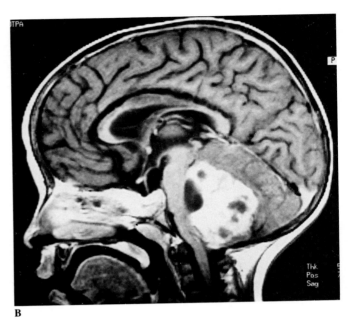

B

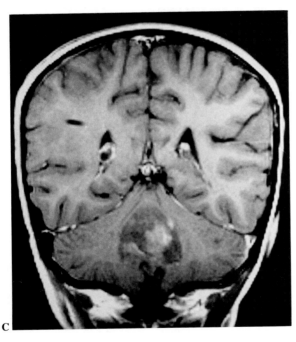

C

Fig. 1-67 Exophytic brainstem glioma. (A) T_1-weighted sagittal MR image shows a heterogeneous, predominantly hypointense, midline posterior fossa mass. The brainstem is compressed along the anterior aspect of the mass, and the cerebellum is compressed posteriorly. The fourth ventricle is obliterated, and the position of the fourth ventricle is not identifiable. (B) There is intense enhancement of the solid components of the mass on this enhanced T_1-weighted sagittal MR image. The cystic or necrotic areas do not enhance and produce low signal intensity. (C) Coronal contrast-enhanced T_1-weighted MR scan shows that the mass conforms to the shape of the fourth ventricle and lies between the cerebellar hemispheres. This exophytic brainstem glioma cannot be reliably differentiated on neuroimaging studies from an ependymoma arising in the fourth ventricle.

rate evaluation of exophytic brainstem lesions than CT. Sagittal images are particularly helpful for defining the position of the fourth ventricle and for tracing the effects of exophytic extension of the tumor. MRI also accurately demonstrates displacement or encasement of the basilar artery by exophytic components of a brainstem glioma.

Nonneoplastic etiologies of brainstem expansion include infection, hemorrhage, edema, syringobulbia, and vascular malformations. Although correlation with the clinical features is essential for accurate differentiation among some of these etiologies, the MR features are often characteristic. Syringobulbia can be differentiated from cystic changes in a brain-stem glioma by lack of signal abnormality adjacent to the fluid collection. The same principle applies for differentiation of isolated hemorrhage associated with a neoplasm. Infection and edema usually produce marked signal abnormality in the brainstem tissues on T_2-weighted images without the focal expansion of the brainstem that usually occurs with a neoplasm.[103,123–125]

Hemangioblastoma

Hemangioblastoma is an uncommon benign tumor of vascular origin that can occur anywhere in the central nervous system. The cerebellum is the most common site. This tumor accounts for 7% to 10% of all posterior fossa tumors and 1% to 2% of all brain tumors. Hemangioblastomas may also occur in the spinal cord and cerebrum. This is usually a tumor of adults; less than 20% occur in children. Approximately 10% of cerebellar hemangioblastomas occur in patients with von Hippel–Lindau disease; these patients often have multiple lesions.

Children with a cerebellar hemangioblastoma may have ataxia, nystagmus, and signs and symptoms of increased intracranial pressure. Polycythemia is present in 10% to 20% of patients who have a cerebellar hemangioblastoma. The hematocrit level usually returns to normal after removal of the tumor.[126]

The most common CT appearance of a cerebellar hemangioblastoma is a small solid tumor nodule in the wall of a larger fluid-filled cyst. Thirty percent to 40% of these tumors are predominantly solid, however. The lesion is most often located in the cerebellar hemisphere, usually near the midline. The attenuation of the solid component of the tumor is usually equal to or slightly lower than that of normal brain on unenhanced CT. High-attenuation areas due to hemorrhage are occasionally present. Contrast-enhanced CT typically demonstrates intense, homogeneous enhancement of the solid portion of the lesion. In some cases, the enhancing tumor nodule is quite small relative to the large, nonenhancing cystic component. The images should be closely inspected for multiple lesions. Occasionally, hemorrhage into the cystic component of a hemangioblastoma results in higher CT attenuation values than clear fluid.

The solid component of a hemangioblastoma is usually slightly hypointense to normal brain on T_1-weighted MR images and hyperintense on T_2-weighted images. Tubular low-signal areas due to enlarged vessels are sometimes visible in the lesion (see Fig. 1-60). The mass typically shows intense, homogeneous enhancement after intravenous administration of paramagnetic contrast material. T_2-weighted images frequently demonstrate a variable degree of high-signal edema in adjacent portions of the cerebellum. If a cystic component is present, this portion most often shows the typical MR characteristics of fluid (ie, low signal on T_1-weighted images and high signal on T_2-weighted images). Hemorrhage into the cyst may alter this pattern, however.[97,127,128]

Supratentorial Neoplasms

The incidence of specific types of supratentorial tumors varies with patient age. The most common lesions in neonates are teratomas, astrocytomas, and primitive neuroectodermal tumors. In infants (ie, those in the age group from 2 months to 2 years), astrocytomas, ependymomas, and primitive neuroectodermal tumors are the most frequently encountered types. In children who are older than 2 years of age, astrocytomas and ependymomas are most common.

Hemispheric Astrocytoma

Hemispheric astrocytoma accounts for approximately 30% of all pediatric supratentorial neoplasms. This tumor occurs at all ages; there is a slight incidence peak at 7 to 8 years of age. The symptoms depend on the location of the tumor. Common presenting symptoms include headache, visual field abnormalities, seizures, focal motor weakness, papilledema, and increasing head size. The symptoms of a hemispheric astrocytoma tend to be of longer duration than those of posterior fossa tumors; this is due at least in part to the earlier onset of obstructive hydrocephalus with the latter lesions.[129]

Various classification schemes have been devised for the pathologic description of hemispheric astrocytomas. The simplest relates increasing degrees of malignancy by describing lesions as low grade, anaplastic, or glioblastoma multiforme. Most hemispheric astrocytomas in children are low-grade lesions, although highly malignant glioblastoma multiforme does occur in pediatric patients. These tumors can also be categorized pathologically according to the cytologic architecture. The most common is the fibrillary pattern, which is usually associated with a low-grade astrocytoma. Pilocytic astrocytomas often resemble cystic cerebellar lesions, in which there is a single large cyst and a mural tumor nodule. Giant cell astrocytoma arises in a subependymal nodule associated with tuberous sclerosis. Anaplastic astrocytomas and glioblastoma multiforme show pleomorphism, mitoses, and other features of high-grade lesions. Hemispheric astrocytoma may arise at any location. There is a tendency for deep locations, such as the basal ganglia or thalamus.[130,131]

A hemispheric astrocytoma may be solid, solid with a central area of necrosis, or cystic with an enhancing mural nodule. On CT, the attenuation of the solid portion of the tumor tends to be equal to or slightly lower than that of normal brain on unenhanced images. High-attenuation areas of hemorrhage, when present, are suggestive of a high-grade lesion. With contrast material, the solid portion may enhance intensely, partially, or not at all (Fig. 1-68). Low-attenuation peritumoral edema is common.[132]

As with CT, there is considerable variation in the appearance of cerebral astrocytoma on MRI. The tumor produces low signal on T_1-weighted images and high signal on T_2-weighted images. Subacute hemorrhage may produce areas of higher signal on T_1-weighted images. Areas of old hemorrhage produce low signal on T_2-weighted images because of hemosiderin. It may be difficult to differentiate cystic from solid components on unenhanced images. As with CT, there is considerable variation in the intensity and homogeneity of paramagnetic contrast material enhancement. The true margins of the tumor may extend beyond the areas of enhancement. Cystic components, necrosis, and edema do not enhance (Fig. 1-69). The imaging features do not allow accurate assessment of histologic grade; as a general rule, however, low-grade astrocytomas tend to be homogeneous, free of hemorrhage, well-circumscribed, and associated with minimal edema. High-grade lesions are most often heterogeneous, are infiltrative, are necrotic, contain areas of hemorrhage, and are surrounded by a moderate amount of edema. A supratentorial mass that has a large cystic component is almost always a high-grade lesion.

Hypothalamic Astrocytoma

Hypothalamic astrocytoma is distinct from other intracranial astrocytomas with respect to its biologic, histologic, and clinical features. These tumors are usually pilocytic neoplasms. The tumor may invade the optic chiasm or extend posteriorly and inferiorly to involve the interpeduncular and

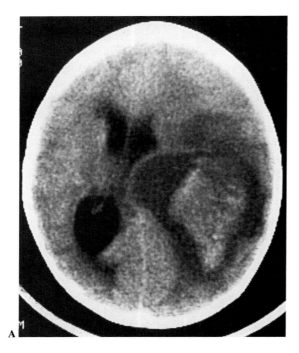
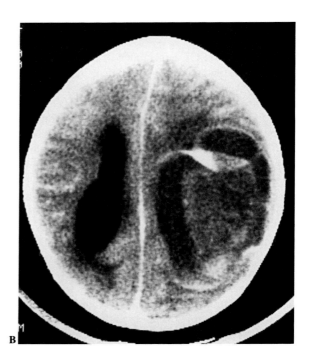

Fig. 1-68 Hemispheric astrocytoma. (**A**) Unenhanced and (**B**) enhanced CT scans show a large mass in the left cerebral hemisphere. The central portion is solid and shows minimal contrast enhancement. The peripheral aspects are cystic, and there is enhancement of the wall of the cyst. The midline structures are displaced toward the right, and there is mild obstructive hydrocephalus. Unlike posterior fossa lesions, cystic supratentorial astrocytomas tend to be aggressive neoplasms.

basal cisternae. It may not be possible to distinguish a large lesion primarily arising in the hypothalamus from one arising in the optic chiasm.

Hypothalamic astrocytomas may produce various endocrinopathies, including failure to thrive, hyponatremia, loss of subcutaneous fat, hypoglycemia, accelerated long bone growth, obesity, diabetes insipidus, and hypogonadism. Involvement of the optic chiasm may produce visual manifestations, such as decreased visual acuity or nystagmus. Infants and young children with hypothalamic astrocytomas may have the diencephalic syndrome. This is a distinct clinical syndrome that is characterized by failure to thrive despite a voracious appetite, pallor, unusual alertness, and hyperactivity. Older patients tend to present with visual symptoms, fever, and an altered (usually depressed) level of consciousness. Signs of obstructive hydrocephalus may develop with extension of the tumor into the region of the foramina of Monro.[133]

A hypothalamic astrocytoma is demonstrated on imaging studies as a mass that obliterates the suprasellar cisterna. The optic chiasm must be visualized separate from the lesion to differentiate a hypothalamic tumor from a primary tumor of the chiasm. The margins of an astrocytoma are often lobulated. Superior extension into the region of the third ventricle is common. On CT, the mass usually is of slightly lower attenuation than normal brain on unenhanced images and shows moderate to marked enhancement on contrast-enhanced

images. Enhancement is often somewhat heterogeneous. Calcification, hemorrhage, and necrosis are uncommon.

On MRI, a hypothalamic astrocytoma is slightly hypointense to normal brain on T_1-weighted images and is hyperintense on T_2-weighted images. Sagittal and coronal images are essential for defining the anatomy of the optic chiasm and optic tracts. Hypothalamic astrocytomas tend to have a more heterogeneous appearance than astrocytomas of the optic chiasm (Fig. 1-70). The lesion shows a pattern of contrast enhancement with paramagnetic contrast material similar to that seen on CT.

Chiasmatic Glioma

Optic chiasm glioma typically presents with bilateral visual abnormalities and optic atrophy. Large tumors may cause hydrocephalus by extension into the third ventricle. The symptoms produced by invasion of the hypothalamus may be similar or identical to those that occur with hypothalamic astrocytomas. There is an increased incidence of chiasmatic gliomas in patients with neurofibromatosis type 1. The peak age at presentation is adolescence.

The usual CT or MR appearance of an optic chiasm glioma is globular enlargement of the chiasm. The mass usually has well-defined contours. Cysts, necrosis, and calcification are rare. Enhancement is usually homogeneous on contrast-enhanced CT or MRI. The mass is isointense or slightly

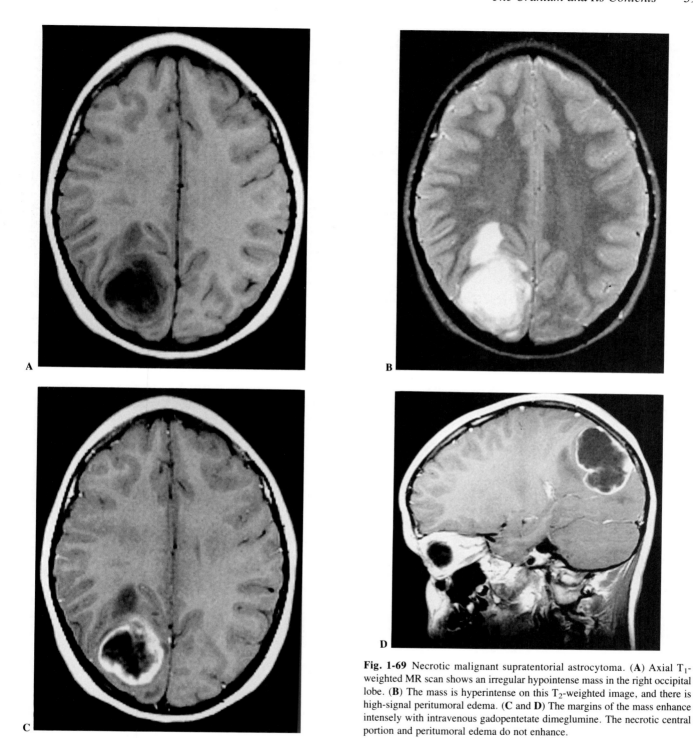

Fig. 1-69 Necrotic malignant supratentorial astrocytoma. (**A**) Axial T_1-weighted MR scan shows an irregular hypointense mass in the right occipital lobe. (**B**) The mass is hyperintense on this T_2-weighted image, and there is high-signal peritumoral edema. (**C** and **D**) The margins of the mass enhance intensely with intravenous gadopentetate dimeglumine. The necrotic central portion and peritumoral edema do not enhance.

hypointense to normal brain on T_1-weighted MR images and hyperintense on T_2-weighted images. The mass may extend into the optic nerves, optic tracts, optic radiations, and (rarely) the hypothalamus (Fig. 1-71). A large chiasmatic glioma with superior extension cannot be reliably differentiated from a hypothalamic tumor; hypothalamic gliomas, however, tend to have a more homogeneous appearance.[134,135]

Hamartoma of the Tuber Cinereum

Hamartoma of the tuber cinereum is a rare benign lesion of the posterior aspect of the hypothalamus. The tumor is composed of nerve cells that are histologically similar to those normally present in the tuber cinereum. The clinical presentation may include seizures, precocious puberty, and behavior

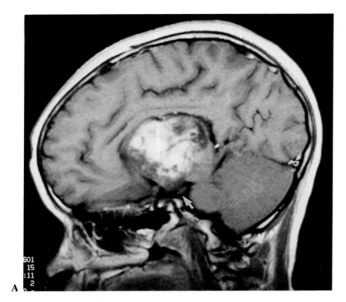
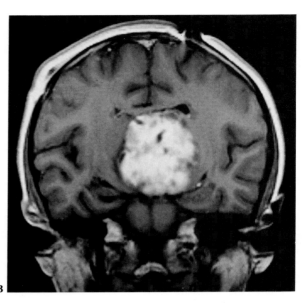

Fig. 1-70 Hypothalamic astrocytoma. (**A**) Contrast-enhanced sagittal and (**B**) coronal T_1-weighted MR scans show an intensely enhancing, heterogeneous hypothalamic mass. The third ventricle is obliterated. The normal optic tract is visible as a linear structure inferior to the lesion (arrow in **A**).

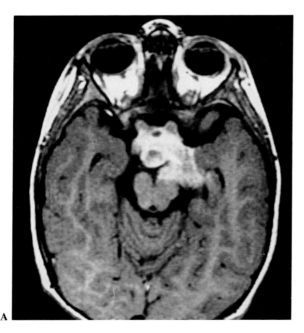
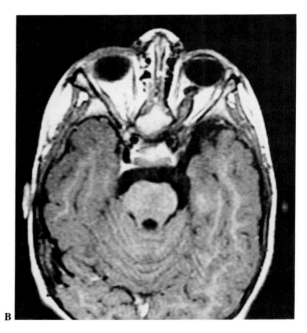

Fig. 1-71 Chiasmatic glioma in a child with neurofibromatosis type 1. (**A**) Contrast-enhanced T_1-weighted axial MR scan shows enhancement and marked enlargement of the optic chiasm. The mass extends into the intracranial portions of the optic nerves and optic tracts. The involvement of the left optic tract is extensive. Most of the mass enhances intensely with paramagnetic contrast material. (**B**) Image of the orbits shows enlargement of the left optic nerve.

disorders. The seizures may be of the gelastic (hysteric laughter) type. Those patients who present with precocious puberty have pedunculated tumors that extend into the suprasellar cisterna. Those patients who present with seizures have lesions that are sessile and broad based with respect to the adjacent hypothalamus.

Imaging studies of hamartoma of the tuber cinereum demonstrate a small homogeneous mass along the posterior aspect of the hypothalamus. The mass usually has sharply defined borders and smooth contours. On CT, the attenuation of the lesion is equal to that of normal brain, and the lesion shows no abnormal contrast enhancement. Uncommonly, the lesion is calcified.[136]

The mass is isointense to gray matter on T_1-weighted MR images. Sagittal and coronal images best display the relationship of the hamartoma to the inferior third ventricle, the

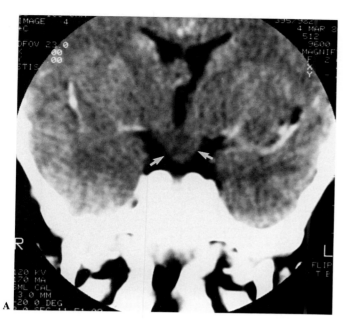

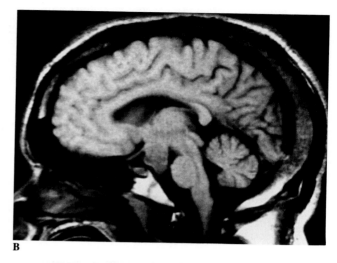

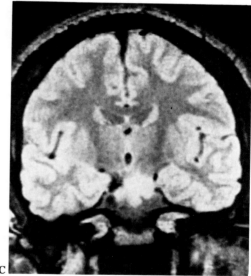

Fig. 1-72 Hamartoma of the tuber cinereum. The clinical presentation of this child was in the form of gelastic seizures. (**A**) Contrast-enhanced coronal CT scan shows a small sessile homogeneous mass (arrows) in the inferior aspect of the hypothalamus. The normal third ventricle is visible superior to the lesion. The attenuation of the mass is equal to that of normal brain, and the lesion does not enhance with intravenous contrast material. (**B**) Sagittal T_1-weighted MR scan shows the homogeneous mass extending inferiorly from the posterior aspect of the hypothalamus. The mass extends into the suprasellar and prepontine cisternae. The optic tract is visible anterior and superior to the lesion. (**C**) Coronal proton-density MR scan shows the mass to be slightly hyperintense to normal brain.

infundibulum, and the mamillary bodies. The lesion may be isointense or hyperintense relative to gray matter on T_2-weighted images (Fig. 1-72).[137]

Giant Cell Astrocytoma

Giant cell astrocytoma is a low-grade neoplasm that is almost always associated with tuberous sclerosis. This tumor occurs in 5% to 10% of patients with tuberous sclerosis. The usual location is the wall of the lateral ventricle, most often in the region of the foramen of Monro. The tumor is thought to arise from a subependymal hamartoma. Most giant cell astrocytomas are discovered incidentally during the imaging evaluation of a patient with tuberous sclerosis. Occasionally, symptoms are produced by obstructive hydrocephalus. The peak incidence of detection is between 5 and 10 years of age.

The typical appearance of a giant cell astrocytoma on imaging studies is a well-demarcated, round to oval lesion in the wall of the lateral ventricle, most often adjacent to the foramen of Monro (Fig. 1-73). Unilateral or bilateral hydrocephalus of the lateral ventricles may be present if the foramen is occluded. On CT, the attenuation of the mass is usually equal to or slightly higher than that of normal brain. There is prominent contrast enhancement, which helps differentiate this lesion from a subependymal hamartoma. On MRI, giant cell astrocytoma is hypointense or isointense to normal brain tissue on T_1-weighted images and hyperintense on T_2-weighted images. There is intense uniform enhancement of the tumor on enhanced images with paramagnetic contrast material.

Craniopharyngioma

Craniopharyngioma is a benign developmental neoplasm that is thought to arise from embryonic squamous cell rests along the pathway of the involuted tract of the hypophyseal pharyngeal duct (pouch of Rathke). Most are located in the suprasellar region. This lesion accounts for about 15% of all pediatric supratentorial tumors and at least 50% of suprasellar tumors. The peak age at diagnosis in children is between 6 and 12 years. There is a second peak in adults in the fourth or fifth decade. The clinical presentation most often consists of visual field defects and signs of anterior pituitary dysfunction. Diabetes insipidus is occasionally seen. With large tumors, signs of increased intracranial pressure may be present.

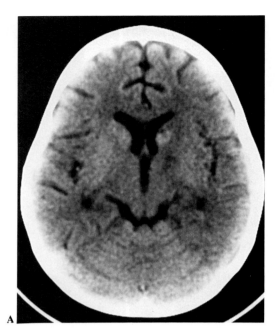
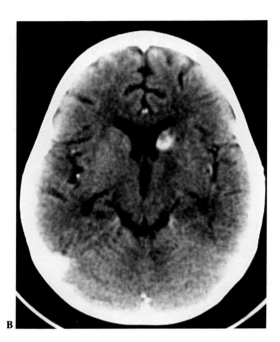

Fig. 1-73 Tuberous sclerosis with giant cell astrocytoma. **(A)** Unenhanced and **(B)** enhanced axial CT scans in a child with tuberous sclerosis demonstrating an intensely enhancing subependymal nodule in the wall of the left lateral ventricle. The lesion contains little or no calcium, as shown on the unenhanced image. An intensely enhancing, noncalcified subependymal mass in a patient with tuberous sclerosis is suggestive of a giant cell astrocytoma. These lesions must be followed closely with sequential imaging studies.

Most craniopharyngiomas are mixed lesions that contain a largely cystic component and a small solid component. Uncommonly, they are entirely solid. There is usually a firm capsule that blends with the surrounding hypothalamus. The cyst contents are often thick, having the consistency of machine oil. Cholesterol crystals are present in the fluid. In some cases, the cyst contents are gelatinous. A chemical meningitis may be produced by spillage of the cyst contents at surgery. The solid components of the tumor often contain foci of calcification or ossification. Craniopharyngiomas occasionally invade adjacent portions of the brain, which evokes a gliotic reaction.

There is considerable variation in the size of craniopharyngiomas. A small tumor may present as a cystic lesion in the tuber cinereum, infundibulum, or sella. Large tumors extend upward into the third ventricle or posteriorly and inferiorly along the dorsum sellae and clivus. At times, the tumor grows into the pituitary fossa. Craniopharyngioma may also occur rarely in an ectopic location in the sphenoid bone, the nasopharynx, the cerebellopontine angle, or the pineal gland.[138]

The typical CT appearance of a craniopharyngioma is a partially calcified mass in the suprasellar region. Ninety percent to 95% of these tumors have one or more cystic components, and some degree of calcification is identified in about an equal percentage. The type of calcification is somewhat variable. Largely cystic lesions tend to have a circumferential rim of calcification. Conglomerate calcification may occur in solid portions of the tumor. Uncalcified solid portions of the lesion

usually show moderate contrast enhancement. Because of the mixed composition of craniopharyngiomas, contrast enhancement is usually heterogeneous.[139,140]

On MRI, the cystic areas in a craniopharyngioma may be of high or low signal intensity with respect to the brain on T_1-weighted images, depending on the contents. Solid components are isointense or hypointense on T_1-weighted images. Both cystic and solid components tend to be of high signal intensity on T_2-weighted sequences, although the cystic areas usually produce higher signal intensity than the solid regions. Fluid-fluid levels are occasionally identified. Calcifications produce signal voids on all imaging sequences. The typical MR appearance of a craniopharyngioma is, therefore, a markedly heterogeneous, multilobulated mass in the suprasellar cisterna (Fig. 1-74). Less than 5% are totally intrasellar. Extension of a suprasellar craniopharyngioma into the posterior fossa (between the clivus and brainstem), middle cranial fossa, or anterior cranial fossa occurs in about one-quarter of cases. Involvement of the third ventricle is fairly common.[141]

Other suprasellar masses that occur in children include optic chiasm glioma, hamartoma of the tuber cinereum, hypothalamic glioma, and pituitary adenoma. In general, the demonstration of calcifications and cysts in the lesion allows a confident diagnosis. The high signal produced by the complex fluid in the cystic components on T_1-weighted MR images is also a helpful diagnostic feature.

Rathke cleft cyst is another pediatric suprasellar mass that produces high signal intensity on T_1-weighted images. This lesion, however, is usually totally intrasellar and uncalcified.

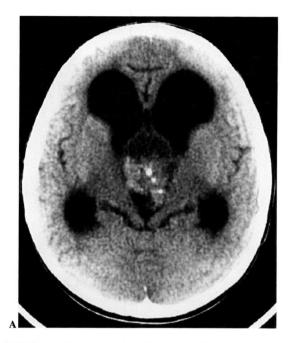

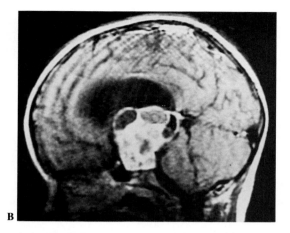

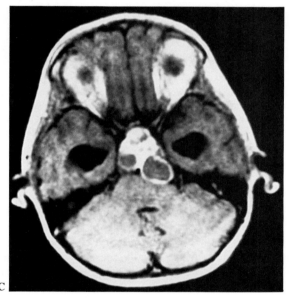

Fig. 1-74 Craniopharyngioma. (**A**) Unenhanced CT scan shows a heterogeneous mass in the suprasellar cisterna obliterating the third ventricle. The mass contains multiple foci of calcification and cystic areas of low attenuation. There is obstructive hydrocephalus. (**B**) T_1-weighted contrast-enhanced sagittal and (**C**) axial MR scans show this heterogeneous mass to occupy the suprasellar cisterna and to displace the third ventricle. There is also extension into the upper aspect of the posterior fossa, causing slight impression on the left side of the pons. Most of the mass enhances intensely, but the calcified and cystic areas do not enhance. The margins of the lesion are somewhat lobulated.

Rathke cleft cyst is a simple epithelial cyst that originates from the cleft between the anterior and intermediate lobes of the pituitary gland. Symptoms may be produced by compression of the pituitary gland or optic chiasm. Most of these cysts contain simple serous fluid and are isointense to cerebrospinal fluid on all MRI sequences. Less commonly, the cyst contains cellular debris and lipid material, such that high signal is produced on T_1-weighted images.

Langerhans Cell Histiocytosis

Langerhans cell histiocytosis commonly involves the central nervous system, but rarely is this the only site of involvement. The usual sites of involvement are the hypothalamic-pituitary axis and the cerebellum. Rarely, the lesion may affect the meninges or the brain parenchyma, usually in the temporal or occipital lobe. This is most often identified in adults. The brain may be involved primarily or from extension of an adjacent calvarial lesion with invasion of the epidural space.

Diabetes insipidus is the most common endocrine manifestation of Langerhans cell histiocytosis. It is due to deficient secretion of antidiuretic hormone. Clinically, these patients present with polydipsia and polyuria. Diabetes insipidus occurs in about 25% of patients with Langerhans cell histiocytosis. It usually develops within 2 years of diagnosis but rarely is found at the time of clinical presentation. It is more common in children with multisystemic disease, especially diseases involving the skull and orbit, and in patients with pulmonary involvement.

On imaging studies, it is uncommon to demonstrate a mass in the inferior hypothalamus or pituitary stalk in patients with Langerhans cell histiocytosis, even among those with diabetes insipidus. In rare cases, the inferior hypothalamus and stalk of the pituitary gland are enlarged. The mass is either isodense or hyperdense with respect to brain on non–contrast-enhanced CT but displays uniform enhancement with intravenous contrast material. On MRI, the mass is isointense to white matter on T_1- and T_2-weighted images (Fig. 1-75). The normal bright signal of the posterior pituitary gland seen on T_1-weighted images is usually not identified in patients with diabetes insipidus. The mass usually shows intense contrast enhancement with paramagnetic contrast material.[142,143]

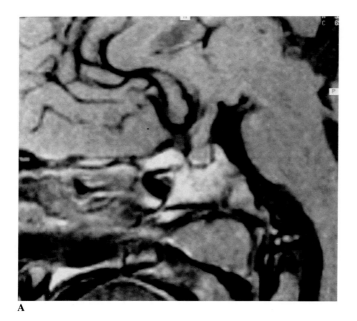
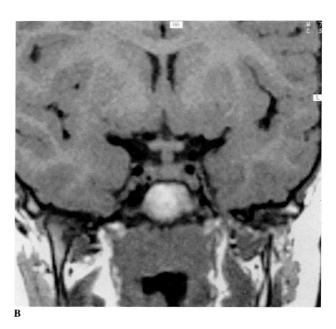

A   B

Fig. 1-75 Langerhans cell histiocytosis. (**A**) Coronal T$_1$-weighted MR scan shows diffuse, symmetric enlargement of the stalk of the pituitary gland. The stalk has uniform signal intensity. The hypothalamus otherwise appears normal. (**B**) Sagittal T$_1$-weighted MR scan confirms enlargement of the stalk of the pituitary gland. The normal high signal of the posterior pituitary gland is lacking. The syndrome of diabetes insipidus occurs in approximately 25% of children with Langerhans cell histiocytosis. Enlargement of the stalk of the pituitary is seen in a minority of children with diabetes insipidus.

Pituitary Adenoma

Pituitary adenomas are rare in children, accounting for 1% of pediatric intracranial tumors. Most are discovered around puberty, generally between 9 and 17 years of age. Pituitary adenomas in children are usually secretory or hormonally active. They may be of any size at the time of clinical presentation. The two most common types of pituitary adenomas are prolactin adenoma and adrenocorticotropic hormone adenoma; growth hormone adenomas are quite rare in children.

Prolactin adenomas typically present with growth deficiency, delay in the onset of puberty, and amenorrhea. Visual disturbances may be produced by compression of the optic chiasm by a large tumor. Laboratory investigation demonstrates increased levels of serum prolactin and decreased levels of growth hormone, thyroid-stimulating hormone, adrenocorticotropic hormone, and gonadotropins.

Adrenocorticotropic adenomas in children are usually quite small and may not be detectable on imaging studies. These children experience obesity, growth delay, hypertension, glucose intolerance, and weakness (Cushing syndrome).

Pituitary adenomas are classified as microadenomas when they are smaller than 1 cm and as macroadenomas when they are larger than 1 cm. In the presence of a macroadenoma, skull radiographs may show enlargement of the sella turcica with thinning and erosion of its walls, a feature shared with other intrasellar mass lesions.

On CT, a prolactin adenoma is most often demonstrated as a low-attenuation pituitary lesion that does not enhance to the same degree as the remainder of the gland with intravenous contrast material. The overall size of the pituitary gland is variable. There is usually a convex configuration of the superior surface. Adrenocorticotropic hormone adenomas are usually quite small and are less well encapsulated than prolactin microadenomas; therefore, these lesions are less reliably identified on CT. A pituitary macroadenoma is demonstrated on CT as a mass greater than 1 cm in diameter that causes enlargement of the sella and shows a variable degree of extension into the suprasellar cisterna. Low-attenuation areas due to cystic or necrotic changes may be present. The solid portions usually show some degree of enhancement with intravenous contrast agents.

On MRI, most pituitary microadenomas are moderately hypointense with respect to normal tissue in the anterior lobe of the pituitary gland on T$_1$-weighted images. Prolactin adenomas tend to have relatively well-defined margins, whereas adrenocorticotropic hormone adenomas are frequently somewhat poorly defined. Necrosis or cyst formation may be present, resulting in further decrease in signal on T$_1$-weighted images. Cystic and necrotic regions are usually hyperintense on T$_2$-weighted images; the solid components, however, usually produce signal similar to that of normal pituitary tissue on T$_2$-weighted images. Paramagnetic contrast-enhanced T$_1$-weighted MR images probably improve the detection rate of small pituitary microadenomas.[144–147]

Ganglioglioma

Ganglioglioma and the closely related tumor ganglioneuroma (gangliocytoma) are composed of both glial and neuronal elements. Gangliogliomas can occur at any age, and the pediatric and adult populations appear to be equally affected. These lesions account for 2% to 3% of pediatric brain tumors and less than 6% of pediatric supratentorial neoplasms. They tend to be relatively slow-growing lesions. There is a predilection for involvement of the temporal lobes. Most patients present with focal neurologic findings. Seizures, which are often bizarre, are common.[148,149]

There is a histologic spectrum of these tumors. If glial elements predominate, the lesion is termed a *ganglioglioma*. If neural elements predominate, the term *ganglioneuroma* or *gangliocytoma* is used. The biologic behavior and imaging features of these two types show no significant differences. The less differentiated types of ganglial neoplasms include ganglioneuroblastoma, anaplastic ganglioglioma, and neuroblastoma.

Gangliogliomas and ganglioneuromas are usually small, slow growing, and well defined. The temporal lobes are the most common locations; other sites, in decreasing order of frequency, include the occipital lobes, frontal lobes, parietal lobes, region of the third ventricle, hypothalamus, and posterior fossa.

Gangliogliomas or gangliocytomas that present in the cerebellum may be either diffuse or focal. Various terms have been applied to this lesion, which in itself reflects the controversy over whether this lesion represents a neoplastic or hamartomatous lesion. Lesions that present in the cerebellum characteristically show a thickening of the cerebellar folia and a loss of normal cerebellar architecture. This extends over only a limited area with a reduction in the amount of normal adjacent white matter.

CT demonstrates a ganglioglioma or ganglioneuroma as a well-demarcated lesion with little or no mass effect. A peripheral location is common, and bone window images may show erosion of the inner table of the calvaria. Calcification is identified in at least 35% of these tumors. Cystic areas may be present, and some of these tumors are predominantly cystic. The attenuation of the solid components may be equal to or slightly lower than that of normal brain. The intensity and pattern of contrast enhancement are quite variable.

As with CT, MRI demonstrates a ganglioglioma or ganglioneuroma as a heterogeneous mass. Predominantly cystic lesions often have well-defined borders, whereas solid tumors tend to have ill-defined borders. T_1-weighted images usually show mixed signal intensity. Cystic areas are sometimes slighly hyperintense on T_1-weighted images, although this is not a consistent finding. Uncalcified portions of the tumor and the peritumoral edema produce moderate or high signal on T_2-weighted images. Enhancement with paramagnetic contrast material is usually heterogeneous (Fig. 1-76). In some cases, MRI shows a large cystic mass that has minimal solid material and margins that enhance only slightly.[150,151]

Supratentorial Ependymoma

About one-third of intracranial ependymomas in children arise in the supratentorial compartment. Supratentorial ependymomas may be located entirely in the lateral or third ventricles, partly intraventricularly, or totally extraventricularly. In contradistinction to ependymomas occuring in the posterior fossa, most supratentorial ependymomas are partially or totally extraventricular. The usual locations, in decreasing

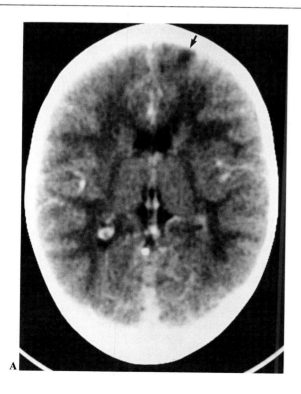

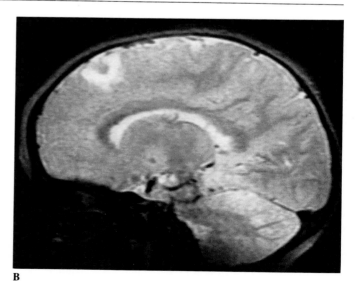

Fig. 1-76 Ganglioglioma. (**A**) Contrast-enhanced CT scan shows a small, low-attenuation lesion in the superficial aspect of the left frontal lobe (arrow). There is no appreciable contrast enhancement. (**B**) Parasagittal T_2-weighted MR scan shows the lesion to be approximately isointense to normal brain, although the affected gyrus is somewhat enlarged. The peritumoral edema produces markedly increased signal intensity.

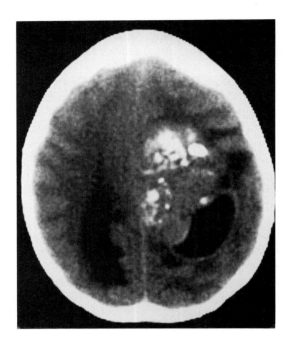

Fig. 1-77 Supratentorial ependymoma. Contrast-enhanced CT scan showing a partially calcified heterogeneous mass in the medial aspect of the left parietal lobe. The noncalcified portions of the mass are of slightly higher attenuation than normal brain. The margins are poorly defined. There is displacement of the left lateral ventricle.

order of frequency, are the frontal, parietal, and temporal lobes. Because of the usual extraventricular location, supratentorial ependymomas are less prone to metastatic spread through cerebrospinal fluid pathways than posterior fossa lesions.

Supratentorial and infratentorial ependymomas are histologically identical. There is a spectrum of histologic grades. There is considerable variability in the gross appearance and composition of these lesions. The clinical presentation may include focal headaches, seizures, and focal motor signs. Common neurologic signs in these children include hemiparesis, hyperreflexia, and visual field abnormalities. These tumors are often quite large at the time of presentation. The peak age at diagnosis is between 1 and 5 years.[118]

The variable composition of ependymomas is reflected in the CT and MR appearances. Most often, the tumor attenuation is approximately equal to that of normal brain on unenhanced CT, although some tumors are hyperdense. Foci of calcification and cystic areas are frequently identified. After contrast agent administration, there is variable enhancement of the solid components of the neoplasm. The lesion is most often identified in a frontal or parietal juxtaventricular location. The most characteristic appearance of a supratentorial ependymoma, therefore, is a heterogeneous, calcified, periventricular, off-midline mass in the frontal or parietal lobe (Fig. 1-77).[122,152]

As with CT, most ependymomas have a heterogeneous appearance on MRI. Mixed signal intensity is usually seen on all imaging sequences as a result of calcifications, cysts, and hemorrhage. A less common, and less specific, appearance is a homogeneous lesion that is isointense or hypointense on T_1-weighted images and hyperintense on T_2-weighted images; in these instances the lesion is indistinguishable from a low-grade astrocytoma.[153]

Supratentorial Primitive Neuroectodermal Tumor

Primitive neuroectodermal tumor is a highly cellular, malignant neoplasm. Histologic examination demonstrates small undifferentiated cells, numerous mitotic figures, areas of vascular endothelial hyperplasia, and necrosis. Small foci of glial or neuronal differentiation may be present but make up only a small part of the cell population. Other primitive neuroepithelial tumors, such as medulloepithelioma, ependymoblastoma, pineoblastoma, and cerebral neuroblastoma, are histologically similar to primitive neuroectodermal tumor, and some investigators include all these lesions under the heading *primitive neuroectodermal tumor*.[100,154]

A supratentorial primitive neuroectodermal tumor is often a large tumor at the time of diagnosis. The most common presenting symptoms are headache, nausea, vomiting, and seizures. Most are identified in children younger than 5 years of age. Primitive neuroectodermal tumor accounts for 4% to 5% of pediatric supratentorial neoplasms. Metastases may occur via the cerebrospinal fluid pathways or hematogeneously; the latter involve other areas of the central nervous system, or the lungs, liver, bone, or bone marrow.[119,155]

Most primitive neuroectodermal tumors have fairly characteristic appearances on imaging studies. The solid portions of the lesion often produce slightly higher attenuation than normal brain on unenhanced CT, reflecting their high cell density. The lesion usually has attenuation similar to that of gray matter. At least 50% of primitive neuroectodermal tumors contain foci of necrosis, cysts, or calcifications, which cause a somewhat heterogeneous appearance. The calcifications may be tiny and diffuse or dense and conglomerate. High-attenuation hemorrhage is occasionally demonstrated. The contrast-enhancement pattern is quite variable among cases, largely depending on the number and size of cysts and the presence of calcification, necrosis, and hemorrhage in the lesion. Homogeneous enhancement is the least common pattern; most of these tumors show heterogeneous or ringlike enhancement (Fig. 1-78).[156]

MRI demonstrates primitive neuroectodermal tumor as a large cerebral mass that has a heterogeneous appearance on all imaging sequences. Calcifications of sufficient size produce signal voids. Cystic areas produce low signal intensity on T_1-weighted images and high intensity on T_2-weighted images. Subacute hemorrhage may produce high-signal areas on T_1-weighted images, and hemosiderin from prior hemorrhage produces signal voids. Peritumoral edema is usually identified on T_2-weighted images. Paramagnetic contrast agent administration results in enhancement of variable intensity and character.[157]

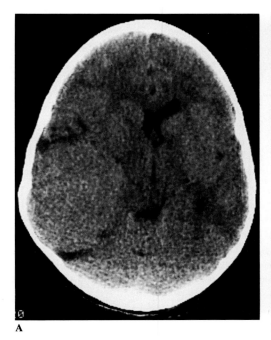
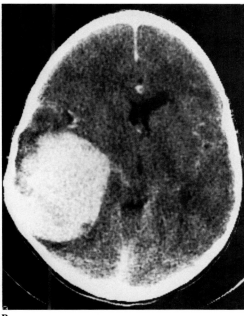

A   B

Fig. 1-78 Primitive neuroectodermal tumor. (**A**) Unenhanced CT scan shows a large solid mass in the right temporal lobe. There are expansion and thinning of the adjacent portion of the calvaria. The mass is of slightly higher attenuation than normal brain. (**B**) Contrast-enhanced CT scan shows intense, fairly homogeneous enhancement of this primitive neuroectodermal tumor.

Choroid Plexus Tumors

Choroid plexus tumors represent about 5% of supratentorial tumors and less than 1% of intracranial tumors in children. These tumors arise from the epithelium of the choroid plexus and may occur as papillomas or carcinomas. Classically, a choroid plexus papilloma presents during infancy with signs of hydrocephalus. The hydrocephalus is due to hypersecretion of cerebrospinal fluid by the tumor. Choroid plexus carcinoma is less common and most often presents between 1 and 5 years of age. Signs and symptoms may be produced by hydrocephalus or local brain involvement.

Most choroid plexus tumors in children occur in the lateral ventricles; the atrium is the most common location. The third ventricle is rarely involved. Bilateral lesions have been reported. There is an unexplained predilection for the left lateral ventricle. In adults, choroid plexus neoplasms, either papilloma or carcinoma, arise more commonly in the fourth ventricle or the cerebellopontine angle cisterna.

These tumors usually have an irregular, frondlike appearance. Papillomas are well defined and are totally intraventricular. Histologically, choroid plexus carcinomas exhibit cellular pleomorphism, mitoses, necrosis, and hemorrhage. These lesions may penetrate the ependymal lining of the ventricle and invade the cerebral parenchyma. Seeding of the cerebrospinal fluid may occur with both benign and malignant histologic types. Extracranial metastases are rare. At times, hemorrhage or calcification is contained in this lesion.[158,159]

Choroid plexus papilloma is demonstrated on CT as an intraventricular mass with frondlike borders. The lesion produces attenuation values that are equal to or slightly higher than those of normal brain parenchyma. Calcifications may be identified. In most cases, there is fairly intense, homogeneous enhancement after infusion of contrast medium. Most choroid plexus papillomas are associated with marked hydrocephalus; occasionally, a large mass in the trigone can cause entrapment of the ipsilateral temporal horn. Rarely, a papilloma will grow through the ependyma and produce changes in the adjacent brain parenchyma.[160,161]

A choroid plexus papilloma is demonstrated on MRI as an intraventricular mass in association with severe hydrocephalus. These lesions may be homogeneous or heterogeneous. Enlarged vessels may be identified in and adjacent to the mass. Foci of hemorrhage or calcification are sometimes present. There is prominent enhancement with paramagnetic contrast agents. The tumor is often best visualized on T_1-weighted images, particularly with intravenous contrast material, because both the tumor and the cerebrospinal fluid produce high signal intensity on T_2-weighted images (Fig. 1-79).[162]

The diagnosis of choroid plexus carcinoma is suggested by the demonstration on CT or MRI of an aggressive intraventricular mass. These lesions usually have irregular contours and grow through the ventricular wall to invade brain parenchyma. On CT, choroid plexus carcinomas typically exhibit a quite heterogeneous composition on both unenhanced and enhanced images. Cysts and areas of hemorrhage are common, as is calcification. This heterogeneous appearance is also reflected on MR images. Hemorrhage and complex material in cystic components frequently result in foci of relatively high signal intensity on T_1-weighted images. There is prominent, heterogeneous contrast enhancement with paramagnetic contrast material (Fig. 1-80).

Colloid Cyst

Colloid cyst is an uncommon intraventricular developmental lesion that is thought to arise from elements of the vestigial

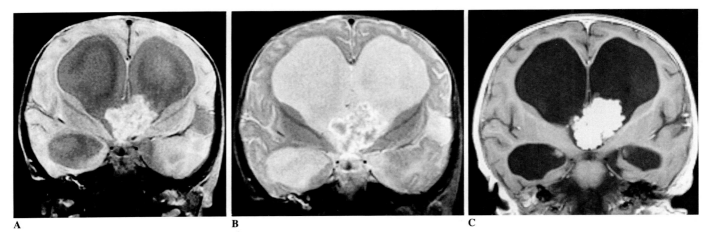

A   B   C

Fig. 1-79 Choroid plexus papilloma. (**A**) Coronal proton-density and (**B**) T_2-weighted MR scans show a heterogeneous, high-signal mass extending from the third ventricle through the foramina of Monro into the lateral ventricles. The lesion is somewhat heterogeneous, particularly on the T_2-weighted image. The borders of the tumor are frondlike. (**C**) The neoplasm enhances intensely with gadopentetate dimeglumine. This choroid plexus papilloma has resulted in severe hydrocephalus from overproduction of cerebrospinal fluid.

paraphysis. This lesion characteristically occurs in the anterior aspect of the third ventricle. Colloid cyst consists of mucinous or dense hyaloid material contained by a smooth fibrous capsule. The cyst wall is attached to the collagenous stroma of the choroid plexus in the third ventricle. Symptoms are produced if the lesion obstructs the ventricular system. The most common clinical findings are headache, gait disturbance, and papilledema. In some cases there are intermittent signs and symptoms of increased intracranial pressure, which is due to a ball-valve effect of the tumor that changes with head position. Although colloid cyst is a developmental lesion, the clinical presentation does not usually occur until early adult life.

Unenhanced CT demonstrates a colloid cyst as a homogeneous, spherical or oval mass in the anterior aspect of the third ventricle. The lesion typically produces high attenuation values on unenhanced CT; uncommonly, the attenuation is equal to or lower than that of normal brain. The cause of the high attenuation values of the contents of the cyst is thought to be related to the presence of hemosiderin, desquamative and secretory products, and microscopic calcifications. The lesion may show minimal or no enhancement with intravenous contrast material.

On MRI, colloid cyst is usually slightly hyperintense to cerebrospinal fluid on T_1-weighted images. On T_2-weighted images, the lesion is hyperintense to brain but may be obscured by surrounding cerebrospinal fluid in the ventricular system. The lesion is often best visualized on proton-density images. Occasionally, there is marked shortening of the T_2-relaxation time in the central portion of the cyst.[163]

Pineal Region Tumors

Tumors of the pineal region account for 3% to 8% of pediatric intracranial tumors. Pineal region tumors may be divided into two groups: pineal parenchymal tumors, and germ cell tumors. Pineal parenchymal tumors are derived from the neuroepithelium of the gland itself. There are three major types of pineal parenchymal tumors: pineoblastoma, pineocytoma, and astrocytoma. The five major types of germ cell tumors that occur in the pineal region are teratoma, germinoma, embryonal carcinoma, choriocarcinoma and endodermal sinus tumor, and mixed germ cell tumors.

In general, the peak incidence of tumors in the pineal region occurs in the 15- to 20-year age group. These lesions are more common in boys than girls. The clinical presentation is quite variable. A relatively specific finding suggestive of a space-occupying lesion in the region of the pineal gland is Parinaud oculoglandular syndrome, which is characterized by paralysis of upward gaze, lack of convergence, and failure of accommodation. Some patients exhibit signs of increased intracranial pressure. Some germ cell tumors secrete α-fetoprotein and β-human chorionic gonadotropin.[164]

Germinoma. Germinoma accounts for greater than 50% of the neoplasms that occur in the region of the pineal gland. Most of these present in adolescents and young adults. Pineal region germinomas are much more common in males, although germinomas arising in the suprasellar region affect both sexes equally. Pineal region germinomas usually present with hydrocephalus or Parinaud syndrome. About one-third of intracranial germinomas arise in the suprasellar region; these usually present with endocrine abnormalities (eg, diabetes insipidus or precocious puberty), which are due to hypothalamic involvement.

Imaging studies demonstrate a pineal region germinoma as a well-defined mass that is usually inseparable from the pineal gland. Rarely, the lesion is identified as lying adjacent to the pineal gland. In a minority of cases, there is evidence of infiltration of adjacent structures, such as the quadrigeminal plate.

Supraseller germinoma is demonstrated as a lobulated mass in the region of the hypothalamus. The optic chiasm and

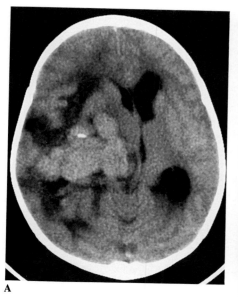
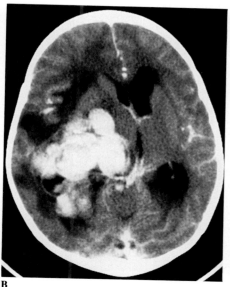
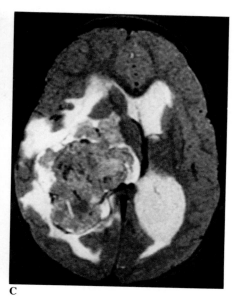

A   B   C

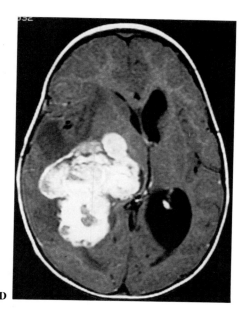

Fig. 1-80 Choroid plexus carcinoma. **(A)** Unenhanced CT scan shows a lobulated mass in the right cerebral hemisphere. The mass is of slightly higher attenuation than normal brain and contains a small focus of calcification. There is extensive peritumoral edema as well as marked mass effect with compression of the right lateral ventricle and minimal hydrocephalus. **(B)** Contrast-enhanced CT scan shows intense enhancement of the neoplasm. A small portion of the temporal horn of the right lateral ventricle is visible at the posterior border of the mass. The frontal horn is displaced anteriorly and toward the left. The third ventricle is shifted across the midline. **(C)** T_2-weighted MR image shows the mass to be heterogeneous. There are tubular areas of flow void in the lesion as a result of prominent vascular structures. There is extensive peritumoral edema. **(D)** Contrast-enhanced T_1-weighted axial MR image shows intense enhancement of most of the mass. The peritumoral edema does not enhance. **(E)** Coronal contrast-enhanced T_1-weighted MR image shows the intraventricular location of this choroid plexus carcinoma.

D

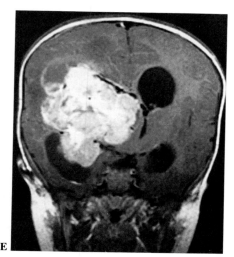

E

pituitary stalk may be displaced or invaded. Superior extension causes displacement of the third ventricle, and there may be evidence of infiltration of the walls of the third ventricle. Metastases via the cerebrospinal fluid pathways may occur with a germinoma in either location.

Unenhanced CT shows a germinoma as a mass whose attenuation is equal to or greater than that of normal brain. Punctate calcifications may be present. Germinoma is hypointense to normal brain on T_1-weighted MR images and hyperintense on T_2-weighted images. Less commonly, relative T_2-relaxation time shortening is present. Germinomas exhibit intense contrast enhancement on both CT and MRI (Fig. 1-81). Cerebrospinal fluid metastases also show intense enhancement. Occasionally germinoma is multifocal, with lesions being located in both the pineal and suprasellar regions. Rarely, germinomas may arise in the basal ganglia or thalamus.[165–168]

Teratoma. Teratoma of the pineal region is much less common than germinoma. As with germinomas, there is a marked male predominance. Most patients present during the second decade of life with Parinaud syndrome or hydrocephalus. Although the pineal region is the most common intracranial

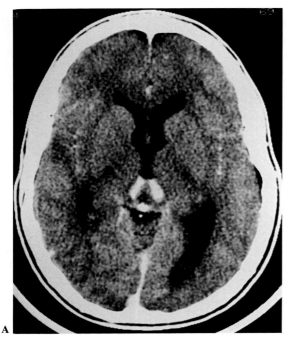

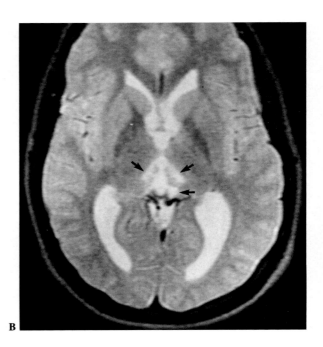

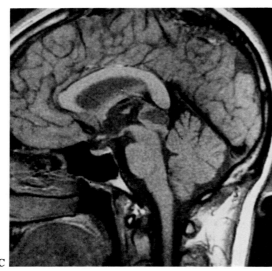

Fig. 1-81 Pineal germinoma. (A) Contrast-enhanced CT scan shows a heterogeneous mass in the region of the pineal gland. Portions of the mass show fairly intense enhancement, whereas others are of relatively low attenuation. There is a slight impression on the posterior aspect of the third ventricle, and the posterior aspect of the mass extends into the quadrigeminal plate cisterna. (B) T_2-weighted axial MR scan also shows a heterogeneous appearance (arrows). Most of the mass is hyperintense, producing signal approximately equal to that of cerebrospinal fluid. (C) Sagittal T_1-weighted MR scan clearly demonstrates the pineal location of the mass. Most of the tumor is hypointense to brain on this T_1-weighted image. There is compression of the aqueduct, although hydrocephalus is not present.

site of teratoma, these tumors may arise in virtually any location, usually in the midline. The suprasellar region is also a fairly common location.

Teratoma in the pineal region is usually demonstrated on CT as a heterogeneous mass. Low-attenuation areas representing fatty components are common, as are dense areas of calcification. A mixture of cystic and solid areas is usually present. Formed elements, such as ossicles or teeth, are occasionally identified. Contrast enhancement is usually minimal. Purely cystic or fatty teratomas may mimic an epidermoid tumor or quadrigeminal plate arachnoid cyst.[169] Malignant germ cell tumors of the pineal region usually show evidence of invasion of adjacent structures and are more apt to show significant contrast enhancement.

As with CT, MRI demonstrates a heterogeneous appearance of most teratomas of the pineal region. Calcifications of sufficient size produce signal voids on both T_1- and T_2-weighted images. Fatty components produce moderate signal on T_1- and T_2-weighted images. Most other solid components produce relatively low signal on T_1-weighted images and high signal on T_2-weighted images. Sagittal MR images are particuarly useful for demonstrating the location of the tumor and its effects on adjacent structures.

Malignant Germ Cell Tumors. Embryonal cell carcinoma, choriocarcinoma, and endodermal sinus tumor are malignant germ cell tumors that can arise in the pineal region. These lesions may also occur in the suprasellar region. They often secrete α-fetoprotein or β-human chorionic gonadotropin, both of which can be used as tumor markers. As with other pineal lesions, the clinical presentation is usually hydrocephalus or Parinaud syndrome.

Malignant germ cell tumors of the pineal region generally show intense contrast enhancement on CT. Nonenhancing areas of hemorrhage or necrosis may be demonstrated. Choriocarcinoma is particularly prone to hemorrhage. Malignant germ cell tumors may demonstrate calcifications.

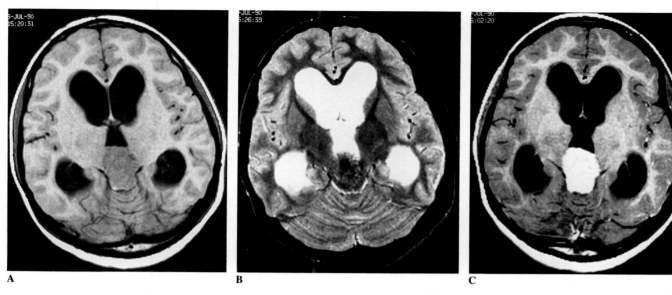

A   B   C

Fig. 1-82 Pineoblastoma. (**A**) T_1-weighted MR image shows a homogeneous, slightly hypointense mass in the region of the pineal gland. There is compression of the posterior aspect of the third ventricle, and a portion of the mass extends into the quadrigeminal plate cisterna. Obstruction of the aqueduct has produced moderate hydrocephalus. (**B**) T_2-weighted MR image shows the mass to be approximately isointense to the thalami. (**C**) Axial and (**D**) sagittal contrast-enhanced T_1-weighted MR scans show homogeneous intense enhancement. The sagittal image clearly demonstrates the pineal location of the tumor and the occlusion of the cerebral aqueduct. Also note the inferior displacement of the colliculi.

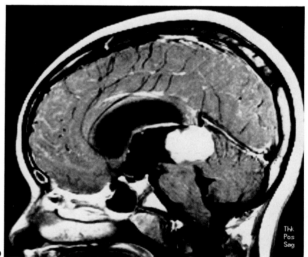

As with CT, MRI usually demonstrates a somewhat heterogeneous appearance of germ cell tumors of the pineal region. Hemorrhage may produce areas of relatively high signal on T_1-weighted images. The tumor is usually significantly hyperintense to normal brain on T_2-weighted images. Areas of old hemorrhage are seen as regions of low signal on T_2-weighted images. In most cases, there is intense enhancement with paramagnetic contrast agents.[165,166,169]

Pineal Parenchymal Tumors. The most common pineal parenchymal tumors are pineoblastoma and pineocytoma. These lesions are derived from the neuroepithelium of the pineal gland. Both these tumors are much less common than germinoma and teratoma.

Pineoblastoma is a highly malignant tumor composed of primitive small round cells. The histologic appearance somewhat resembles that of medulloblastoma. Local invasion and seeding via the cerebrospinal fluid are common. This tumor is most often diagnosed in the pediatric age group.

Pineocytoma is a rare tumor composed of relatively mature cells. These lesions are usually slow growing and noninvasive, although there are uncommon cases in which metastases occur. Pineocytoma may present at any age.

Imaging studies show pineoblastoma as a lobulated pineal gland mass. There may be anterior and lateral extension into the third ventricle or inferior extension into the posterior fossa.

Unenhanced CT occasionally demonstrates calcifications in or adjacent to the neoplasm. Cystic areas, which are of low attenuation on CT and produce low signal on T_1-weighted MR scans, are sometimes present. Solid components of the lesion are hypointense or isointense on T_1-weighted MR images and hyperintense or isointense on T_2-weighted images. There is usually intense enhancement on CT and MRI with intravenous contrast material (Fig. 1-82). Cerebrospinal fluid metastases are best demonstrated on MR images enhanced with gadopentetate dimeglumine.

In contradistinction to pineoblastoma, pineocytoma often contains dense calcifications. Noncalcified portions of the tumor may be isodense or hyperdense to normal brain on unenhanced CT scans. Cystic components are occasionally present. The solid portions of pineocytoma are hypointense on T_1-weighted MR images and hyperintense on T_2-weighted images. Sagittal images are particularly helpful for precise

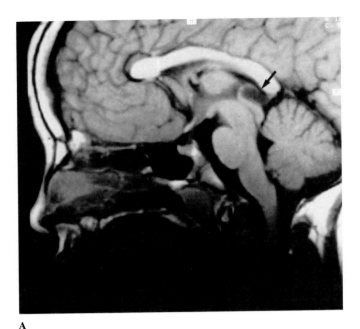

A

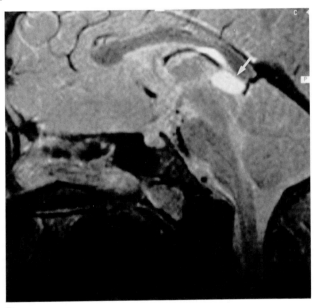

B

Fig. 1-83 Pineal cyst. **(A)** T_1-weighted and **(B)** T_2-weighted sagittal MR images demonstrate a homogeneous, oval mass (arrow) in the region of the pineal gland. The signal characteristics are those of proteinaceous fluid, so that there is slightly higher signal than cerebrospinal fluid on T_1-weighted images and moderately higher signal on T_2-weighted images.

localization of the tumor. Contrast-enhanced CT or MRI usually demonstrates mild to moderate enhancement of the solid components of the lesion. Pineocytomas rarely show evidence of invasion of adjacent structures.[170]

Pineal Cysts. Pineal gland cysts are fairly common incidental findings in patients of all ages. These are small nonneoplastic lesions that are not associated with symptoms. Pineal cysts are identified in approximately one-third of spec-

imens. On CT, pineal cysts are isointense to cerebrospinal fluid on both unenhanced and enhanced images. On MRI, these lesions are typically isointense to cerebrospinal fluid on T_1-weighted images and are slightly hyperintense to cerebrospinal fluid on proton-density and T_2-weighted images (Fig. 1-83). The lesion is often best visualized on proton-density–weighted images. Rarely, there is high signal intensity on T_1-weighted images as a result of hemorrhage.

Oligodendroglioma

Oligodendroglioma accounts for approximately 1% of pediatric brain tumors. This is a low-grade gliomatous tumor, although dissemination via the cerebrospinal fluid pathways may occur. Most oligodendrogliomas are histologically pure. Of the remainder, the diagnosis of oligodendroglioma is made if the predominant cell type is the oligodendroglial cell. The cerebral hemispheres are the most common location of these tumors. The frontal lobes are most often involved. Rarely the lesion may occur in the cerebellum.

The great majority of oligodendrogliomas presents clinically with seizures. Other clinical signs and symptoms are largely determined by the location of the tumor in the cerebral hemisphere. Because the tumor is slow growing, there may be a protracted clinical course before diagnosis.

CT demonstrates an oligodendroglioma as a hemispheric mass, most commonly involving the cortex and subcortical white matter. There is a predilection for involvement of the frontal lobes. Rarely, this tumor may occur in the region of the third ventricle or the cerebellum. Calcification is present in at least 50% to 60% of oligodendrogliomas and may be nodular, shell-like, or linear. Low-attenuation cystic areas are also common. Most of the tumor usually has attenuation values approximately equal to or lower than those of normal brain on unenhanced CT, and contrast enhancement is variable. Contrast enhancement is sometimes most prominent along the outer borders of the mass. Mass effect and surrounding edema are usually minimal. Bone window images may show erosion of the inner table of the skull.[171]

The solid components of an oligodendroglioma produce low signal intensity on T_1-weighted MR images and high signal intensity on T_2-weighted images. Calcification produces areas of low signal intensity on all imaging sequences. Cystic components have variable signal characteristics, depending on the cyst contents. Solid portions of the tumor show contrast enhancement (Fig. 1-84).[172]

Miscellaneous Cranial and Intracranial Tumors

Dermoid and Epidermoid Tumors

Dermoid and epidermoid tumors are developmental lesions that may arise in virtually any portion of the body. The posterior fossa is the most common intracranial location. Intracranial and intraspinal dermoids and epidermoids are usually extra-axial tumors. These lesions are thought to arise

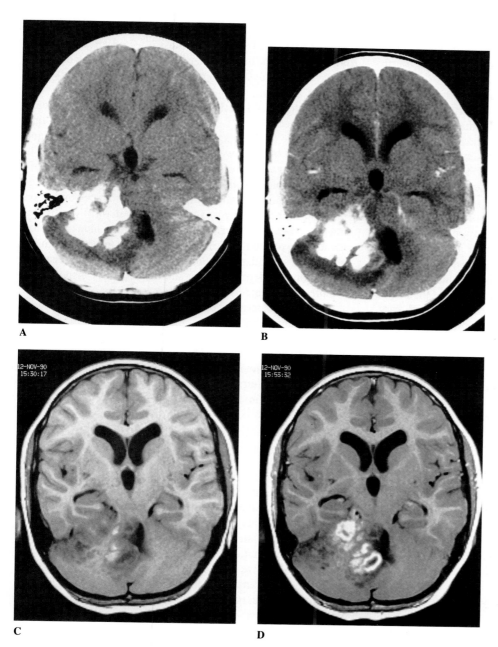

Fig. 1-84 Oligodendroglioma. **(A)** Unenhanced CT scan in a child with right hearing loss shows a densely calcified mass in the right cerebellar hemisphere and moderate surrounding edema. **(B)** Contrast-enhanced CT scan shows minimal enhancement of the periphery of this lesion, especially adjacent to the fourth ventricle. **(C)** Axial T_1-weighted MR image shows the mass to be heterogeneous. There are areas of low signal interspersed with areas of high signal. The areas of high signal are due to subacute hemorrhage. **(D)** Contrast-enhanced MR image shows intense enhancement of most of the lesion. Nonenhancing areas are due to hemorrhage, necrosis, calcification, and cyst formation.

from congenital cell rests that result from incomplete separation of the neuroectoderm from the cutaneous ectoderm during closure of the neural tube. Epidermoids are composed of epidermal elements; dermoids contain epidermal and mesodermal elements. Both these lesions are often cystic.

Intracranial epidermoid tumors are more common than intracranial dermoids. Epidermoids may be intradural-extra-axial, extradural, or intraventricular; most are intradural. The most frequent intracranial location of an epidermoid is the cerebellopontine angle cisterna. Other relatively common sites include the region of the sella turcica, the middle cranial fossa, and the fourth ventricle. These lesions usually do not present in childhood but are most commonly encountered during the fourth or fifth decade of life. Clinically, epidermoids in the cerebellopontine angle are often associated with symptoms of cranial nerve dysfunction, especially of the facial or auditory nerves. Epidermoids in the region of the sella turcica may cause hydrocephalus. Lesions in the middle cranial fossa are often clinically silent unless there is leakage of material from the cystic tumor to cause a chemical meningitis.

Intracranial dermoid tumors exhibit a predilection for midline locations. These lesions are most often located in the posterior fossa near the fourth ventricle; midline locations adjacent to the base of the brain are also common. Most intracranial dermoid tumors are associated with a complete or incomplete dermal sinus. There may also be an associated sinus tract to the fourth ventricle. Dermoid cysts that occur in the posterior fossa may be extradural or contained in the fourth ventricle.

Dermoid tumors are the result of incomplete separation of the epithelial ectoderm from the neural ectoderm. The wall is composed of epidermis and dermis and may contain hair follicles, sweat glands, and sebaceous glands. These lesions enlarge slowly and become filled with desquamated epithelium, sweat, and sebaceous material. On rare occasions, the lesion ruptures and produces a chemical meningitis. A dermoid cyst is the most common intracranial lesion to undergo rupture, either spontaneously or in response to trauma. More frequently, repeated bouts of septic meningitis lead to the discovery of an occipital dimple and an adjacent sinus tract that leads to the lesion in the posterior fossa.

On CT, an intracranial epidermoid is demonstrated as a well-defined, low-attenuation mass. The contour of the lesion is often lobulated. The attenuation values of epidermoids vary somewhat among cases, according to the composition. The two major components are keratinized cellular debris and cholesterol. Most often, the mass produces CT attenuation values similar to those of cerebrospinal fluid. Occasionally, sufficient lipid material is present to produce negative attenuation values. Less often, the keratinized debris is calcified, thereby producing high attenuation values; mural calcification may also occur. Epidermoids do not enhance with intravenous contrast material. Because the wall of an epidermoid is usually quite thin, an intradural lesion that has attenuation values similar to those of cerebrospinal fluid may be difficult to identify on CT. Extradural dermoids often produce bone erosion, which is demonstrated on skull radiographs or bone window CT scans as a well-marginated, lucent defect in the skull base or diploë.

On MRI, an epidermoid appears as a lobulated extra-axial mass that produces low signal intensity on T_1-weighted images and high signal on T_2-weighted images. As with CT, these tumors often have a signal intensity similar to that of cerebrospinal fluid. Inspection of images obtained with various imaging parameters, however, usually confirms slight variation from cerebrospinal fluid signal. In addition, the characteristic lobulated appearance, displacement without invasion of adjacent structures, and lack of edema are helpful signs in the diagnosis of these tumors. Epidermoids that contain a large amount of lipid material may produce moderate to high signal on both T_1- and T_2-weighted images, in which case the lesion cannot be reliably differentiated from a lipoma or dermoid.[173]

Skull radiographs may reveal a defect in the occipital bone that has densely sclerotic margins if there is a dermal sinus that connects the skin to a posterior fossa dermoid. If there is no sinus tract, skull radiographs are normal. On CT, a dermoid tumor is demonstrated as a relatively low-attenuation extra-axial mass near or in the midline. If sufficient lipid material is present, the lesion will have negative attenuation values. Peripheral calcifications are sometimes present. Rarely, an intracranial dermoid cyst will be uniformly high in attenuation on unenhanced CT scans.[174] Unless infected, these lesions do not show contrast enhancement. With infection, the periphery of the dermoid cyst may enhance intensely with intravenous contrast material.

The extra-axial location of most dermoid tumors is clearly demonstrated on MRI. Because these lesions contain lipid material, the mass typically produces moderate to high signal intensity on both T_1-weighted and T_2-weighted images. The MR appearance, therefore, is frequently identical to that of a lipoma or lipid-containing epidermoid tumor. Occasionally, there is a nonlipid cystic component that produces low signal on T_1-weighted images and high signal on T_2-weighted images. Mural calcifications produce signal voids. Enhancement with paramagnetic contrast material is lacking in the absence of secondary infection. The extracranial soft tissues in the region of a dermoid tumor should be closely inspected for the presence of a dermal sinus tract.

Rupture of a dermoid cyst results in spillage of the contents into the subarachnoid spaces or ventricular system. In these cases, CT and MRI may show fatty droplets or fat-fluid levels in the intracranial spaces. This material may be demonstrated to be mobile by imaging with the head in a decubitus or prone position. Intraventricular spillage of the contents of a dermoid cyst may result in obstructive hydrocephalus.[175,176]

Neurinoma

Intracranial neurinoma is quite rare in children. These are benign tumors that arise from the Schwann sheath cells of the cranial nerves. Acoustic neurinomas occur in association with neurofibromatosis type 2. Neurinomas of other cranial nerves are often associated with neurofibromatosis type 1. The clinical manifestations of neurinoma of cranial nerve VIII include progressive hearing loss. With large tumors, signs of increased intracranial pressure, facial nerve palsy, and cerebellar dysfunction may be identified. After cranial nerve VIII, neurinomas most often involve cranial nerves V or IX. Involvement of other nerves is extremely rare. Clinical manifestations of neurinoma of cranial nerve V include facial pain and paresthesias.

On CT, most neurinomas have attenuation values approximately equal to or lower than those of normal brain. Calcifications are occasionally present. Hemorrhage or necrosis may rarely occur in large lesions. Nonnecrotic portions of the tumor usually show appreciable enhancement with intravenous contrast material. Skull radiographs and bone window CT images usually show enlargement of the bony canal of the affected nerve.

Most neurinomas are isointense or slightly hypointense to brain on T_1-weighted MR images and hyperintense to brain on T_2-weighted images (Figs. 1-85 and 1-86). Large lesions may be somewhat heterogeneous and may show evidence of intratumoral hemorrhage. Typically, significant enhancement is identified with paramagnetic contrast media.[177–181]

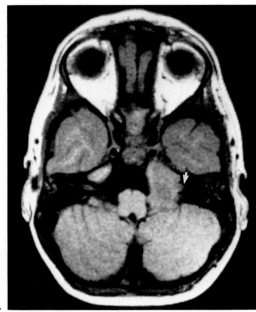

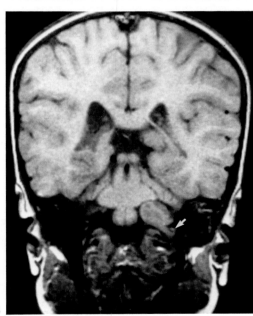

Fig. 1-85 Acoustic neurinoma. (A) Axial and (B) coronal T$_1$-weighted MR scans demonstrate a homogeneous mass in the left cerebellopontine angle cisterna. A portion of the mass lies in the left internal auditory canal (arrows).

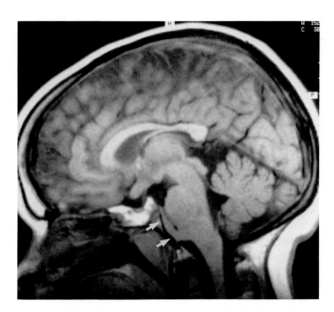

Fig. 1-86 Neurinoma of cranial nerve VI. Sagittal T$_1$-weighted MR image in a child with neurofibromatosis type 1 showing a fusiform mass (arrows) in the prepontine cistern extending from the anterior surface of the upper medulla. A chiasmatic glioma is also seen in the suprasellar region.

Teratoma

Intracranial teratomas account for 1% to 2% of intracranial tumors in children. Many of these lesions are discovered during infancy. Teratomas are benign developmental tumors that are derived from totipotential germ cells. In general, these tumors show a predilection for midline locations throughout the body. Although less common, malignant germ cell tumors may also occur intracranially.

Slightly less than half of intracranial teratomas arise in pineal and parapineal regions. Other relatively common sites include the third ventricle (particularly in the floor), the posterior fossa, the pituitary gland, and the hypothalamus. The clinical presentation is determined by the effects of the tumor on the adjacent structures; these include endocrine abnormalities (such as precocious puberty) from effects on the pituitary gland or visual compromise by compression of the optic chiasm and tracts. Posterior fossa teratomas may produce hydrocephalus or cerebellar signs.[182]

Teratomas are composed of elements of all three germ cell layers. The composition of individual tumors is quite variable from case to case. Components that may be present include fat, soft tissue, hair, calcification, and ossification. Benign teratomas are well marginated and cause displacement, but not invasion, of adjacent structures. Malignant germ cell tumors are more often invasive. These malignant lesions often produce α-fetoprotein and β–human chorionic gonadotropin; these can be measured in both cerebrospinal fluid and serum.

The characteristic appearance of a teratoma on imaging studies is a midline heterogeneous mass that contains fat and calcium. CT is the most sensitive technique for the identification of calcification and ossification in these tumors. MRI is often the superior technique for demonstrating the site of origin of the lesion and for defining the effects on adjacent structures. The fatty components produce moderate to high signal intensity on both T$_1$- and T$_2$-weighted images. Calcification or ossification of sufficient size produces signal voids. Large cystic components may be present in teratomas (Fig. 1-87). In comparison to benign teratomas, malignant germ cell tumors more often show evidence of necrosis and invasion of adjacent structures and are less likely to contain a large amount of fat or calcification.[169,176,183]

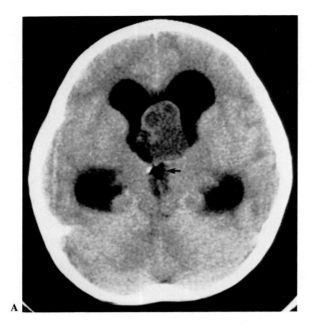

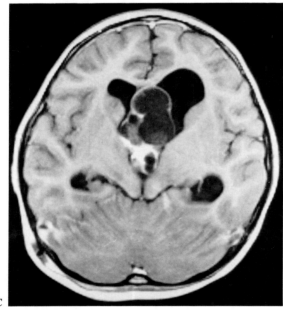

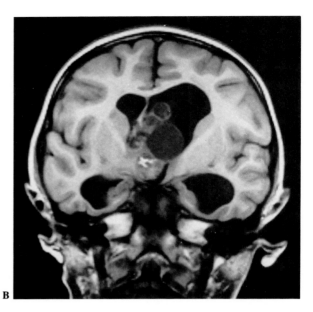

Fig. 1-87 Benign intraventricular teratoma. (**A**) Unenhanced CT scan shows a well-defined midline mass lying between the frontal horns of the lateral ventricles. The mass is of lower attenuation than normal brain but has higher attenuation than clear cerebrospinal fluid. There is a small fatty component (arrow) along the posterior aspect of the mass. Obstruction of the third ventricle and foramina of Monro has resulted in moderate hydrocephalus. (**B**) T_1-weighted coronal MR image shows the mass to be composed of several cystic components that have various signal characteristics. The fatty portion produces relatively high signal. The mass predominantly occupies the third ventricle and extends into the frontal horn of the left lateral ventricle. The septum pellucidum is displaced to the right. (**C**) Contrast-enhanced T_1-weighted axial MR image shows enhancement of the cyst walls and of the solid components of the mass.

Intracranial lipomas are easily demonstrated on either CT or MRI. Most often, the lesion is homogeneous and shows the typical imaging characteristics of fat (see Fig. 1-24). The margins are fairly well defined, and the tumor tends to conform to adjacent tissue planes and produces little or no mass effect. Calcifications may be present in the wall of the lesion, particularly with lipomas that lie adjacent to the corpus callosum. Contrast enhancement does not occur.

Meningioma

Meningiomas are relatively uncommon in children, accounting for 1% to 3% of pediatric intracranial tumors. The frequency of these lesions increases after the age of 10. About one-quarter of pediatric cases of meningioma are associated with neurofibromatosis type 2. There is some evidence that low-dose cranial irradiation may induce intracranial meningiomas. In children, meningiomas occur with approximately equal frequency in boys and girls.[185,186]

In comparison to adults, a greater proportion of meningeal tumors in children are malignant meningiosarcomas. Also, a high percentage of pediatric meningiomas are intraventricular. The clinical signs and symptoms are determined by the size and location of the tumor. Common findings include seizures,

Lipoma

Intracranial lipoma is a rare tumor that is thought to be due to abnormal inclusion of mesodermal elements early in gestation. It is, therefore, a developmental lesion. Most intracranial lipomas are located at or near the midline. The most frequently involved structures are the corpus callosum, the cerebellopontine angle cisterna, and the quadrigeminal plate cisterna. Other less common potential sites include the brainstem, cerebral hemispheres, cranial nerve roots, ventral diencephalon, dorsal midbrain, and choroid plexus. Intracranial lipomas are often associated with other developmental anomalies, such as cranium bifidum, agenesis of the corpus callosum, cephalocele, myelomeningocele, and agenesis of the cerebellar vermis.[184]

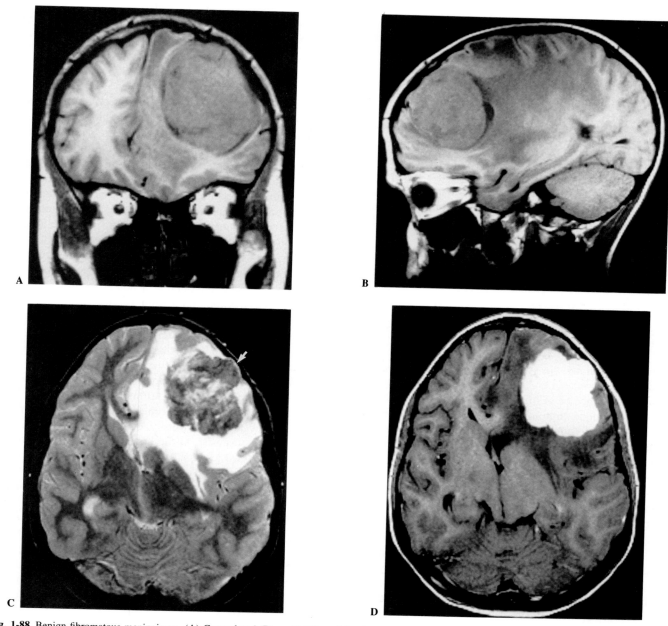

Fig. 1-88 Benign fibromatous meningioma. **(A)** Coronal and **(B)** sagittal T_1-weighted MR images show a slightly heterogeneous extra-axial mass that causes marked mass effect on the adjacent left cerebral hemisphere. The lesion is clearly differentiated from brain tissue. There is decreased signal intensity of the left hemispheric white matter as a result of edema. **(C)** T_2-weighted MR image shows the mass to be quite heterogeneous. There is extensive edema in the adjacent portions of the left hemisphere. There are marked midline shift and a suggestion of dural attachment of the mass along the peripheral aspect (arrow). **(D)** Contrast-enhanced T_1-weighted MR image shows intense, homogeneous enhancement.

signs of increased intracranial pressure, and focal neurologic signs. Meningiosarcomas tend to be large, aggressive lesions and are associated with a poor prognosis. Central nervous system metastases may occur.

The usual CT appearance of a benign fibromatous meningioma is a well-defined mass whose attenuation is approximately equal to or slightly higher than that of normal brain. Calcifications are present in the lesion in approximately half the cases. Bone window images show hyperostosis in the adjacent portion of the skull in approximately half the cases.

With intravenous contrast material, most meningiomas show intense homogeneous contrast enhancement. Nonenhancing cystic or necrotic areas are occasionally present but are probably more common in malignant lesions. Rarely, large cysts are contained in a meningioma.[187]

On MRI, most meningiomas are approximately isointense to gray matter on all imaging sequences. Calcifications, cysts, and necrosis may alter this appearance somewhat. Solid portions of the tumor show intense uniform enhancement with paramagnetic contrast media (Fig. 1-88). Linear enhancement of the dura mater that is continuous with or emanates from the dural margins of a meningioma is commonly seen on contrast-enhanced MR images. This is termed the glove or tail sign.[188]

Although imaging studies do not allow accurate differentiation between benign and malignant meningeal tumors, most meningiosarcomas are large and heterogeneous neoplasms. Unenhanced CT scans show a large mass with poorly defined borders, with the tumor itself consisting of areas of differing attenuation values. Calcifications are common. There is often extensive peritumoral edema. After administration of intravenous contrast material, there is intense enhancement of the solid portions of the neoplasm. Nonenhancing areas due to cysts, calcification, or necrosis are common. The heterogeneous composition of the lesion is also well demonstrated on MRI.

The classic arteriographic appearance of a meningioma is a round mass with a fairly intense homogeneous tumor blush. In most cases, the vascular supply is demonstrable as originating from meningeal vessels.[156,189,190]

Brain Lymphoma

Primary central nervous system lymphoma is an uncommon disorder. It represents only 2% of all brain tumors. There is an increased incidence of primary central nervous system lymphoma in immunocompromised patients. The single largest group is those with acquired immunodeficiency syndrome, but primary brain lymphoma also occurs with increased incidence in patients receiving immunosuppressive therapy for organ transplantation and with inherited immunodeficiency disorders such as Wiskott-Aldrich syndrome, severe combined immunodeficiency, and X-linked immunodeficiency.

With the growing acquired immunodeficiency syndrome epidemic, many rare central nervous system lesions such as toxoplasmosis and primary brain lymphoma are becoming increasingly more common. Each of these disorders may have similar clinical and imaging presentations. Currently, primary brain lymphoma affects 2% to 5% of all patients with acquired immunodeficiency syndrome.

Some patients with primary brain lymphoma have a solitary, hyperdense, uniformly enhancing lesion on CT. Most patients, especially immunocompromised individuals, have multiple lesions located throughout the brain. Any portion of the neuraxis may be involved. These lesions demonstrate multiple patterns of differing contrast enhancement. The most commonly identified pattern is ring enhancement. Rarely, gyral-like enhancement has been observed. The lesions are usually surrounded by significant edema. It is not unusual for several different contrast enhancement patterns to occur simultaneously in the same patient (Fig. 1-89).

An important problem in the differential diagnosis is differentiating between primary central nervous system lymphoma and toxoplasmosis. Both can cause mass lesions in patients with acquired immunodeficiency syndrome. On the basis of CT imaging features, the location, size, multiplicity, and pattern of contrast enhancement are indistinguishable between primary brain lymphoma and toxoplasmosis.[191-194]

Metastases

The brain and meninges may be involved with metastatic disease by a number of mechanisms. Epidural extension from calvarial metastatic infiltration, such as in neuroblastoma, is one mechanism. Central nervous system tumors may spread through the intracranial cerebrospinal fluid pathways; the most common of these are medulloblastoma, pineoblastoma, retinoblastoma, and ependymoma. Meningeal infiltration occurs in some cases of leukemia and lymphoma. Intracranial metastasis due to hematogenous spread of extracranial solid tumors is quite rare in children, although the potential for this complication exists with virtually every malignant tumor. The most common extracranial neoplasms to cause focal brain metastases include lymphoma, rhabdomyosarcoma, Wilms tumor, osteosarcoma, and neuroblastoma.

On CT, epidural metastases from neuroblastoma characteristically produce high attenuation. The appearance may mimic acute epidural hemorrhage. Skull radiographs and bone window CT images, however, demonstrate permeative destruction of the adjacent portion of the skull. Rarely, epidural metastases from neuroblastoma may become quite large and cause significant displacement of adjacent intracranial structures (Fig. 1-90). Rarely, neuroblastoma can hematogenously metastasize to the brain parenchyma to produce one or more focal lesions.

Leukemic infiltration of the meninges may be demonstrated on CT or MRI as abnormal contrast enhancement of the meninges. Occasionally, small nodular lesions are visible. Lymphomatous metastases to the brain parenchyma are demonstrated on CT as isodense or hyperdense masses that typically enhance significantly with intravenous contrast agents. On MRI, these usually are slightly hypointense to normal brain on T_1-weighted images and hyperintense on T_2-weighted images. Contrast enhancement may also be demonstrated on MRI.

Cerebrospinal fluid seeding is a potential mechanism for metastasis of several central nervous system tumors. This may occur in the form of one or more nodules in the subarachnoid spaces of the head or spine or as diffuse meningeal infiltration. CT and MRI may demonstrate sulcal and basilar cisterna obliteration and enhancement, ependymal-subependymal enhancement, gyral enhancement, and ventricular dilatation. Large nodules are sometimes demonstrable as enhancing masses. The most sensitive method for the detection of subarachnoid metastasis is contrast-enhanced MRI (Figs. 1-91 and 1-92).[195]

Brain metastases from distant solid organ neoplasms are usually demonstrated on CT as one or more round masses whose attenuation is equal to or lower than that of normal brain on unenhanced CT scans and that show a variable degree of contrast enhancement. Peritumoral edema is commonly pres-

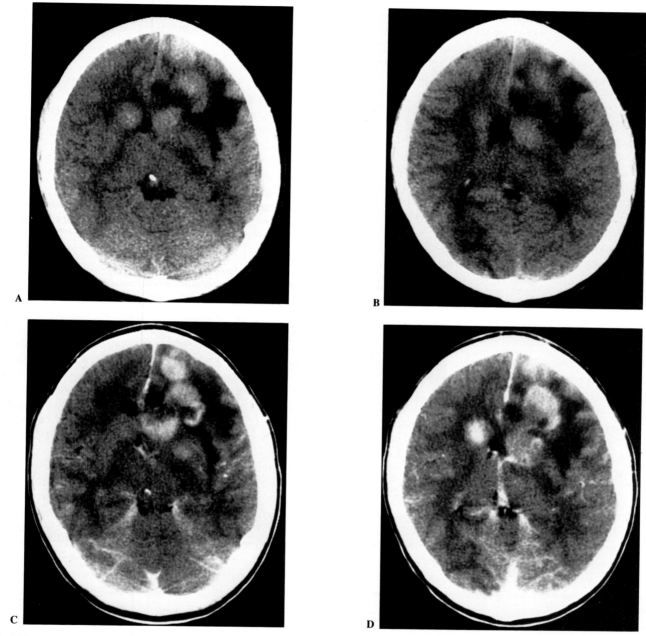

Fig. 1-89 Primary brain lymphoma. (**A** and **B**) Unenhanced and (**C** and **D**) enhanced CT scans of a child with hemophilia and acquired immunodeficiency syndrome show multifocal enhancing masses in both hemispheres. The lesions are of slightly higher attenuation than normal brain on the unenhanced images and are predominantly confined to the white matter. There is extensive peritumoral edema. The lesions enhance intensely but inhomogeneously. One lesion shows ring enhancement.

ent. Likewise, MRI shows these lesions to be isointense or hypointense to brain on T_1-weighted images and variably hyperintense on T_2-weighted images.[196,197]

Skull Tumors

Primary skull tumors are extremely rare in children. The principles of the radiographic diagnosis of these lesions are the same as those for the remainder of the skeletal system.

Osteochondromas may arise from cartilaginous segments of the skull base, usually in the anterior portion near the cribriform plate. Osteomas are rare in children. They may occur in the paranasal sinuses as a part of Gardner syndrome. Chondromas are extremely rare in children.

Angiomas and neurofibromas of the scalp may involve the underlying skull and cause bone defects, bone deformities, or regional increased bone deposition. Cavernous hemangiomas of the skull are characterized radiographically by round areas

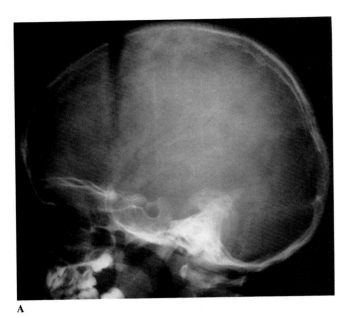

A

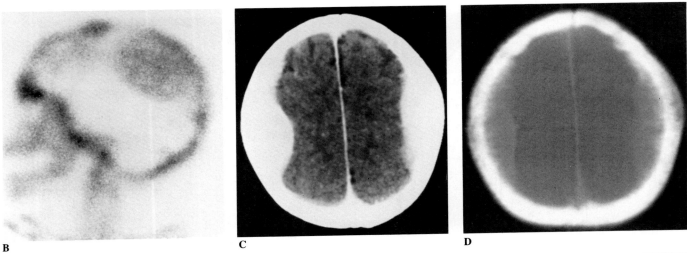

B

C

D

Fig. 1-90 Large epidural metastases from neuroblastoma. (**A**) Lateral skull radiograph in a child with neuroblastoma demonstrates diastasis of the coronal sutures. There are ill-defined, mixed lytic and sclerotic changes in the parietal bones. (**B**) Bone scintigraphy shows increased tracer accumulation in the parietal and frontal bones as well as in the skull base. (**C**) Contrast-enhanced CT scan shows large, lentiform-shaped, extra-axial masses causing impression on the parietal lobes. (**D**) Bone window image shows that these masses are associated with permeative changes in the calvaria.

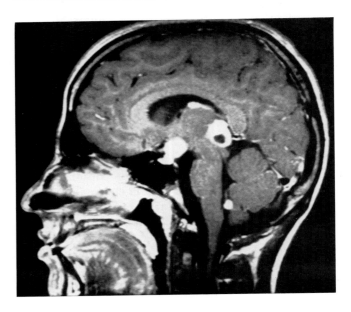

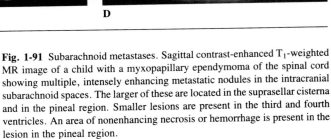

Fig. 1-91 Subarachnoid metastases. Sagittal contrast-enhanced T_1-weighted MR image of a child with a myxopapillary ependymoma of the spinal cord showing multiple, intensely enhancing metastatic nodules in the intracranial subarachnoid spaces. The larger of these are located in the suprasellar cisterna and in the pineal region. Smaller lesions are present in the third and fourth ventricles. An area of nonenhancing necrosis or hemorrhage is present in the lesion in the pineal region.

of diminished bone density in which there may be a honeycomb or radial pattern of greater density, which is caused by spiculation. These lesions usually do not displace or affect the inner table. Cranial lymphangiomas are extremely rare. They may involve the calvaria to produce radiologic findings that are similar to those of a cephalohematoma. The two conditions can be differentiated on clinical grounds.

Epidermoids are ectodermal rests or inclusions that may be located in the scalp, in the diploic space, or between the inner

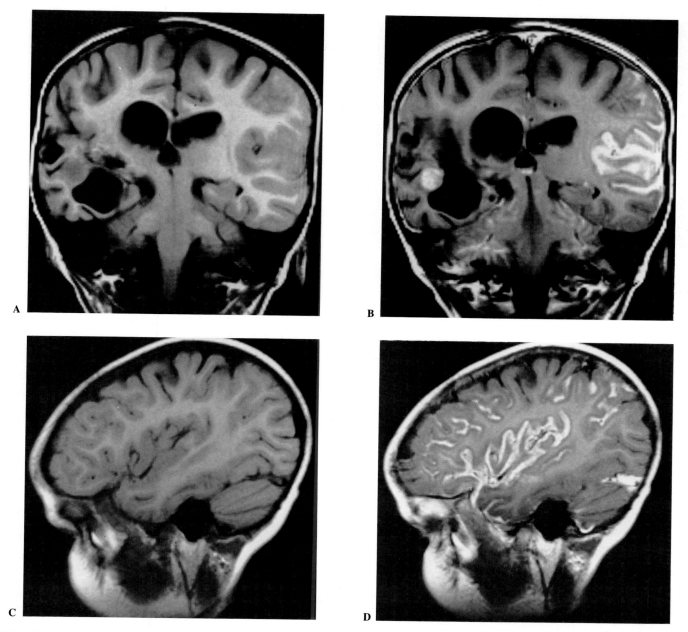

Fig. 1-92 Subarachnoid metastases. (**A**) Coronal unenhanced and (**B**) enhanced T$_1$-weighted MR scans show an enhancing nodule in the right temporal lobe at the site of a partially resected malignant astrocytoma. There are encephalomalacia in the adjacent portions of the temporal lobe and atrophic enlargement of the right lateral ventricle. There is extensive meningeal enhancement in the left temporal and parietal regions as a result of metastatic meningeal infiltration. (**C**) Unenhanced and (**D**) enhanced parasagittal T$_1$-weighted images show the extensive abnormal meningeal enhancement in the left hemisphere.

table and dura. These developmental lesions are usually benign and grow slowly, if at all. Rarely, they can protrude into the cranial cavity and cause cerebral symptoms. When an epidermoid grows in the bone or impinges on it, there is local destruction of bone that is demonstrated radiographically as a well-defined region of diminished density that is surrounded by a sclerotic rim (Fig. 1-93). The margin is due to flaring of the edge of the bone into the marginal ridge. Scalloping of the calvaria is occasionally identified in the region of the lesion.

Dermoid Tumors

A dermoid tumor is a developmental lesion that results from inclusion of extra elements during closure of the neural tube. A dermoid tumor contains sebaceous material in addition to keratin and epithelial debris. Hair may also be present in a dermoid tumor. Dermoid tumors are relatively common in children. Approximately 25% are noticeable at birth, and the remainder become apparent during childhood. Dermoid

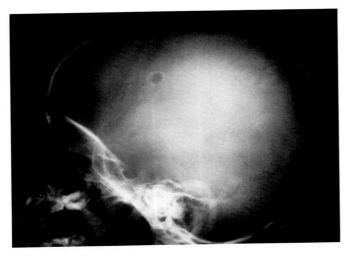

Fig. 1-93 Epidermoid. Lateral skull radiograph showing a well-defined, round, radiolucent lesion in the parietal bone that is surrounded by a sclerotic rim. This is the typical appearance of an epidermoid of the skull.

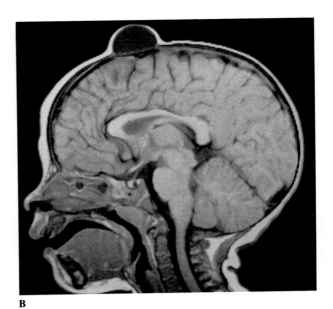

B

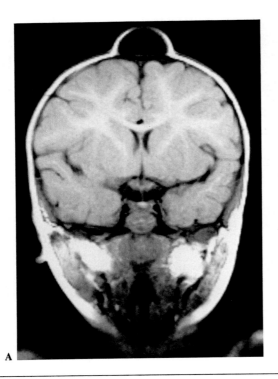

A

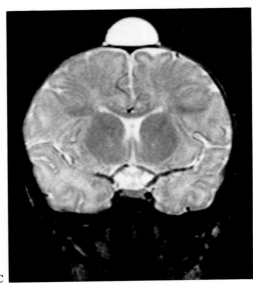

C

Fig. 1-94 Extracranial dermoid cyst. (A) Coronal and (B) sagittal T_1-weighted MR images show a well-defined extracranial mass in the region of the anterior fontanelle. The intact dura deep to the mass is visualized as a hypointense linear structure. The subcutaneous fat forms a hyperintense rim around the periphery of the lesion. (C) T_2-weighted coronal image shows the mass to be hyperintense and homogeneous. The hypointense dura lies between the mass and the subarachnoid space.

tumors are usually located adjacent to a cranial suture. They are most common about the orbit. In the skull, dermoid tumors are most common in the midline, frequently in the region of the anterior fontanelle.

On CT, a dermoid tumor is a mass of low attenuation. It is well demarcated and frequently is surrounded by a well-defined capsule. The low-density nature of the lesion is due to lipids in the cyst contents. On T_1-weighted MR images, the lesions often have moderate signal intensity as a result of their fat content; they show moderate to high signal intensity on T_2-weighted images (Fig. 1-94).

Clivus Tumors

Chordoma. Intracranial chordomas are extremely rare tumors in children. These most often arise from the clivus, presumably from osseous notochordal remnants. Patients with clivus chordoma may present with cranial neuropathies or, in

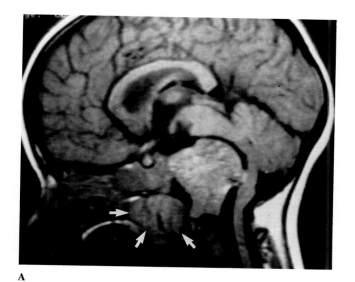

A

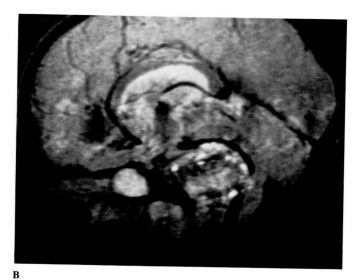

B

Fig. 1-95 Clivus chordoma. (**A**) T_1-weighted and (**B**) T_2-weighted sagittal MR scans demonstrate a large mass arising from the clivus. Posteriorly, the mass causes marked displacement and narrowing of the brainstem. A portion of the tumor extends into the pharynx (arrows in **A**). The signal characteristics are heterogeneous, particularly on the T_2-weighted image. Sclerotic bone produces a hypointense region in the central portion of the mass. (**C**) Lateral vertebral angiogram shows marked posterior displacement of the basilar artery.

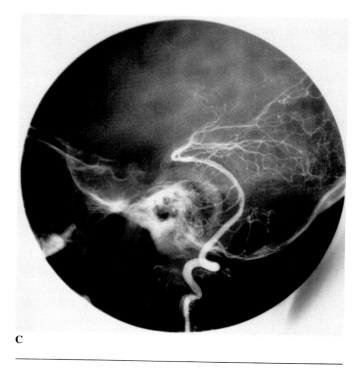

C

the presence of intrasellar extension, with endocrine abnormalities. Chordomas are benign, slow-growing, locally infiltrative neoplasms.[198]

Imaging studies demonstrate a clivus chordoma as a large mass associated with destructive changes in the clivus. The mass typically has attenuation values approximately equal to those of normal brain tissue on CT. Calcifications may be present. Contrast enhancement is heterogeneous. On MRI, these lesions usually are hypointense on T_1-weighted images and hyperintense on T_2-weighted images. Clivus chordomas usually extend significantly from the bone of origin to involve the prepontine cisterna, nasopharynx, sphenoid sinuses, or middle cranial fossa (Fig. 1-95). With a large tumor, the site of origin may not be clear.[199,200]

Chondroma. Intracranial chondroma is a rare tumor that usually develops from the spheno-occipital synchondrosis. The clinical and imaging features of this lesion closely mimic those of chordoma. Chondroma tends to be less hyperintense on T_2-weighted MR images, however.[201,202]

METABOLIC AND DESTRUCTIVE DISORDERS

White Matter Diseases

White matter pathology may be caused by a broad range of metabolic, autoimmune, infectious, ischemic, and traumatic disorders. Many of these processes involve the gray matter concomitantly. In general, white matter diseases can be separated into four broad categories. (1) Dysmyelinating diseases include conditions in which there is abnormal formation or maintenance of myelin. (2) The myelinoclastic or demyelinating diseases include those disorders in which there is breakdown of normally formed myelin. (3) Delay of myelination may occur in developmentally delayed children and in association with various metabolic, toxic, nutritional, and idiopathic disorders. (4) Finally, white matter disease of unknown origin is identified on imaging studies in some children. These classifications are somewhat arbitrary, and some diseases have features that overlap types of white matter abnormalities.[203]

Dysmyelinating Diseases

The dysmyelinating diseases predominantly comprise the leukodystrophies. These are inherited diseases in which there is failure of formation or maintenance of the myelin sheaths. Most or all of these disorders are due to enzymatic defects. These enzymatic defects may produce their effect by causing failure of formation of one of the components of myelin or by causing deficient catabolism of the constituents of the complex proteins found in the myelin sheaths. Specific enzyme deficiencies have been identified for several of these disorders. With the exception of globoid cell leukodystrophy and metachromatic leukodystrophy, the leukodystrophies do not affect the peripheral nervous system.

Alexander Disease. Alexander disease is a rare degenerative disorder of the central nervous system of unknown etiology. The histologic hallmark of Alexander disease is the presence of eosinophilic hyaline bodies in hypertrophied astrocytic cells. There is variable loss of myelin. Specific biochemical defects have not been identified as yet for Alexander disease.

Three clinical syndromes of Alexander disease are recognized. It is not known whether these are different expressions of the same disease or distinct pathophysiologic processes that have similar features. The infantile form of Alexander disease is most common. Clinical presentation may occur from shortly after birth to 2 years of age, with the average age at onset being 6 months. The clinical findings include macrocephaly, spasticity, seizures, hydrocephalus, and psychomotor retardation. The juvenile form of Alexander disease is less common than the infantile form. These patients usually present between 7 and 14 years of age. These children usually do not have significant intellectual dysfunction. The predominant features include swallowing dysfunction, nystagmus, tongue atrophy, facial diplegia, generalized spasticity, weakness, and ataxia. The adult form of Alexander disease is quite rare. The clinical features include spasticity, nystagmus, blurred vision, and dysarthria.[204,205]

CT in cases of Alexander disease shows decreased attenuation of the cerebral white matter. There is often relative sparing of the subependymal regions of white matter. The findings tend to be most prominent in the frontal lobes. There may be subtle increased attenuation of the corpus striatum and the columns of the fornices. The findings of megalencephaly may be noted. Abnormal contrast enhancement may be identified in the white matter adjacent to the frontal horns, particularly early in the disease. Contrast enhancement may also be noted in the caudate nuclei and thalami.

MRI is more sensitive than CT for the demonstration of the white matter abnormalities of Alexander disease. T_2-weighted images show symmetric high-signal abnormality in the white matter; usually this is most prominent in the frontal lobes (Fig. 1-96). Rarely, the findings may be asymmetric. A variable degree of ventricular enlargement may be identified. Late in the course of the disease the corpus callosum and brainstem may become atrophic, and cystic changes may occur in the frontal lobes.[206-208]

Canavan Disease. Canavan disease, also termed spongy degeneration or van Bogaert disease, is a degenerative central nervous system disorder of unknown etiology. Pathologically, the white matter in these patients contains innumerable fluid-containing vacuoles that produce a spongy appearance. These changes are most marked in the subcortical regions; the internal capsule is relatively spared. There is a lesser degree of involvement of the cortical gray matter. The brainstem and cerebellum may also be involved. The vacuoles are thought to result from metabolic disturbances of astrocytes, possibly related to mitochondrial abnormalities. The precise biochemical mechanisms are unknown. There is evidence that a deficiency of aspartoacylase (an enzyme in the myelin synthesis pathway) may be involved in the pathogenesis.

Three clinical variants of Canavan disease have been identified. The infantile form is most common. This type occurs with increased incidence in Jewish people of northeastern European heritage. Clinical presentation occurs during the first few months of life with hypotonia, macrocephaly, and poor head and neck control. After approximately 6 months of age, the hypotonia is replaced by spasticity. Visual disturbances and seizures may occur. The infantile form of Canavan disease is usually inherited as an autosomal recessive disorder.[209,210]

The neonatal form of Canavan disease is rare. The clinical features include lethargy, hypotonia, respiratory difficulties, and swallowing dysfunction. These neonates usually die during the first few weeks of life.

The juvenile form of Canavan disease is also rare. By definition, the clinical presentation occurs after 5 years of age. The usual findings include tremor, ataxia, and mental deterio-

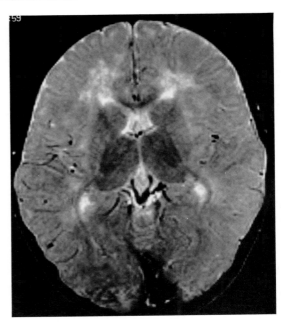

Fig. 1-96 Alexander disease. Axial T_2-weighted MR image showing abnormal high signal in the frontal white matter bilaterally with lesser involvement of the temporal white matter. This is due to dysmyelination of the hemispheric white matter in a child with the infantile form of Alexander disease.

ration. Subsequent findings include signs of cerebellar dysfunction, spasticity, dysarthria, and visual deterioration. This type is usually sporadic.[211]

CT and MRI in children with Canavan disease show diffuse symmetric white matter disease. CT shows decreased attenuation values of cerebral white matter; MRI shows abnormally low signal intensity on T_1-weighted images and high signal intensity on T_2-weighted images. Early in the course of the disease the white matter appears edematous, and the lateral ventricles may appear small and compressed. As the disease progresses, the lateral ventricles become somewhat enlarged, there is progressive white matter demyelination, and small cavities that have the imaging characteristics of cerebrospinal fluid appear in the white matter. Severe cerebral atrophy eventually occurs. Vacuolization and spongy degeneration of the cerebral white matter can also occur in other metabolic disorders, such as 3-hydroxy-3-methylglutaryl coenzyme A lyase deficiency, phenylketonuria, homocystinuria, and maple syrup urine disease.[212–215]

Krabbe Disease. Krabbe disease, also termed globoid cell leukodystrophy, results from β-galactocerebrosidase deficiency. There is marked demyelination, particularly in the posterior aspect of the centrum semiovale and the cerebellar white matter, with dense fibrous astrocytic proliferation and the presence of numerous perivascular multinucleated cells, which are termed globoid cells. There is severe brain atrophy and marked decrease in the volume of white matter. The gray matter is somewhat thin but histologically appears otherwise normal.

Krabbe disease usually becomes manifest between 3 and 8 months of life, before which growth and development may be normal. In the initial stages of the disorder, the infant is hyperirritable and may experience feeding difficulties, psychomotor abnormalities, and seizures. Subsequently, the infant develops spasticity and hyperactive deep tendon reflexes. In the later stages of the disorder, occurring several months after the initial presentation, the deep tendon reflexes become depressed. The affected child is usually deaf and blind and exhibits opisthotonos. Most children die by 2 to 3 years of age. The disorder is inherited as an autosomal recessive trait.[216–218]

Imaging studies in young infants with Krabbe disease may initially be normal. Subsequently, CT and MRI show white matter abnormalities consisting of decreased attenuation on CT and prolongation of T_1- and T_2-relaxation times on MRI. The earliest detectable lesions may be small symmetric areas of abnormality in the posterior aspect of the centrum semiovale. These may also occur in the cerebellum, brainstem, thalami, caudate nuclei, and periventricular areas. In the later stages of the disease the entire white matter is involved, and the appearance is similar to that of other end-stage dysmyelinating diseases. Atrophic changes may be identified.[219–221]

Metachromatic Leukodystrophy. Metachromatic leukodystrophy includes several closely related disorders in which there is deficiency of arylsulfatase A (cerebroside sulfatase A).

This disease results in the abnormal accumulation of sulfatides in the central and peripheral nervous systems as well as in the kidneys, pancreas, adrenal glands, liver, and gallbladder. Sulfatide accumulation in the white matter results in demyelination. Neuropathologic examination demonstrates severe white matter demyelination, eventually leading to focal cavitation. Myelin sheath destruction is accompanied by the accumulation of metachromatic granules of sulfatide-rich lipid material.

The different forms of metachromatic leukodystrophy are clinically classified according to the usual age of presentation. The late infantile form usually presents between 1 and 2 years of age. The initial manifestations include ataxia, hypotonia, and diminished deep tendon reflexes. Subsequently, there is intellectual deterioration, progressive hypotonia, and bulbar and pseudobulbar palsies. The juvenile form of metachromatic leukodystrophy usually presents between 4 and 10 years of age. These previously normal children develop ataxia, a spastic gait, intellectual impairment, and hyperactive deep tendon reflexes. Progressive mental deterioration follows the clinical presentation.

The adult form of metachromatic leukodystrophy most often presents between the ages of 20 and 40. Findings with this type include dementia and signs of corticobulbar, corticospinal, and cerebellar dysfunction.[222–224]

Imaging studies may be normal in the early stages of metachromatic leukodystrophy. As with other white matter diseases, CT demonstrates areas of decreased attenuation in the white matter, and MRI shows prolongation of T_1- and T_2-relaxation times (Fig. 1-97). These changes are probably due to both demyelination and edema from tissue injury. Most often, there are diffuse changes in the cerebral white matter (Fig. 1-98). In the early stages, white matter involvement may be most marked in the frontal regions with subsequent posterior progression. In the late stages, the findings of cerebral atrophy may be present.[225]

Sudanophilic Leukodystrophy. Sudanophilic leukodystrophy, also termed Pelizaeus-Merzbacher disease, refers to a group of disorders in which there are patchy areas of white matter demyelination and perivascular islands of preserved myelin. Histologic examination demonstrates accumulation of sudanophilic droplets that contain cholesterol and triglycerides. The underlying biochemical abnormalities are poorly understood, but there is evidence of deficient synthesis of proteolipid protein in the white matter. Classically, five types are recognized; some investigators include Cockayne syndrome as a sixth variant. The genetic characteristics of the various types of sudanophilic leukodystrophy are somewhat variable. Types 1 and 2 occur predominantly in boys and usually follow an X-linked recessive pattern of inheritance. Type 3 usually occurs as a sporadic disorder. Type 4 appears to be an autosomal dominant disorder.

Type 1 sudanophilic leukodystrophy is the classic form of Pelizaeus-Merzbacher disease. The onset is usually within the first few months of life with nystagmus and head tremor. There are delayed motor development, axial hypotonia, spasticity of

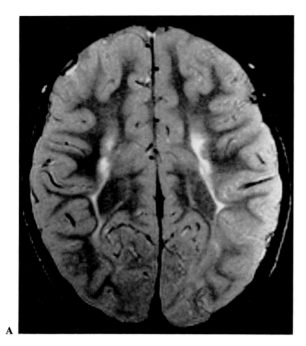

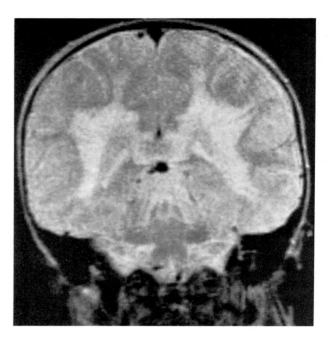

Fig. 1-98 Metachromatic leukodystrophy. Coronal T_2-weighted MR image in a 5-year-old child with the late infantile form of metachromatic leukodystrophy showing high-signal abnormality involving virtually all the cerebral white matter. Signs of cortical atrophy have not yet developed.

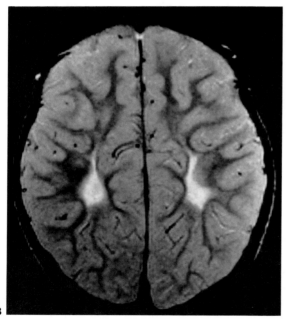

Fig. 1-97 Metachromatic leukodystrophy. (A and B) Axial T_2-weighted MR images showing high-signal abnormality in the periventricular hemispheric white matter in a child with the late infantile form of metachromatic leukodystrophy. Cerebral atrophy is not present in this young child.

the limbs, and progressive microcephaly. Type 2 sudanophilic leukodystrophy presents at birth with severe psychomotor abnormalities. Type 3 has a clinical severity intermediate between types 1 and 2, with the predominant features including nystagmus, tremor, spasticity, and mental retardation. Type 4 occurs in adulthood and has a slower course than types 1 through 3. Movement disorders and ataxia are the usual manifestations. Type 5 includes variants with features that do not allow assignment to types 1 through 4.[226,227]

Imaging studies in cases of sudanophilic leukodystrophy may be normal early in the course of the disease. Focal areas of deficient white matter myelination may be identified in longstanding disease. These appear to be most common in the periventricular regions. The abnormalities are multifocal, with islands of intact myelination remaining (Fig. 1-99). In the late stages, cerebral or cerebellar atrophy may be identified. Also, decreased signal in the basal ganglia and thalami on T_2-weighted images may result from iron deposition.[228–230]

Cockayne Syndrome. Cockayne syndrome shares some features with sudanophilic leukodystrophy. The predominant features of cerebral involvement are patchy demyelination and preserved islands of myelin. In contradistinction to the other forms of sudanophilic leukodystrophy, however, Cockayne syndrome also involves the skin, joints, and endocrine system.

Infants with Cockayne syndrome are usually normal at birth. A photosensitive dermatitis usually develops within the first 6 months of life and is followed by growth retardation, kyphosis, microcephaly, mental retardation, and retinitis pigmentosa. Subsequently, cerebellar dysfunction and signs of upper motor neuron abnormalities develop. Many cases of Cockayne syndrome are sporadic; autosomal recessive inheritance has been identified in some cases.

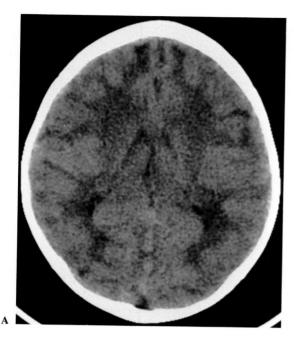

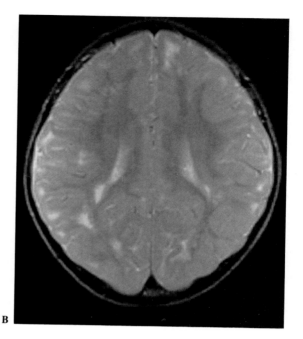

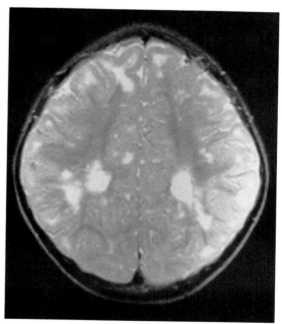

Fig. 1-99 Type 1 sudanophilic leukodystrophy. (**A**) Axial unenhanced CT scan shows ill-defined patchy areas of low attenuation in the cerebral white matter bilaterally. (**B** and **C**) These regions produce high signal on T_2-weighted MR images. These findings indicate multifocal white matter demyelination.

CT in cases of Cockayne syndrome may demonstrate small calcifications in the basal ganglia and cerebellar nuclei. The earliest MR finding is a delayed myelination pattern for age. Subsequently, patchy areas of deficient white matter myelination may be present. Occasionally, there are areas of high-signal abnormality on T_2-weighted images in the periventricular white matter. The findings of cerebral atrophy may develop.[231,232]

Adrenoleukodystrophy. Adrenoleukodystrophy includes several generalized metabolic disorders that are characterized by abnormal lipid storage resulting from peroxisomal abnormalities. A number of organ systems may be involved, including the brain, peripheral nervous system, adrenal gland, and testes. The predominant cerebral effect is demyelination.

X-linked adrenoleukodystrophy is the most common type of adrenoleukodystrophy and occurs almost exclusively in boys. The clinical presentation most often occurs between 4 and 8 years of age. Signs and symptoms of central nervous system involvement in these patients include dementia, memory disorders, emotional lability, seizures, and motor disturbances. The motor and sensory deficiencies may be asymmetric. Visual disturbances are common. Adrenoleukomyeloneuropathy is the second most common form of adrenoleukodystrophy. The great majority of these patients present as adults.

Neonatal adrenoleukodystrophy is a rare disorder that appears to have an autosomal recessive pattern of inheritance.

These neonates exhibit severe hypotonia and seizures. There is severe retardation of growth and development. Microcephaly, nystagmus, optic atrophy, truncal hypotonia, hyperreflexia, and visual and hearing abnormalities may be identified.

Pathologically, X-linked adrenoleukodystrophy produces prominent white matter loss, which is most marked in the parietal, occipital, and posterior temporal lobes. The cerebellum and spinal cord may also be involved. In comparison, the demyelination of neonatal adrenoleukodystrophy tends to be more diffuse and less intense. Cerebellar demyelination appears to be more prominent with this form.[233]

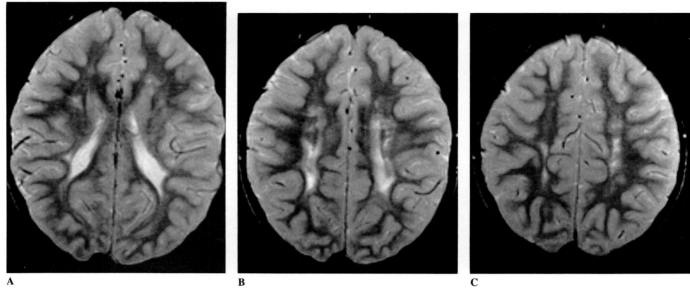

A   B   C

Fig. 1-100 X-linked adrenoleukodystrophy. (**A, B**, and **C**) T_2-weighted axial MR scans in a 5-year-old boy with X-linked adreno leukodystrophy showing patchy areas of demyelination in the cerebral white matter. These are demonstrated as areas of abnormally high signal intensity. The parietal lobes are the most severely involved.

The findings on imaging studies in cases of X-linked adrenoleukodystrophy are somewhat variable. The most common pattern is grossly symmetric areas of hemispheric demyelination (Fig. 1-100). The demyelination may be most prominent around the ventricular trigones in the occipital lobes, joining in the splenium of the corpus callosum. Irregular bands of contrast enhancement may be identified along the anterior edges of these areas. The splenium of the corpus callosum may be atrophic. Less common imaging patterns include predominantly unilateral involvement, predominantly frontal and occipital involvement, or predominantly frontal disease. CT sometimes demonstrates calcifications in the parietal or occipital regions. These variations are most often identified early or late in the course of the disease.

CT and MRI in cases of neonatal adrenoleukodystrophy most often demonstrate diffuse cerebral white matter abnormality and severe cerebral atrophy. The corpus callosum is extremely small. The head is microcephalic.[234–237]

In cases of adrenoleukomyeloneuropathy, CT is usually normal. On MRI, the imaging features are similar to those of adrenoleukodystrophy, with areas of high signal in the white matter surrounding the ventricles. The involvement is greatest in the occipital and parietal lobes. Areas of demyelination are also identified in the pons and upper cervical spine; these are seen as areas of high signal on T_2-weighted images.[238]

Myelinoclastic Diseases

Multiple Sclerosis. Multiple sclerosis is a demyelinating disease of the central nervous system of unknown etiology. Multiple sclerosis is, for the most part, a disease of adults, with only 2% of all patients presenting during childhood. Most pediatric cases become manifest during the second decade of life, with only 20% of children having symptoms before 10 years of age. Compared to the situation with adults, multiple sclerosis presenting in adolescents shows a more striking female predominance and more severe clinical manifestations. Immune mechanisms appear to be involved in the pathogenesis of multiple sclerosis.

The symptoms of multiple sclerosis are primarily due to focal involvement of a portion of the white matter, producing acute symptoms. This is followed by a period of remission and often by a subsequent acute episode involving a different area of white matter. The signs and symptoms may reflect involvement of the white matter of the cerebrum, cerebellum, brainstem, or spinal cord. The deficiencies may involve motor, sensory, or visual systems. Potential clinical manifestations include optic neuritis, nystagmus, brainstem and spinal cord dysfunction, cerebellar abnormalities, hemiplegia, sphincter dysfunction, dysesthesia, paraplegia, and meningeal signs. Fever is fairly common in children.[239,240]

The basic lesion of multiple sclerosis consists of a localized area of myelin breakdown, which is referred to as a plaque. Most plaques are less than 1.5 cm in diameter, but there is considerable variation. Acutely, a plaque of demyelination in multiple sclerosis is demonstrated on CT as a small, well-delineated area of abnormally low attenuation in the white matter. Contrast enhancement may be identified during the acute phase. The enhancement is often delayed and may be shown to be most marked approximately 1 hour after contrast agent administration. Large plaques may show evidence of mass effect. The enhancement pattern ranges from homogeneous to peripheral to central. The enhancement usually becomes less apparent during remission or during steroid therapy. In the chronic phases of the disorder, glial scarring of a plaque may produce a well-defined, low-attenuation lesion in the deep white matter.[241-243]

MRI is much more sensitive than CT for the detection of the plaques of multiple sclerosis. The lesion appears as a hyperintense white matter lesion on T_2-weighted images (Fig. 1-101). The cerebral white matter is the most common location, particularly the periventricular regions. Concomitant lesions may be identified in the posterior fossa. Cerebellar and brainstem involvement appears to be more common in children than in adults. Cerebral atrophy and abnormal iron deposition are uncommon in children with multiple sclerosis.[244,245]

Central Pontine Myelinolysis. Central pontine myelinolysis is a demyelinating disorder of uncertain etiology that primarily affects the pons. This is, for the most part, a disease of adults, but pediatric cases have been reported. Central pontine myelinolysis is usually associated with one of several potential underlying disorders, including chemotherapy, brain tumors, adrenal insufficiency, leukemia, sickle cell disease, sepsis, renal transplantation, Hodgkin disease, and liver disease. It is hypothesized that this disorder may be related to a rapid rise in serum sodium, which causes osmotic injury to endothelial cells. Endothelial cell injury may cause increased capillary permeability and edema and may also release enzymes that cause demyelination.

Imaging with CT in cases of central pontine myelinolysis may demonstrate one or more foci of decreased attenuation in the pons. MRI is of greater sensitivity and shows areas of high signal intensity on T_2-weighted images.[246-248] The lesion is most often located in the central portion of the pons, with an intact rim of normally myelinated tissue being preserved at the margins of the pons. Occasionally, there is extension into the medial menisci or into the midbrain. There are also uncommon instances in which there is extrapontine involvement of the temporal lobes, basal ganglia, internal capsule, thalamus, or cerebral cortex.[249-251]

Leukoencephalopathy. Leukoencephalopathy is a potential complication of therapy for acute lymphoblastic leukemia. This complication is most often identified in patients who have received cranial radiation with or without chemotherapy. Leukoencephalopathy may also occur in association with intrathecal methotrexate therapy.

CT early during the course of radiation- and chemotherapy-associated leukoencephalopathy demonstrates multiple low-attenuation areas in the centrum semiovale and periventricular regions. These areas may show some degree of contrast enhancement. Dense calcifications eventually develop in the white matter and basal ganglia (Fig. 1-102). The ventricles may become somewhat enlarged.[252]

Acute Disseminated Encephalomyelitis. Acute disseminated encephalomyelitis is an autoimmune disorder of the central nervous system that is usually associated with a viral illness. Four types are recognized on the basis of presumed etiology: postinfectious (most often associated with measles,

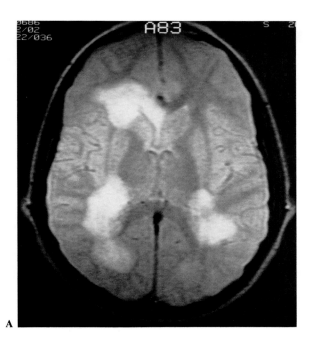

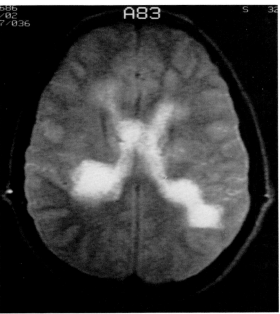

Fig. 1-101 Multiple sclerosis. (**A** and **B**) Axial proton-density MR images in a 14-year-old girl with multiple sclerosis showing multiple demyelinating plaques in the hemispheric white matter. These produce large, asymmetric regions of high signal intensity. There is extensive involvement of the corpus callosum.

mumps, varicella, rubella, pertussis, and Epstein-Barr virus infection), spontaneous or associated with a nonspecific respiratory infection, allergic (postvaccination), and fulminating. It is presumed that the precipitating condition induces a host-antibody response against a central nervous system antigen. This results in confluent areas of demyelination.

The clinical presentation of acute disseminated encephalomyelitis is usually in the form of seizures and focal neu-

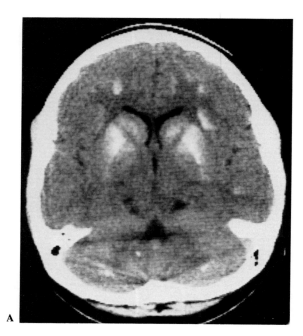

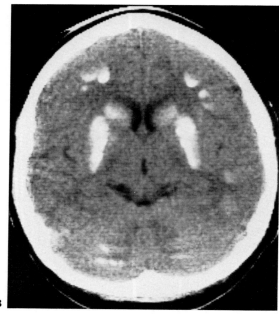

Fig. 1-102 Leukoencephalopathy. (**A** and **B**) Unenhanced CT scans in a child with leukemia several months after cessation of intrathecal chemotherapy and cranial radiation therapy show dense areas of calcification at the gray matter–white matter junctions in the cerebral hemispheres and cerebellum as well as dense calcifications in the basal ganglia.

rologic signs, which develop 1 to 2 weeks after the clinical onset of the predisposing condition. Rarely, visual symptoms due to cystic nerve involvement are present. In most patients, there is gradual complete resolution. Permanent neurologic damage occurs in 10% to 20% of cases.[253,254]

CT and MRI in cases of acute disseminated encephalomyelitis show patchy areas of edema in one or more regions of the central nervous system. These are demonstrated as areas of abnormally low attenuation on CT and prolongation of the T_1- and T_2-relaxation times on MRI (Fig. 1-103). The lesions are most often located in the subcortical white matter. The adjacent portions of the gray matter and white matter tracts in the basal ganglia, brainstem, and cerebellum may also be involved. Sequential studies may demonstrate a fleeting nature of the lesions, with some areas improving while new areas of abnormality appear.[255]

Delayed Myelination

Delayed myelination may occur in infants in association with a number of conditions. As described previously, failure of normal formation of myelin is a component of many of the dysmyelinating disorders. There is also a wide variety of metabolic, nutritional, toxic, and idiopathic disorders that cause delayed or deficient myelination.

From an imaging standpoint, the common feature that is shared by these disorders is a delay in the normal orderly progression of brain myelination. With MRI, standards have been developed for assessing normal brain myelination in infants and young children. On the basis of MRI, the child may be assigned a white matter age that can be correlated with the chronologic age.

In infants younger than 6 months of age, T_1-weighted images are usually most useful. Myelination of the cerebellum indicates a white matter age of 3 to 4 months, myelination of the splenium of the corpus callosum indicates a white matter age of 4 to 6 months, and myelination of the genu indicates a white matter age of greater than 6 months. In children older than 6 months of age, T_2-weighted images with long repetition and echo times are most helpful. The order of myelination of various structures, which can be used to assign white matter age, is as follows: splenium, 6 to 8 months; genu, 8 to 11 months; anterior limb of the internal capsule, 11 to 14 months; frontal white matter, 14 to 18 months; peripheral extension and fine arborization in the centrum semiovale, greater than 18 months (Fig. 1-104).[256–258]

Diseases That Affect the Basal Ganglia

The basal ganglia may be involved in various metabolic, toxic, and ischemic abnormalities (Table 1-6). Preferential involvement of the basal ganglia in these disorders may be due to the structural, biochemical, and vascular features that make the basal ganglia unique from the remainder of the brain. The detection and characterization of basal ganglia abnormalities is usually best achieved with MRI, although CT is most sensitive for the identification of calcifications.

Huntington Chorea

Huntington chorea is a hereditary progressive encephalopathy. The brain appears to be the only organ involved. Pathologic findings include severe atrophy of the caudate nucleus and putamen, cerebral cortical atrophy, and generalized neu-

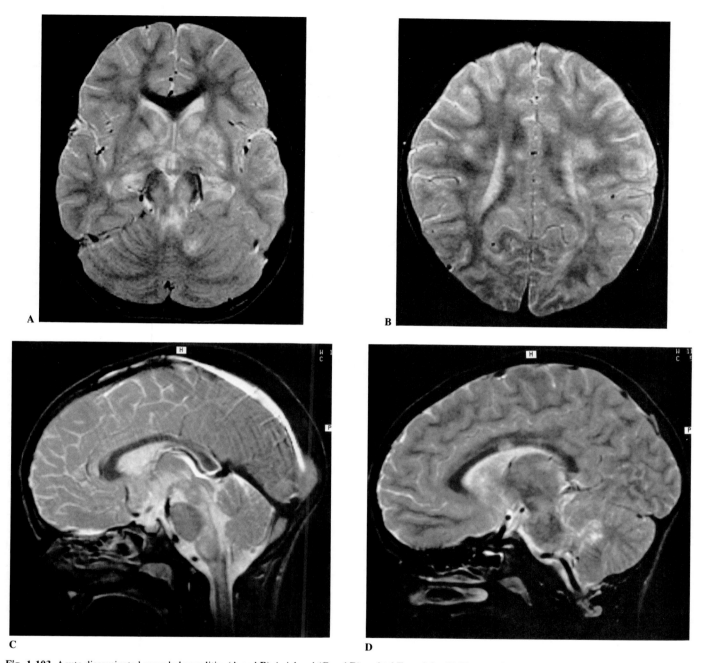

Fig. 1-103 Acute disseminated encephalomyelitis. (**A** and **B**) Axial and (**C** and **D**) sagittal T_2-weighted MR scans show multiple ill-defined areas of high signal intensity in the hemispheric white matter, cerebellar white matter, basal ganglia, thalami, brainstem, and corpus callosum. Imaging in this child was performed for the evaluation of seizures that developed 15 days after a viral illness. Follow-up imaging 2 months later (not shown) demonstrated complete resolution of the central nervous system lesions.

ronal loss and gliosis. Other structures may also be affected, such as the hypothalamus, subthalamus, red nucleus, tegmentum of the brainstem, and cerebellum. Huntington chorea is inherited as an autosomal dominant trait.

In most cases, the age at presentation of Huntington chorea is middle adulthood. Even so, approximately 5% of patients develop symptoms before 14 years of age. The predominant symptom is slowly progressive rigidity. Other findings include progressive dementia, seizures, choreoathetosis, and ataxia.

Mental deterioration and behavior disorders are frequent. The chorea forms of Huntington disease are due to neuronal loss in the corpus striatum. There is marked neuronal loss in the caudate nuclei and lesser involvement of the putamina. The mental changes in this disease are related to a neuronal loss in cortical cells, there being especially marked involvement of layers 3, 5, and 6.

CT and MRI in cases of Huntington chorea show slight enlargement of the frontal horns of the lateral ventricles as a

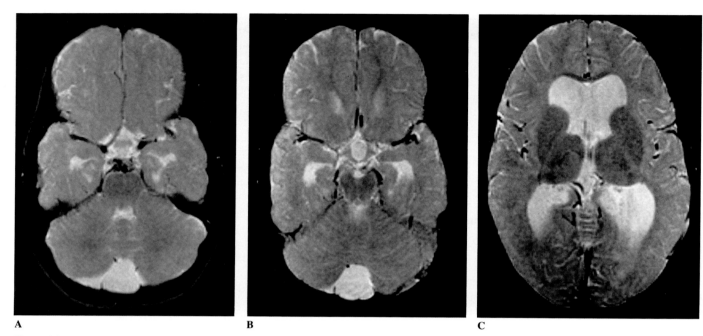

A   B   C

Fig. 1-104 Delayed myelination. (**A** and **B**) T_2-weighted axial MR images of a 5-year-old child with severe developmental delay show virtually complete lack of myelination of the cerebral and cerebellar white matter. (**C**) On the most superior image, the anterior aspect of the corpus callosum produces slightly decreased signal, indicating some degree of myelination. There is moderate ventriculomegaly. The white matter age in this child is less than 3 months.

result of thinning of the caudate nuclei. MRI is probably the most sensitive technique for demonstrating caudate nucleus atrophy. The putamina may also be atrophic. Significant cortical atrophy is usually not identifiable until adulthood. Because imaging studies are usually normal before clinical presentation of this disease, CT and MRI do not provide early preclinical diagnosis in the offspring of an affected adult.[259–262]

Sydenham Chorea

Sydenham chorea is a clinical syndrome that has multiple causes. It is most commonly a sequela of streptococcal infection (rheumatic-related chorea). Other potential causes include pregnancy, systemic lupus erythematosus, thyrotoxicosis, myeloproliferative disorders, rubella and pertussis infection, and drug interactions. Most patients developing Sydenham chorea are young, with 75% presenting between the ages of 7 and 12 years. The latency period for onset of rheumatic-related chorea after acute streptococcal infection may vary from 1 to 6 months.[263]

Symptoms of Sydenham chorea may be unilateral (approximately 20%) or bilateral. They are characterized by choreoathetoid movements that vary from purposeless, sudden jerking motions to more prolonged, grotesque posturing that is superimposed on volitional movements. Associated neurologic symptoms may include dysarthria, encephalopathy with personality changes, emotional lability, disorientation and confusion, weakness, and reflex changes. It is not uncommon to see rheumatic-related chorea in the absence of signs or symptoms of associated joint or heart involvement.

MRI demonstrates increased signal in the corpus striatum contralateral to the symptomatic side if unilateral symptoms are present. The greatest degree of involvement is in the head of the caudate nucleus; there is lesser involvement of the putamen. The lesions show moderate contrast enhancement after intravenous administration of paramagnetic contrast material. The MR findings correlate with anatomic regions that have been described to be susceptible to cross-reaction with immunoglobulin G antibodies formed in association with streptococcal infection. The findings are reversible with time. It is important to recognize this disease clinically and radiographically because it has a benign nature and an excellent prognosis.[264]

Table 1-6 Bilateral Basal Ganglia Abnormalities: Differential Diagnosis

Wilson disease
Leigh disease
Hallervorden-Spatz disease
Mitochondrial encephalomyelopathy
Carbon monoxide poisoning
Hydrogen sulfide poisoning
Barbiturate intoxication
Hypoglycemia
Striatonigral degeneration
Cyanide poisoning
Huntington chorea

Wilson Disease

Wilson disease is an autosomal recessive disorder in which brain degeneration and cirrhosis of the liver are the dominant features. The basic pathophysiologic abnormality in Wilson disease is extensive deposition of copper in the liver, brain, and other tissues. In the brain, the predominant abnormalities are localized in the basal ganglia, particularly in the putamina. Spongy degeneration may occur in the putamina, occasionally in the cortex of the frontal lobes, and less often in the brainstem, dentate nuclei, and substantia nigra. Some degree of cerebral cortical atrophy may be present, particularly in the frontal lobes.

During the first several years of life, the predominant signs and symptoms are usually due to liver involvement; these include jaundice, acute hemolytic anemia, and portal hypertension. Older children more often exhibit neurologic symptoms. Dystonia often develops between 5 and 10 years of age. These children may also exhibit tremor, speech impairment, abnormal limb posture, and retraction of the upper lip. Other children may exhibit dysarthria and tremor.

CT and MRI in cases of Wilson disease often show mild or moderate dilatation of the ventricular system, particularly the frontal horns. Cerebral white matter atrophy of variable severity is usually present. The basal ganglia, and less often the thalami, are of abnormally low attenuation on CT and show prolongation of T_1- and T_2-relaxation times on MRI. Occasionally, focal areas of high-signal abnormality on T_2-weighted images are identified in the cerebral hemispheric white matter.[265–267]

Leigh Disease

Leigh disease, also termed subacute necrotizing encephalomyelopathy, is a rare autosomal recessive degenerative disorder of the central nervous system. The pathologic changes include disruption of myelin sheaths, disintegration of the ground substance, microcysts, necrotic changes, and proliferation of small blood vessels. The necrotizing changes occur symmetrically throughout the entire brainstem. The hypothalamus, thalamus, lenticular nucleus, caudate nucleus, and posterior column of the spinal cord may also be involved. The most marked changes are usually identified in the globus pallidus, red nucleus, substantia nigra, and dorsal tegmentum of the midbrain and pons. Leigh disease is thought to be caused by one or more abnormalities in energy metabolism, which probably involve disorders of pyruvate metabolism. The most common are cytochrome C oxidase deficiency, pyruvate carboxylase deficiency, and pyruvate dehydrogenase complex defect.[268,269]

The clinical onset of Leigh disease is before 2 years of age in at least two-thirds of patients; neonatal presentations have been reported. Most often, there is an insidious onset with retarded motor and intellectual development. Occasionally, there is an acute onset with respiratory distress and metabolic alterations. Other potential findings in these children include swallowing difficulties, vomiting, weakness, ophthalmoplegia, seizures, ataxia, dystonia, and peripheral neuropathy. Many affected children die within 6 months of diagnosis.[270]

The imaging findings in Leigh disease consist of regions of abnormally decreased attenuation on CT and prolongation of T_1- and T_2-relaxation times on MRI. In the early stages of the disorder, imaging studies most often show these edemalike abnormalities in the basal ganglia (particularly the putamina) and the adjacent portions of the frontal lobes. There may be slight contrast enhancement at the borders of these lesions. As the disease progresses, the lesions may diminish in size somewhat and become more well defined. The abnormalities are most often located in the putamina, caudate nuclei, periaqueductal gray matter, occasionally the hemispheric gray matter, and rarely the cerebellum. In the late stages of Leigh disease, ventricular enlargement and cortical atrophy develop and may be severe (Fig. 1-105).[271–274]

Mitochondrial Encephalomyelopathies

The mitochondrial encephalomyelopathies are characterized by functional or structural abnormalities of the mitochondria. These are multisystem diseases that usually affect all organ systems to some extent. Central nervous system involvement is demonstrated on CT and MRI as edematous changes in the basal ganglia, particularly the putamina, and hemispheric white matter. Diffuse cerebral atrophy may be present.[275,276]

Hallervorden-Spatz Disease

Hallervorden-Spatz disease is a rare metabolic disorder that predominantly involves destructive changes in the globus pallidus and substantia nigra. These structures contain elevated concentrations of iron, calcium, copper, and zinc. The accumulation of toxic metabolites causes abnormal synthesis of myelin or destruction of synthesized myelin sheaths. Edema and destruction of axons also occur. These changes predominantly involve the globus pallidus and substantia nigra, although more peripheral portions of the cerebral cortex may also be affected.[274]

Hallervorden-Spatz disease usually presents during the first decade of life. The initial manifestations usually consist of motor dysfunction, dystonia, muscular rigidity, choreoathetosis, dysarthria, and hyperreflexia. The subsequent clinical course is quite variable. This disorder appears to be transmitted as an autosomal recessive trait.[277,278]

CT in cases of Hallervorden-Spatz disease may show either increased or decreased attenuation values of the globi pallidi. It is presumed that the decreased attenuation is due to edema and tissue destruction and that the high attenuation is produced by deposition of iron and calcium. The high attenuation pattern appears to be more common.

MRI usually shows abnormal hypodensity of the globi pallidi on T_2-weighted images, presumably as a result of iron and calcium deposition. Similar changes may also be noted in

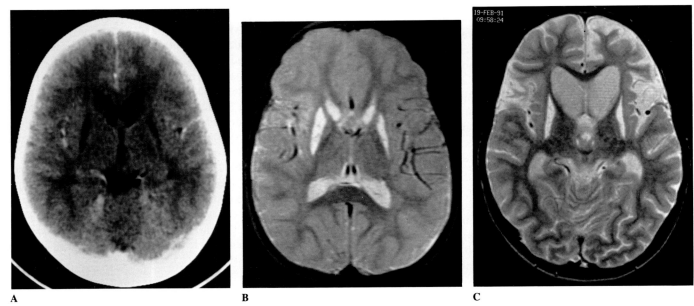

A   B   C

Fig. 1-105 Leigh disease. (**A**) Axial contrast-enhanced CT scan of this 12-month-old child shows markedly decreased attenuation of the caudate nuclei and the putamina. (**B**) T_2-weighted axial MR scan at the same age shows markedly high signal abnormality in these same portions of the basal ganglia. No areas of signal abnormality are visible in the cortex. (**C**) T_2-weighted MR scan 2 years later shows interval development of moderate ventriculomegaly. High-signal abnormality remains in the basal ganglia. Areas of increased signal have developed in the hemispheric gray matter in the anterior aspect of the left frontal lobe and the posterior aspect of the right frontal lobe. There are also areas of high signal in the periaqueductal gray matter.

the substantia nigra. Destructive changes and gliosis may result in high-signal foci in the globi pallidi on T_2-weighted images. Atrophy of the brainstem and cerebellum may be identified.[279,280]

Fahr-Volhard Disease

Fahr-Volhard disease is a hereditary condition in which there is calcium deposition in the walls of the blood vessels of the dentate and lenticular nuclei. Although some patients present during childhood, the peak age at presentation is between 30 and 50 years of age. The usual findings include seizures, dementia, and generalized rigidity. Imaging studies show irregular calcifications in the lenticular and dentate nuclei (Fig. 1-106). Clinical correlation is required in the differentiation of this entity from Cockayne syndrome and hypoparathyroidism.

Carbon Monoxide Toxicity

Carbon monoxide poisoning may produce brain injury by three basic mechanisms. Carbon monoxide has a higher affinity for hemoglobin than oxygen; this results in hypoxemia. It also impairs the ability of hemoglobin to release oxygen to the tissues; this results in tissue hypoxia. Carbon monoxide also has a direct toxic effect on mitochondria because of binding of carbon monoxide to cytochrome a_3. This impairs cellular oxidative metabolism.

The clinical manifestations of carbon monoxide poisoning roughly correlate with the carboxyhemoglobin level. Patients

with mild cases (indicated by carboxyhemoglobin levels of less than 20%) may exhibit headache, dyspnea, decreased visual acuity, and subtle neurologic dysfunction. Moderate toxicity (carboxyhemoglobin levels between 20% and 40%) may produce irritability, visual impairment, nausea, fatigability, and intellectual impairment. Severe intoxication (carboxyhemoglobin concentrations greater than 40%) may be manifested by ataxia, shock, severe intellectual impairment, and coma. Concentrations of carboxyhemoglobin higher than 60% are usually fatal.

The pathologic manifestation of brain injury with carbon monoxide poisoning is in the form of focal areas of necrosis. The most commonly involved areas are the globi pallidi. Other areas of brain injury may include the cerebral white matter, cerebral cortex, and the hippocampus, particularly the horn of Ammon. These lesions are demonstrated on CT as areas of decreased attenuation. MRI is more sensitive than CT and shows areas of prolongation of T_1- and T_2-relaxation times. Most often, there is symmetric involvement of the globi pallidi and variable involvement of other portions of the brain (Fig. 1-107).[281,282]

Metabolic Disorders That Predominantly Involve the Cortical Gray Matter

There are several metabolic diseases that primarily affect cortical gray matter. These are often termed poliodystrophies. Because gray matter disease primarily affects neurons, the

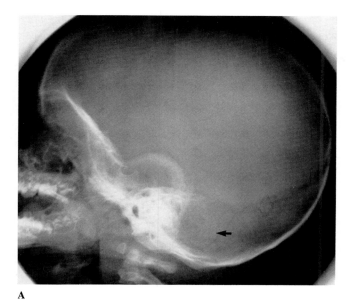

A

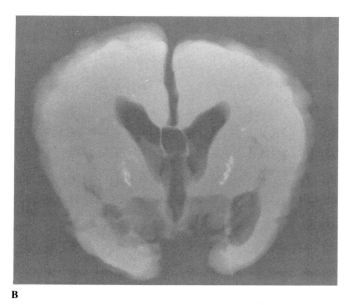

B

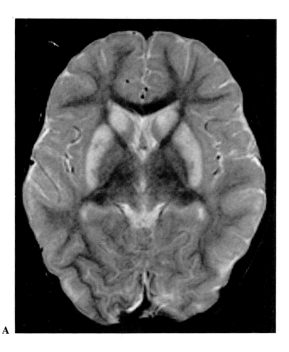

C

Fig. 1-106 Fahr-Volhard disease. (**A**) Lateral skull radiograph shows small, irregular calcifications in the dentate nuclei (arrow) and scattered in the central portions of the hemispheres. (**B**) Radiograph of a coronal section of the brain shows slight ventricular enlargement. There are focal areas of calcification in the putamina. (**C**) Radiograph of a coronal section of the cerebellum shows punctate areas of calcification in the dentate nuclei.

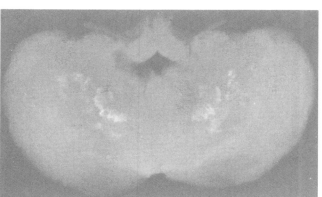

A

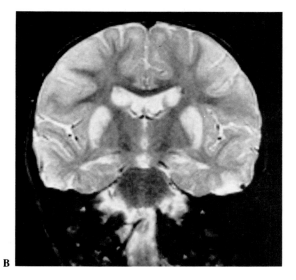

B

Fig. 1-107 Carbon monoxide poisoning. (**A**) Axial and (**B**) coronal T_2-weighted MR scans of a child after smoke inhalation in a fire showing high-signal abnormality involving the putamina and caudate nuclei bilaterally.

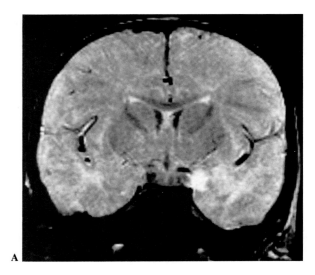

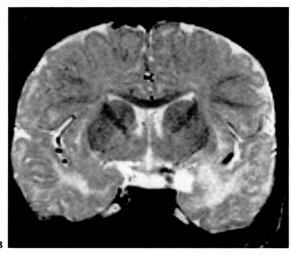

Fig. 1-108 Mesial temporal sclerosis. (**A** and **B**) Coronal T$_2$-weighted MR images show irregular high signal in the region of the hippocampal gyrus on the left. In addition, there is intense high signal in the extreme medial aspect of the left temporal lobe. This lesion enhanced only slightly with gadopentetate dimeglumine. The patient had partial complex epilepsy.

early symptoms reflect neuronal dysfunction. This may produce seizures, intellectual deterioration, and visual changes. White matter diseases, in comparison, more often produce ataxia, spasticity, or loss of motor skills. Imaging studies in these gray matter diseases are usually nonspecific and show diffuse cerebral atrophy. Attempts at classifying disease as primarily affecting gray matter, white matter, or both are somewhat arbitrary. The most important diseases that primarily affect the gray matter include Alper disease, Menkes kinky hair disease, ceroid lipofuscinosis, Rett syndrome, and various lysosomal diseases.[283,284]

Mesial temporal sclerosis is the best recognized cause of partial complex epilepsy. This condition involves the horn of Ammon of the hippocampus. Similar sclerosis may also involve the amygdala and the parahippocampal gyrus.

Patients who develop mesial temporal sclerosis frequently have a history of febrile convulsions in infancy and early childhood. Patients who have early-onset seizures with severe generalized tonic-clonic seizures accompanied by a high frequency of temporal lobe attacks have a poor prognosis. It is generally accepted that prolonged febrile convulsions in early life may cause hippocampal sclerosis that subsequently results in complex partial epilepsy.

MRI is the most sensitive method for detecting mesial temporal sclerosis. The findings are best seen on coronal T$_2$-weighted images. The lesion appears as an area of high signal in the medial aspect of the temporal lobe adjacent to the temporal horn of the lateral ventricle. There may be minimal edema in the adjacent white matter. The lesion may enhance with paramagnetic contrast material (Fig. 1-108).[285,286]

Disease Predominantly Localized to the Cerebellum

Ataxia-telangiectasia is an autosomal recessive neurocutaneous disorder in which the predominant feature is cerebellar cortical atrophy. Histologic studies show degeneration of both Purkinje and internal granule cells. There is demyelination of the posterior columns and dorsal spinal cerebellar tracts. There may also be neuronal loss in the substantia nigra and hemosiderin deposits in the globi pallidi.[287]

The clinical presentation of ataxia-telangiectasia may occur in infancy with cerebellar signs. Most often, ataxia becomes apparent early in childhood or infancy. This is usually in the form of progressive truncal ataxia, which is followed by incoordinated limb movements. Ocular disorders are common. Cutaneous telangiectasias usually become apparent between 3 and 6 months of age. These patients often have recurrent sinopulmonary infections and are at increased risk for the development of neoplasia such as Hodgkin disease, leukemia, lymphoma, basal cell carcinoma, gastric adenocarcinoma, and brain tumors.[288,289]

The predominant abnormality in cases of ataxia-telangiectasia as demonstrated on CT and MRI is cerebellar cortical atrophy. This produces an overall decrease in cerebellar size, increased prominence of the sulci, and enlargement of the fourth ventricle. Intracranial hemorrhage may result from rupture of cerebral telangiectasias. Also, shunting through pulmonary vascular malformations may result in embolic cerebral infarcts.[96]

Miscellaneous Metabolic Disorders

Mucopolysaccharidoses

The mucopolysaccharidoses are a group of hereditary disorders in which there is a deficiency of a specific lysosomal enzyme involved in the degradation of mucopolysaccharides. Incompletely degraded mucopolysaccharides accumulate in various tissues. Also, mucopolysaccharide deposits in the lysosomes interfere with the degradation of other macromolecules, resulting in the accumulation of other materials in the lysosomes. The mucopolysaccharidoses that have significant central nervous system involvement include types I-H (Hurler), I-H/S (Hurler-Scheie), II (Hunter), III-A-D (Sanfilippo), and VII (Sly). Genetic transmission of the mucopolysaccharidoses is autosomal recessive, with the exception of type II, which is an X-linked recessive disorder.

The typical neuropathologic manifestations of the mucopolysaccharidoses include lysosomal storage bodies in cortical neurons, astrocytes, and capillary pericytes. The periadvential spaces in the white matter are dilated and filled with fluid and mesenchymal cells. Meningeal involvement is also present in the form of abnormal collagen deposition. This may result in arachnoid cysts (most often in the parasellar region) or communicating hydrocephalus.[290,291]

Central nervous system involvement in the mucopolysaccharidoses is demonstrated on CT and MRI as variable degrees of atrophy and white matter abnormalities. The white matter changes consist of diffuse, low-attenuation areas on CT and areas of hyperintensity on T_2-weighted MR images. These may be most marked in the parietal regions. Such a finding is thought to be due to cavitation and dilatation of the perivascular spaces (the spaces of Virchow-Robin). Meningeal involvement may be seen as thickening of the tentorium and dura. Hydrocephalus is not uncommon.[292,293]

Infantile Neuroaxonal Dystrophy

Infantile neuroaxonal dystrophy is an autosomal recessive disease of unknown etiology. The presentation usually occurs between 6 months and 2 years of age. The clinical findings may include intellectual and motor abnormalities, progressive hypotonia, visual disturbances, and pyramidal tract signs. There is usually progressive deterioration that eventually leads to death. CT and MRI demonstrate rapidly progressive cerebral, cerebellar, and brainstem atrophy.[294]

FETAL AND NEONATAL BRAIN INJURY

There is a broad spectrum of stresses to which the fetus and neonate may be subjected that may ultimately produce significant brain injury. These include asphyxia, congenital infection, maternal drug abuse, anesthesia, prescription drug use, metabolic disorders, hematologic disorders, and birth trauma. It is estimated that intrapartum abnormalities account for 10% to 15% of cases of cerebral palsy or severe mental retardation. In 1985, it was estimated that in the United States there were 750,000 children with cerebral palsy and 850,000 children with mental retardation.[295–297]

Hypoxic-ischemic disturbances are the most common causes of prenatal and perinatal cerebral damage. There are numerous pathophysiologic mechanisms that may produce cerebral injury in the presence of circulatory abnormalities. These include acute fetal circulatory failure, acute fetal hypovolemia, acute fetal anoxia, increased fetal blood viscosity, cerebral emboli, chronic fetal anemia, and chronic placental insufficiency. The most common cause of cerebral emboli in neonates is right-to-left shunting in cases of congenital cyanotic heart disease. Acute fetal hypovolemia or circulatory failure can be produced by hemorrhage or fetomaternal transfusion. The most common cause of neonatal cerebral ischemia is perinatal asphyxia.

The neuropathologic changes associated with hypoxic-ischemic insults can be divided into those reflecting primary cellular damage and those due to hemorrhage. The pathologic changes vary according to the gestational age of the infant, the characteristics of the primary insult, and the nature of therapeutic intervention. Periventricular or intraventricular hemorrhage is the most common central nervous system manifestation of hypoxic-ischemic injury in preterm infants. White matter disease is probably the next most common abnormality in these children; this is followed by necrotic changes in the deep gray nuclei and the brainstem. These children may also have cerebellar necrosis and cortical infarctions. Intraventricular hemorrhage may also occur in term infants, but the pathogenesis is somewhat different than in preterm infants. The most common neuropathologic manifestations of hypoxic-ischemic injury in term infants are cortical infarctions and necrosis of the deep gray nuclei and brainstem.

Periventricular or intraventricular hemorrhage occurs in up to 40% of infants weighing less than 1500 g or younger than gestation week 32. The hemorrhage arises from the germinal matrix, usually at the junction of the head of the caudate nucleus and the choroid plexus in the floor of the lateral ventricle. The germinal matrix disappears by the end of normal gestation; therefore, the germinal matrix is present only in premature infants. This highly vascular structure contains thin-walled vessels that are fragile and susceptible to injury.

The pathogenesis of germinal matrix hemorrhage due to cerebral hypoxia-ischemia is thought to involve endothelial injury and impaired autoregulation of cerebral blood flow. Platelet and coagulation disturbances, alterations in systemic blood pressure, and increased cerebral venous pressure may also be involved. The friable vessels of the germinal matrix are particularly sensitive to fluctuations of the local arterial and venous pressure. The hemorrhage may range from a small area of bleeding in the subependymal region to massive intraventricular or intraparenchymal hemorrhage. Many large intraparenchymal hemorrhages in preterm neonates are secondary hemorrhages into ischemic hemispheric brain tissue rather than extensions from a germinal matrix hemorrhage.[298,299]

Intraventricular hemorrhage in term infants usually arises from the choroid plexus. Trauma is thought to be a common etiologic factor, although an identifiable cause is not clear in approximately one-quarter of these cases. Minor subarachnoid hemorrhages are relatively common as a consequence of childbirth. Many go undetected.[300]

A number of white matter changes are relatively common in preterm infants with cerebral hypoxia-ischemia. An increase in the number of reactive astrocytes in the white matter (perinatal telencephalic leukoencephalopathy) occurs in up to 15% to 40% of these children. This gliosis may interfere with normal myelin development. A second white matter lesion that may occur in preterm infants is abnormal deposition of lipids. The third type of white matter pathology commonly identified is periventricular leukomalacia. True periventricular leukomalacia consists of focal nodular or linear areas of coagulation necrosis in the periventricular white matter, sometimes with minimal petechial hemorrhage. These foci are most often located in the corona radiata, adjacent to the occipital and temporal horns of the lateral ventricles, and anterior to the frontal horns of the lateral ventricles. With time, these lesions become cystic and may eventually contract into gliotic scars. Lesions similar to the periventricular leukomalacia of preterm infants may be identified in term infants with congenital heart disease or a coagulopathy.[301–304]

Cortical injury due to a hypoxic-ischemic insult may be produced by interruption of venous flow, arterial flow, or both. Watershed infarction may be produced by global decrease in cerebral blood flow. Isolated arterial occlusions most often involve term infants; the middle cerebral artery is most frequently involved. Superficial cortical infarcts, sometimes hemorrhagic, may be produced by venous occlusions of the dural sinuses or major cortical veins.[305,306]

Hemorrhagic and necrotic lesions of the basal ganglia, thalamus, and diencephalon may accompany hypoxic-ischemic insults in both full-term and preterm neonates. Similar changes may occur in the brainstem, sometimes selectively involving brainstem nuclei.

In the cerebellum, the Purkinje cells are most vulnerable to ischemic injury. The most marked changes usually occur at the boundaries of the superior and inferior cerebellar arterial zones and in the foliar cortex. White matter edema and small hemorrhages may also occur.[307]

During the first two trimesters of gestation, the ventriculofugal cerebral blood vessels (ie, those vessels coursing peripherally from the central portions of the brain) are relatively poorly developed. At this stage of development, most of the blood supply to the cortex and cerebral white matter is provided by ventriculopetal flow through vessels that extend centrally from the surface of the brain. Therefore, during this stage of gestation, the watershed areas that are most susceptible to ischemia are the periventricular regions. Term infants, on the other hand, show a watershed pattern more akin to that of adults as a result of their more fully developed ventriculofugal vascular system.[308,309]

On imaging studies, germinal matrix hemorrhage can be divided into four grades of severity. With grade I, there is isolated germinal matrix hemorrhage with minimal or no intraventricular hemorrhage. With grade II, the germinal matrix hemorrhage is accompanied by significant intraventricular hemorrhage, although ventricular size is normal. Grade III is defined as subependymal hemorrhage, intraventricular hemorrhage, and hydrocephalus. Grade IV refers to significant extension of subependymal hemorrhage into one or both cerebral hemispheres. The higher grades of germinal matrix hemorrhage according to this classification system portend an increased incidence and greater severity of long-term neurological sequelae.[272,310]

Germinal matrix hemorrhage of prematurity most often occurs during the first 3 days of life. About 36% occur on day 1, 32% on day 2, and 18% on day 3.[311] Most often, the hemorrhage is a single event, although some neonates show evidence of progressive hemorrhage over a 2-day period. The demonstration of progression of hemorrhage on imaging studies carries a poor prognosis. Rarely, subependymal hemorrhage may occur between 1 week and 3 months of age.[302,312]

On sonography, germinal matrix (subependymal) hemorrhage is demonstrated as a focus of increased echogenicity. In general, the hemorrhage must be at least 4 to 5 mm in size to be detected sonographically. The hemorrhage may occur anywhere in the subependymal germinal matrix of the lateral ventricle, although the most common site is the region of the head of the caudate nucleus. The hyperechoic focus is usually well marginated and may be unilateral or bilateral. Coronal images usually show the focus to lie inferior and lateral to the floor of the frontal horn (Fig. 1-109). Occasionally, the hemorrhage is large enough to compress the frontal horns or bodies of the lateral ventricles. Parasagittal images show the area to lie immediately anterior to the foramen of Monro; this is helpful in differentiating the lesion from the normally echogenic choroid plexus, which should only be visualized posterior to the foramen of Monro. Also, the normal choroid plexus tapers anteriorly in the caudothalamic groove. More extensive subependymal hemorrhage may conform to the shape of the lateral ventricle.

Acute grade II hemorrhage is demonstrated sonographically as intensely echogenic material in the lateral ventricle (Fig. 1-110). In some cases, layering of blood in the dependent portion of the ventricle is identified. A small grade II hemorrhage may be difficult to differentiate from an isolated subependymal hemorrhage. This distinction is of little importance from a clinical standpoint because the prognosis is similar (Fig. 1-111).

Occasionally, intraventricular hemorrhage originates from the choroid plexus without concomitant germinal matrix hemorrhage. This is a more common abnormality in term than in premature infants. Isolated choroid plexus hemorrhage is quite difficult to recognize sonographically because the choroid plexus is normally echogenic. Features suggestive of this abnormality include enlargement and an irregular contour of the echogenic choroid plexus and loss of the normal tapering of the choroid plexus anteriorly. In some cases, free blood is identified in the dependent portion of the ventricle.

Grade III hemorrhage is demonstrated sonographically as dilatation of the ventricles with echogenic blood. The hemorrhage may be unilateral or bilateral and may extend into the third and fourth ventricles. In some cases, the echogenic blood predominantly occupies the middle and posterior portions of

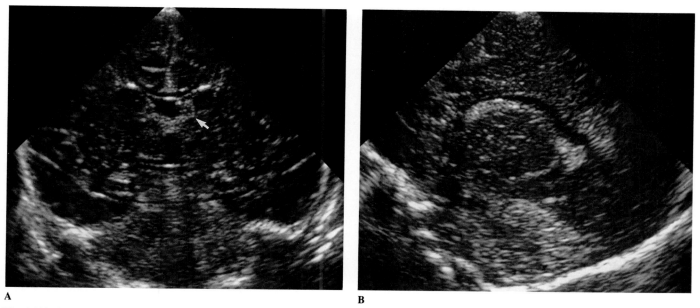

Fig. 1-109 Grade I subependymal germinal matrix hemorrhage. (**A**) Coronal and (**B**) sagittal neural sonograms of a 2-day old premature infant show a focus of increased echogenicity in the subependymal region of the left lateral ventricle (arrow in **A**). The lesion lies anterior to the foramen of Monro.

the dilated lateral ventricle; in others the ventricle is completely filled with echogenic blood.

The intraparenchymal component of an acute grade IV hemorrhage is demonstrated sonographically as an intensely echogenic lesion in the deep white matter of the centrum semiovale. The frontal and parietal lobes are the most common locations. There is usually extensive coexistent subependymal and intraventricular hemorrhage. During the acute phase, the parenchymal hematoma has irregular margins. Signs of mass

effect are usually present; this aids in the differentiation from nonhemorrhagic parenchymal edema.

Sequential sonographic examinations usually demonstrate progressive stages of resolution of subependymal-intraventricular hemorrhage. During the acute stage, the hemorrhage is homogeneously hyperechoic. Over the next few weeks, the central portion becomes less echogenic while the peripheral aspect remains hyperechoic. Subsequently, there is a progressive decrease in the diameter of the lesion. Small

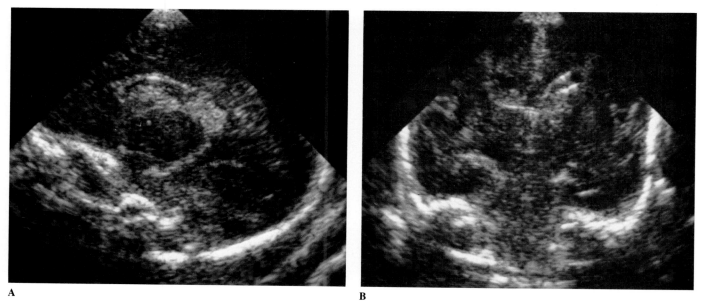

Fig. 1-110 Grade II subependymal intraventricular hemorrhage. (**A**) Coronal sonogram shows bilateral hyperechoic subependymal hemorrhages, the left being larger than the right. (**B**) Sagittal image shows irregular hyperechoic hemorrhage in the lateral ventricle. The ventricle is not dilated.

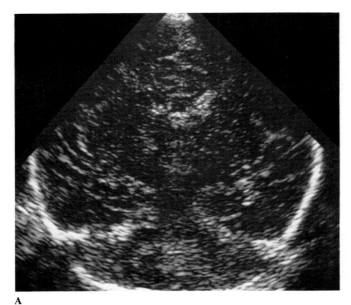

A

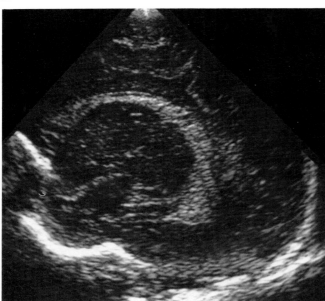

B

Fig. 1-111 Grade II unilateral germinal matrix hemorrhage. **(A)** Coronal and **(B)** sagittal sonograms show hyperechoic subependymal germinal matrix hemorrhage along the course of and within the left lateral ventricle. On the sagittal image, the hyperechoic abnormality extends anterior to the foramen of Monro.

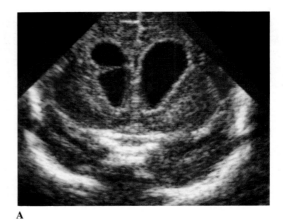

A

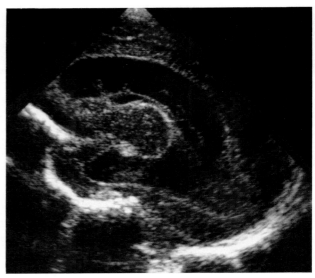

B

Fig. 1-112 Resolution of intraventricular clot. **(A)** Coronal and **(B)** sagittal sonograms in an infant 3 weeks after a grade III germinal matrix hemorrhage show increased echogenicity of the ventricular walls and moderate dilatation of the lateral ventricles. Linear hyperechoic adhesions are present as residuals from the intraventricular clot.

germinal matrix hemorrhages eventually resolve completely in most cases. Others result in the formation of a small subependymal cyst.

Intraventricular clot also tends to become well defined and less echogenic over the first few weeks after the acute event. At this point, the clot is less echogenic than the normal choroid plexus. As the clots retract, cerebrospinal fluid surrounds the hypoechoic clot to produce a ventricle-in-a-ventricle appearance. Residual bands or septations in the ventricle are common. Increased echogenicity of the ventricular walls may

be identified for some time during the resolution phase. Posthemorrhagic hydrocephalus occurs in about 75% of infants with intraventricular hemorrhage, although the hydrocephalus is progressive in only 25% (Fig. 1-112).

Follow-up evaluation of an intraparenchymal component shows the central portion of the hemorrhage to become progressively less echogenic. Liquefaction usually occurs within 1 to 2 weeks of the hemorrhage, resulting in a hypoechoic appearance and a well-defined echogenic rim. The overall size of the clot may decrease because of clot retraction (Fig. 1-113). A large hemorrhage may eventually (2 to 3 months) form a porencephalic cyst or cystic encephalomalacia.[313–315]

On CT, acute germinal matrix hemorrhage is demonstrated as a focus of relatively high attenuation that is usually located adjacent to the lateral ventricle near the head of the caudate nucleus. An intraventricular component may be demonstrated as a well-defined, high-attenuation clot or as free blood that

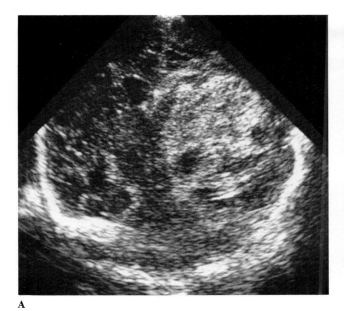

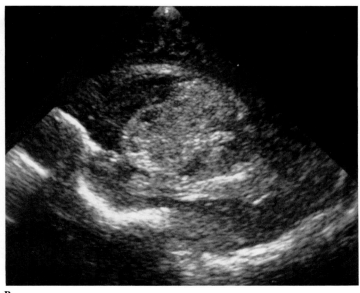

Fig. 1-113 Grade IV germinal matrix hemorrhage. (**A**) Coronal and (**B**) sagittal sonograms of a premature infant demonstrate hyperechoic subependymal hemorrhage on the left. There is extension into the left lateral ventricle as well as a large, hyperechoic, intraparenchymal hematoma extending into the left parietal and temporal lobes. There is shift of the midline to the right. (**C**) Follow-up examination 1 week later shows that the central portion of the intraparenchymal hematoma is now hypoechoic. The margins of the hematoma remain hyperechoic, and hyperechoic intraventricular clot is still visible. There is less midline shift than on the previous studies.

layers in the dependent portion of the ventricular system. The attenuation values decrease as the hemorrhage resolves. MRI is also quite sensitive and specific for the demonstration of acute germinal matrix hemorrhage (Fig. 1-114).

Other types of intracranial hemorrhage in preterm and term neonates are usually related to a traumatic delivery. Subdural hematomas in these children tend to occur in the interhemispheric fissures or adjacent to the tentorium. Convexity subdural and epidural hematomas may occur with skull fractures. Subarachnoid hemorrhage may be produced by traumatic delivery or by a diffuse ischemic insult.

Subarachnoid hemorrhage is not well demonstrated on sonography, although a large hemorrhage may be identified as hyperechoic material in the sylvian fissures on coronal images. Likewise, epidural and subdural blood collections are visualized only if they are fairly large. These extra-axial hemorrhages are best demonstrated on CT.

Some infants with severe neonatal lung disease, such as occurs in meconium aspiration syndrome, are placed on extracorporeal membrane oxygenation to place the lungs at rest. This requires systemic anticoagulation, which places these neonates at significant risk for intraparenchymal hemorrhage in the brain. The infants are monitored with sequential sonography. The hemorrhages that occur in these infants tend to be large and to arise in the substance of the brain. Germinal matrix hemorrhages are uncommon because most of these infants are term or near term (Fig. 1-115).

The usual sonographic finding in cases of periventricular leukomalacia is diffuse, ill-defined, increased echogenicity in the periventricular regions (Fig. 1-116). The most common locations are the posterior periventricular white matter adjacent to the lateral aspect of the trigone and the white matter adjacent to the foramina of Monro. The echogenic appearance is due to edema and petechial hemorrhage. The abnormality is usually bilateral but may be asymmetric. There is little or no mass effect, which helps differentiate this lesion from the parenchymal component of a germinal matrix hemorrhage. It is important that the abnormality be visualized in both coronal and sagittal views because mildly increased echogenicity is often seen in the periatrial regions as a normal variation on sagittal sonographic images. The sonographic appearance of acute periventricular leukomalacia is similar or identical to

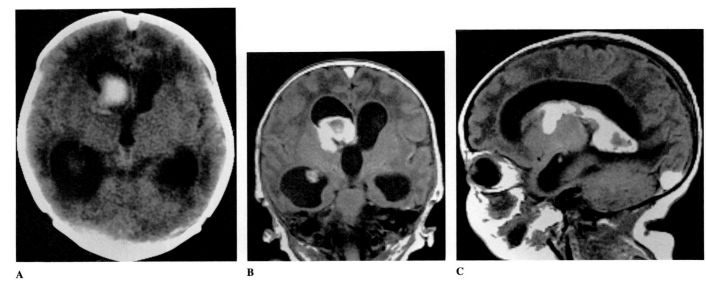

A   B   C

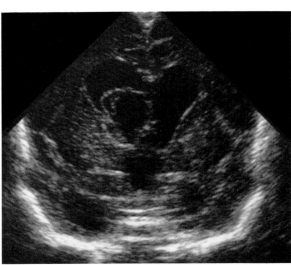

D

Fig. 1-114 Grade III subependymal-intraventricular germinal matrix hemorrhage. **(A)** Axial CT scan of a 4-day-old premature infant demonstrates high-attenuation, acute hemorrhage in the subependymal region on the right as well as a large clot in the right lateral ventricle. There is moderate dilatation of the ventricular system and decreased attenuation in the periventricular white matter as a result of transependymal flow of cerebrospinal fluid. Also, there is high-attenuation, acute thrombosis of the superior sagittal sinus. **(B)** T_1-weighted coronal and **(C)** sagittal MR scans at 7 days of age demonstrate extension of high-signal hemorrhage from the right subependymal region into the right lateral ventricle. The intraventricular component of the clot extends posteriorly into the occipital and temporal horns. Most of the clot produces high signal intensity. The central portions produce lower signal intensity as a result of the presence of deoxyhemoglobin. There is moderate dilatation of the ventricular system. The coronal image shows high-signal clot in the superior sagittal sinus. **(D)** Coronal and **(E)** parasagittal sonograms at 10 days of age show liquefaction of the intraventricular component of the clot; this is seen as hypoechoic material surrounded by a thin, irregular margin.

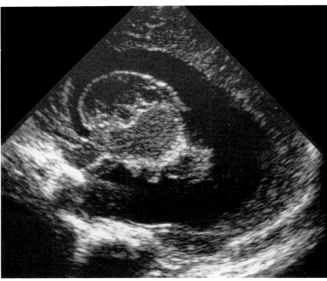

E

that of perinatal telencephalic leukoencephalopathy (white matter gliosis) and acute cerebral infarction.[316–319]

Over a period of 2 to 3 weeks, small anechoic cysts develop in the hyperechoic regions of periventricular leukomalacia. These small cysts usually coalesce into larger cystic lesions, producing a multicystic appearance (Fig. 1-117). Eventually, the cysts collapse and coalesce and are replaced by glial scars. At this point, sonography is usually normal aside from slight enlargement of the adjacent portions of the lateral ventricles. If the insult has been severe, the brain may become replaced by numerous cysts of variable size surrounded by glial scars. The ventricles are usually mildly dilated.[302,305]

During the acute phase of periventricular leukomalacia, CT may be normal or show a subtle, low-attenuation abnormality in the periventricular region despite obvious sonographic abnormalities. In those cases of periventricular leukomalacia that contain significant hemorrhage, however, CT shows a high-attenuation abnormality in the periventricular white mat-

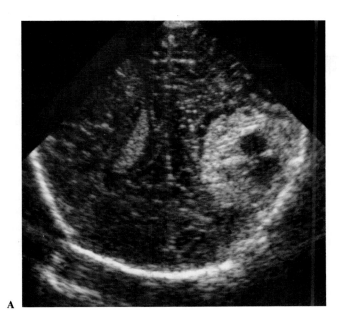

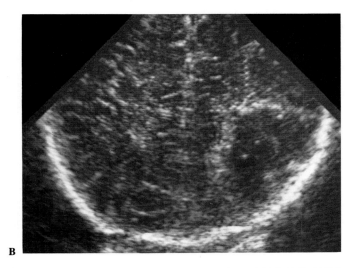

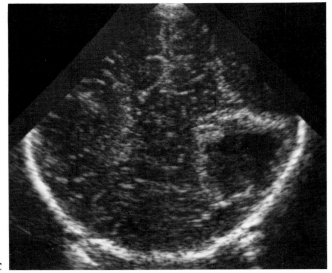

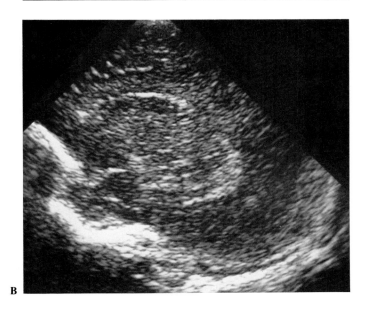

Fig. 1-115 Intraparenchymal hemorrhage. (**A**) Coronal sonogram of a neonate on extracorporeal membrane oxygenation shows a large, predominantly hyperechoic intraparenchymal hematoma in the left parietal lobe. The central portion of the hemorrhage is slightly hypoechoic. There is mass effect adjacent to the hematoma. (**B**) Follow-up examination 2 days later shows the hematoma to be isoechoic to hypoechoic with respect to brain. There is a remaining thin, hyperechoic rim surrounding the clot. (**C**) Four days later there has been further liquefaction of the clot, seen here as an anechoic central area. The overall size of the hematoma has also decreased in the interval.

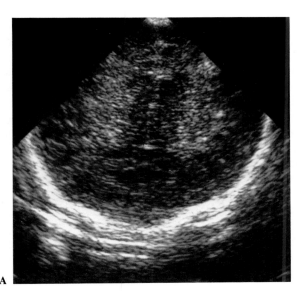

Fig. 1-116 Periventricular leukomalacia. (**A**) Coronal and (**B**) parasagittal sonograms of a premature infant with a history of perinatal asphyxia demonstrate bilateral, ill-defined, increased echogenicity of the hemispheric white matter. There is no mass effect. This hyperechoic appearance of the white matter is due to edema and petechial hemorrhage.

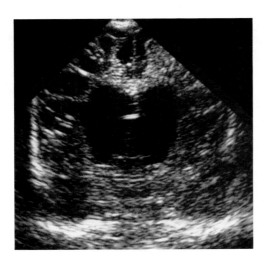

Fig. 1-117 Multicystic encephalomalacia. Coronal sonogram approximately 3 weeks after the acute onset of periventricular leukomalacia demonstrating anechoic cystic areas in the right frontal and temporal lobes as sequelae of periventricular leukomalacia. There is subtly decreased echogenicity in the left hemisphere, although macroscopic cystic lesions are not visible on the left. There is dilatation of the ventricles, and a shunt catheter is present.

ter. This can be differentiated from a parenchymal component of germinal matrix hemorrhage because the hemorrhage of periventricular leukomalacia is not contiguous with the subependymal or intraventricular regions. During the subacute phase of periventricular leukomalacia, cysts of sufficient size may be detected on CT as low-attenuation lesions in the periventricular distribution. The end-stage glial scarring is also usually not demonstrable on CT unless it is extensive. CT will, however, usually show slight enlargement of the lateral ventricles and thinning of white matter in the region of previous periventricular leukomalacia. This is demonstrated as mild ventriculomegaly with an irregular outline of the body and trigone of the lateral ventricles. The periventricular white matter is reduced in quantity in the region of the trigones, and severe cases show involvement of more extensive portions of the centrum semiovale. After severe periventricular leukomalacia, CT may show prominent sulci that extend nearly to the ventricular margins with little or no interposed white matter.[320]

MRI is rarely performed during the acute phase of periventricular leukomalacia. At this stage, T_1-weighted images show periventricular areas of low signal intensity. The abnormality may be difficult to differentiate from normal unmyelinated white matter on T_2-weighted images. During the subacute cystic stage, T_1-weighted MR images show multiple, round, low-signal abnormalities in the periventricular white matter. On T_2-weighted images, these cysts produce high signal intensity and are surrounded by a low-signal rim, which presumably is due to deposition of hemosiderin. MRI is probably the single best imaging modality for demonstration of the late sequelae of periventricular leukomalacia. The residual glial scarring is demonstrated as abnormally high signal on T_2-weighted images in the periventricular region, typically adjacent to the trigone. This area of signal abnormality usually abuts the ventricular wall and often extends into the subcortical white matter with a flame-shape appearance. There is often thinning of the posterior body and splenium of the corpus callosum, which presumably is due to degeneration of transcallosal fibers. White matter thinning and ventricular enlargement are also demonstrated.[321]

In mild cases of periventricular leukomalacia, the MR appearance may be difficult to differentiate from that of normal unmyelinated white matter. With periventricular leukomalacia, however, the signal abnormality directly abuts the ventricular wall; normal unmyelinated white matter is usually separated from the ventricular wall by a thin band of normally myelinated white matter in the splenium of the corpus callosum.[322,323]

Benign small cysts of uncertain etiology may occur in the periventricular regions and may be confused with the cystic stage of periventricular leukomalacia. These benign cysts, however, may be identified as early as the first week of life. They tend to be located adjacent to the frontal horns near the caudate nuclei. These cysts are small and have thin walls. The surrounding brain parenchyma is normal. Sequential studies usually show that the cysts remain stable in size for several weeks and then slowly involute.[324]

In term infants who have experienced a hypoxic-ischemic insult, the watershed area that is most susceptible to infarction comprises a band of tissue at the margins of the anterior and middle cerebral artery distributions and the middle and posterior cerebral artery distributions. In these children, imaging studies may demonstrate discrete infarctions in the watershed areas between the major vascular territories. These are most common in the frontal and parieto-occipital regions. Both the cortex and white matter are involved. If large enough, these infarcts are demonstrated on sonography as regions of abnormally increased echogenicity. CT shows abnormally low attenuation; this may be difficult to appreciate in neonates, however, because there is normally poor gray matter–white matter differentiation on CT. MRI is probably the most sensitive technique for the demonstration of these focal infarcts. T_1-weighted images demonstrate an infarct as a hypointense lesion of the cortex and subjacent white matter. The lesions produce high signal intensity on T_2-weighted images but may be difficult to differentiate from the normal high signal intensity of poorly myelinated neonatal brain tissue. The lesions may be regional or wedge shaped. Local atrophy may become evident in the late stages.[325]

A number of abnormalities may be demonstrated in severe diffuse hypoxic-ischemic brain injury in preterm or term neonates. In the acute stage there is diffuse cerebral edema, which is shown on sonography as an abnormal heterogeneous appearance of the brain parenchyma. The diencephalon may appear to have increased echogenicity, and the ventricular system is small and compressed. Doppler studies show decreased flow velocity in the major cerebral vessels. Follow-up sonography over the few weeks after the acute event may

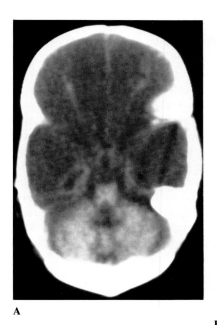

A

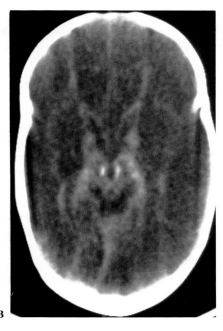

B

Fig. 1-118 Severe end-stage multicystic encephalomalacia. Axial CT scans in a 1-month-old child who experienced severe perinatal asphyxia show marked decrease in the attenuation of the entirety of both cerebral hemispheres, which have the appearance of multicystic leukoencephalomalacia. There is also moderate atrophy of the brainstem and cerebellum.

show return to a nearly normal appearance of the brain. In other cases, cystic parenchymal changes and progressive atrophy are identified.

In the acute stages of severe global ischemia, CT demonstrates diffuse, symmetric decreased attenuation of the cerebrum. Gray matter–white matter differentiation is lost. The diencephalon is frequently spared. The ventricular system is compressed, as are the extra-axial spaces. The cerebellum usually retains normal attenuation characteristics. Progression to cystic encephalomalacia is demonstrated on CT as a low-attenuation abnormality involving a fairly large portion of the cerebral hemispheres, usually symmetrically. Some portions of the cortex may be relatively spared and may have more normal attenuation values. The low-attenuation regions may progress to true cyst formation. Some degree of ventricular enlargement usually occurs but is usually not massive. With severe end-stage multicystic encephalomalacia, cystic degeneration replaces most of the cerebral hemispheres (Fig. 1-118).

Although not usually performed in the acute phases of severe global ischemia, MRI shows prolongation of T_1- and T_2-relaxation times of the parenchyma as a result of edema. As with CT, relative preservation of the diencephalon and cerebellum may be observed. The ventricles are small and compressed. The subsequent changes of cystic encephalomalacia are often best demonstrated on T_1-weighted images as areas of abnormally decreased signal intensity. These regions are often criss-crossed by bands or septations of gliosis.

The pattern of structural brain damage in asphyxiated preterm neonates differs from that in asphyxiated term neonates. This can be demonstrated on MRI. Neonates experiencing asphyxia at 24 to 26 weeks of gestational age usually show localized ventricular enlargement and irregular ventricular margins. There is only minimally increased signal in the surrounding white matter as a result of gliosis. With asphyxia occurring at later stages of gestation, there are greater degrees of gliosis. In asphyxiated term neonates, MRI shows marked thinning and prolongation of the T_2-relaxation time in the hemispheric white matter and cerebral cortex. These changes are usually most marked in the parasagittal watershed regions. In postterm neonates with asphyxia, there tends to be relative sparing of the periventricular white matter.[326]

With severe neonatal asphyxia, there may be hypoxic damage to the basal ganglia. This causes injury to the neuronal bodies and myelinating axons that course through this region. The resulting gliosis and neuronal loss in the basal ganglia and thalamus in combination with interspersed bundles of myelinated fibers are referred to pathologically as status marmoratus. This may be demonstrated on T_1-weighted MR images as spotty areas of higher signal intensity in the hypointense basal ganglia and thalami.[325]

In newborn infants, there is normally greater perfusion of the apices of the gyri than of the more central portions. Therefore, there may be greater damage in the central portions of the gyri than in the peripheral aspects in the face of a hypoxic event. This phenomenon is termed ulegyria. Ulegyria is demonstrated on MRI as tissue loss in the depths of the sulci with relative preservation of the gyri.

In most instances of asphyxic brain injury, there is relative preservation of the posterior fossa structures and diencephalon. Occasionally, however, there is disproportionate involvement of the thalamus and dorsal brainstem. This is thought to be most common in cases in which there is a short episode of complete anoxia. The sequelae of this injury are demonstrated on MRI as a decrease in size of the basal ganglia and slight dilatation of the third ventricle.[327,328]

CRANIAL TRAUMA

Head trauma is the most common cause of death due to trauma during infancy and is a major cause of morbidity in children of all ages. In neonates, head injury during delivery is an important cause of cranial and intracranial abnormalities. In infants, 90% to 95% of serious head injuries are the result of child abuse, with most of the remainder being due to motor vehicle accidents. In older children, motor vehicle accidents and falls account for approximately 50% of cases and child abuse for another 25%.[329–331]

There is a spectrum of intracranial manifestations of cranial trauma. The most minor abnormality is a concussion, in which there are only minimal anatomic changes in the brain and only transient neurologic manifestations. A contusion consists of gross or microscopic hemorrhage and edema in a focal area of the brain. A laceration refers to actual physical disruption of brain tissue and is usually associated with a penetrating injury or depressed skull fracture. Shearing injuries may be produced by sudden acceleration or deceleration of the skull, resulting in shearing of the axons and vessels in the central portions of the brain, including the corpus callosum, internal capsule, brainstem, fornices, or anterior commissure.

The syndrome of malignant cerebral edema, or hyperemia with secondary edema, occurs in up to 50% of children with severe cranial trauma. These edematous changes predominantly involve the subcortical white matter and the centrum semiovale and potentially may cause uncal herniation. The overall intracranial pressure is markedly increased.[332]

The most common areas of intracranial hemorrhage in association with cranial trauma are in the extradural spaces. Subdural hematomas are usually due to tearing of cortical veins, and epidural hematomas are more often associated with arterial hemorrhage. Minor degrees of subarachnoid hemorrhage are also common with head trauma. Aside from petechial hemorrhages in association with a contusion, significant intracerebral hemorrhage is a relatively uncommon sequela of trauma.

A stroke is an uncommon potential complication of cranial trauma. A stroke in these cases may be due to vasospasm of one or more major cerebral arteries. Posttraumatic cerebral edema also interferes with blood supply, either because of direct compression of cerebral vessels or because of generalized interference with perfusion by increased intracranial pressure. Blunt or penetrating trauma to the neck may cause direct damage to the carotid or vertebral arteries.

In general, CT is the imaging modality of choice for the evaluation of cranial trauma. CT is quite sensitive for the detection of acute intracranial hemorrhage and allows evaluation of the skull for depressed fractures. MRI has greater sensitivity for the detection of subtle areas of edema and may be helpful for the subsequent evaluation of the long-term sequelae of head trauma. Sonography may be useful in the evaluation of neonates after birth trauma. Skull radiographs are the most sensitive technique for the detection of injury of the calvaria. There is, however, little or no correlation between the presence or absence of a skull fracture and the probability of an intracranial injury.[333–335]

Birth Trauma

Head injuries acquired during childbirth differ significantly from those in older children with respect to the mechanisms of injury, the most common types of injury, and the pathologic effects on the immature brain, meninges, and calvaria. Sonography in these cases may be helpful for demonstrating large intracranial hematomas and for detecting cerebral edema or hydrocephalus. CT, however, is the most sensitive technique for the detection of acute intracranial hemorrhage. MRI may be helpful for evaluating the sequelae of trauma in the subacute and chronic stages.

Extracranial Injury

Traumatic subperiosteal hemorrhage, or cephalohematoma, occurs in approximately 1% of vaginal deliveries. The incidence is much higher for forceps deliveries. The hemorrhage is usually clinically evident at the time of delivery and may increase somewhat during the perinatal period. Palpation demonstrates a tense mass. Spontaneous resolution occurs over a period of weeks to months, depending on the size of the lesion. Because the blood is confined externally by the periosteum, it does not cross cranial sutures. Skull radiographs demonstrate a homogeneous extracranial mass and show the underlying calvaria to be intact. During the acute and subacute phases, a cephalohematoma is demonstrated on sonography, CT, or MRI as a crescent-shaped extracranial mass. The character of the contents of the lesion as evaluated on cross-sectional imaging will correspond to the age of the hematoma. On CT, the blood is hyperdense acutely and then gradually decreases in attenuation value. During the subacute phase, the lesion produces high signal intensity on both T_1- and T_2-weighted MR images. Subsequently, the lesion exhibits prolonged T_1- and T_2-relaxation times as well as hypointense areas of hemosiderin deposition and calcification. Because a cephalohematoma results in elevation of the periosteum, the lesion usually calcifies (Fig. 1-119). Nevertheless, even densely calcified lesions usually disappear completely as skull growth and remodeling occur.

Another common variety of extracranial hemorrhage due to childbirth is caput succedaneum. This consists of hemorrhagic edema in the superficial soft tissues of the scalp resulting from the trauma that occurs during vaginal delivery. This complication is readily identified clinically and can be differentiated from cephalohematoma by its superficial nature and the fact that the abnormality crosses suture lines.

The third common type of extracranial birth trauma is subgaleal hemorrhage. This refers to a hematoma confined externally by the aponeurosis covering the scalp beneath the occipitofrontalis muscle. As with caput succedaneum, the hemorrhage crosses suture lines. In some cases, there is dis-

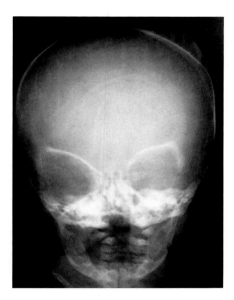

Fig. 1-119 Cephalohematoma. Frontal skull radiograph of a 3-week-old infant showing a partially calcified left parietal cephalohematoma. Note that the lesion does not cross the sagittal suture. The underlying calvaria is intact.

section of blood into the subcutaneous tissues of the neck. Imaging studies are not useful in the evaluation of this type of hemorrhage.

Skull Fracture

Skull fracture is a potential, but uncommon, complication of forceps delivery. Also, a depressed skull fracture may occur during unassisted delivery as a result of compression of the head against the pelvis. These injuries may be evaluated with routine skull radiographs. CT may be helpful in those cases in which there is evidence of depression. The thin neonatal calvaria is susceptible to ping-pong ball fractures, in which the bone collapses inward without a radiographically visible fracture line.

Intracranial Injury

Subdural hematoma is probably the most common symptomatic type of intracranial hemorrhage due to head trauma during childbirth. Small subarachnoid hemorrhages are also common (Fig. 1-120). In neonates experiencing particularly severe head trauma during childbirth, a number of other intracranial injuries may occur, including contusion, hemorrhagic contusion, and intraparenchymal hemorrhage (Fig. 1-121). Posterior fossa subdural hemorrhages due to birth trauma may be produced by either occipital osteodiastasis or a tentorial laceration. Occipital osteodiastasis refers to traumatic separation of the squamous portion of the occipital bone from the exoccipital portion. Mild occipital osteodiastasis is common during vaginal deliveries; with marked separation, however, the dura and venous sinuses may be torn, thereby producing a large subdural hemorrhage in the posterior fossa.[336]

Distortion of the cranium during childbirth may also result in stresses on the tentorium. This may cause tearing of small infratentorial veins or large tentorial lacerations accompanied by rupture of the vein of Galen, straight sinus, or transverse sinus. Supratentorial veins or the falx cerebri may also be damaged. The type of hemorrhage produced by these injuries is determined by the location and size of the damaged vascular structures. Therefore, there may be infratentorial (most common) or supratentorial hematomas (or both).

Posterior fossa subdural hematoma may produce signs of increased intracranial pressure, such as bulging of the fontanelles, sutural diastasis, lethargy, and vomiting. Most of these neonates have a history of difficult delivery, including forceps delivery in half the cases and breech presentation in one-fourth of the cases.[336] If a large vascular structure is ruptured, a large, rapidly expanding subdural hematoma can cause fatal compression of the brainstem.[337]

Supratentorial subdural hematomas may be produced by avulsion or tearing of superficial cortical veins or by laceration of the falx cerebri. Superficial cortical vein disruption causes a convexity subdural hematoma, which is usually unilateral. Subarachnoid blood is usually present as well. There may also be evidence of parenchymal brain injury, such as a contusion that is adjacent to a subdural blood collection. Laceration of the falx cerebri tends to occur near its junction with the tentorium, resulting in injury to the inferior portion of the sagittal sinus. The resulting subdural hematoma is usually located in the inferior aspect of the interhemispheric fissure.

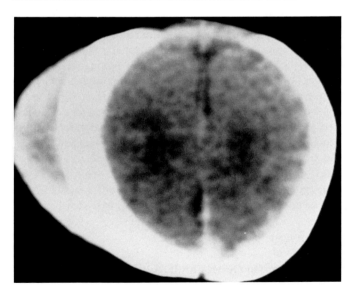

Fig. 1-120 Unenhanced axial CT scan of a 1-day-old child after forceps delivery showing high-attenuation, acute hemorrhage in the extracranial soft tissue of the right parietal region due to a cephalohematoma. Note that the subperiosteal hemorrhage does not cross the suture lines. There is a small, high-attenuation, acute hemorrhage in the subarachnoid spaces along the anterior interhemispheric fissure and the sulci of the left parietal lobe. Subsequent clinical and neuroimaging studies showed no evidence of permanent neurologic sequelae.

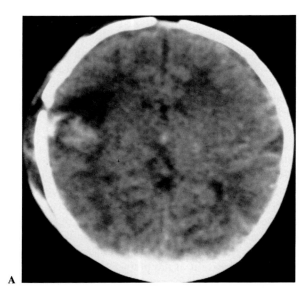
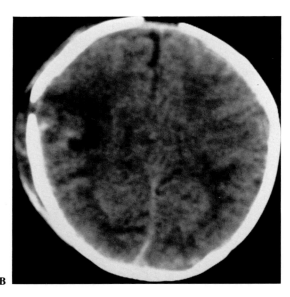

A   B

Fig. 1-121 (A and **B)** Unenhanced axial CT scans of a newborn after traumatic delivery showing a slightly diastatic right parietal skull fracture. There is an intraparenchymal hematoma in the right parietal lobe, with edematous changes surrounding the hematoma. There is also evidence of acute subarachnoid hemorrhage adjacent to the skull fracture and extending along the anterior interhemispheric fissure. There is a small extracranial subperiosteal hemorrhage adjacent to the fracture.

Large subdural hematomas in the newborn may be detected on sonography. CT and MRI, however, are more sensitive and specific. Coronal views are often helpful on CT, and coronal and sagittal views should be performed with MRI. An infratentorial subdural hematoma is demonstrated as a homogeneous mass with a linear superior margin and a crescentic inferior margin. There may be extension inferior and posterior to the cerebellar hemisphere in the occipital subdural space. Occasionally, supratentorial and infratentorial subdural hematomas coexist. A supratentorial hemispheric subdural hematoma is demonstrated as a crescentic, homogeneous mass adjacent to the inner table of the skull that produces a variable degree of mass effect on the adjacent portion of the cerebral hemisphere. Because the right and left subdural spaces do not freely communicate, the lesion is usually unilateral. An interhemispheric subdural hematoma shows homogeneous, irregular thickening along the course of the falx cerebri. In most cases, the blood collection remains confined to one side of the falx, producing a triangular mass. This is differentiated from subarachnoid hemorrhage by the lack of extension into the sulci.

Head Trauma in Older Children

Skull Fracture

Skull fractures in children are usually linear and asymptomatic. There is an increased incidence of fracture diastasis in infants and young children compared to adults. The presence of a simple linear skull fracture does not indicate an increased incidence of significant intracranial injury; likewise, the absence of a skull fracture is of no value in assessing the probability or severity of intracranial injury. Skull fractures are best evaluated with routine radiographs. Tangential views should be obtained to evaluate for depression (Fig. 1-122). In those cases in which the clinical or radiographic evaluation suggests the presence of a significantly depressed fracture, CT should be performed.

Basal skull fractures are relatively uncommon in children. Clinically, a basal skull fracture is suggested by the presence of periorbital and periauricular ecchymoses and by hemorrhage in the nasopharynx and ear. Basal skull fractures are usually not demonstrable on routine skull radiographs or routine CT. Thin-section axial or coronal CT may be utilized to demonstrate the fracture, but the clinical management is usually not affected by the information provided by this examination.

An acute skull fracture is demonstrated radiographically as a linear radiolucent defect that has sharp, well-defined, nonsclerotic margins. Within 1 to 2 weeks of the acute traumatic event, the margins of the skull fracture become less distinct on radiographs as bone resorption and remodeling occur (Fig. 1-123). In infants, simple skull fractures usually heal completely within several months. In older children, healing usually occurs within 1 year. This compares to a healing time of 2 to 3 years in adults and adolescents.

Leptomeningeal cyst is an uncommon complication of a skull fracture. This develops in cases in which a diastatic fracture occurs in association with a laceration of the underlying dura. In these cases, the meninges can herniate through the dural defect and into the fracture site. The interposition of this tissue prevents normal healing of the dura and bone. Cerebrospinal fluid pulsations may cause progressive enlargement

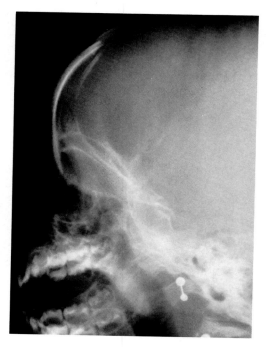

Fig. 1-122 Depressed skull fracture. Lateral skull radiograph showing a slightly comminuted, depressed fracture of the frontal bones in this child with blunt trauma to the forehead. There is a linear area of increased density due to overlapping of fracture fragments.

of the fracture and an increase in size of the fluid-filled meningeal sac that contains the leptomeningeal cyst.

Skull radiographs in the presence of a leptomeningeal cyst show a diastatic fracture with ill-defined, beveled, or sclerotic margins (Fig. 1-124). If the cyst is of sufficient size, it may be demonstrated as an extracranial soft tissue mass. CT and MRI show extension of cerebrospinal fluid or a combination of cerebrospinal fluid and brain tissue through the calvarial defect (Fig. 1-125). Posttraumatic encephalomalacia of the underlying portion of the brain is common.

Contusion

Cerebral contusions may be associated with loss of consciousness, seizures, focal neurologic deficits, and signs of increased intracranial pressure. Contusions may be hemorrhagic or nonhemorrhagic. A large contusion may produce significant mass effect. Contusions are most often due to impact injuries in which the surface of the brain contacts the inner table of the skull either at the site of impact or in a contrecoup location.

On CT, a contusion is demonstrated as an area of decreased attenuation in the cortex, usually involving both gray and white matter. The margins are usually poorly defined. Small contusions may be difficult to appreciate on CT. Hemorrhagic components may be located in the subpial or corticosubcortical regions. These produce ill-defined, often subtle areas of high attenuation during the acute phase of the injury.

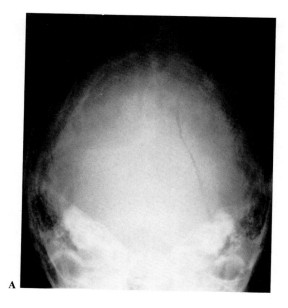

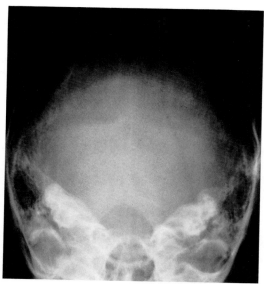

Fig. 1-123 Linear skull fracture. **(A)** Skull radiograph demonstrates a linear left occipital fracture without evidence of diastasis or depression. Note the sharp, nonsclerotic margins of the fracture line. **(B)** Follow-up radiograph 3 weeks later shows the fracture margins to be less distinct as a result of bone resorption and fracture healing.

MRI has greater sensitivity than CT for the detection of small contusions. The lesion is shown as an area of high signal intensity involving the gray and white matter, usually in a relatively superficial location (Fig. 1-126). Petechial hemorrhage usually does not significantly alter this appearance. In the subacute phase, hemorrhage of sufficient size may be identified as producing moderate to high signal intensity on both T_1- and T_2-weighted images.

Follow-up imaging with CT and MRI in cases of cerebral contusion shows progressive resolution of edema and hemorrhage over the first few weeks after the traumatic event. Mass

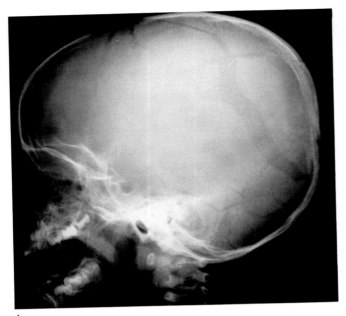

A

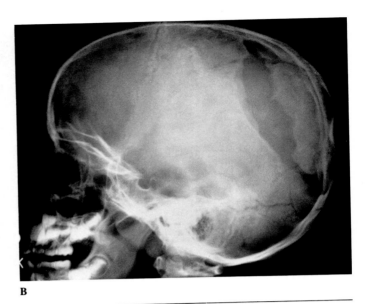

B

Fig. 1-124 Leptomeningeal cyst. (**A**) Lateral radiograph of a child after a severe fall shows a comminuted, widened parietal skull fracture. (**B**) Radiograph 1 year later shows interval healing of some of the components of the fracture. The main fracture line is enlarged and has smooth sclerotic margins, however. A pulsatile, fluid-filled meningeal sac was palpable at the site of the leptomeningeal cyst.

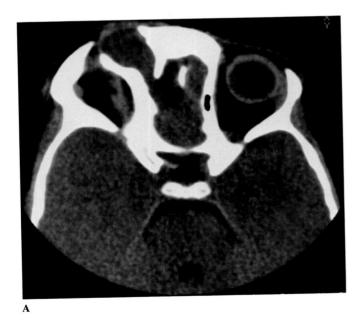

A

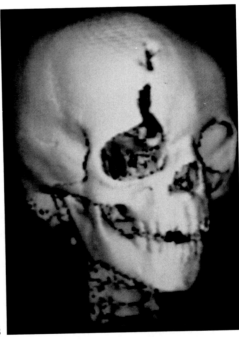

B

Fig. 1-125 Leptomeningeal cyst. (**A**) Axial CT scan of an 8-year-old child 6 months after a right frontal bone fracture shows protrusion of meninges and cerebrospinal fluid through a defect in the inferior aspect of the right frontal bone. The margins of the bone are sclerotic and smooth. (**B**) Oblique three-dimensional CT reformation shows the course of the fracture through the right frontal bone and into the roof of the right orbit. Intraorbital extension of this leptomeningeal cyst caused inferior displacement of the right globe.

effect usually disappears in a matter of days. Eventually, signs of focal atrophy (posttraumatic encephalomalacia) may develop in the region of the contusion, as evidenced by shrinkage of the gyri, enlargement of the pericerebral subarachnoid spaces, and enlargement of the adjacent portion of the lateral ventricle.[338]

Diffuse Cerebral Swelling

Diffuse cerebral swelling occurs in up to 50% of children after a severe head injury. It is most common among children with posttraumatic coma. It is thought to be due to edema and increased cerebral blood volume related to a decrease in cere-

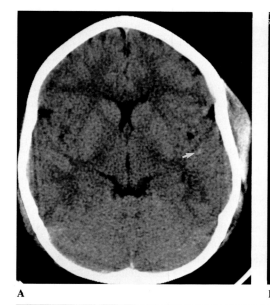
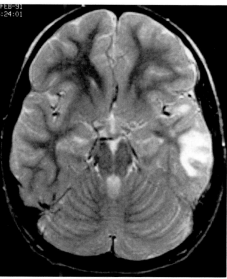

Fig. 1-126 Parenchymal contusion. **(A)** Axial CT scan in a child after blunt trauma to the left side of the head shows an extracranial hematoma in the soft tissues of the left temporoparietal region. A small focus of intraparenchymal hemorrhage is identified in the left temporal lobe (arrow). **(B)** T$_2$-weighted MR scan is much more sensitive for demonstrating the extensive area of involvement of the temporal lobe. This is shown as high signal intensity involving the superficial portions of the gray and white matter in the left temporal lobe.

brovascular resistance. The syndrome of malignant cerebral edema is apparently unique to the pediatric age group. The mean age is about 6 years. It is unknown whether this is a form of injury or a phenomenon occurring in response to injury. It does not appear to be entirely due to cerebral edema, but it is probably due in part to a loss of cerebral autoregulation with hyperemia. The inciting events include trauma, hypotension, and hypercarbia.

CT usually shows collapse of the ventricles and obliteration of the extra-axial subarachnoid spaces. With edema of rapid onset, compression of the aqueduct and third ventricle may prevent complete collapse of the lateral ventricles. There is an overall decrease in the attenuation values of the supratentorial structures and loss of the normal gray matter–white matter differentiation. The edematous changes are usually most marked in the peripheral aspects of the hemispheres, but there may be relative sparing of the basal ganglia, thalami, and posterior fossa structures (Fig. 1-127). In infants, the increased intracranial pressure causes spreading of the cranial sutures. Follow-up examinations may show the intracranial structures to return to normal or, more commonly, to develop diffuse atrophy.[304,339]

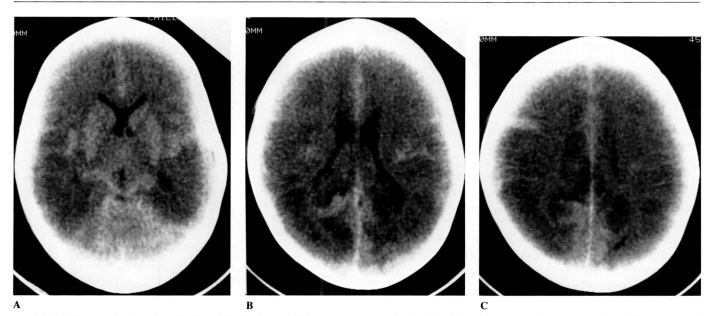

Fig. 1-127 Diffuse cerebral swelling. **(A, B, and C)** Unenhanced CT scans in a child who had sustained blunt head trauma 8 hours earlier show diffuse, decreased attenuation of the hemispheric white and gray matter. The attenuation characteristics of the basal ganglia, cerebellum, and small patches of hemispheric gray matter are preserved. The basal cisternae and pericerebral subarachnoid spaces are compressed. Compression of the aqueduct and third ventricle by the cerebral edema has prevented collapse of the lateral ventricles.

Shearing Injuries

Parenchymal shearing injuries are produced by severe rotational forces. Shearing injury is a major cause of unexplained deep coma or a persistent vegetative state in patients sustaining severe head trauma. This is due to axial stretching and disruption of nerve fiber tracts. These forces appear to be most commonly caused by high-speed motor vehicle accidents with rapid deceleration. They result in disruption of groups of axons and occasionally their accompanying blood vessels. These injuries tend to produce relatively severe neurologic consequences, often despite minimal abnormalities on imaging studies.

CT and MRI demonstrate ill-defined areas of edema with or without petechial hemorrhages. Occasionally, clefts can be identified in the white matter on T_1-weighted MR images. Shear injuries tend to occur at the junction of gray and white matter. The regions most often involved include the corpus callosum, deep white matter of the centrum semiovale, the internal capsule, and the basal ganglia. There may be ventricular and cisternal compression. Subarachnoid hemorrhage is occasionally present. Follow-up studies often demonstrate atrophic changes, which presumably are due to wallerian degeneration.[340]

Brainstem Injuries

Traumatic brainstem injuries may be produced by shearing forces or direct laceration between the clivus and tentorium. The resultant areas of edema or petechial hemorrhage are often too small to be visualized on CT. They may also be obscured by artifact from bone. MRI is the most sensitive imaging modality in these cases.

Patients with brainstem injury have the most severe impairment of consciousness. They usually have multiple other lesions, most often diffuse axonal injury (white matter shear). Brainstem injuries are rarely hemorrhagic.

Epidural Hematoma

Epidural hematomas are uncommon in children and rare in infants. In contradistinction to the situation in adult patients, many epidural hematomas in children are due to tears of dural veins rather than middle meningeal artery lacerations. At least 25% of pediatric epidural hematomas are of venous origin, with hemorrhage being derived from diploic veins or dural sinuses. Because of this, the time course over which the hematoma enlarges may be somewhat slower, and the symptoms may be more delayed.

Classically, an epidural hematoma is characterized clinically by a relatively asymptomatic interval after the traumatic event with subsequent rapid deterioration, in which there is progressive loss of consciousness and the onset of focal neurologic signs. This pattern is most often identified in adults and adolescents. In infants and young children, there is often a longer delay between the trauma and the onset of neurologic findings. Also, the clinical onset may be less precipitous. This is due at least in part to the presence of open sutures, which allow for an increase in head size in response to the enlarging hematoma. In more than half the cases in infants and young children, there is no loss of consciousness. In young infants, an epidural hematoma may produce hypovolemic shock and anemia. In the pediatric age group as a whole, acute epidural hematomas are accompanied by a fracture of the squamous portion of the temporal bone in 65% to 70% of cases.[341,342]

CT and MRI demonstrate an acute epidural hematoma as a homogeneous, convex (lens-shaped) hematoma adjacent to the inner table of the skull (Fig. 1-128). Temporal and temporoparietal locations are most common. About 4% of epidural hematomas in children occur in the posterior fossa. An epidural hematoma in the frontal area tends to be of larger size. CT shows the high-attenuation characteristics of acute hemorrhage, and MRI usually shows isointensity on T_1-weighted images and hypointensity on T_2-weighted images. As with other intracranial hematomas, the CT and MR characteristics of the lesion change with time (Fig. 1-129).[343,344]

Acute Subdural Hematoma

A subdural hematoma results from tears of the cortical veins that course through the subdural space and communicate with the dural sinuses. Motor vehicle accidents and falls are the usual causes in most pediatric patients. In these cases, the hematoma is usually unilateral, and the symptoms are dictated by the location and size of the hematoma. With a large acute subdural hematoma, the findings may include signs of increased intracranial pressure, seizures, an altered level of consciousness, or focal neurologic defects. In neonates, the

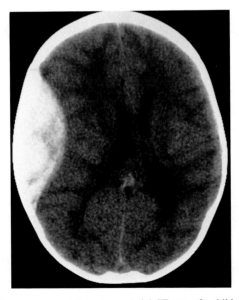

Fig. 1-128 Acute epidural hematoma. Axial CT scan of a child who experienced blunt trauma to the right side of the head showing a lens-shaped, high-attenuation hematoma in the epidural space of the right parietal region. There is compression of the underlying brain with contralateral shift of the midline.

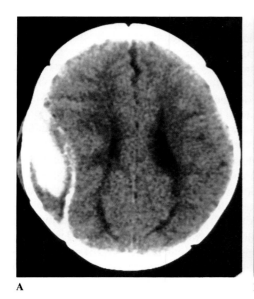 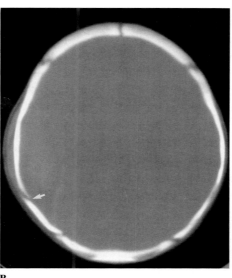

Fig. 1-129 Acute epidural hematoma. **(A)** Axial CT scan 24 hours after blunt trauma to the right side of the head demonstrates a right temporoparietal epidural hematoma. There is a mixed-attenuation character of the lesion because of clot lysis and retraction. **(B)** Bone window image shows a minimally depressed skull fracture (arrow) adjacent to the hematoma.

A   B

subdural hematomas associated with birth trauma are often bilateral and are usually located over the frontoparietal convexities. Interhemispheric subdural hematomas are common in infants who have been subjected to physical abuse.[345,346]

CT and MRI typically demonstrate an acute subdural hematoma as a crescent-shaped extracranial blood collection as opposed to the biconvex or lens shape that is characteristic of an epidural hematoma. In general, the margins of the subdural hematoma tend to be more irregular and less clearly defined than those of an epidural hematoma. Because the right and left subdural spaces do not freely communicate, the falx is often visible as a limiting margin of the hematoma. Interhemispheric fissure subdurals tend to be located along only one side of the falx, producing a triangular configuration. A small convexity subdural hematoma sometimes cannot be differentiated from an epidural lesion on imaging studies.[347,348]

Acutely, subdural hemorrhage is of high attenuation on CT. The attenuation values gradually decrease, such that the hemorrhage is approximately isodense to normal brain at some point within 1 to 3 weeks of the injury. A small isodense subdural hematoma may be difficult to detect on CT unless there are secondary signs such as mass effect. The lesion is readily demonstrated, however, after contrast agent administration because the hematoma itself does not enhance and because there may be an enhancing inner membrane. Approximately 2 to 3 weeks after the acute injury, the hematoma becomes lower in attenuation than brain parenchyma, and eventually the attenuation may approach that of cerebrospinal fluid. These chronic subdural hematomas often show a thick, enhancing inner membrane on contrast-enhanced CT. Delayed contrast opacification of the hematoma itself (4 to 6 hours after injection) is sometimes observed. Occasionally, during the subacute or chronic phases, fluid-fluid or fluid-debris levels are visible. In general, axial CT is sufficient for the evaluation of most hematomas. Tentorial subdural hema-

tomas are best visualized on coronal CT images, however.[349,350]

The MR signal characteristics of subdural and other hematomas vary according to the time period that has elapsed since the acute bleed. The changes in signal intensity are due to loss of oxygen from hemoglobin molecules, which is followed by oxidation of hemoglobin to methemoglobin and the latter's subsequent breakdown into paramagnetic materials, primarily hemosiderin. Hematomas imaged in the first 24 hours after the ictus are mildly hyperintense on T_1-weighted images and hyperintense on T_2-weighted sequences (stage 1). Over the next 24 to 48 hours, the hematoma becomes isointense or hypointense on T_1-weighted images and markedly hypointense on T_2-weighted images (stage 2). There is significant variability in the appearance of the hemorrhage among patients 3 to 7 days after the ictus. The hematoma usually becomes markedly hyperintense on T_1-weighted sequences beginning on about day 4. It again becomes hyperintense on T_2-weighted images beginning on day 5 or 6 (stage 3). Usually by the end of the first week, the hematoma is hyperintense on all pulsing sequences (stage 4).[351] The signal intensity of the hematoma on T_1-weighted images gradually decreases as it enters the chronic phase, although it remains hyperintense with respect to cerebrospinal fluid. Hemosiderin at the margin of the hematoma may produce areas of low signal intensity on both T_1- and T_2-weighted images. A chronic subdural hematoma usually is surrounded by membranes that will enhance with paramagnetic contrast material.[352]

Subarachnoid Hemorrhage

A variable degree of subarachnoid hemorrhage is common with head trauma of sufficient severity to produce brain injury. CT demonstrates high-attenuation material in the cisternae, pericerebral subarachnoid spaces, or interhemispheric fissure.

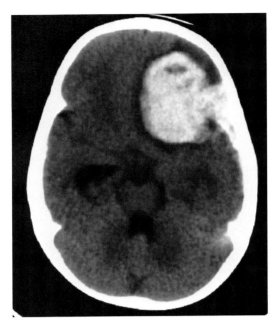

Fig. 1-130 Intracerebral hematoma. Unenhanced axial CT scan of a boy with hemophilia who sustained a minor blow to the head showing a large intracerebral hematoma in the left frontal lobe. There is also a small adjacent acute subdural hematoma.

Interhemispheric subarachnoid hemorrhage is distinguished from an interhemispheric subdural hematoma or a normal hyperdense falx by the irregular appearance of the blood collection and extension of the blood into the cerebral sulci.[353,354]

Intracerebral Hematoma

Although petechial hemorrhage in association with cerebral contusion or shear injuries is common, large space-occupying intercerebral hematomas due to trauma are unusual in children. CT and MRI show a homogeneous mass with the imaging characteristics of acute hemorrhage. There is much greater mass effect than that usually associated with a hemorrhagic contusion (Fig. 1-130). Subsequent imaging studies show alterations in the characteristics of the hematoma with time, similar to the findings with extra-axial hematomas. In the chronic phase, MRI often demonstrates regions of low signal intensity that are due to hemosiderin deposition.[355]

Long-Term Complications and Sequelae of Head Trauma

Chronic Subdural Hematoma

Chronic subdural hematomas may occur as sequelae of previous trauma or as a result of various other insults, such as meningitis. In infants with this abnormality, the clinical manifestations may include irritability, failure to thrive, fever, macrocephaly, and a bulging fontanelle. The identification of a chronic subdural hematoma in an infant without a clear history of etiology should raise clinical suspicion of child abuse.

Imaging studies show a chronic subdural hematoma as a crescentic, extra-axial fluid collection that causes mass effect on the adjacent brain parenchyma. In infants, the lesions are often bilateral. On CT, the fluid collection is isodense or hypodense to brain parenchyma but usually has higher attenuation than cerebrospinal fluid. A thick, enhancing membrane may be visualized on images after contrast material administration. The MR appearance of a chronic subdural hematoma is also somewhat variable, depending on the contents. Most often, the fluid is hypointense with respect to brain and slightly hyperintense with respect to cerebrospinal fluid on T_1-weighted images and hyperintense to brain on T_2-weighted images. Occasionally, the fluid is slightly hyperintense to brain on T_1-weighted images. As with CT, contrast-enhanced MRI often shows an enhancing membrane (Fig. 1-131).

Subdural Hygroma

A subdural hygroma contains fluid with a composition similar to that of cerebrospinal fluid. In most cases, this lesion is thought to arise from a traumatic arachnoid tear that allows leakage of cerebrospinal fluid into the subdural space. A chronic subdural hematoma from which cellular debris has been absorbed is clinically and radiologically indistinguishable from this lesion. CT and MRI demonstrate a crescentic, subdural fluid collection with imaging characteristics identical to those of cerebrospinal fluid.

Posttraumatic Hydrocephalus

Posttraumatic hydrocephalus may be produced by adhesions in the ventricles or extra-axial subarachnoid spaces. This complication is most often associated with posterior fossa or intraventricular hemorrhages. Imaging studies demonstrate dilatation of the third and lateral ventricles and sometimes the fourth ventricle, depending on the location of the obstruction. Because severe head trauma is often associated with some degree of atrophy, ventricular enlargement due to atrophy may be difficult to differentiate from hydrocephalus in some cases. Hydrocephalus should be suspected when ventricular enlargement is out of proportion to the prominence of the extra-axial subarachnoid spaces. Also, the ventricles tend to assume a more rounded configuration than is seen with atrophic enlargement. Most important are clinical features such as enlarging head size and a bulging fontanelle. In some cases, radionuclide cisternography may be helpful for evaluating the cerebrospinal fluid flow dynamics.

Child Abuse

Intracranial injury is a relatively common and potentially devastating occurrence in physically abused children. Significant head trauma is estimated to occur in 15% to 25% of

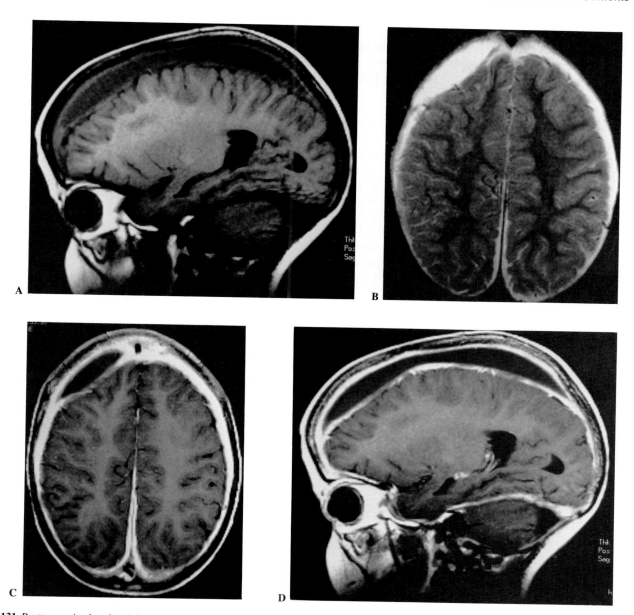

Fig. 1-131 Posttraumatic chronic subdural hematoma. **(A)** Right parasagittal T_1-weighted MR scan shows a large, crescentic, subdural fluid collection that is hypointense to brain and slightly hyperintense to cerebrospinal fluid. A membrane that has slightly higher signal intensity encompasses the fluid collection. **(B)** Axial T_2-weighted MR scan shows the right subdural fluid collection to be of high signal intensity. There is also generalized high signal intensity in the thickened meninges. **(C)** Contrast-enhanced axial T_1-weighted MR scan shows diffuse enhancement of the meninges. The subdural fluid collection does not enhance and remains hypointense. **(D)** Sagittal contrast-enhanced T_1-weighted MR scan shows the crescentic, subdural fluid collection surrounded by enhancing margins.

physically abused children. Child abuse is the single most common cause of serious intracranial injury in infants younger than 1 year of age. Intracranial injury is the major cause of death in abused children, and serious long-term neurologic deficits are common sequelae among survivors. Some series have indicated that significant intracranial injury is as common or more common than skeletal injuries.[329,356–358]

Billmire and Myers[329] evaluated 84 infants between 3 weeks and 11 months of age who were admitted with the diagnosis of head injury or with CT findings of head injury. They found that 95% of serious intracranial injuries in these

infants were the result of physical abuse. They reported that 64% of all the head injuries, excluding uncomplicated linear skull fractures, were due to intentional injury.

Pathogenesis

The mechanical forces involved in head trauma can be broadly classified into two types: translational and rotational. Translational force is produced by a direct impact to the head with transmission of forces directly to the soft tissues and skull and potentially to the underlying intracranial structures. Rotational forces are produced by sudden acceleration or deceleration of the head, usually with rotation on the axis of the upper cervical vertebrae. The whiplash phenomenon produces high rotational forces. Impact injuries may produce both translational and rotational forces.

There are several important morphologic and physiologic characteristics of the immature skull and brain that influence the pathogenesis of childhood intracranial injuries. The calvaria and meninges have greater flexibility than those in older children and adults, thereby decreasing the likelihood of skull fracture but providing less protection to the underlying brain. The prominent pericerebral subarachnoid spaces and increased cerebral plasticity of infants help protect the brain from direct injury. These factors, however, also permit increased movement and distortion of the brain in response to rotational forces. This motion of the brain in the skull may apply shearing stress on the small bridging cerebral veins that extend to the dural sinuses. Impact injuries that produce predominantly translational forces tend to cause extra-axial hemorrhage, brain contusion, cerebral hemorrhage, infarction, or generalized edema. Rotational forces may produce subdural hemorrhage, parenchymal shear injuries, or generalized edema.

In addition to these morphologic factors, there are physiologic considerations that are important in the response of the immature brain to trauma. Infants and young children often exhibit a predisposition to cerebral edema after head trauma. This is thought to be due, at least in part, to increased cerebral vasoreactivity and a high metabolic rate. Also, brain perfusion may be compromised by the increased intracranial pressure that occurs with diffuse cerebral edema. Occasionally, perfusion is compromised as a result of direct trauma to cerebral or cervical vessels.[350,359]

Severe manual shaking is a common etiology of intracranial injury in abused children. When the child is grasped by the torso and severely shaken, the head is subjected to severe rotational forces. Infants are particularly prone to this type of injury because of the relatively large head size in comparison to the size of the body and the relative weakness of the neck muscles. Compression of the cervical spinal cord may lead to high cervical cord contusion or extra-axial hemorrhage at the cervicomedullary junction.[360] Extremity injuries may also occur in these cases as a result of violent flailing of the arms and legs.[361]

It has been clearly demonstrated in animal models that severe intracranial injuries can be produced by rotational forces without a direct blow to the head.[362] Also, clinical studies have documented significant intracranial injuries such as subdural hemorrhage in patients without skull fractures or soft tissue injuries of the face or head. Infants subjected to severe shaking may show bruises or rib fractures—especially of the posterior segments—as a result of the grasping of the torso during shaking.

Although severe manual shaking clearly is an important cause of intracranial injury in child abuse, impact injuries are also identified in many children. The relative incidence of brain injury due to these two mechanisms is unknown. In many cases, both forms of injury may be present. It is essential to recognize, however, that a severe intracranial traumatic injury may be present in an abused child without clinical evidence of soft tissue injury in the face or head and with skull radiographs that show no fractures.[362–366]

Skull and Scalp Injuries

Children with a significant impact injury to the head frequently exhibit swelling of a portion of the scalp. A large subgaleal hematoma may be produced by an impact or hair pulling. A large subgaleal hematoma may be identified on skull radiographs or CT scans. The identification of this finding should prompt a careful search for an underlying skull fracture.[367]

It is essential that the absence of a skull fracture not be taken to indicate that intracranial injury related to child abuse is not present. Radiographic demonstration of one or more skull fractures, however, provides firm documentation that a significant impact force has been applied to the calvaria. The demonstration of a skull fracture is not in and of itself proof of abuse; nevertheless, correlation between the alleged mechanism of injury and the radiographic findings is essential in all infants and young children with skull fractures.

Most large series have reported a 10% to 13% frequency of detection of skull fractures in physically abused children. Of those abused children with clinical or radiographic evidence of head trauma, 23% to 48% have been reported to have skull fractures.[357,359,362,363,368,369] As with injuries elsewhere in the skeletal system, the great majority of skull fractures in abused children occur during infancy; 80% to 85% occur in children younger than 2 years of age.

Most skull fractures related to physical abuse are single linear fractures. The parietal bone is most frequently involved. The occipital bone is probably the next most common site. Although a simple linear fracture is the most common type in abused children, this is also the most common skull fracture that occurs with accidental trauma. There are, however, a number of radiographic patterns of skull fractures that, when identified, suggest severe or unusual trauma and indicate the need for close correlation with the alleged mechanism of injury. These patterns include fractures that are multiple, complex, depressed, or diastatic or that cross one or more sutures (Fig. 1-132). The presence of a depressed fracture, particularly when there is a stellate configuration with the fracture lines radiating from a central point, suggests that there has been direct impact with a sharp or pointed object. The identification of a depressed occipital bone fracture is virtually pathognomonic of abuse. A diastatic or growing fracture is also suggestive of severe trauma.

Various studies have been performed in attempts to correlate the usual mechanisms of injury with the type of skull fracture in infants and children with accidental injuries. Hobbs[370] reported that most accidental skull fractures in children are due to falls from heights of 3.5 to 5.5 ft (107 to

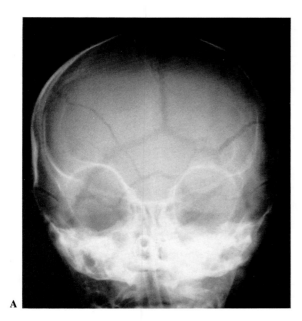

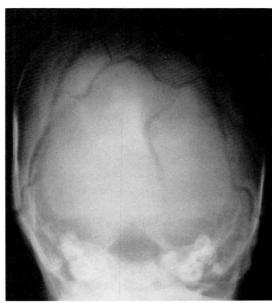

Fig. 1-132 Skull fracture due to child abuse. (**A** and **B**) Skull radiographs in a physically abused infant showing several fracture lines in the occipital and parietal bones. Several of the fractures cross a suture; most are diastatic. There is also widening of the cranial sutures as a result of cerebral edema. Physical examination demonstrated extracranial findings suggestive of head trauma.

or less. These data are helpful in correlating the radiographic findings with the alleged mechanism of injury in questionable cases.[372] Kleinman[373] has proposed that all cases of children with complex skull fractures or neurologic findings occurring after a fall from a height reported to be less than 2.9 ft (90 cm) should be regarded as possible instances of abuse.

When skull radiographs demonstrate a severe or complex skull fracture, CT should be performed for evaluation of the intracranial structures. The absence of radiographic evidence of a skull fracture, however, should in no way be taken to imply that significant intracranial injury has not occurred. Because of the relatively high incidence of intracranial damage in physically abused children and the potential severity of long-term sequelae, a high index of suspicion for clinical signs of intracranial injury should be maintained in the care of all children in which there is a question of physical abuse.

Intracranial Injuries

Subdural hemorrhage is probably the most common acute intracranial abnormality in physically abused children. CT is the imaging modality of choice in most of these cases; MRI may also be useful for evaluating shear injuries and the long-term sequelae of serious head injury.

Subdural hemorrhage may be produced by an impact injury but is probably more often due to tearing of bridging cortical veins in response to rotational forces produced by severe shaking. In some cases, a small or moderate-size pericerebral subdural hematoma is identified. This is shown on CT as a crescentic peripheral zone of high attenuation adjacent to the brain surface without interdigitation into the sulci. The inner margin of the blood collection is concave, and the outer margin adjacent to the inner table of the skull is convex. The falx serves as a relative barrier to the spread of the subdural fluid from one side to the other.

Subdural hemorrhage in the interhemispheric fissure is generally acknowledged to be more common in cases of child abuse than pericerebral subdural hemorrhages. Hemorrhage in this location is due to rupture of bridging veins between the cortex and the superior sagittal sinus. Manual shaking is the etiology in the great majority of cases. These acute interhemispheric subdural hematomas occur almost exclusively in the parieto-occipital region and are most often unilateral.[359]

An acute interhemispheric subdural hematoma is demonstrated on CT as a crescentic or triangular, high-attenuation blood collection in the parasagittal region. The blood collection has a flat medial border where it is in contact with the falx, and the lateral border tends to be convex (Fig. 1-133). There is often some degree of extension into the adjacent pericerebral subdural space. Also, because most interhemispheric subdural hematomas occur in the parieto-occipital region, the hematoma frequently extends along the subdural spaces of the superior aspect of the tentorium. A tentorial subdural hematoma usually produces a band of increased attenuation on CT, but this may be difficult to identify on axial images. Coronal images in these cases clearly demonstrate the high-attenua-

167 cm). The great majority of falls from this distance usually do not cause a fracture, and when a fracture is present it is typically linear and nondiastatic. More severe fractures in this series were produced from falls down stairs or from heights greater than 6 ft (182 cm). Kravitz and coworkers[371] reported that only 2% of infants experiencing accidental falls from heights between 2 and 5 ft (61 to 154 cm) sustained a skull fracture. Helfer and colleagues[372] reported three skull fractures in 246 children who fell from a height of 4.9 ft (150 cm)

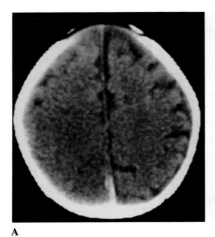 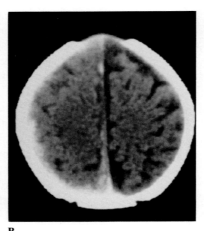

Fig. 1-133 Acute interhemispheric subdural hematoma in child abuse. (**A** and **B**) Unenhanced CT scans showing a triangular, high-attenuation blood collection on the right side of the interhemispheric fissure. This is an acute interhemispheric subdural hematoma produced by severe manual shaking in an abused child. There are also subtle signs of edema in the parietal lobes with compression of the sulci and poor gray matter–white matter differentiation.

A   B

tion, crescentic blood collection along the surface of the tentorium.

A small interhemispheric subdural hematoma may be quite subtle on CT, and maintaining a high index of suspicion is important. Even the presence of a small area of hemorrhage indicates that significant intracranial trauma has occurred and severe neurologic sequelae may ensue. Also, clear documentation of acute intracranial hemorrhage is important from a medical-legal aspect. The specific finding of high-attenuation blood may disappear within a few days when the hematoma is small. A small interhemispheric subdural hemorrhage may produce only subtle asymmetric thickening of the posterior falx on CT. The hemorrhage may be differentiated from the normal high-attenuation falx by noting that the blood collection usually is unilateral and somewhat irregular in comparison to the normally linear, well-defined falx. The demonstration of extension of blood into the subdural space of the tentorium, when present, is helpful as a confirmatory sign. Also, serial CT examinations may be performed to document clearing of the hemorrhage.

MRI is quite helpful for confirming the presence of hemorrhage in cases in which the CT findings are subtle or inconclusive. MRI is most specific during the subacute stage, when the blood produces relatively high signal intensity on T_1-weighted images. Small subdural blood collections can be accurately localized on MRI. Sagittal images are particularly helpful for demonstrating involvement of the tentorial subdural space (Fig. 1-134).

Serial neuroimaging examinations are also helpful for the identification of other findings of intracranial injury that may have a delayed appearance on CT, such as cerebral edema or infarction (Fig. 1-135). Zimmerman and coworkers[359] reported a 100% incidence of subsequent cerebral atrophy in cases of large interhemispheric subdural hematomas. Interhemispheric or convexity hematomas may become chronic, in which case CT demonstrates low-attenuation, crescentic subdural fluid collections and MRI shows high signal on T_2-weighted images and moderate or low signal on T_1-weighted

images. Because subdural fluid collections in abused children may be due to repeated episodes of injury, imaging at the time of presentation may demonstrate the presence of both chronic and acute subdural hematomas. When present, this finding is quite suggestive of nonaccidental trauma.

Subarachnoid hemorrhage is less common than subdural hemorrhage in child abuse. In these cases, subarachnoid hemorrhage usually occurs in association with a parenchymal brain injury. A large subarachnoid hemorrhage is demonstrated on CT as high-attenuation blood accumulating in the cerebral cisternae and extending into the cerebral sulci. A smaller hemorrhage may be manifested only as high-attenuation blood in the interhemispheric fissure. This finding on CT may cause confusion with a normal hyperdense falx or an interhemispheric subdural hematoma. The high attenuation produced by subarachnoid blood in the interhemispheric fissure has a wider and more irregular appearance than a normal dense falx (Fig. 1-136). Although interhemispheric subdural hematomas tend to occur in the posterior portion of the fissure and have flat medial borders and crescentic lateral borders, interhemispheric subarachnoid blood more often occurs anteriorly and occupies both sides of the fissure. Also, an interhemispheric subdural hematoma in the anterior portion of the fissure is limited internally by the margin of the falx, whereas subarachnoid blood extends more centrally toward the genu of the corpus callosum.[359]

An acute epidural hematoma is uncommon in child abuse. Unlike subdural hematomas, an epidural hematoma usually is the result of a direct blow and is often associated with a skull fracture. A large epidural hematoma typically has a lenticular shape on axial CT or MRI. A smaller epidural blood collection, however, may be indistinguishable from a small subdural hematoma.[374]

A number of parenchymal brain injuries may result from head trauma in child abuse. These include cerebral edema, contusions, shear injuries, and intraparenchymal hematomas. Cerebral edema in these children may result from various mechanisms, but in many cases it is probably an indirect

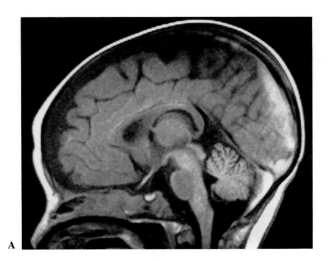

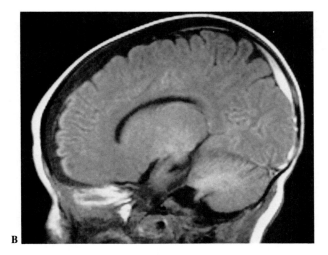

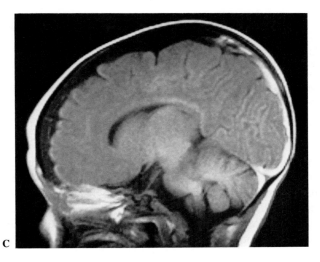

Fig. 1-134 Intracranial hemorrhage in child abuse. (**A**) Sagittal T_1-weighted MR scan at the midline shows high-signal acute hemorrhage in the posterior interhemispheric fissure. There is inferior extension into the subdural space along the tentorium. Subacute subdural hemorrhage is also seen posterior to the cerebellum. (**B** and **C**) Parasagittal images to the right of the midline also show acute hemorrhage in the posterior pericerebral subdural spaces. Anteriorly, there is a hypointense chronic subdural hematoma. This combination of acute and chronic subdural hematomas in an infant without a clear history of significant accidental head trauma is virtually pathognomonic of child abuse.

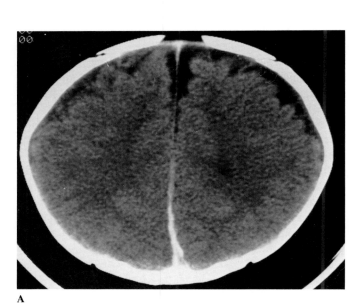

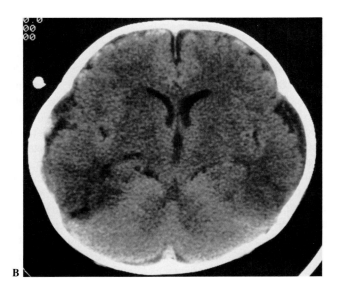

Fig. 1-135 Intracranial hemorrhage in child abuse. (**A**) Unenhanced axial CT scan of an infant who presented with a history of seizures and irritability shows an acute posterior interhemispheric subdural hematoma. There is also a small subacute or chronic hematoma in the right frontal parietal region. No intraparenchymal brain abnormalities are identified. (**B**) Follow-up unenhanced CT scan 1 week later shows diffuse cerebral edema. The child's parent subsequently admitted to having severely shaken the infant. Follow-up studies showed progressive cerebral atrophy.

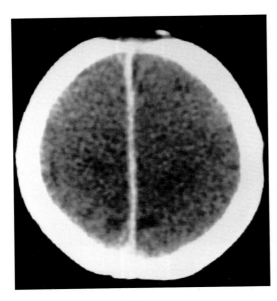

Fig. 1-136 Subarachnoid hemorrhage in child abuse. Unenhanced axial CT scan of a physically abused child with head trauma showing high-attenuation acute hemorrhage in the subarachnoid spaces of the interhemispheric fissure. There is also decreased attenuation of the brain parenchyma and obliteration of the sulci by cerebral edema.

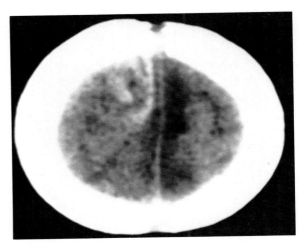

Fig. 1-137 Cerebral contusion in child abuse. Axial unenhanced CT scan in the superior parietal region showing a heterogeneous area of mixed increased and decreased attenuation in the right superficial aspect of the right parietal lobe. This is a hemorrhagic contusion in an abused child.

pathophysiologic response to head trauma. Posttraumatic cerebral edema may be focal, multifocal, or diffuse. CT demonstrates areas of decreased attenuation, which may be subtle. Localized edema may produce mass effect; diffuse edema usually causes a decrease in the size of the ventricular system and obliteration of the extra-axial cerebrospinal fluid spaces. MRI is much more sensitive than CT for the demonstration of edema but is often not practical in the acutely injured child. In some cases of severe diffuse edema, CT shows diminished attenuation throughout the cortical gray and white matter with relative preservation of the attenuation characteristics of the thalamus, brainstem, and cerebellum; this has been termed the reversal sign because of the relatively higher attenuation of the central regions of the brain compared with the peripheral aspects of the hemispheres.[375]

Cerebral contusions or hematomas may be produced by direct translational forces in an impact injury or from shearing of superficial or deep cerebral tissues induced by severe rotational forces. The appearance of a cerebral contusion on CT is somewhat variable, depending on the presence and degree of petechial hemorrhage. Contusions without hemorrhage are imaged as areas of heterogeneous decreased attenuation, usually involving both gray and white matter. If it is large enough, there may be signs of mass effect. More often, the contusion is demonstrated as a heterogeneous area of mixed high and low attenuation (Fig. 1-137). After the first 24 hours postinjury, the high-attenuation component progressively decreases as the hemorrhage resolves. Contusions typically have poorly defined margins with the adjacent, more normal portions of the brain. Cerebral contusions, often multiple, may be produced

at the gray matter–white matter junctions as a result of shearing injuries (Fig. 1-138). Contusions are particularly well demonstrated on MRI, which shows areas of abnormal prolongation of the T_1- and T_2-relaxation times.[376]

A large intracerebral hematoma is uncommon in child abuse. CT demonstrates a well-marginated, homogeneous area of high attenuation in the brain parenchyma. There is usually surrounding low-attenuation edema. MRI is also quite sensitive for detecting and characterizing an intracerebral hematoma; the signal characteristics vary according to the age of the hemorrhage.

Gross intraventricular hemorrhage may occur with massive intracranial injury. CT is quite sensitive for the detection of acute intraventricular hemorrhage because the high-attenuation blood is easily differentiated from cerebrospinal fluid. The blood usually layers in the dependent portions of the ventricular system.

Imaging studies may reveal various long-term sequelae of head trauma in child abuse. As described previously, chronic subdural fluid collections are the most common sequelae. Cerebral atrophy is also common. Other findings may include encephalomalacia, porencephaly, or leptomeningeal cyst (Fig. 1-139).[357] Posttraumatic hydrocephalus is occasionally identified.

CENTRAL NERVOUS SYSTEM INFECTIONS

Infections of the central nervous system represent a heterogeneous group of diseases. Clinical evaluation and laboratory studies are of paramount importance for the diagnosis and treatment of these disorders. For the most part, imaging studies serve complementary or supportive roles. There are occasional instances, however, in which central nervous system

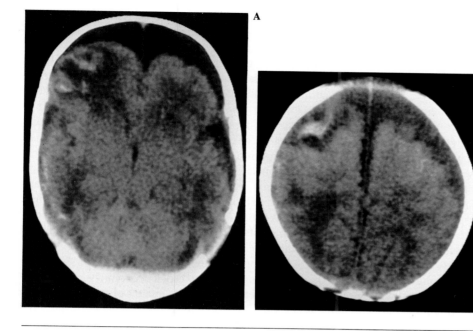

Fig. 1-138 Intracranial injury in child abuse. (**A** and **B**) Unenhanced axial CT scans of a 2-month-old infant showing a large hemorrhagic contusion on the right frontal lobe. There are also edema and minimal hemorrhage in the right temporal and parietal lobes. Low-attenuation chronic subdural hematomas are present in the bifrontal regions. This infant had been subjected to severe shaking. The hemorrhagic contusions in this child are probably due to shearing injuries produced by severe rotational forces.

infection is initially detected with neuroradiologic studies. Imaging studies also can provide clues to the specific etiologic diagnosis.

Meningitis

Meningitis is the most common form of central nervous system infection. Meningitis may be caused by a variety of infectious agents. There is considerable variation with respect to the pathophysiologic consequences of infection with different organisms. Also, patient age strongly influences the epidemiologic factors and pathophysiologic effects of these infections.

Viral Meningitis

Viral meningitis is the most common and clinically the most benign form of central nervous system infection. Viral men-

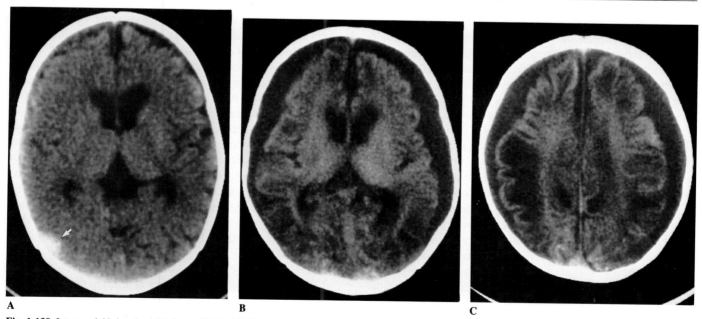

Fig. 1-139 Intracranial injury in child abuse. (**A**) Axial CT scan in a physically abused infant (severe shaking injury) shows a small acute subdural hematoma along the superior surface of the tentorium on the right (arrow). There are small subacute or chronic subdural hematomas in the frontal regions. There is poor gray matter–white matter differentiation in both hemispheres as a result of cerebral edema. (**B** and **C**) Follow-up CT scans 1 month later show large, bilateral, chronic subdural hematomas. There are severe cerebral atrophy and encephalomalacia.

ingitis is included under the broader term *aseptic meningitis*, which includes noninfectious inflammatory conditions that evoke a meningeal response. These include collagen vascular diseases, leukemia, central nervous system tumors, and intrathecal chemotherapy.

The most common etiologic agents responsible for viral meningitis and aseptic meningitis are the enteroviruses. A large number of other viruses may also produce meningitis; among the more common are herpes simplex type 2 (usually in older children), mumps virus, and lymphocytic choriomeningitis virus. Some of these viruses may also produce an acute encephalitis either concomitantly with or separately from the meningeal infection; the most common of these are herpes simplex virus types 1 and 2 and mumps virus.

Aseptic meningitis is typically characterized by an abrupt onset, a relatively short duration, and a favorable outcome. The usual clinical findings include fever, headache, vomiting, and neck stiffness. Lumbar puncture demonstrates mild spinal fluid pleocytosis, with the type of cellular response varying with the stage of the infection and the specific etiologic agent. Gradual recovery usually occurs within days to weeks of the onset of symptoms.

Imaging studies are not required in uncomplicated cases of viral meningitis. When performed, CT or MRI is normal or shows minimal prominence of extra-axial fluid surrounding the convexities. In those cases of viral meningitis in which there is an associated encephalitis, CT may show subtle low-attenuation parenchymal brain abnormalities. MRI is much more sensitive and demonstrates the areas of edema as regions of abnormal high signal intensity on T_2-weighted images.

Bacterial Meningitis

Acute bacterial meningitis is an important cause of acquired neurologic disease in infants and children. This infection is most often the result of hematogenous spread of organisms from a remote focus directly to the meninges or via the choroid plexus. Other potential mechanisms of infection include rupture of superficial cortical abscesses and contiguous spread from an adjacent extracranial source, such as the paranasal sinuses, middle ear cavities, or mastoid air cells. Different species of bacteria exhibit different abilities to pass from the blood into the meninges.

As a meningeal infection becomes established, polymorphonuclear cells migrate from the bloodstream into the cerebrospinal fluid, and the meninges become inflamed with a polymorphonuclear infiltrate. Further spread of infection may occur along the leptomeningeal sheaths of penetrating cortical vessels in the Virchow-Robin spaces. In the early stages of the infection, the endothelial cells of these cortical vessels become edematous and cause the vessel lumina to narrow. Inflammatory cells may also infiltrate the vessel walls, and foci of necrosis may occur. These changes may progress to the point of causing thrombosis of cortical arteries and veins. This septic thrombosis may also serve as a pathway for extension of infection into the superficial portions of the brain.

The initial signs and symptoms of bacterial meningitis are due to leptomeningeal inflammation and increased intracranial pressure. The findings may include fever, irritability, fullness of the fontanelle, lethargy, stiff neck, headache, seizures, and focal neurologic deficits. Fever may be absent in small infants or debilitated children. Specific signs of meningeal irritation may be absent in young infants. In older children, there is often a history of a preceding upper respiratory or gastrointestinal infection. Because the initial presentation may be subtle or nonspecific, and because of the potential for severe neurologic sequelae of delayed treatment, a high degree of clinical suspicion is essential in the care of all infants and young children exhibiting one or more of the potential signs and symptoms of bacterial meningitis. The diagnosis is readily confirmed in most cases with cerebrospinal fluid obtained by lumbar puncture.[377,378]

The epidemiology of bacterial meningitis shows significant age, seasonal, geographic, and socioeconomic variation. The incidence peaks between 6 and 12-months of age. Only 25% of cases occur after 2 years of age. The prevalence of bacterial meningitis in the United States for children younger than 5 years of age is approximately 87 cases per 100,000 children per year, and for individuals older than 5 years of age the rate is approximately 2.2 cases per 100,000 persons per year. *Hemophilus influenzae* type B meningitis peaks in spring and fall; virtually all other types of bacterial meningitis are more common during the winter months. Significant neurologic sequelae from bacterial meningitis are more common in infants and young children than in adults.[379,380]

The incidence of neonatal meningitis (ie, onset during the first month of life) is approximately 0.4% of live births. There is an increased incidence with prematurity or complicated labor or delivery and in cases of maternal infection. Species of enterobacteria are the most common etiologic agents, particularly *Escherichia coli*, *Proteus mirabilis*, *Klebsiella* species, and *Pseudomonas aeruginosa*. Group B streptococci are the next most common etiologic bacteria. Coagulase-negative staphylococci have emerged as important pathogens, particularly among low–birth weight infants who had intravascular catheters. These infants often demonstrate an insidious onset of signs and symptoms, with the usual findings consisting of irritability, drowsiness, anorexia, and vomiting. Fever may or may not be present and is often minimal and transient.[381]

Beyond the neonatal period, *H influenzae* type B is the most frequent pathogen in childhood bacterial meningitis. *Neisseria meningitidis* and *Streptococcus pneumoniae* are the next most common etiologic agents. *N meningitidis* and *S pneumoniae* are more common than *H influenzae* in children after the age of 10 years.[380,382]

In general, neuroimaging studies are not performed in cases of meningitis unless there are clinical findings that suggest the presence of complications. These clinical findings may include persistent or recurrent fever, focal neurologic deficits, prolonged seizures, signs of increased intracranial pressure, persistence of positive cerebrospinal fluid cultures, or unusual alteration in level of consciousness. In general, CT is suffici-

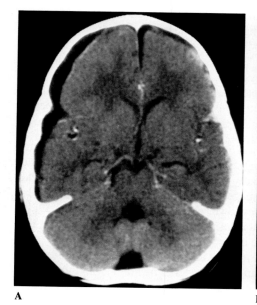
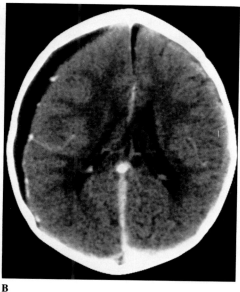

A   B

Fig. 1-140 Subdural effusion in meningitis. (**A** and **B**) Contrast-enhanced CT scans of a child 5 days into the course of treatment for *Hemophilus influenzae* meningitis showing a right subdural fluid collection. A smaller subdural effusion is present in the left frontal region that extends into the interhemispheric subdural space. There is a thin, enhancing membrane along the medial aspect of the right subdural effusion, and there are dilated cortical veins in this region.

ent for evaluation of these children, although MRI is more sensitive for several of the potential complications.

In uncomplicated cases of bacterial meningitis, CT and MRI are usually normal. The most common finding is small, transient, extra-axial fluid collections surrounding the cerebral convexities. Also, contrast-enhanced CT or MRI may show diffuse or focal meningeal enhancement; MRI is of greater sensitivity for this finding than CT. Occasionally, the lateral ventricles appear somewhat small and compressed in the early stages of bacterial meningitis.

Accumulation of fluid in the subdural spaces surrounding the cerebral convexities in cases of bacterial meningitis is most often identified in infants and young children and is less common in older children. It is usually seen during the first week of the illness. The fluid is serosanguineous, has a high protein content, and contains polymorphonuclear cells. In the great majority of cases, the fluid is sterile and therefore represents an effusion rather than an empyema. The fluid collections are usually bilateral but may be somewhat asymmetric. Most often, follow-up neuroimaging examinations show resolution of these subdural effusions. Less commonly, there is progressive enlargement, fibrin organization, or progression to a chronic fluid collection. Rarely, an empyema or extra-axial abscess may develop.

Most subdural effusions in cases of bacterial meningitis are shown on CT as small, extra-axial subdural fluid collections. The effusions usually have attenuation values slightly higher than those of cerebrospinal fluid and are sometimes isodense to brain. Contrast-enhanced images usually show slight enhancement of the underlying meninges (Fig. 1-140). There may also be slight prominence of subarachnoid fluid surrounding the convexities. Although not required in most cases, MRI shows the subdural fluid collections to have the characteristics of complex fluid with high signal intensity on T_2-weighted images and slightly higher intensity than cerebrospinal fluid on

T_1-weighted images. Images obtained after intravenous administration of paramagnetic contrast material frequently show enhancement of an inflammatory membrane along the medial aspect of the fluid collection.[383,384]

One of the important potential complications of bacterial meningitis is hydrocephalus. This complication is probably more common in neonates than older children. Secondary hydrocephalus is most common with meningitis due to *S pneumoniae*, *Staphylococcus aureus*, and enterobacteria and is uncommon with meningococcal and *H influenzae* infections. Communicating hydrocephalus may develop as a result of accumulation of fibropurulent exudate in the basilar cisternae or over the cerebral convexities. If sufficient exudate accumulates in the cerebral aqueduct or the foramina of Luschka and Magendie, noncommunicating hydrocephalus results. Hydrocephalus may also be related, at least in part, to compromised function of the arachnoid villi due to inflammation and narrowing of the sylvian aqueduct due to proliferation of ependymal and glial cells. In some cases hydrocephalus is mild and transient, whereas in others it may progress to the point of requiring diversionary shunting.[385,386]

Concomitant ventriculitis occurs in up to 90% of neonates with bacterial meningitis. This complication occurs in approximately 30% of older children with bacterial meningitis. Ventriculitis is demonstrated on CT or MRI as ventricular dilatation and intense contrast enhancement of the ependyma. Occasionally, fluid-fluid levels are identified in the ventricular system (Fig. 1-141). Intraventricular septations may develop, sometimes causing localized ventricular dilatation.[381,387,388]

The most common parenchymal brain changes in cases of bacterial meningitis are small superficial infarcts that are due to septic thrombophlebitis. Although both arteries and veins may be involved, venous infarcts are probably more common. These small superficial areas of edema may be difficult to demonstrate on CT, on which they are shown as ill-defined,

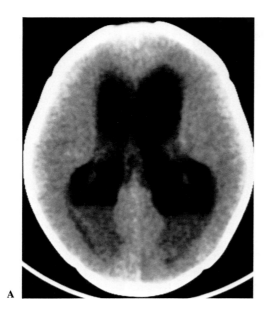

A

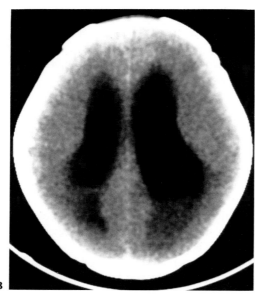

B

Fig. 1-141 Pyocephalus. (**A** and **B**) Unenhanced axial CT scans of a child being treated for *Escherichia coli* meningitis showing moderate hydrocephalus. Fluid-fluid levels are present in the lateral ventricles; these are due to severe ventriculitis. There are subtle areas of decreased attenuation in the frontal periventricular regions as a result of transependymal flow of cerebrospinal fluid. There is evidence of increased intracranial pressure with compression of the cerebral sulci and spreading of the cranial sutures.

ment of the clot and intense enhancement of dural collateral vessels, producing the delta sign. On MRI, venous sinus thrombosis is usually demonstrated as abnormally high signal on T_1-weighted images. During the acute phase, however, the thrombus produces lower signal intensity but can usually be differentiated from the absent signal of flowing blood. The diagnosis may be confirmed on angiography.[391]

Large cerebral infarcts are uncommon but potentially devastating complications of bacterial meningitis. In most cases, these are presumably caused by septic thrombosis or vascular spasm of major cerebral arteries. CT and MRI demonstrate sharply marginated regions of edema that conform to an arterial vascular territory. Also, smaller lacunar infarcts may be identified in the brainstem and basal ganglia; these are due to involvement of the smaller peripheral vessels. Subsequent studies in children with large arterial infarcts may show the development of regional atrophy or porencephaly. Occasionally, calcifications may develop in the areas of ischemia.[392]

Progression of septic thrombophlebitis to cerebritis and brain abscess is a rare complication of bacterial meningitis. Cerebritis is demonstrated on CT and MRI as an irregular area of edema and heterogeneous contrast enhancement. A brain abscess is demonstrated as a heterogeneous mass that causes displacement of adjacent structures. This is usually best demonstrated on contrast-enhanced images, which show irregular contrast enhancement and edema surrounding the nonenhancing central fluid component.[393]

Tuberculous Meningitis

Tuberculous meningitis is now an uncommon disease in the developed countries but remains an important cause of central nervous system infectious disease in many parts of the world. Tuberculous meningitis is most often due to hematogenous dissemination of tubercle bacilli from a primary tuberculous lesion elsewhere in the body, usually in the lung. Meningeal involvement may also result from rupture of a tuberculoma in the meninges or superficial portion of the cerebral cortex. The meninges become thickened and infiltrated, and a gelatinous exudate fills the basal cisternae. The exudate is often particularly prominent in the prepontine cisterna and may cause extraventricular obstructive hydrocephalus. The meninges, brain, choroid plexus, and ependyma may contain multiple small tuberculomas. In approximately 50% of cases, a perivasculitis involves the lenticulostriate and thalamoperforating arteries.[394]

The incidence of tuberculous meningitis roughly parallels the prevalence of tuberculosis in the community. The inci-

low-attenuation areas involving peripheral gray and white matter. There may be evidence of mild mass effect. Contrast enhancement in the region is sometimes identified. Petechial hemorrhage is visible in the lesion in some cases. MRI is quite sensitive for the detection of superficial infarcts, demonstrating ill-defined areas of edema with prolonged T_1- and T_2-relaxation times.[389,390] Follow-up scans may show a return to a normal appearance or the development of localized areas of peripheral atrophy.

Thrombosis of larger venous structures, such as the superior sagittal sinus, is much less common. During the acute phase, thrombosis of an intracranial venous sinus is identified on CT as an abnormal high-attenuation appearance of the sinus. Over the next few days, the thrombus becomes isodense to brain. Contrast-enhanced scans at this point show lack of enhance-

dence is highest during the first 5 years of life, although tuberculous meningitis is rare before 3 months of age. Involvement of the central nervous system is the most common cause of death due to tuberculosis.[395]

The initial manifestations of tuberculous meningitis are often vague and nonspecific. Many children exhibit several weeks of prodromal symptoms such as apathy, anorexia, or headache. This may be followed by alteration of consciousness, low-grade fever, nausea, vomiting, headache of increasing severity, and abdominal pain. During the more advanced stages, the clinical findings may include coma, seizures, cranial nerve palsy, and cardiac or respiratory alterations. The mortality due to tuberculous meningitis approaches 10% to 20%. Permanent neurologic sequelae such as cranial nerve dysfunction are common.[396]

The predominant finding on imaging studies in cases of tuberculous meningitis is filling of the basal cisternae by fibropurulent exudate. In the acute stage, CT shows homogeneous material of moderate attenuation values filling the basal cisternae. This usually shows marked contrast enhancement. The abnormality may extend into the sylvian fissures and cortical sulci. This exudate is usually best demonstrated with MRI on T_1-weighted images, on which it is shown as material that is of higher signal intensity than clear cerebrospinal fluid. As with CT, intense enhancement usually occurs with intravenous paramagnetic contrast material. CT and MRI frequently show some degree of hydrocephalus due to obstruction of the extra-axial cerebrospinal fluid pathways by the thick exudate.[397,398]

Some element of parenchymal brain involvement is common in cases of tuberculous meningitis. Miliary tuberculous emboli tend to be located at the gray matter–white matter junctions in the brain. These are shown on CT as small, ill-defined, low-attenuation areas that enhance with intravenous contrast agents. MRI is of greater sensitivity for the detection of these lesions and demonstrates T_1 and T_2 prolongation and enhancement with paramagnetic contrast material. One or more large parenchymal tuberculomas are occasionally present. Supratentorial tuberculomas tend to be multiple; posterior fossa tuberculomas are usually solitary. There is usually evidence of significant mass effect, although surrounding edema is typically minimal. On CT, tuberculomas may mimic a cerebral neoplasm. The appearance is somewhat variable. Tuberculomas less than 2 cm in diameter typically are solid and show uniform contrast enhancement. Those that are greater than 2 cm in diameter tend to have a somewhat heterogeneous necrotic center and a thick peripheral rim of enhancement. Similar findings are demonstrated on MRI, with the lesion producing prolongation of T_1- and T_2-relaxation values and viable portions enhancing fairly intensely with paramagnetic contrast material.[399,400]

Involvement of the lenticulostriate and thalamoperforating arteries in cases of tuberculous meningitis frequently leads to small infarcts in the basal ganglia and thalamus. These appear as nonenhancing, low-attenuation areas on CT. MRI is much more sensitive for the detection of these infarcts and demonstrates areas that are hypointense on T_1-weighted images and hyperintense on T_2-weighted images. Similar lesions may be identified elsewhere in the brain; these are due to cortical infarcts from thrombosis of cortical vessels.

Subdural and Epidural Abscesses

Pyogenic infection in the subdural or epidural spaces is termed an empyema. In children, it is usually produced by direct extension from a contiguous source, such as purulent sinusitis or otitis media. Peripheral extension of a bacterial meningitis may also cause empyema. Other potential sources include orbital cellulitis, penetrating trauma, osteomyelitis of the skull, hematogenous dissemination in sepsis, congenital osseous defects allowing contamination from external organisms, and secondary infection of a subdural effusion. An epidural abscess is the most common intracranial complication of bacterial sinusitis. The clinical manifestations of subdural or epidural abscesses may include focal neurologic findings, seizures, or signs of increased intracranial pressure.

On CT, a subdural or epidural abscess is usually demonstrated as a crescentic, extra-axial fluid collection that most often has attenuation values slightly higher than those of cerebrospinal fluid but lower than those of normal brain. On MRI, the fluid collection most often is slightly hyperintense to cerebrospinal fluid on both T_1- and T_2-weighted images. After infusion of contrast material for CT or MRI, there is often an enhancing capsule or pseudocapsule along the internal margin of the lesion (Fig. 1-142). In general, a localized subdural effusion due to meningitis cannot be reliably differentiated from an empyema with imaging studies.

Frequently, imaging studies may not allow precise localization of the abscess to the subdural or epidural spaces. If the fluid collection is near the midline, parafalcine extension indicates a subdural location. An empyema in the frontal epidural space frequently crosses the midline anterior to the falx, whereas a subdural fluid collection in a similar location will be restricted by the falx at the midline.[398,401,402]

Bacterial Cerebritis and Brain Abscess

Bacterial infection of the brain parenchyma may occur by one of three mechanisms: hematogenous inoculation from a distant site of infection; extension from a contiguous infection of the meninges, skull, or paranasal sinuses; or inoculation via a penetrating head wound. Children with a right-to-left intracardiac shunt or left heart endocarditis are at increased risk for cerebritis and brain abscess.

Cerebritis due to hematogenous inoculation tends to be localized at the junction of the gray and white matter. Lesions due to direct spread from an adjacent focus tend to be located superficially and adjacent to the extracerebral infectious abnormality.

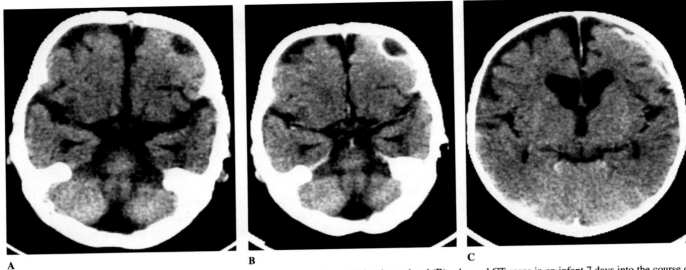

A   **B**   **C**

Fig. 1-142 Acute subdural abscess as a complication of bacterial meningitis. **(A)** Unenhanced and **(B)** enhanced CT scans in an infant 7 days into the course of treatment for *Hemophilus influenzae* meningitis show a nonenhancing, low-attenuation, left subdural fluid collection. There is intense enhancement of the meninges surrounding this lesion. **(C)** More superior image shows thickened, intensely enhancing meninges adjacent to the left frontal and temporal lobes. The extra-axial spaces are prominent in the right frontal region as well, although there is no abnormal enhancement in this area.

Once organisms gain access to the brain parenchyma, the initial lesion is cerebritis or septic encephalitis. The brain tissue becomes edematous and infiltrated with inflammatory cells. Petechial hemorrhages may be present. In the absence of therapeutic intervention, the center of the infected area becomes necrotic, and a cavity is formed. The walls of the cavity are at first poorly formed but gradually become thicker and more solid. There may be extensive cerebral edema surrounding the capsule. The outer layer of the capsule consists of thin inflammatory granulation tissue that progressively becomes thicker with time. Eventually, a thick collagenous capsule develops. Brain abscesses often exhibit a tendency to enlarge medially into the softer and less vascularized white matter, and the medial aspect of the capsule may be less well formed than the peripheral aspect. Occasionally, the abscess will rupture into the ventricular system. In neonates and young infants, there tends to be relatively poor capsule formation in response to a cerebral abscess.[403,404]

A number of signs and symptoms may be produced by cerebritis or brain abscess. Frequently, there is subacute development of headache, confusion, and a depressed level of consciousness. Nuchal rigidity may occur if there is meningeal inflammation. Seizures, papilledema, and focal neurologic signs may occur. Fever, if present, is often minimal or transient. Anaerobic bacteria account for approximately 70% of brain abscesses, and multiple organisms may be present. Common bacterial pathogens include microaerophilic or anaerobic streptococci, *Staphylococcus aureus, Streptococcus pneumoniae, Proteus* species, *Hemophilus influenzae, H aphrophilus,* and *Bacteroides fragilis.*

Neonates and young infants with cerebritis or brain abscess tend to present with one of two clinical syndromes. Most often, there is an acute or subacute appearance of signs of increased intracranial pressure. Less often, there is an acute onset of the signs and symptoms of fulminating bacterial meningitis. The most common organisms isolated from neonates with brain abscess are *Citrobacter* and *Proteus* species. Most are located supratentorially, with the frontal lobes being most often affected. An abscess in the cerebellum may accompany severe otitis media or be associated with a dermal sinus.[405,406]

Neuroimaging is essential in both diagnosing and monitoring cerebritis and brain abscess. In the early stages of cerebritis, CT demonstrates an ill-defined, heterogeneous area of low attenuation in the brain parenchyma. There is usually evidence of mass effect. Irregular contrast enhancement is common. In the later stages, CT may show a ring-enhancement pattern, even though a true abscess cavity may not have formed. Within 4 to 6 weeks of the initial infection, liquefaction and encapsulation usually occur. At this point, CT shows a heterogeneous area that is usually of lower attenuation than normal brain. The peripheral aspect enhances intensely with intravenous contrast medium, and there is usually considerable edema surrounding the enhancing portion (Fig. 1-143). A fluid-fluid level is sometimes demonstrated (Fig. 1-144). Occasionally an abscess is multilocular, or contiguous satellite abscesses are identified. Classically, cerebral abscesses develop at the gray matter–white matter junction. The inner margin of the capsule tends to be smooth and regular, and the peripheral aspect has a more irregular appearance. In about 50% of cases, the medial aspect of the capsule is thinner than the peripheral aspect.[407–410]

On MRI, cerebritis is identified as an area of somewhat heterogeneous hyperintensity on T_2-weighted images. In the later stages of cerebritis, the peripheral aspect of the lesion tends to be relatively hyperintense on T_1-weighted images and

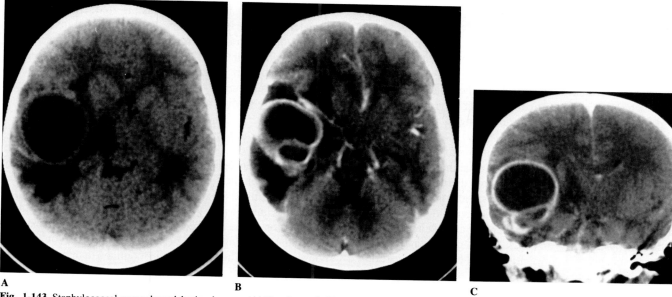

Fig. 1-143 Staphylococcal parenchymal brain abscess. (**A**) Unenhanced CT scan in a child with cyanotic heart disease demonstrates a well-defined, low-attenuation mass in the right temporal lobe surrounded by a thin rim that is of slightly higher attenuation. There are marked edema in the adjacent portions of the brain and significant mass effect. (**B** and **C**) Contrast-enhanced CT scans show intense enhancement of the periphery of the abscess. There is a septation inferiorly and posteriorly that produces a multilocular configuration.

slightly hypointense on T_2-weighted images; the central portion is heterogeneous and produces high signal intensity on T_2-weighted images. During the early formation of a true abscess, the wall is often hyperintense on both T_1- and T_2-weighted images, and the center is uniformly hypointense on T_1-weighted images and hyperintense on T_2-weighted images.

With a mature abscess, the wall is isointense on T_1-weighted images and markedly hypointense on T_2-weighted images. The necrotic central portion is isointense or slightly hypointense on T_1-weighted images and hyperintense on T_2-weighted images. The contrast enhancement pattern of cerebritis and cerebral abscesses with paramagnetic contrast material is similar to that identified with CT.[411,412]

Encephalitis

Viral Encephalitis

Encephalitis may result from a great variety of viruses. Brain involvement may occur in conjunction with meningitis, as an isolated infection, or as a component of a systemic infection. Also, encephalitis may be produced by direct viral cytotoxicity or as a secondary phenomenon related to the immunologic reaction of the host to the virus. This last phenomenon is termed viral leukoencephalitis.

The most common type of direct cytotoxic viral infection of the central nervous system is herpes simplex encephalitis. In newborns, this is most often due to infection with type 2 herpes simplex virus; type 1 herpes simplex encephalitis is usually seen in older children and adults. Type 2 herpes simplex encephalitis is usually a multisystem disease, with intracranial dissemination occurring via a hematogenous route. Type 1 herpes simplex encephalitis more often occurs as an isolated infection.

There are a number of epidemic encephalitides, most of which are arthropod borne. These usually show a seasonal distribution and are most common during the summer and fall.

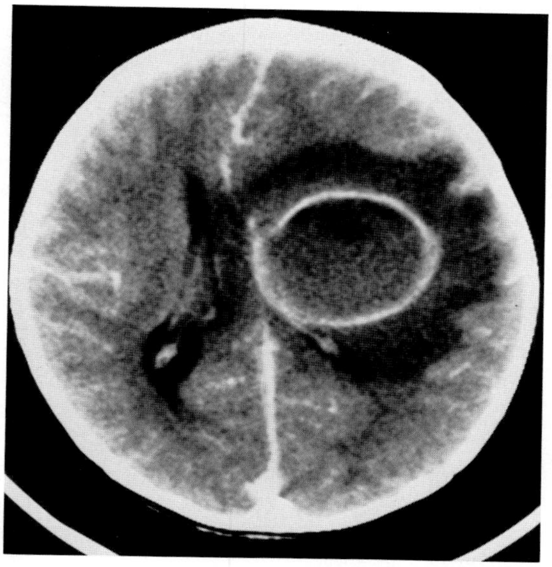

Fig. 1-144 Contrast-enhanced CT scan showing a parenchymal brain abscess in the left parietal lobe. There are an intensely enhancing pseudocapsule and extensive edema in the parietal lobe adjacent to the mass. Layering of debris in the dependent portion of the abscess produces the appearance of a fluid-fluid level. *Staphylococcus aureus* was isolated from the abscess cavity.

The epidemic encephalitides are usually caused by arboviruses and Bunyamwera viruses.

Encephalitis occurring as a complication of viral meningitis (ie, meningoencephalitis) tends to be relatively benign and usually carries a good prognosis. These viral meningoencephalitides are often associated with the childhood exanthems, such as mumps or varicella. Coxsackievirus, nonparalytic polio, and lymphocytic choriomeningitis may also produce viral meningoencephalitis.

Viral encephalitis with coexistent meningitis may be clinically indistinguishable from aseptic meningitis. With sufficient involvement of brain parenchyma, there may be severe alterations in the level of consciousness, abnormal behavior, emotional lability, seizures, and focal neurologic signs. In some cases, there is a period of irritability and excitement that is followed by lethargy or coma. Signs of increased intracranial pressure are often present. Signs of brainstem dysfunction occasionally occur. Some viruses, such as the herpes zoster varicellosus virus, may preferentially involve the cerebellum and produce ataxia. Other viruses that may cause a localized cerebellitis include mumps virus, polio virus, Epstein-Barr virus, coxsackievirus, echoviruses, enteroviruses, and measles virus.[413]

Viral encephalitis is demonstrated on CT as one or more ill-defined regions of decreased attenuation in the brain parenchyma (Fig. 1-145). MRI is much more sensitive for detecting these subtle edematous changes and demonstrates regions of high signal intensity on T_2-weighted images. With herpes simplex type 1 encephalitis, the abnormality tends to be localized to the anteromedial portion of the temporal lobe. Extension into the insular cortex is common. The lenticular nucleus tends to be spared. The orbital surface of the frontal lobe, particularly the gyrus rectus, is frequently involved. Unilateral disease is most common, but bilateral involvement may occur. A gyral pattern of contrast enhancement may be identified on either CT or MRI. Occasionally, unenhanced CT shows small foci of high attenuation, which are due to petechial hemorrhage. After resolution of the acute infection, neuroimaging studies may show regional atrophy.[414–417]

Rasmussen Encephalitis

Rasmussen encephalitis is a rare disease characterized by chronic encephalitis, progressive neurologic deficits, and focal intractable seizure activity. Although the precise etiology is unknown, a viral etiology is suspected. Histologic examination of the affected portion of the brain demonstrates inflammatory changes with perivascular lymphocytic infiltration and gliosis. These findings are confined to or predominant in one hemisphere.

The median age at diagnosis of Rasmussen encephalitis is 5 years; presentation occurs during the first decade of life in approximately 85% of patients. There is a history of an infectious or inflammatory illness in the patient or one or more close family members immediately before the clinical presentation in about two-thirds of cases. The predominant clinical finding is intractable seizure activity. The seizures are usually unilateral, and there may be progressive hemiparesis. Other clinical findings may include hemianopsia, dysphagia, and mental deterioration.

Neuroimaging in cases of Rasmussen encephalitis demonstrates progressive unilateral cerebral atrophy. The lateral ventricles in the involved hemisphere become progressively enlarged, and the sulci become increasingly prominent. MRI

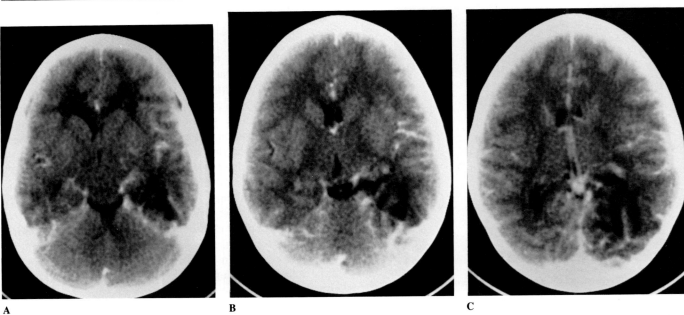

A   **B**   **C**

Fig. 1-145 Herpes simplex type 1 encephalitis. (**A**, **B**, and **C**) Contrast-enhanced CT scans showing low-attenuation edematous changes in the left occipital and temporal lobes. The basal ganglia are not involved. There is slight mass effect with shift of the midline structures toward the right.

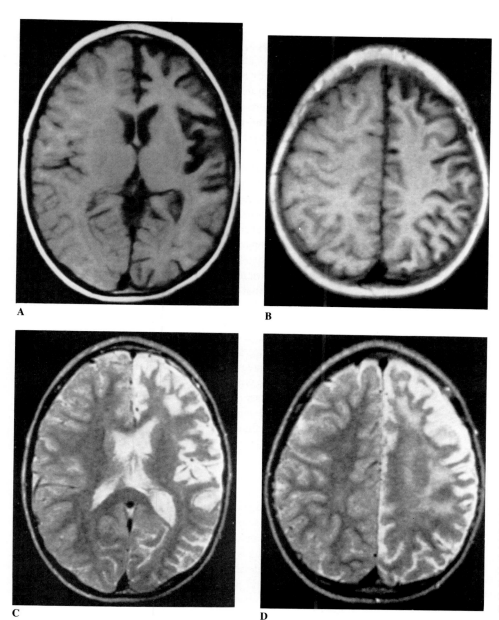

A

B

C

D

Fig. 1-146 Rasmussen encephalitis. (**A** and **B**) T_1-weighted axial MR scans demonstrate prominence of the sulci and the left cerebral hemisphere, reflecting atrophy. The right hemisphere is normal. (**C** and **D**) T_2-weighted axial MR scans show slight atrophic enlargement of the left lateral ventricle. There is high signal from cerebrospinal fluid in the prominent sulci from atrophy. There is also high-signal abnormality in the white matter of the left hemisphere.

shows increased signal intensity in white and gray matter in the affected hemisphere on T_2-weighted images (Fig. 1-146). Iodine-123–labeled iofetamine used as a tracer in brain imaging with single-photon emission CT shows decreased accumulation in the involved hemisphere. Potentially, a hypermetabolic seizure focus can produce increased tracer accumulation; this finding has been demonstrated on positron emission tomography.[418]

Subacute Sclerosing Panencephalitis

Subacute sclerosing panencephalitis is a rare disease that appears to be a reactivation of measles virus infection years after the initial illness or years after vaccination with the modified measles virus. The age at onset ranges from 3 to 20 years with a mean of approximately 7 years. In most patients, there is a history of prior measles infection, most often before the age of 3 years. Subacute sclerosing panencephalitis is characterized clinically by the insidious onset of behavior changes and mental deterioration. Speech and sleep disorders are also frequent early signs. Subsequently, ataxia, myoclonus, pyramidal and extrapyramidal hypertonia, and seizures may develop. Cerebrospinal fluid obtained by lumbar puncture demonstrates the presence of antibodies to measles virus.

Neuroimaging studies in cases of subacute sclerosing panencephalitis are nonspecific and are frequently normal during the early phases of the disorder. Ill-defined foci of low attenuation on CT and of high signal intensity on T_2-weighted MR images may be identified in the periventricular and subcortical

Table 1-7 Fungal Pathogens in Central Nervous System Disease

Pathogens in Normal Hosts	Pathogens in Immunocompromised Hosts
Blastomyces dermatitidis	Cryptococcus neoformans
Coccidioides immitis	Actinomyces israelii
Cryptococcus neoformans	Aspergillus fumigatus
Histoplasma capsulatum	Candida albicans
Nocardia asteroides	Phycomycosis (mucormycosis)
Paracoccidioides brasiliensis	

white matter within a few weeks of the clinical onset. During the acute phases, CT and MRI may show ventricular compression and obliteration of the cortical sulci. No areas of abnormal contrast enhancement are identified. Eventually, generalized cerebral atrophy is identified.[419–421]

Fungal Infections

Central nervous system involvement with fungal infections (Table 1-7) may be in the form of meningitis, cerebritis, brain abscess, or granulomatous disease. The type of infection produced in individual patients is related to the intensity and type of exposure, the virulence of the organism, and the resistance of the host. In general, fungal infections of the central nervous system can be divided into two major categories: disease caused by fungi that are capable of infecting previously healthy individuals, and disease caused by saprophytes in individuals whose resistance to infection is compromised. Opportunistic infections of the central nervous system with saprophytic fungi may occur in children with chronic diseases such as a neoplasm or diabetes or in conjunction with the prolonged use of chemotherapy, corticosteroids, or antibiotics. They also occur with increased incidence among children with acquired immunodeficiency syndrome. In many cases, the clinical manifestations of central nervous system fungal infections are quite subtle.[422]

Cryptococcosis

Cryptococcosis (torulosis) is the most prevalent fungal infection of the central nervous system. It is rarely seen in otherwise healthy individuals. It most often occurs as an opportunistic infection in immunosuppressed patients, debilitated individuals with cancer or diabetes, those treated with corticosteroids or chemotherapy, and, most commonly, patients with acquired immunodeficiency syndrome. *Cryptococcus neoformans* is an encapsulated yeast that is often harbored in bird feces, particularly that of pigeons. Human exposure is usually via inhalation or ingestion. The lung is the initial site of disease, after which hematogenous dissemination may occur to a number of organs and systems, including the central nervous system. The involvement of the central nervous system is most often in the form of meningitis, but abscess formation or granulomatous disease may also occur.

The clinical features of cryptococcosis are often nonspecific and include nausea, vomiting, headache, and, in about 60% of patients, fever. Central nervous system involvement is most often suggested by meningeal signs, although these manifestations are not identified in up to half the patients. Other findings may include signs of increased intracranial pressure, focal neurologic signs, or cranial nerve palsies. The diagnosis is established by laboratory analysis of the cerebrospinal fluid.[423,424]

Cryptococcal meningitis typically produces a thick exudate that is most prominent in the basilar cisternae. CT and MRI may show thickened tissue in the basal cisternae that exhibits marked enhancement with intravenous contrast materials. Hydrocephalus is common. Vascular involvement may result in ischemic changes, as are identified with other forms of severe meningitis. The choroid plexus is commonly involved, resulting in ventriculitis. This is imaged as ventricular enlargement and abnormal ependymal enhancement. Intraventricular septations may be identified. Cryptococcosis occasionally produces trapping of the temporal horn. Rarely, a brain abscess or intraparenchymal granuloma is identified; this is demonstrated as a parenchymal mass that may enhance throughout or have a peripheral ring pattern of enhancement. In some patients with cryptococcosis, intraparenchymal gelatinous pseudocysts occur. They have a predilection for occurring in the basal ganglia. On MRI, they appear as multilocular cystic masses that have prolonged T_1- and T_2-relaxation times.[424–427]

Coccidioidomycosis

Coccidioidomycosis is caused by the fungus *Coccidioides immitis*. The disease is acquired by inhalation of spore-laden dust or transcutaneously after skin disruption. Infection of the central nervous system is an uncommon complication acquired secondarily via hematogenous spread of a systemic infection. Central nervous system involvement appears to be particularly common with skin lesions about the nose. Endemic areas for coccidioidomycosis include the southwestern United States, northern Mexico, and portions of Central and South America. Symptoms in the presence of central nervous system coccidioidomycosis include headache, low-grade fever, weight loss, obtundation, and meningeal signs.[428]

Involvement of the central nervous system with coccidioidomycosis is in the form of meningitis. The leptomeninges become thickened and congested, and multiple granulomas develop. Osteomyelitis of the skull may occur.

The imaging findings in meningeal coccidioidomycosis are relatively nonspecific. CT and MRI show thickened meninges and exudate filling the basal cisternae and a variable degree of involvement of other cisternal spaces. There is usually marked contrast enhancement in these areas. Hydrocephalus is common and results from either extraventricular obstruction of the cisternal spaces or intraventricular obstruction due to ependymitis. The identification of parenchymal brain lesions is

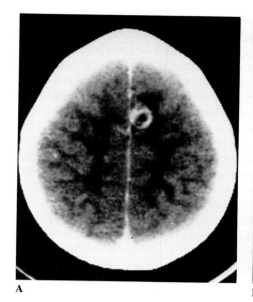
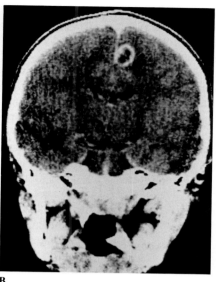

A   B

Fig. 1-147 Blastomycosis. (**A**) Axial and (**B**) coronal contrast-enhanced CT scans show a small, low-attenuation abscess in the left hemisphere adjacent to the falx. There is an irregular, intensely enhancing rim and minimal adjacent edema. This abscess is due to hematogenous dissemination of pulmonary blastomycosis.

unusual. Small infarcts due to vasculitis may occur, but these are relatively rare.[429]

Blastomycosis

Blastomycosis is caused by the dimorphic saprophytic fungus *Blastomyces dermatitidis*. Human infection occurs after inhalation of airborne spores from contaminated soil, which reach the lower respiratory tract. They become converted to the yeast form after a long incubation period and establish a primary pulmonary infection. Dissemination can occur from a focus of chronic pulmonary infection.

The central nervous system is rarely involved in blastomycosis. When it is involved, the infection is most often in the form of a small, localized brain abscess or intraparenchymal granuloma. The signs and symptoms are nonspecific and include fever, which may be low grade, and seizures.

Neuroimaging studies in cases of central nervous system blastomycosis may demonstrate an abscess as a small- to moderate-size area of low density on CT and of low signal on T_1-weighted and high signal on T_2-weighted MR images. Lesions usually show intense enhancement with contrast material, often in a ringlike fashion (Fig. 1-147).

Candidiasis

Involvement of the central nervous system in candidiasis may occur in the form of meningitis; brain abscess; or large, small, or miliary granulomas. Central nervous system candidiasis is usually a sequela of disseminated disease in a debilitated patient. In children, it is most often seen as a complication of immune suppression, prolonged antibiotic or corticosteroid therapy, extensive burns, or surgery. Neonates and young infants are at increased risk for the development of candidal infection in the presence of congenital anomalies, shunted hydrocephalus, meconium ileus, or infected venous catheters.[430,431]

Neuroimaging studies in cases of central nervous system candidiasis show various findings, depending on the nature of the disease. Candidal meningitis is shown on CT and MRI as thickened meninges and exudate in the basal cisternae and marked enhancement of these areas with intravenous contrast media. Cerebral candidiasis in debilitated patients may produce a diffuse cerebritis and widespread microabscesses. These are demonstrated on CT and MRI as multiple, ill-defined areas of edema with or without appreciable contrast enhancement. When the fungus invades the brain primarily, it often progresses to gross abscess formation; this is imaged as a thick-walled abscess with poorly defined margins.

Rickettsial Disease

The important rickettsial diseases include Rocky Mountain spotted fever, epidemic typhus, murine typhus, Q fever, rickettsialpox, and scrub typhus. With the exception of Q fever, which is airborne, the rickettsial diseases are transmitted by arthropod vectors. Rodents and humans are reservoirs for the organism. Most of these infections are accompanied by a skin eruption. Involvement of the central nervous system occurs in more than 90% of rickettsial infections. The clinical manifestations and pathologic changes of central nervous system rickettsial infections are virtually identical with all the rickettsial species, differing only in severity.[432]

Rocky Mountain spotted fever is the most prevalent rickettsial disease in North America. The infecting organism, *Rickettsia rickettsii*, gains access to the circulation of the host from a tick bite. After entering the body, the rickettsiae multiply and disrupt the endothelial cells of capillaries and arteries. Small vessel involvement in the brain results in subarachnoid hemorrhage and microscopic cerebral infarctions. Meningeal irritation also occurs. With healing, fibrotic and gliotic changes occur, and focal nodules develop in the white matter.

Rocky Mountain spotted fever is prevalent across wide geographic areas. It has been identified throughout North and South America and is particularly common in the Rocky Mountain and Piedmont regions. The symptoms are quite variable. Fever, malaise, lethargy, and headache are common. A petechial rash is present at some point during the course. Some patients have only mild symptoms, whereas in others there is a rapid and fatal course. With fulminating disease, patients may experience shock, coma, and general or focal neurologic impairment. MRI demonstrates focal or multifocal edema as areas of high signal intensity on T_2-weighted images.[433,434]

Parasitic Infections

The central nervous system may be involved in a number of parasitic infections. In some cases, there is direct invasion from the circulatory or lymphatic systems, resulting in inflammation, edema, or granuloma formation. Involvement of the central nervous system may also occur in the form of immunologic or hypersensitivity effects.[435]

Parasitic infections of the central nervous system may be produced by various organisms (Table 1-8). These parasitic organisms are divided into four broad classifications on the basis of morphology. The protozoa are monocellular organisms. The trematodes (flukes) are nonsegmented worms that possess a digestive tract. The cestodes are tapeworms that have no epidermis or digestive tract. The nematodes are cylindric, nonsegmented worms.

Cysticercosis

Cysticercosis is caused by ingestion of the larvae of the pork tapeworm *Taenia solium*. About two-thirds of cases are due to *Cysticercus cellulosae* and one-third to *C racemose*. The ingested ova hatch in the stomach, and the organisms are transported into the intestine, where they pierce the intestinal wall and gain access to the circulation. They enter the larval

stage in subcutaneous tissue, muscle, and brain. Infection of the brain may occur in the meninges, ventricles, or brain parenchyma. The larvae, or cysticerci, may cause cyst formation in the ventricles, cisternae, or brain parenchyma. The meninges may become edematous and thickened, and a purulent exudate may form when one or more cysts rupture and the contents initiate an intense inflammatory response.

Cysticercosis occurs worldwide but is rare in the United States and Canada. The disease is most common in Mexico, Latin America, eastern Europe, Asia, Africa, Spain, and Portugal. The clinical presentation is somewhat variable, and neurologic manifestations of the disease may be delayed for years after the initial infection. Seizures are the most common manifestation of brain involvement, occurring in up to 90% of patients. Other findings may include occipital headache, vomiting, vertigo, and progressive obtundation. Papilledema, hemiparesis, and sensory disturbances have also been reported.[436–438]

Leptomeningitis due to central nervous system cysticercosis is demonstrated on neuroimaging studies as meningeal thickening, predominantly in the basilar cisternae. There is marked enhancement on contrast-enhanced scans. As with other forms of severe leptomeningitis, extraventricular obstructive hydrocephalus and small cerebral infarcts may be identified.

Intracranial cysticerci are most often located in the brain parenchyma. They can be either solid or cystic. CT often demonstrates punctate calcifications in the presence of a solid lesion. A cystic lesion is demonstrated as a relatively low-attenuation center with a rim of prominent enhancement on both CT and MRI. On unenhanced MRI, the cystic component is hypointense on T_1-weighted images and hyperintense on T_2-weighted images. When the cysticerci die, the lesion usually exhibits homogeneous enhancement. Both solid and cystic cysticerci tend to be located in the gray matter. There is often surrounding edema that is best visualized on MRI (Fig. 1-148). A dead cysticercus larva may eventually become completely calcified, and, as the local inflammatory process subsides, contrast enhancement will no longer be identified. It is estimated that this process of calcification may take up to 4 to 7 years.[439,440]

Intraventricular cysticerci may produce acute ventricular obstruction. The CT and MR characteristics of the contents of the cyst usually are nearly identical to those of the adjacent cerebrospinal fluid. The cyst wall is usually quite thin. The scolex of the parasite produces a nodule of soft tissue density in the cyst. The scolex is often best visualized on T_1-weighted MR scans.

Multilobular nonviable cysts may occur in the cerebral cisternae. These are termed racemose cysts. Although these cysts lack an organism with a scolex and are sterile, they may progressively increase in size. Racemose cysts may measure up to several centimeters in diameter. These lesions are most often located in the suprasellar region, the cerebellopontine angle cisterna, and the basilar cisternae. CT demonstrates one or more large cystic lesions that may enhance with intravenous contrast media. There are multiple septations in the cyst that

Table 1-8 Parasites That May Cause Central Nervous System Disease in Children

Protozoa	Trematodes	Cestodes	Nematodes
Toxoplasma gondii	*Schistosoma* spp	*Taenia* spp	*Toxocara* spp
Entamoeba histolytica	*Paragonimus* spp	*Diphyllobothrium* spp	*Angiostrongylus* spp
Trypanosoma spp		*Multiceps* spp	*Trichinella* spp
Naegleria spp		*Echinococcus* spp	
Plasmodium spp			
Babesia spp			

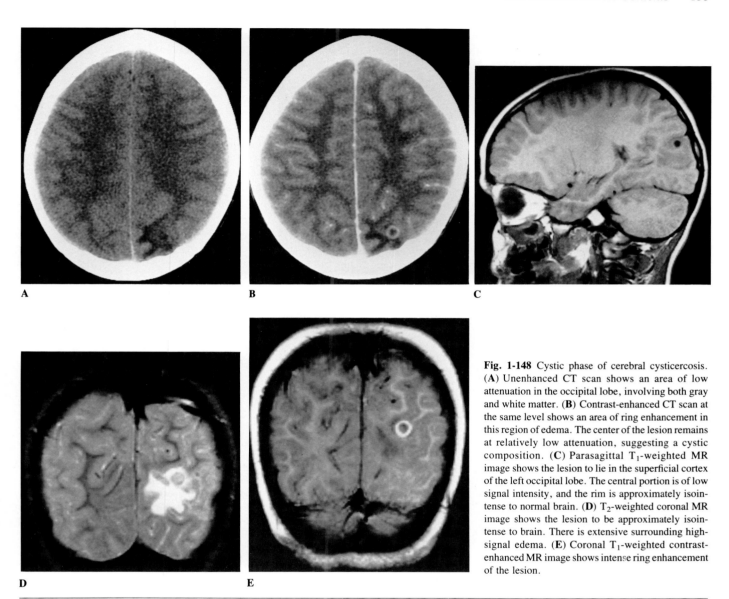

Fig. 1-148 Cystic phase of cerebral cysticercosis. (A) Unenhanced CT scan shows an area of low attenuation in the occipital lobe, involving both gray and white matter. (B) Contrast-enhanced CT scan at the same level shows an area of ring enhancement in this region of edema. The center of the lesion remains at relatively low attenuation, suggesting a cystic composition. (C) Parasagittal T_1-weighted MR image shows the lesion to lie in the superficial cortex of the left occipital lobe. The central portion is of low signal intensity, and the rim is approximately isointense to normal brain. (D) T_2-weighted coronal MR image shows the lesion to be approximately isointense to brain. There is extensive surrounding high-signal edema. (E) Coronal T_1-weighted contrast-enhanced MR image shows intense ring enhancement of the lesion.

are often best identified on T_1-weighted MR scans. Chronic meningitis may result from cyst rupture and meningeal inflammation.[439–441]

Echinococcosis

Echinococcosis, or hydatid disease, is an important health problem that occurs throughout the world. There are two major forms, both of which result in the formation of cystic lesions in one or more organ systems. *Echinococcus granulosus* infestation usually results in the formation of a unilocular cyst, and *E multilocularis* infestation causes formation of a multiloculated cyst. *E multilocularis* is most prevalent in Canada, Alaska, Germany, central Europe, Italy, the Soviet Union, and Switzerland. *E granulosus* is distributed globally. Canines are the definitive hosts for *Echinococcus* organisms; humans are accidental intermediate hosts.

Cerebral involvement occurs in only 2% to 3% of cases of echinococcosis. Cerebral infection is much more frequent in children than in adults, however. Cerebral involvement most often occurs in the form of a solitary hydatid cyst that is usually located in the white matter. Mild inflammatory and gliotic reaction occurs in the cerebral tissue adjacent to the cyst. Cerebral hydatid cysts are often quite large at the time of diagnosis. There is generally a slow rate of growth, and the onset of signs and symptoms may be insidious. Mass effect from the cyst may produce signs of increased intracranial pressure or focal neurologic impairment. Most pediatric cases of cerebral hydatid cyst are diagnosed after the age of 6 years.[442,443]

CT and MRI demonstrate a cerebral hydatid cyst as a homogeneous round or oval mass, most often in the hemispheric white matter. The contents of the cyst have imaging characteristics similar to those of cerebrospinal fluid. On CT,

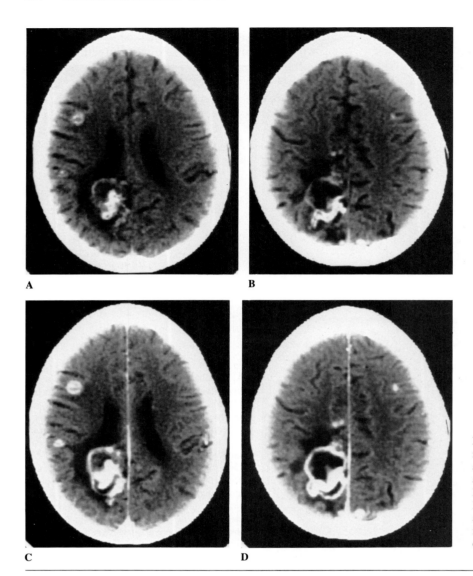

A

B

C

D

Fig. 1-149 Multiple brain abscesses due to toxoplasmosis in an immunosuppressed child with leukemia. (A and B) Unenhanced CT scans show multiple, high-attenuation lesions in both cerebral hemispheres. The larger lesion in the posterior right parietal lobe also has a low-attenuation component, and there is edema in the adjacent white matter. (C and D) Images obtained after intravenous administration of contrast material show enhancement of the solid components of these lesions.

the surrounding compressed cerebral tissue may show slightly higher attenuation values than normal brain. Also, there may be slight enhancement in this region with intravenous contrast medium. Increased attenuation of the cyst contents suggests hemorrhage or superinfection. Rarely, a multiloculated hydatid cyst is identified. Multiple cysts are rare. Calcifications occasionally occur in the wall of the cyst.[444,445]

Toxoplasmosis

Encephalitis due to *Toxoplasma gondii* infestation is most often now observed as a recrudescence of latent central nervous system infection in patients with acquired immunodeficiency syndrome or those who have received immunosuppressive therapy for malignancies. It is estimated that up to 10% of patients with acquired immunodeficiency syndrome will develop *Toxoplasma* encephalitis. This has also been reported in children, although it is much less common than in

adults, presumably reflecting the lower incidence of latent *Toxoplasma* infection in this age group. The predominant neurologic symptoms are headache, disorientation, and drowsiness. The central nervous system lesions behave as mass lesions.

The CT appearance of central nervous system toxoplasmosis is single or multiple mass lesions that have surrounding edema. The periphery of the lesions may be calcified. Ring or nodular enhancement is most common, but homogeneous enhancement or nonenhancement also occurs, although uncommonly (Fig. 1-149).

MRI is more sensitive than CT in the detection of focal mass lesions, especially in the cortex and subcortical deep gray matter. MRI commonly detects more lesions than CT. The lesions produce low signal intensity on T_1-weighted images and intermediate to high signal intensity on T_2-weighted images. The lesions are round or oval in shape and are usually multiple. High signal from surrounding edema may obscure the margins of the lesions on T_2-weighted images. The lesions usually show intense but often heterogeneous enhancement with intravenous paramagnetic contrast material.[446]

Congenital Infections

Congenital infections may be produced by two basic pathways by which organisms gain access to the fetus. Bacterial infections are usually due to the ascent of organisms from the cervix into the amniotic fluid. The organisms responsible for most types of congenital infections of the central nervous system, however, are usually transmitted transplacentally. The most common organisms involved in congenital infections of the central nervous system are cytomegalovirus, rubella virus, *Toxoplasma gondii*, human immunodeficiency virus, and herpes zoster varicellosus virus. The age of the fetus at the time of the infection of the developing central nervous system is of great importance in determining the sequelae. As a general rule, central nervous system infections occurring during the first two trimesters most often cause malformations, and infections occurring during the third trimester tend to produce destructive lesions.

Maternal infections contracted during pregnancy may or may not result in significant deleterious effects on the fetus. Potential adverse effects due to maternal infection include fetal death, intrauterine growth retardation, and congenital infection. Neonates with congenital infection may be symptomatic at birth, or the manifestations of the infection may not become clinically evident until later in life. Neurologic involvement is a source of major long-term sequelae in infants with congenital infection.

Congenital Cytomegalovirus Infection

Cytomegalovirus is the most common cause of congenital infections. The incidence of congenital cytomegalovirus infection ranges from 0.2% to 2.2% of live births.[447] Congenital cytomegalovirus infection can result either from a primary maternal infection or from reactivation of a maternal infection contracted before the pregnancy. Primary maternal infections appear to be associated with more severe neonatal manifestations. Those that occur early in pregnancy are more often associated with severe manifestations of disease in the neonate.[448,449]

More than 90% of neonates with congenital cytomegalovirus infection are asymptomatic at birth. A minority of these infants subsequently show evidence of long-term sequelae of these asymptomatic infections. It is estimated that between 13% and 17% of these children will have permanent sensorineural hearing loss. Approximately 2000 children are born each year in the United States who have cytomegalovirus-induced sensorineural hearing loss. There are also weak indicators that some of these children may have impaired intellectual development and behavioral problems.[450–452]

The clinical manifestations that may be identified in neonates with congenital cytomegalovirus infection include hepatomegaly, splenomegaly, jaundice, petechiae, microcephaly, and chorioretinitis. Central nervous system sequelae attributed to cytomegalovirus infection include mental retardation, developmental delay, learning disorders, behavioral disorders, seizures, neuromuscular disorders, and defects in hearing and vision. The great majority of neonates with symptomatic cytomegalovirus infection have permanent neurologic sequelae.[452,453]

The pathologic changes that may occur with congenital cytomegalovirus infection of the brain include porencephaly, cerebellar hypoplasia, polymicrogyria, periventricular parenchymal brain calcifications, and hydranencephaly. The periventricular distribution of calcifications is thought to be due to an affinity of the virus for the rapidly growing cells of the germinal matrix. The association with polymicrogyria may result from vascular alterations and disturbances in neuronal migration that occur late during the second trimester. Ocular abnormalities that may occur with congenital cytomegalovirus infection include microphthalmia, chorioretinitis, cataracts, and optic disc anomalies.

The changes due to congenital cytomegalovirus infection have been identified on prenatal sonography. These studies demonstrate a pattern of bilateral periventricular calcifications that may be preceded by hypoechoic periventricular ringlike zones. These findings appear to be specific for intrauterine infection with cytomegalovirus. This disease may also result in widespread cerebral destruction.[454]

Skull radiographs in cases of congenital cytomegalovirus infection may show curvilinear calcifications in a pattern that conforms to the margins of the lateral ventricles. The calcifications are best detected on CT and may be difficult to identify on MRI unless they are quite prominent. In mild cases, CT may show slight prominence of the cerebral sulci and slight generalized prominence of the ventricular system with small scattered periventricular calcifications. In addition to ventricular enlargement, MRI may show areas of high-signal abnormality on T_2-weighted images in the brain parenchyma; usually these are most prominent in the periventricular regions. In severe cases of congenital cytomegalovirus infection, CT and MRI show marked ventriculomegaly, microcephaly, and extensive cortical calcifications. Neuronal migration abnormalities may be identified as a smooth appearance of the brain surface and shallow, vertically oriented sylvian fissures (Fig. 1-150). Sequential neuroimaging procedures may show that areas of edema in the neonatal period progress to encephalomalacia or porencephaly. Progressive cerebral atrophy may also be identified.[455–458]

Congenital Toxoplasmosis

Toxoplasmosis is caused by the protozoan *Toxoplasma gondii*. This parasite infects a wide range of birds and mammals, especially cats. Human infection is usually acquired by

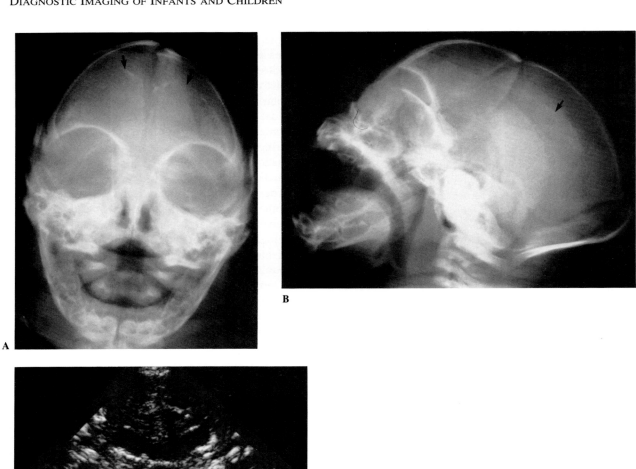

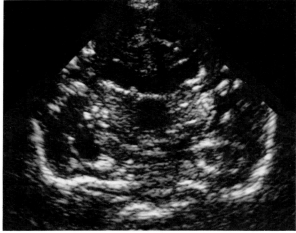

Fig. 1-150 Congenital cytomegalovirus infection. (A) Anteroposterior and (B) lateral skull radiographs show severe microcephaly. There are curvilinear and punctate intracranial calcifications (arrows). (C) Coronal sonogram shows ventricular dilatation and multiple hyperechoic foci scattered throughout the brain. (D and E) Unenhanced CT scans show dense calcifications throughout the brain, including the cerebellum. The brain surface is relatively smooth, reflecting pachygyria. The cerebellum is atrophic, and there is a large cisterna magna. There is marked ventriculomegaly due to severe cerebral atrophy.

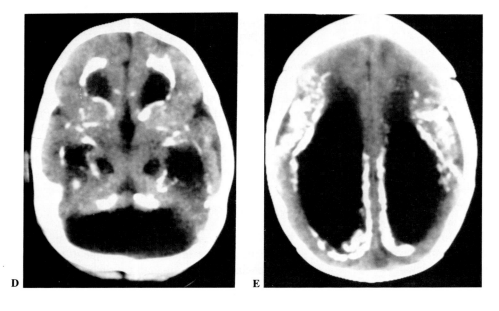

the ingestion of oocytes through exposure to cat feces or in undercooked, contaminated meat. Infection in normal adults may be asymptomatic or produce mild, nonspecific symptoms. Fetal infection is associated with a broad clinical spectrum of severity. The incidence of congenital toxoplasmosis in the United States is approximately 1 in 1000 live births, and the incidence may be as high as 1% of all pregnancies when stillborns are included.[459,460]

Most infants infected in utero with *T gondii* are asymptomatic at birth. Some of these infants manifest sequelae such as chorioretinitis or impaired intellectual performance at a later age. These sequelae may not become clinically evident until several years after birth. The incidence of neurologic sequelae in children with subclinical congenital toxoplasmosis is unknown, but careful evaluations usually demonstrate one or more sequelae of variable severity in most of these children.[461,462]

About 20% of neonates who have congenital infection with *T gondii* are symptomatic at birth. Evidence of involvement of the central nervous system is almost always present in these symptomatic infants. The severity and type of clinical manifestations roughly correlate with the gestational age at which fetal infection occurred. Severe forms resulting from early infection may present in the neonate; the most common neurologic manifestations include microcephaly, macrocephaly due to hydrocephalus, and signs of meningoencephalitis. Fetal infection occurring during the third trimester may result in chorioretinitis as the sole manifestation. The overall mortality of infants with symptomatic congenital toxoplasmosis is approximately 10% to 15%. The long-term sequelae include mental retardation in 85%; seizures, spasticity, and other neurologic abnormalities in 75%; severe visual impairment in 50%; and deafness in 10% to 15%.[463]

The predominant neuropathologic lesions of congenital toxoplasmosis include diffuse inflammation of the meninges, meningeal granulomatous lesions, and inflammation and necrosis of areas of brain parenchyma. The parenchymal brain abnormalities predominate in the basal ganglia, deep white matter, and areas adjacent to the cerebral aqueduct. Inflammation and necrosis tend to occur in the periventricular regions. At birth, calcifications are usually identifiable in the areas of parenchymal brain involvement on pathologic examination. The calcifications may increase during the first few months of life. Enlargement of the ventricles may result from occlusion of the aqueduct or reflect atrophy due to resorption of necrotic brain tissue. With early fetal infections, developmental lesions such as polymicrogyria and hydranencephaly may occur.[464]

Skull radiographs in cases of congenital toxoplasmosis may show multiple small calcifications in a periventricular distribution. Calcifications are detected with greater sensitivity on CT. Calcifications may occur in the periventricular regions, basal ganglia, and cerebral cortex.

As with cytomegalovirus infection, the neuroimaging findings with congenital toxoplasmosis roughly correlate with the gestational age at which fetal infection occurs. Early infection (before gestation week 20) may cause ventriculomegaly, por-

encephaly, and extensive dense calcifications, particularly in the basal ganglia. Ventricular dilatation is usually most marked in the posterior aspects of the lateral ventricles. Ventricular enlargement may occur from generalized atrophy or localized areas of brain necrosis. In particularly severe forms, CT and MRI may show polymicrogyria, hydranencephaly, or multiple large porencephalic cysts. Microphthalmia and ocular calcifications may also be identified. Infection occurring later during pregnancy is usually associated with less severe clinical and imaging abnormalities. With mild cases, imaging studies may be normal or show only small periventricular and intracerebral calcifications.[465]

Neonatal Herpes Simplex Virus Infection

As opposed to most other types of congenital infections, herpes simplex virus infection is usually due to exposure of the fetus to the virus at the time of delivery. Neonatal infection with herpes simplex virus can be caused by either herpes simplex virus type 1 or type 2. More than two-thirds of these infections are due to type 2. Most often, the infant is exposed to the virus at the time of delivery as a result of a genital infection of the mother. The risk of infection of the newborn is greater in cases of maternal primary genital herpes (>50%) than in cases of recurrent or reactivated genital herpes simplex virus infection (<8%). Intrauterine herpes simplex virus infection of the fetus appears to be quite rare.[466-469]

Overall, approximately 30% of neonates with herpes simplex virus infections show evidence of central nervous system involvement. Early antiviral therapy significantly decreases the incidence of neurologic sequelae, however. The most common clinical manifestation of neonatal herpes simplex virus infection is vesicular mucocutaneous lesions. Without treatment, about 75% of these infants progress to disseminated or encephalitic forms of infection; with early antiviral therapy, neurologic sequelae occur in only 10%. Neonates with disseminated herpes simplex virus infection usually present during the first several days of life with fever and signs of sepsis. These infants may have thrombocytopenia, hepatitis, pneumonia, and encephalitis. The mortality, even with treatment, approaches 50%. Encephalitis due to herpes simplex type 1 carries a better prognosis than that due to type 2. Those infants with evidence of encephalitis during the acute phase of the illness usually have permanent neurologic sequelae.

The onset of encephalitis in neonates with herpes simplex virus infection usually occurs at about 2 weeks of age; the range is 1 to 6 weeks. The clinical findings may include poor feeding, lethargy, fever, and seizures. Analysis of the cerebrospinal fluid most often demonstrates a mild pleocytosis and elevated protein with normal or decreased levels of glucose. The long-term sequelae may include hemiparesis, spasticity, psychomotor retardation, and microcephaly.

Intrauterine herpes simplex virus infection usually results in fairly severe abnormalities that are evident at birth. Most of these neonates have widespread cutaneous lesions. The central nervous system manifestations include microcephaly, hydranencephaly, cerebral atrophy, and chorioretinitis. Profound psychomotor retardation is universal among those neonates who survive.

CT and MRI may be normal during the first few days of life in neonates with herpes encephalitis. The earliest finding is the demonstration of focal regions of edema. These are most often in the temporal lobes but may also be present in the frontal lobes, in the parietal lobes, or throughout an entire cerebral hemisphere. Petechial hemorrhages in these areas are rare. A variable degree of contrast enhancement may occur on the peripheral aspects of these areas, often with a meningeal pattern. Prolonged retention of iodinated contrast material in areas of infection with herpes simplex virus have been reported with CT. The ventricles may be compressed because of edema. The areas of parenchymal edema progress to focal atrophy or porencephaly; this progression may be quite rapid and is often identified as early as the third week of life. Also, with progression of the disease, there is often an increase in the attenuation values of cortical gray matter on CT; this finding may persist for weeks to months. Eventually, CT and MRI demonstrate diffuse cerebral atrophy, sometimes with areas of porencephaly. Punctate or gyriform calcifications usually develop in both cortex and white matter. Cerebellar involvement occurs in about 50% of patients with herpes simplex encephalitis.[470,471]

Congenital Rubella

Congenital rubella is extremely rare in the developed countries because of childhood immunization and screening techniques performed on pregnant women. Many young adult women remain susceptible to rubella, however, because of either a lack of childhood immunization or failure of development of adequate immunity. The viremic phase of maternal rubella infection often results in placental infection. The risk of transmission of infection to the fetus and the severity of effects on the developing fetus roughly correlate with the gestational age at which the maternal infection occurs. The highest risk occurs during the first 8 weeks of gestation, during which the incidence of transmission may be as high as 90%. The frequency of fetal infection decreases to about 10% by gestation week 24.

Overall, only 5% to 10% of infected fetuses exhibit manifestations of congenital rubella syndrome at birth. Only occasionally does an initially asymptomatic patient later develop symptoms in infancy or childhood. The risk of clinically evident abnormalities due to congenital rubella syndrome is approximately 85% in cases in which the infection occurs during gestation weeks 1 to 8, 52% at gestation weeks 9 to 12, and 16% at gestation weeks 13 to 20. Fetal rubella infection occurring beyond gestation week 20 is almost always asymptomatic in the neonatal period; the risk of late-onset sequelae is low.[472,473]

Early fetal rubella infection frequently causes damage of the vascular endothelium. This results in stenotic lesions of the pulmonary artery and aorta. Both early and late infections tend to be associated with hearing dysfunction and ocular abnor-

malities, such as microphthalmia, cataracts, and glaucoma. Some children exhibit subtle signs of neurologic sequelae, often evidenced by delays in language and psychomotor development. Occasionally, there is evidence of an active meningoencephalitis at birth. With severe early intrauterine infections, there may be microcephaly at birth.

Common clinical manifestations of congenital rubella at birth include hypotonia, lethargy, and a bulging fontanelle. During the first few months of life, irritability, vasomotor instability, and photophobia may be identified. Seizures occur in about 25% of these children. Occasionally, there are neonates who show evidence of a syndrome of progressive encephalitis with progressive neurologic deterioration.

Severe congenital rubella is manifested pathologically as microcephaly, hydrocephalus, and severe cerebral atrophy. Calcification and foci of necrosis may occur in the periventricular white matter, basal ganglia, and brainstem. These foci of necrosis may be due to vasculitis. The meninges show evidence of chronic inflammation.[474]

Skull radiographs and CT scans in cases of congenital rubella with brain involvement may show foci of calcification in the periventricular white matter and basal ganglia. Occasionally, calcifications are present in the brainstem. In those neonates with active infection, CT and MRI may show generalized or focal areas of edema that may progress to necrosis and atrophy. In severe cases, atrophy and microcephaly are present.

Congenital Varicella

Clinical manifestations of intrauterine infection are identified in less than 5% of infants born to mothers who have had varicella during pregnancy. Almost all reported cases of congenital varicella syndrome have been associated with maternal infection during the first trimester of pregnancy. Immunologic evidence of intrauterine herpes zoster varicellosus virus infection has been identified in some asymptomatic neonates.

In those uncommon cases in which maternal varicella is associated with symptomatic congenital varicella syndrome, neurologic manifestations such as microcephaly and chorioretinitis are usually present. A number of autonomic disorders including neurogenic bladder and gastroesophageal reflux may occur. Other findings may include cicatricial cutaneous scars, limb atrophy, and rudimentary digits. Neuroimaging studies may show cerebral atrophy of variable severity.

Infants born to mothers who acquire varicella during the last few days of pregnancy may develop the clinical manifestations of acute varicella. These infants are at risk for disseminated infection, including encephalitis. The infection usually begins with the typical cutaneous exanthem, occurring between 5 and 10 days of life. The disease may progress to pneumonia, encephalitis, hepatitis, and bleeding disorder. The onset of encephalitis is indicated clinically by the development of seizures. Studies of the cerebrospinal fluid show pleocytosis and increased protein. Neuroimaging studies show the findings of acute encephalomyelitis.[475–477]

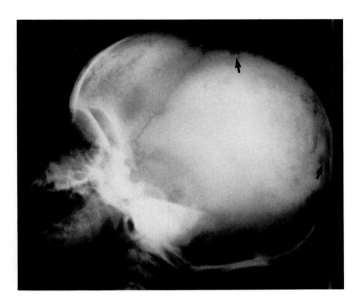

Fig. 1-151 Congenital syphilis. Lateral skull radiograph of an infant with congenital syphilis showing extensive, ill-defined, lytic abnormalities of the calvaria. Button sequestra are visible in several of these lytic areas (arrows).

Congenital Human Immunodeficiency Virus Infection

Infants born to mothers infected with human immunodeficiency virus are at risk for the development of acquired immunodeficiency syndrome. The overall risk of intrauterine infection is not known at this time. Neonates infected with this virus usually develop clinical manifestations of the disease during the first year of life. The clinical findings may include one or more of the following: failure to thrive, hepatosplenomegaly, diffuse lymphadenopathy, chronic interstitial pneumonitis, oral candidiasis, protracted diarrhea, thrombocytopenia, and other recurrent infections. A number of neurologic complications may occur from encephalitis due to the virus, various opportunistic infections, or neoplasia. The neuroimaging findings of advanced human immunodeficiency virus encephalopathy include calcifications of the cerebrum, cerebellum, and pons; diffuse cerebral atrophy; and ventricular enlargement.[478–481] Opportunistic infections of the brain and neoplasia associated with infection with this virus are discussed elsewhere in this chapter.

Congenital Syphilis

Congenital syphilis results from transplacental transmission of the spirochete *Treponema pallidum*. The risk of transplacental transmission varies with the stage of maternal illness. Untreated pregnant women with primary and secondary syphilis who have spirochetemia are more likely to transmit the infection to their unborn infants. Transmission may occur throughout pregnancy but is most likely to occur in the third trimester. Because the infection is usually acquired late, brain formation is usually normal.

Infants born with congenital syphilis frequently have hepatosplenomegaly. Bone involvement is common. The most frequent sites of involvement are the long bones, especially about the wrists, elbows, ankles, and knees. There is often dense periostitis of the long bones. The skull is involved in a minority of cases. The lesions in the calvaria show ill-defined areas of radiolucency. They may have central dense areas that look like buttons, representing button sequestra in the chronic osteomyelitis that is due to congenital syphilis (Fig. 1-151).

CEREBROVASCULAR DISEASES AND MALFORMATIONS

Cerebrovascular disease (Table 1-9) is uncommon in the pediatric age group. Unlike the situation in adults, cerebrovascular disease is rarely caused by atherosclerosis, hypertension, or the complications of diabetes mellitus. Congenital vascular anomalies and secondary abnormalities related to underlying medical conditions are the most common causes of cerebrovascular disease in children. Excluding trauma, infec-

Table 1-9 Classification of Cerebrovascular Disease in Children

Developmental Cerebrovascular Abnormalities	Acquired Cerebrovascular Diseases
Vascular malformations	Neonatal medical conditions
Capillary telangiectasia	Preterm infants
Cavernous malformations	Subependymal/
Arteriovenous malformations	intraventricular hemorrhage
Venous anomalies	Term infants
Sturge-Weber disease	Perinatal trauma
Aneurysms	Disseminated intravascular
Fibromuscular dysplasia	coagulation
Carotid and vertebral artery	Placental infarcts or emboli
anomalies	Polycythemia
Spontaneous dissection	Vascular occlusive diseases
Angiodysplasia and	Thromboembolism
proliferative vasculopathy	Atherosclerosis
	Inflammatory necrotizing vasculitis
	Infectious vasculitis
	Necrotizing vasculitis
	Systemic lupus erythematosus
	Vascular lesions associated with metabolic diseases
	Homocystinuria
	Sickle cell disease
	Collagen vascular disease
	Leigh disease
	Menkes kinky hair disease
	Miscellaneous etiologies
	Radiation therapy
	Blood dyscrasias
	Trauma
	Cardiac disease

tion, and perinatal medical problems, the annual incidence of cerebrovascular disease in children in the United States is estimated to be 2.5 cases per 100,000 population.[482]

There are two basic pathophysiologic mechanisms by which cerebrovascular disease affects the brain: interruption of adequate blood flow to a part of the brain, and blood vessel rupture with hemorrhage into the brain parenchyma. Different parts of the brain exhibit significant differences in susceptibility to and manifestations of cerebrovascular disease. Also, there are important physiologic and anatomic differences in the developing brain at different ages.

Most cerebrovascular accidents in children are caused by interruption of arterial blood flow as a result of thrombosis or embolism. This circulatory impairment causes a rapid onset of neuronal compromise due to a lack of oxygen and glucose. If the interruption in blood supply is severe and sustained, irreversible damage follows swiftly. Metabolic acidosis develops rapidly in the affected area, and the adjacent blood vessels become dilated, resulting in luxury perfusion. Localized edema results from breakdown of the blood-brain barrier and neuronal and glial cell damage. Neuronal death and perivascular edema and hemorrhage are followed by an influx of polymorphonuclear leukocytes and, subsequently, mononuclear cells and macrophages. The necrotic cerebral tissue is removed, resulting in an area encephalomalacia. Glial scarring is produced by a proliferation of astrocytes.

Occlusion of cerebral veins may initiate a pathophysiologic response similar to that described for arterial occlusions. Because of the increased venous pressure proximal to the occlusion, there is a greater tendency for blood vessel rupture and hemorrhage. With occlusion of large cerebral veins, there is often a marked increase in intracranial pressure.

A large intraparenchymal hemorrhage also produces neuronal death and regional damage to the blood-brain barrier that leads to edema. Mass effect from a large hematoma can accentuate increases in intracranial pressure. The presence of blood and blood breakdown products in the subarachnoid spaces may produce vascular spasm that can accentuate the ischemic abnormalities. Interference with the flow of cerebrospinal fluid and absorption may result in hydrocephalus.

The presence of potential collateral pathways of circulation in different portions of the brain is an important factor in the consequences of vascular occlusions. The brain receives virtually all its blood supply from the carotid and vertebral-basilar circulations. Anastomoses between these circulations occur at the circle of Willis and, to a lesser extent, in small vessels in the leptomeninges. Vascular occlusions proximal to the circle of Willis, therefore, are often compensated by these anastomoses, particularly when the occlusion develops relatively slowly. Certain regions of the brain, however, are supplied by end arteries and are therefore particularly susceptible to arterial occlusions. One such region is the diencephalon. Also, watershed zones of the cerebral cortex that lie between the most distal portions of the vascular distribution of two major arterial systems are particularly vulnerable to damage when there is a decrease in cerebral perfusion pressure.

The brain is particularly susceptible to ischemic damage because of a virtual complete lack of oxygen reserve. The relatively high cerebral metabolic rate is also an important factor. Symptoms of cerebral hypoxia generally occur when the oxygen tension falls below 40 torr. Brain metabolic activity requires a relatively high cerebral blood flow. There are important variations in cerebral blood flow at different ages. In adults, the cerebral flow is approximately 50 mL per 100 mg of brain per minute; children between the ages of 3 and 10 years have cerebral blood flow values of approximately 105 mL per 100 mg of brain per minute.

Cerebral blood flow is constantly adjusted by various autoregulating mechanisms that respond to the metabolic needs of the brain. Autoregulation provides an increase in cerebral blood flow in response to increased neuronal activity. Cerebral blood flow is also affected by intracranial pressure, perfusion pressure, and vascular resistance. Increased concentrations of carbon dioxide result in increased cerebral blood flow by causing dilatation of the intracranial vessels. These autoregulatory mechanisms are less effective in neonates, particularly in preterm infants.[483,484]

Cerebrovascular Disease in Neonates

By far the most common form of cerebrovascular disease in preterm infants is subependymal hemorrhage. The highly vascular subependymal germinal matrix is susceptible to hemorrhage in these infants. The hemorrhage may extend into the ventricular system or deep cerebral white matter. The pathogenesis of subependymal hemorrhage may be related to hypoxia, impaired autoregulation of the cerebrovascular system, and episodes of hypotension and subsequent hypertension. Risk factors for subependymal hemorrhage include prolonged labor, low Apgar scores, intrapartum trauma, blood pressure fluctuations, episodes of apnea and bradycardia, large patent ductus arteriosus, sepsis, coagulopathy, pneumothorax, and rapid volume expansion with intravenous fluids. Detection and characterization of subependymal hemorrhage are readily provided by real-time sonography.[485–487]

In term neonates, intracranial hemorrhage is most often due to birth trauma. Focal ischemic lesions are also sometimes identified in term neonates. These may be due to placental infarcts or emboli, direct trauma to cervical arteries, hypotension, disseminated intravascular coagulation, and polycythemia. Intracranial hemorrhage in the newborn is best evaluated on CT. Focal ischemic lesions are demonstrated as abnormal hyperechoic foci on sonography and as foci of decreased attenuation on CT.[488]

Cerebrovascular Malformations

A number of congenital malformations of the cerebrovascular system may occur in infants and children. These malformations may primarily involve arteries, capillaries, or venous structures. Various classification schemes have been developed for cerebrovascular malformations. Most divide these lesions into four major types: arteriovenous malformations, cavernous malformations, venous malformations, and capillary telangiectasias. Occasionally, the pathologic features of a lesion may overlap somewhat among these types.

Although these vascular malformations are congenital lesions, the clinical presentation may occur at any time throughout life, and some lesions remain asymptomatic throughout adulthood. Most often, these lesions become clinically apparent as a result of bleeding or seizures. There are also neurocutaneous syndromes in which specific types of vascular malformations are associated components.

Arteriovenous Malformation

An arteriovenous malformation consists of a compact collection of abnormal, thin-walled vessels (the nidus) that connect dilated arteries to veins without intervening capillaries. Rapid arteriovenous shunting occurs through these vessels. The neural tissue that is intermingled with the abnormal vessels undergoes secondary abnormalities, such as acute necrosis with hemorrhage or chronic necrosis with gliosis and hemosiderin-laden macrophages. The vascular walls in the anomalous vessels may show hyalinization, fibrosis, and ectasia. Intimal damage in the draining veins may progress to stenosis or occlusion, resulting in progressive dilatation of the venous structures proximally and an increased potential for hemorrhage. Rapid blood flow through the arteriovenous malformation may also lead to formation of arterial aneurysms in the circle of Willis or the feeding arteries adjacent to the malformation.

Most arteriovenous malformations are located in the subarachnoid space and may or may not have an intracerebral component. Purely intracerebral arteriovenous malformations may also occur. These lesions may be located in any region of the central nervous system. About 90% of arteriovenous malformations are located supratentorially and involve the cerebral hemispheres; 10% are located in the cerebellum or brainstem. Superficial cortical lesions are more common than deep lesions. Only about 10% of supratentorial arteriovenous malformations are located in the deep portions of the hemispheres, involving the basal ganglia, thalamus, or corpus callosum. Superficial hemispheric arteriovenous malformations tend to have a conical shape, with the base being located on the cortical surface and the apex being directed internally. Arteriovenous malformations may undergo a variable degree of enlargement with age. There may also be progressive dilatation of the feeding arteries and draining veins.[489,490]

Approximately 20% of arteriovenous malformations become symptomatic before the age of 20 years. The most common clinical presentation is due to intracranial hemorrhage. Arteriovenous malformations are the single most common cause of spontaneous intracranial hemorrhage in children, accounting for approximately 40% of cases. These lesions are also responsible for about 20% of all strokes in children. The incidence of rupture of an arteriovenous malformation as an etiology for intracranial hemorrhage is approximately 1 per 100,000 children per year. A large central nervous system arteriovenous malformation in a neonate may present with signs of high-output congestive heart failure.[482]

Characteristically, rupture of an arteriovenous malformation produces intracerebral hemorrhage, although a superficial lesion may cause subarachnoid hemorrhage. A deep arteriovenous malformation may cause intraventricular hemorrhage. Other signs and symptoms associated with arteriovenous malformations include seizures, progressive neurologic deficits, and chronic recurrent headache. Headaches are most often identified with arteriovenous malformations that receive their blood supply from external carotid artery branches or are located in the parieto-occipital region and receive their blood supply from the posterior cerebral artery. Seizures occur at some point in 60% to 70% of patients with arteriovenous malformation.[491,492] A seizure is the presenting manifestation in only about 15% of arteriovenous malformations in children, however; recurrent headache is the presenting symptom in only 3% to 5% of cases.[489] Progressive neurologic deficits occur in only a small number of children with arteriovenous malformation. This finding is most often associated with a large lesion that involves the motor cortex. The mortality associated with the initial rupture of an arteriovenous malformation is approximately 10%. Children appear to be at higher risk than adults for recurrent hemorrhage from an arteriovenous malformation.

The clinical presentation of an infratentorial arteriovenous malformation is also most often related to spontaneous hemorrhage. Infratentorial lesions may result in an altered level of consciousness, meningeal signs, and a number of clinical signs of cerebellar, brainstem, long tract, or cranial nerve involvement. Rupture into the fourth ventricle system is usually associated with rapidly deepening stupor.

On unenhanced CT, an arteriovenous malformation of sufficient size is usually demonstrated as a heterogeneous area of slightly higher attenuation than normal brain. Small calcifications may be present. There may also be adjacent areas of encephalomalacia due to ischemia or prior hemorrhage. A large area of high attenuation is usually due to a spontaneous hemorrhage. Contrast-enhanced CT shows marked enhancement of the arteriovenous malformation and its feeding arteries and draining veins. The malformation itself is demonstrated as an area of dense enhancement from which dilated tortuous veins arise. Deep malformations tend to have a rounded configuration, and peripheral lesions are more often triangular. There is usually little mass effect associated with an arteriovenous malformation (Fig. 1-152).

Unenhanced CT after hemorrhage from an arteriovenous malformation demonstrates subarachnoid, parenchymal, or intraventricular bleeding. In many cases, the resultant hematoma obscures the arteriovenous malformation itself. The hematoma associated with an arteriovenous malformation undergoes temporal changes that may be demonstrated on CT. In the acute stage, the hematoma is of high attenuation and is

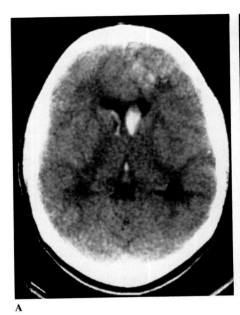
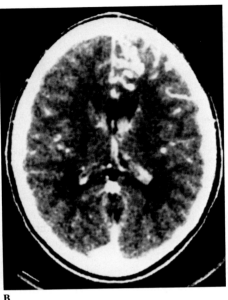

A   B

Fig. 1-152 Parenchymal arteriovenous malformation. **(A)** Unenhanced CT scan in a child with acute onset of severe headache and vomiting shows high-attenuation acute hemorrhage in the ventricular system. There is an ill-defined triangular zone of slightly higher attenuation than normal brain in the left frontal lobe. **(B)** Contrast-enhanced CT scan shows multiple, large vascular structures in this region. This parenchymal arteriovenous malformation has undergone spontaneous intraventricular hemorrhage. There is no appreciable mass effect associated with the lesion.

relatively homogeneous. In the following days, the attenuation values progressively diminish, particularly at the periphery of the clot. There is often low-attenuation edema in the adjacent brain tissue. This adjacent edematous tissue may show ringlike contrast enhancement in the subacute phase. Eventually the hematoma is absorbed, and there is residual encephalomalacia. Calcifications may be present.[493,494]

On MRI, the fast-flowing blood in an arteriovenous malformation produces low signal intensity on spin-echo sequences. The nidus of the malformation is demonstrated as a tangle of curvilinear structures with flow void. The feeding arteries and draining veins are also well demonstrated as tubular structures with flow void. Hemosiderin or calcification from previous hemorrhages may be demonstrated as areas of low signal intensity adjacent to the malformation on both T_1- and T_2-weighted images. An acute hematoma is usually isointense to brain on T_1-weighted images and hypointense on T_2-weighted images; this is due to the presence of deoxyhemoglobin in the erythrocytes within the hematoma. Subsequently, the hematoma develops high signal intensity on T_1-weighted images, beginning in the periphery of the lesion and progressing centripetally with time. This high signal intensity is first visible on T_1-weighted images and later occurs on T_2-weighted images as well (Fig. 1-153). This developing high signal intensity is due to the conversion of deoxyhemoglobin to methemoglobin. As the blood breakdown products are resorbed, the signal intensity of the hematoma on T_1-weighted images diminishes, until the lesion is isointense to cerebrospinal fluid on both T_1- and T_2-weighted sequences.[495–498] Later, decreased signal on T_2-weighted sequences is seen as a result of hemosiderin formation.

Angiography is required for precise delineation of the anatomy of an arteriovenous malformation. Angiography is most useful for defining the feeding arteries and draining veins for therapeutic planning. The typical angiographic appearance of an arteriovenous malformation is a tangle of small, irregular vessels supplied by enlarged, tortuous feeding arteries and drained by rapidly filling, dilated veins (Fig. 1-154). Rarely, one or more aneurysms are identified in feeding arteries or draining veins (Fig. 1-155). A large aneurysm may obscure the nidus of the malformation.

Cavernous Malformations

A cavernous malformation is a vascular anomaly composed of a cluster of abnormal, dilated blood vessels. The vessels in the lesion vary in diameter and wall thickness. Some vessels may be occluded by thrombus. Calcifications may occur in the vessel wall. The feeding arteries and draining veins associated with a cavernous malformation are typically normal in caliber. Unlike most arteriovenous malformations, there is usually little or no neural tissue contained in a cavernous malformation. Most are located in the brain parenchyma, but a subarachnoid component may be present. Multiple lesions are fairly common.[499,500]

The clinical presentation of cavernous hemangioma most often occurs during adulthood, although presentation during childhood does occur. The most common clinical manifestation is seizures. These are most often partial motor or partial complex seizures. Symptoms are sometimes produced by acute hemorrhage in the malformation. Small subclinical hemorrhages may also occur. Cerebral cavernous malformation occasionally occurs with a familial pattern; this is most common in Hispanic individuals.[501,502]

Skull radiographs in cases of cavernous hemangioma are usually normal but occasionally demonstrate one or more small, round calcifications. The identification of calcifications is much more common in adults than in children. CT may show small calcifications that are not visible on skull radio-

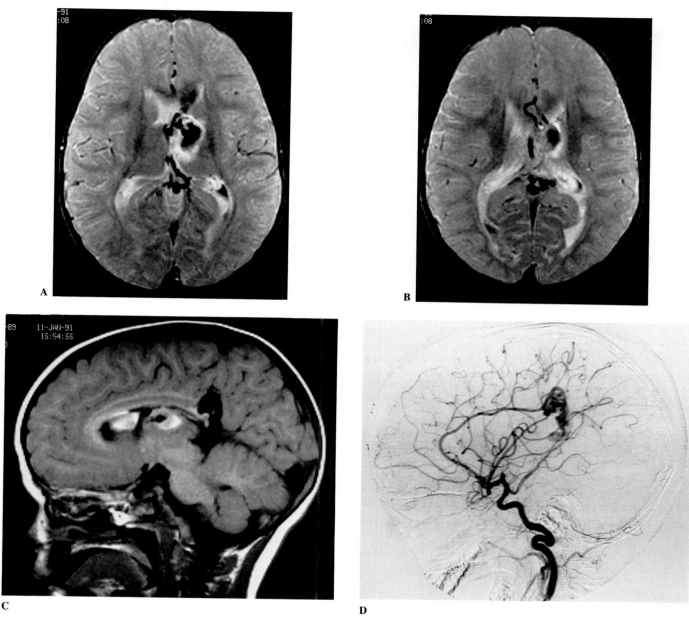

Fig. 1-153 Arteriovenous malformation. (**A and B**) Proton-density axial MR scans show two deep left hemispheric arteriovenous malformations. There are tangles of enlarged vessels that exhibit flow void. Enlarged feeding arteries and draining veins are also demonstrated. The posterior lesion lies in the region of the splenium of the corpus callosum and drains into the vein of Galen and the straight sinus. The anterior lesion lies in the region of the left thalamus and basal ganglia. There are hypointense areas of hemosiderin deposition from prior hemorrhage in the central portion of this lesion. The more peripheral aspect of the lesion produces moderate signal intensity as a result of subacute hemorrhage. Hypointense acute hemorrhage is visible in the frontal horn of the left lateral ventricle. (**C**) Parasagittal T_1-weighted MR scan shows high-signal subacute hemorrhage in the left lateral ventricle, the basal ganglia, and the thalamus adjacent to the anterior lesion. Signal void is visible in enlarged, tortuous vascular structures in the region of the more posterior lesion. (**D**) Early arterial-phase left cerebral angiogram shows opacification of the posterior arteriovenous malformation from branches arising from the anterior and posterior cerebral artery circulations. The more anterior lesion filled only on the right cerebral angiogram (not shown).

graphs. A cavernous hemangioma is usually demonstrated on CT as a spherical or lobulated, well-demarcated mass. On unenhanced images, the lesion may be hypodense, isodense, or hyperdense to normal brain. The intensity of contrast enhancement is also somewhat variable, ranging from marked to minimal. Occasionally, contrast enhancement is heterogeneous or ringlike.[502,503]

Cavernous hemangiomas are usually angiographically occult. Rarely, a faint capillary blush or one or more early draining veins are observed. Another rare angiographic sign of this lesion is sedimentation of contrast material in the large cavernous spaces.[504]

MRI demonstrates cavernous hemangioma as a well-defined parenchymal brain mass. The most characteristic fea-

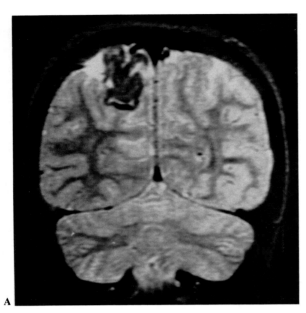

A

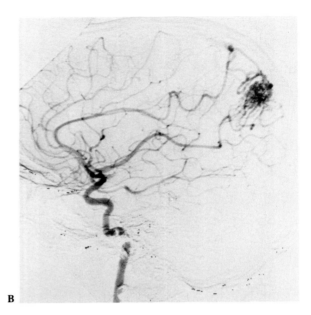

B

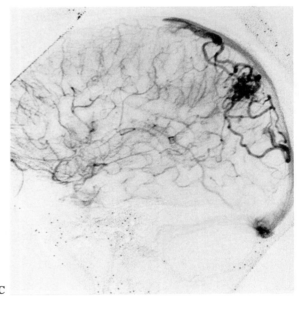

C

Fig. 1-154 Arteriovenous malformation. (**A**) T_2-weighted coronal MR scan shows a superficial right occipital arteriovenous malformation. The irregular, tortuous vascular structures that form the nidus of the lesion contain flow voids. There is little mass effect. Cerebral angiography in (**B**) the early arterial and (**C**) early venous phases shows the arteriovenous malformation as a tangle of irregular vascular structures that compose the nidus. There are enlarged feeding arteries that arise from the anterior and middle cerebral artery systems. There are multiple enlarged, tortuous early draining veins.

ture is evidence of recent and old hemorrhage. There is usually a peripheral hypointense rim on T_2-weighted images; this is due to hemosiderin deposition. The stagnant blood in the large vascular spaces produces low signal intensity on T_1-weighted images and high signal intensity on T_2-weighted images.[505,506]

Venous Malformations

Venous malformations are composed solely of veins. The lesion most often consists of a radiating array of enlarged subcortical or periventricular medullary veins that drain centripetally to a dilated venous trunk. The large draining vein courses through the brain parenchyma to empty into either the deep or the superficial venous system. The group of veins that make up a venous malformation are separated by histologically normal brain parenchyma. The central draining vein or veins have a varicose appearance, and the walls are usually thickened and hyalinized. There is no arterial or capillary component to a venous malformation. In those cases in which there is only a single dilated vein without the radiating small veins, the lesion is termed a varix.[507]

Intracranial venous malformations rarely cause symptoms. Most often, the lesion is identified on neuroradiographic procedures performed for unrelated indications. Some patients experience severe, recurrent, migrainelike headaches. Venous malformations rarely hemorrhage; hemorrhage appears to be somewhat more common with posterior fossa lesions than with cerebral lesions.[508,509]

The dilated draining vein of an intracranial venous malformation may be demonstrated on contrast-enhanced CT. The vein may drain either peripherally into the superficial venous system or centrally into the deep venous system. MRI shows a tuft of small vessels that coalesce to form a single large vein (Fig. 1-156). MRI is probably more sensitive and specific for the diagnosis than CT. Evidence of hemorrhage on CT or MRI is a rare finding with a venous malformation.

Angiography in cases of intracranial venous malformation demonstrates a group of multiple, slightly enlarged medullary veins that drain in an umbrellalike pattern into a large draining vein (Fig. 1-157). These vessels are opacified during the early venous phase of the study. Opacification of the draining vein may persist for up to 2 minutes after the injection.[510,511]

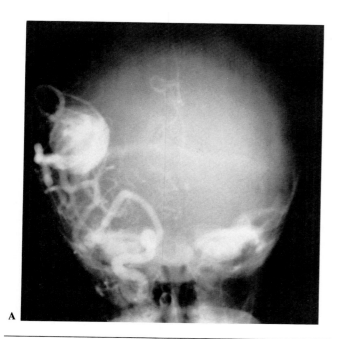

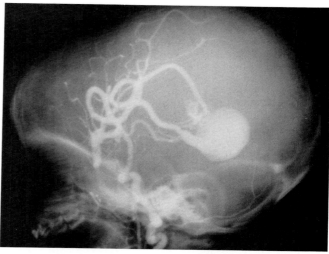

Fig. 1-155 Arteriovenous malformation. (**A** and **B**) Arterial phase of right cerebral angiograms showing a right temporal arteriovenous malformation that is supplied by markedly enlarged middle cerebral artery branches. A large aneurysm is present in the malformation.

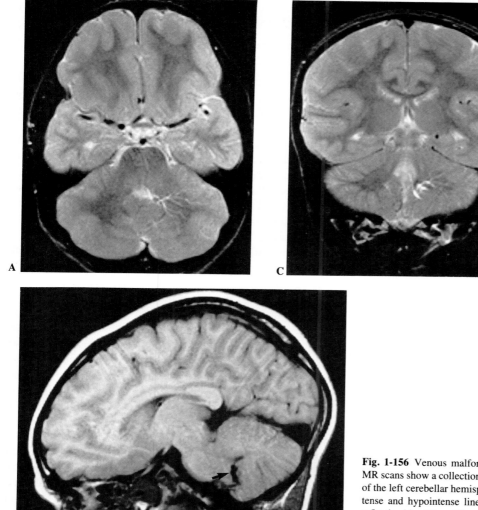

Fig. 1-156 Venous malformation. (**A**) Axial and (**B**) coronal T$_2$-weighted MR scans show a collection of small vascular structures in the central portion of the left cerebellar hemisphere. This is seen as alternating parallel hyperintense and hypointense lines that are due to spatial misregistration artifact reflecting blood flow. These vascular structures converge medially. (**C**) Sagittal T$_1$-weighted MR image shows a single prominent draining vein (arrow) from this cerebellar venous malformation.

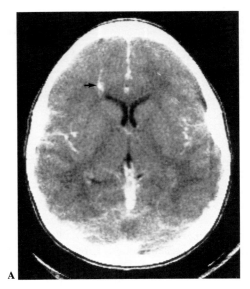

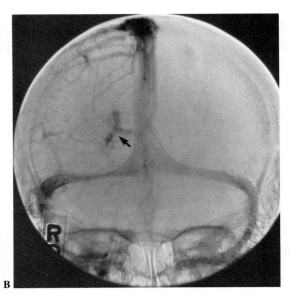

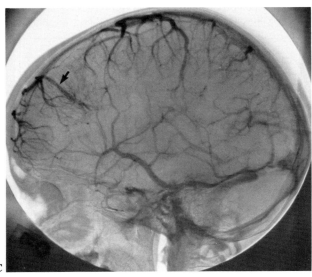

Fig. 1-157 Venous malformation. (A) Contrast-enhanced CT scan shows a linear area of abnormal enhancement in the right frontal lobe (arrow). (B) Anteroposterior and (C) lateral venous-phase angiograms demonstrate numerous small medullary veins that drain in an umbrellalike pattern into a single large draining vein (arrow). This is the characteristic angiographic appearance of a venous malformation.

Capillary Telangiectasia

Capillary telangiectasias are composed of clusters of moderately dilated capillaries that are separated by normal brain parenchyma. There are no enlarged feeding arteries or draining veins. The pons appears to be the most common location of capillary telangiectasias. Multiple meningeal or parenchymal telangiectatic lesions of the central nervous system may occur as part of Osler-Weber-Rendu disease.

Capillary telangiectasias of the central nervous system are of little clinical significance. These lesions are almost always asymptomatic. They are not space-occupying lesions and only rarely cause hemorrhage. Capillary telangiectasias are not demonstrable on neuroimaging studies.

Vein of Galen Malformation

Vein of Galen malformation is a term that is used to describe the condition of a heterogeneous group of patients who have an uncommon congenital anomaly of the cerebrovascular circulation. In a vein of Galen malformation, enlarged deep venous structures of the galenic venous system are fed by abnormal arteriovenous communications that lie in the midline. The feeding arteries most often arise from the thalamoperforator, choroidal, or anterior cerebral systems. The connections with the vein of Galen may be in the form of large, direct fistulae or multiple small connections. Some investigators have proposed that intrauterine thrombosis or failure of formation of the straight sinus is involved in the pathogenesis of vein of Galen malformation.[512]

Patients with vein of Galen malformations can be categorized into three types on clinical grounds: the neonate presenting with intractable congestive heart failure and a loud intracranial bruit; the infant presenting with hydrocephalus, seizures, or both; and the older child or adult presenting with headaches and signs of subarachnoid hemorrhage.[513] More than 90% of these lesions present during the neonatal period.

Although the shunt produced by a vein of Galen malformation develops in utero, significant cardiac failure does not occur until after birth because of hemodynamic differences between the fetal and postnatal circulation. In the fetus, circulation through the placenta competes with the intracranial malformation for cardiac output; therefore, there is less blood flow through the intracranial arteriovenous shunt. Also, the intracranial circulation in the fetus is primarily supplied by the left ventricle, whereas the right ventricle supplies the placenta and lower portion of the body. This results in a sharing of the circulatory overload between the two ventricles. After birth,

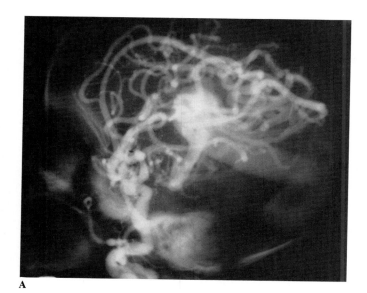

A

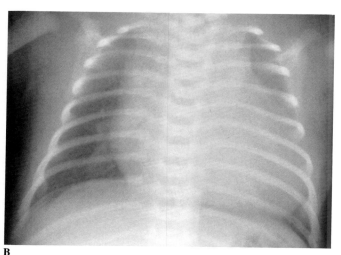

B

Fig. 1-158 Vein of Galen malformation. (**A**) Chest radiograph of a neonate with clinical findings of severe heart failure shows marked cardiomegaly and central pulmonary vascular prominence. There is widening of the superior mediastinum due to enlarged vascular structures. (**B**) Cerebral angiogram shows a large vein of Galen malformation. The malformation is supplied by numerous, enlarged, tortuous vessels from the anterior and middle cerebral artery circulations. The drainage is via a markedly dilated vein of Galen that connects to an enlarged parafalcine vein. The straight sinus is absent.

The clinical presentation of vein of Galen malformation is determined by the severity of shunting through the fistula. The clinical presentation differs in cases in which an arteriovenous fistula supplies the malformation as opposed to those in which the nidus of an arteriovenous malformation supplies the vascular malformation. Patients with a fistula present in the neonatal period; most present before 1 month of age. In those patients with a nidus, the median age at diagnosis is approximately 9 months. Among infants with arteriovenous fistula, the most common clinical signs are congestive heart failure and hydrocephalus. Among those with a nidus, the presenting clinical symptoms are evenly distributed among those referable to congestive heart failure, hydrocephalus, ophthalmologic abnormalities, and other less specific signs such as developmental delay.[517]

Those cases that present during the neonatal period usually have multiple fistulae that shunt at least 25% of the cardiac output. Clinical presentation later during infancy is usually associated with a smaller shunt, often having only one fistulous connection or a nidus. Signs of heart failure may or may not be present in these infants. The dilated vein of Galen may occlude the aqueduct and posterior third ventricle to produce hydrocephalus. Older children and adults usually have comparatively slow flow throughout an angiomatous network supplying the dilated vein of Galen. The clinical presentation is usually due to intracranial hemorrhage or, less commonly, hydrocephalus. The intracranial hemorrhage may occur into the subarachnoid space or into the brain parenchyma.

Skull radiographs in cases of vein of Galen malformation may show macrocrania and spreading of the cranial sutures. Only rarely are calcifications visible in the wall of the dilated vascular structures. Chest radiographs in symptomatic neonates show evidence of congestive heart failure (Fig. 1-158).

Sonography of an affected neonate may be utilized to demonstrate the markedly dilated vein of Galen. Echogenic thrombus may be present in the lesion. The tangle of feeding vessels usually produces ill-defined regions that are mildly hyperechoic. Rapid, turbulent flow is seen on color Doppler sonography.[518]

On unenhanced CT, the dilated vein of Galen is identified as a round mass whose attenuation is equal to or slightly greater than that of normal brain. Calcification in the walls of the vein is rare. The mass is located in the posterior incisural region and may extend rostrally and anteriorly to displace the third ventricle. Areas of parenchymal brain infarction, sometimes with petechial hemorrhages, may be observed. White matter cal-

the ventricles function in series, and the burden of flow on each ventricle is increased. With removal of the placental circulation, there is an abrupt increase in flow through the intracranial fistula. Cardiac output and blood volume increase in response to opening of the pulmonary capillary bed and lowered peripheral resistance caused by the fistula. This causes pulmonary hypertension. The large venous return to the right atrium, which is due to the presence of the intracranial fistula, augments right-to-left shunting at the atrial level through the foramen ovale. Pulmonary hypertension may also cause right-to-left shunting through the ductus arteriosus. These effects may combine to produce cyanosis. These infants also have reduced coronary blood flow because of low diastolic pressure and high left ventricular intracavitary pressure. All these factors contribute to progressive and intractable heart failure in neonates with a large vein of Galen malformation. The high flow through the fistula may also steal blood supply from brain parenchyma and cause ischemic parenchymal brain damage.[514–516]

cifications due to chronic ischemia are occasionally identified. Obstruction of the aqueduct may produce hydrocephalus. Images obtained after injection of contrast material show intense enhancement of the malformation. The contours of the lesion are smooth and well defined. Occasionally, nonenhancing areas of thrombosis are visible in the lesion.[519]

On MRI, vein of Galen malformation is typically hypointense on both T_1- and T_2-weighted images because of the rapidly flowing blood. Thrombus of variable age is often identified lining the wall of the varix. Areas of acute thrombosis are isointense to brain on T_1-weighted images and hypointense on T_2-weighted images; subacute thrombus is hyperintense on both T_1- and T_2-weighted sequences.

The feeding arteries supplying a vein of Galen malformation can often be visualized on MRI and are definitively identified on cerebral angiography (Fig. 1-159). The angiographic patterns tend to vary somewhat according to the age of the patient at clinical presentation. In neonates, the feeding vessels usually arise from the anterior cerebral arteries, the lenticulostriate arteries, the thalamoperforating arteries, and both the anterior and the posterior choroidal arteries. The feeding vessels tend to enter the malformation along its anterosuperior border. The malformation drains into a markedly enlarged accessory falcine sinus and lateral sinuses. The straight sinus is usually absent. In those cases in which the clinical presentation occurs later during infancy, the feeding vessels often consist only of one posterior choroidal artery that enters the varix inferiorly and laterally. In those cases that present late during childhood, the feeding vessels tend to arise from the posterior choroidal arteries and anterior cerebral arteries and enter along the anterior and superior aspects of the varix. In older children and young adults, the feeding vessels of the malformation consist of an angiomatous network of vessels that arise predominantly from the posterior choroidal arteries and the thalamoperforating arteries.[516]

Dural Arteriovenous Malformation

Dural arteriovenous malformations account for 10% to 15% of intracranial arteriovenous malformations. Although these are congenital lesions, most are asymptomatic. Congenital dural arteriovenous malformations are thought to be due to abnormal development of arteriovenous plexi that communicate with emissary channels, which drain extracranial structures medially into the dural sinuses during embryonic and early fetal development. It is also proposed that some dural arteriovenous malformations are acquired lesions resulting from thrombosis of a dural vein or sinus or from trauma.

Although most dural arteriovenous malformations are asymptomatic, the presence of such a lesion may be suggested clinically by the identification of a cranial bruit in a patient with a history of seizures. Affected children may show signs of hydrocephalus and developmental delay. A large dural arteriovenous malformation may present in infancy with heart failure, macrocephaly, and scalp vein distention. High-flow dural arteriovenous malformations may produce increased intracranial pressure and communicating hydrocephalus as a result of chronic elevation of pressure in the superior sagittal sinus. Rarely, a dural arteriovenous malformation may be associated with thrombosis of the sagittal sinus, resulting in a further increase in intracranial venous pressure and ventricular pressure. Dural arteriovenous malformations located in the anterior cranial fossa or tentorium drain into cortical veins and, therefore, are associated with a higher incidence of hemorrhage.[520–522]

The external carotid artery provides most of the feeding vessels that supply dural arteriovenous malformations. Posterior fossa lesions are most frequently supplied by the occipital artery. Posterior meningeal branches of the ascending pharyngeal artery may supply lesions in the middle or posterior cranial fossae. The meningohypophyseal trunk is the most frequent internal carotid artery branch that supplies a dural arteriovenous malformation. Anterior and posterior meningeal branches from the extracranial portion of the vertebral artery may supply posterior fossa lesions. Posterior fossa dural arteriovenous malformations usually drain into the transverse and sigmoid sinuses.

Because of the variable arterial supply, the complete angiographic evaluation of a dural arteriovenous malformation requires injections into the external carotid arteries, the internal carotid arteries, and both vertebral arteries. As with cerebral arteriovenous malformations, enlarged, tortuous feeding arteries and draining veins are identified; the malformation itself is composed of a tangle of small, irregular vessels. Its peripheral location is clearly evident.[523,524]

A dural arteriovenous malformation of sufficient size may be demonstrated on CT as an area of abnormal enhancement adjacent to the inner table of the skull, with multiple prominent vascular structures coursing into and away from the lesion. Occasionally, there may be an intraparenchymal component of the lesion. Evidence of hemorrhage, local mass effect, and prominent vascular grooves along the inner table of the calvaria may be visible. The major route of venous drainage is usually dilated. Impaired venous drainage may lead to hydrocephalus. Local impairment of venous drainage adjacent to the lesion may cause patchy areas of edema in the subjacent white matter. Retrograde venous drainage through cortical or diploic collateral vessels may result in regions of patchy enhancement.[525]

The rapidly flowing blood in a dural arteriovenous malformation and the supplying vessels produces signal voids on MRI. This is the most sensitive technique for demonstrating the precise location of the lesion and for defining any intraparenchymal components. Local areas of white matter edema due to impaired venous drainage adjacent to a dural arteriovenous malformation are demonstrated on T_2-weighted images as patchy areas of high signal intensity.

Carotid-Cavernous Fistula

Carotid-cavernous fistula is an arteriovenous communication in the region of the cavernous sinus. This is a rare condition in children that may develop either spontaneously or as a consequence of trauma. The lesion causes increased

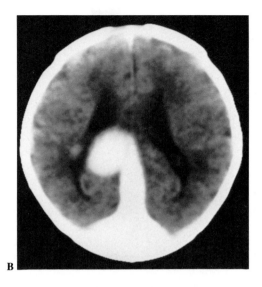

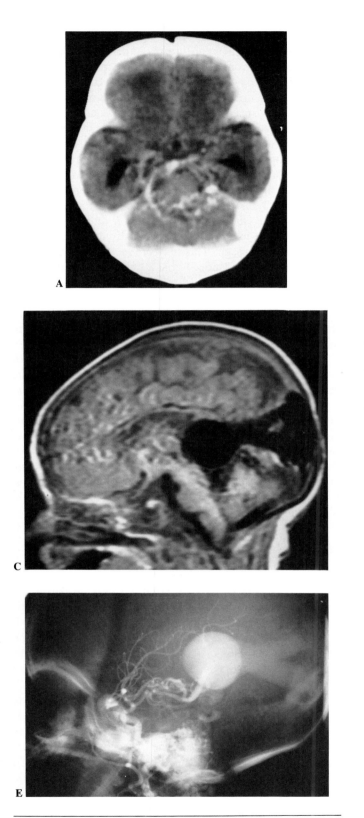

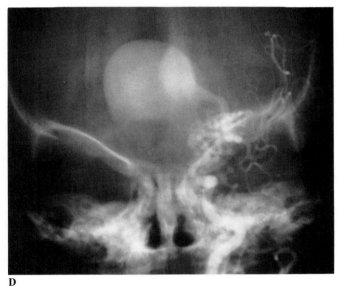

Fig. 1-159 Vein of Galen malformation. (**A** and **B**) Contrast-enhanced CT scans of a neonate who presented with signs of congestive heart failure show massive dilatation of the vein of Galen and parafalcine sinus. There are tortuous feeding arteries surrounding the upper brainstem and tentorium. (**C**) Sagittal T_1-weighted MR scan shows flow void in the massively dilated vein of Galen and venous sinuses. The straight sinus is absent. Smaller tortuous feeding arteries are visible inferior to the vein of Galen. (**D**) Antero-posterior and (**E**) lateral cerebral angiograms show multiple, dilated, tortuous arteries arising from the right middle and posterior cerebral arteries and draining into a massively dilated vein of Galen and dilated venous sinuses.

venous pressure in the orbital venous drainage system, resulting in pulsating exophthalmos, chemosis, diminution of vision, and an intracranial bruit. Carotid-cavernous fistulae in children are almost always due to trauma.

The size, location, and major supplying and draining vascular structures of carotid-cavernous fistulae can be demonstrated angiographically. Most often, the arterial supply arises from both the internal and the external carotid arteries. The meningohypophyseal trunk is the most common contributor from the internal carotid artery, and the middle meningeal branch is the most common feeding vessel arising from the external carotid artery. The venous drainage usually is into the

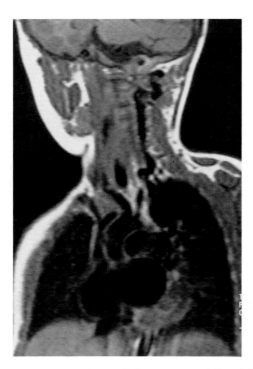

Fig. 1-160 Vertebral artery fistula. Oblique paracoronal T₁-weighted MR image shows an enlarged and tortuous left vertebral artery. Axial images (not shown) showed communication of the fistula with a dilated jugular vein.

posterior cavernous sinus and subsequently into the superior ophthalmic vein. Alternatively, the inferior ophthalmic vein, petrosal sinuses, or clival venous plexi may provide venous outflow.[526,527]

Vertebral Artery Fistulae

Vertebral artery fistulae are abnormal connections between the vertebral artery and the surrounding paravertebral venous plexus. This lesion may be due to trauma, or it may arise as a developmental anomaly. The clinical presentation may include neck pain and a bruit. Rarely, a large lesion may cause a steal phenomenon that produces neurologic manifestations. A large vertebral artery fistula may be demonstrated on CT or MRI as marked enlargement of the vertebral artery to the level of the lesion and multiple, tortuous, dilated veins draining away from the lesion (Fig. 1-160). A more precise depiction of the pathologic anatomy is provided by angiography.[528,529]

Intracranial Aneurysms

Saccular Aneurysms

Although intracranial saccular aneurysms are congenital lesions, they rarely present in the pediatric population. Less than 1% to 2% of intracranial aneurysms are identified in children younger than 15 years of age. There is an increased incidence of intracranial aneurysms in patients with coarctation of the aorta. Compared to the situation in adults, pediatric intracranial aneurysms are more often of the large (giant) type and more often arise peripheral to the circle of Willis. Most cerebral aneurysms occur at the crotch of an arterial bifurcation and are usually due to congenital defects in the media of the artery. Hemodynamic forces are probably also important in the pathophysiology of these lesions. In children, approximately 50% of intracranial saccular aneurysms arise from the internal carotid bifurcation, 25% from the anterior cerebral artery, and 12.5% from the posterior cerebral artery.[530–534]

As in adults, the clinical presentation of an intracranial saccular aneurysm in childhood is usually due to acute subarachnoid hemorrhage. This may produce severe headache, vomiting, and obtundation. About 20% of these children have a history of recurrent headaches. A giant aneurysm may produce focal neurologic signs and symptoms as a result of mass effect on the adjacent brain. Mass effect or extension of thrombus from an aneurysm may occlude the artery of origin and lead to an acute stroke.

At the time of clinical presentation, CT in most cases of saccular intracranial aneurysm demonstrates evidence of acute subarachnoid hemorrhage. If the aneurysm is of sufficient size, it may be visualized as a blood-filled saccular structure. Usually, the aneurysm enhances intensely after intravenous contrast agent administration; this appearance varies somewhat, however, depending on the presence and degree of thrombus in the lesion. MRI is also useful for demonstrating an aneurysm of sufficient size (Fig. 1-161). Angiography is essential, however, for defining the neck of the lesion and in identifying multiple aneurysms.[534]

Mycotic Aneurysm

A mycotic aneurysm is a focal arterial dilatation that is due to an infectious process. This lesion is a rare but potentially life-threatening complication of an underlying infectious disease. These lesions account for between 2% and 5% of all cerebral aneurysms and, in a relative sense, are more common in children than adults. Between 27% and 55% of patients with mycotic aneurysms are identified in the pediatric age group.[535–537]

The most common cause of intracranial mycotic aneurysm is an underlying infective endocarditis. Rupture of a mycotic aneurysm may be the presenting manifestation of subacute infective endocarditis. Mycotic aneurysms related to endocarditis may result from septic emboli that lodge in the lumen of a cerebral vessel or from hematogenous bacterial invasion through the vasa vasorum of the vessel wall. A focal arteritis occurs that leads to septic degeneration of the elastic lamina and muscularis, producing fusiform aneurysmal dilatation. These aneurysms most often arise beyond the circle of Willis in the distal branches of the intracranial circulation; the middle cerebral artery system is the most frequent site. Children at

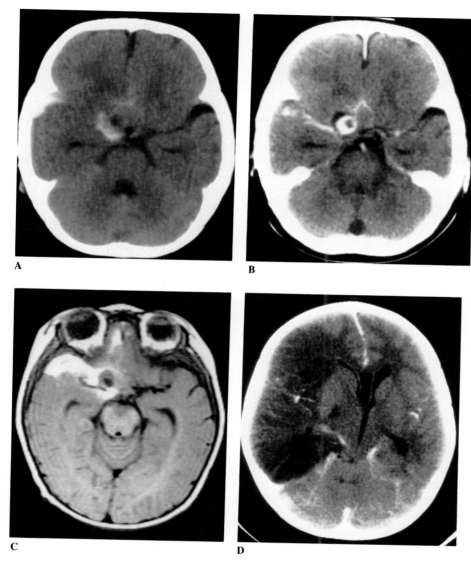

Fig. 1-161 Saccular aneurysm. **(A)** Unenhanced CT scan shows acute subarachnoid hemorrhage in the right suprasellar cisterna and in the subarachnoid spaces anterior to the right temporal lobe. **(B)** Enhanced CT scan shows an enhancing saccular aneurysm adjacent to the origin of the right middle cerebral artery. Nonenhancing thrombus is visible in the aneurysm. **(C)** T_1-weighted MR image shows the subacute hemorrhage as high-attenuation material in the subarachnoid spaces anterior to the right temporal lobe. The saccular aneurysm lies anterior to the proximal right middle cerebral artery. The aneurysm has mixed signal characteristics because of slowly flowing blood and thrombus. **(D)** Contrast-enhanced CT scan several months later shows an acute stroke in the right middle cerebral artery territory. There are decreased attenuation and mass effect in the involved portion of the right hemisphere as a result of extension of the thrombus from the aneurysm into the middle cerebral artery.

greatest risk for endocarditis include those with congenital heart disease (particularly right-to-left intracardiac shunts and prosthetic cardiac valves) and rheumatic heart disease.

In addition to endocarditis, another important etiology of mycotic aneurysms in children is local invasion of an intracranial vessel from an adjacent infection. Infectious diseases of the head and neck that can be complicated by mycotic aneurysm include middle ear infection, paranasal sinus infection, meningitis, osteomyelitis of the skull base, septic cavernous thrombophlebitis, cervical lymphadenitis, and retropharyngeal abscess. In these cases, there is direct spread of the infectious process into the arterial wall with initial involvement of the adventitia and subsequent invasion of the muscularis and internal elastic lamina. The focal arteritis may progress to thrombosis or degeneration and dilatation of the arterial wall. Occasionally, multiple aneurysms are present in

the area of infection. Mycotic aneurysms are usually fusiform and involve the entire vessel circumference.

In cases of mycotic aneurysm that are attributable to infective endocarditis, the most common presenting signs and symptoms are due to subarachnoid or intracerebral hemorrhage. Because multiple septic emboli may occur in these children, there may also be signs of cerebral ischemia. Seizures, headache, and signs of bacterial meningitis or brain abscess may also occur in these children. In those cases of mycotic aneurysm occurring in association with a contiguous infectious process, the underlying infection usually dominates the clinical picture, and the aneurysm itself may be asymptomatic. Ischemic signs may occur if there is thrombosis of the involved vessel.[535,538]

Mycotic aneurysms of sufficient size can be demonstrated on CT or MRI. Associated lesions, such as focal cerebritis, brain abscess, edema, hemorrhage, or infarction, may also be demonstrated. Angiography is required for definitive characterization of the lesion. These aneurysms usually have a fusiform configuration. Those that are due to septic emboli in association with infective endocarditis are usually located peripherally in the cerebral vasculature, most often in the distribution of the middle cerebral artery. Those lesions resulting from direct extension of an adjacent infectious process are usually located in the region of the skull base or neck. In these instances, cross-sectional imaging with CT, MRI, or sonography is quite helpful for defining the extent of the infectious process and the relationship to the involved artery.[539,540]

Cerebrovascular Obstruction

Cerebrovascular obstruction may occur at the arterial, venous, or capillary levels. The obstruction may occur as an acute event or as a slowly progressive or recurrent phenomenon. Cerebrovascular obstruction can be associated with a wide variety of etiologic or predisposing conditions. The obstruction may occur in the form of thrombosis, vascular spasm, extrinsic compression, embolism, trauma, and intrinsic vessel narrowing (Table 1-10).

Arterial Obstruction

Acute arterial obstruction in the cerebrovascular system leads to permanent sequelae within several minutes of the acute event. Initially, edematous changes occur in the ischemic gray and white matter. Neuropathologic changes include disintegration of the nerve cells, myelin sheaths, and oligodendroglia and the appearance of numerous polymorphonuclear cells in the perivascular spaces. If this area becomes revascularized during this phase, the damaged capillary and arterial walls may allow extensive plasma leakage and hemorrhage. In the subacute phase, the infarcted area accumulates mononuclear cells and macrophages, and astrocytic infiltration occurs. After several weeks, a cystic space bordered by astrocytes may form.

The clinical manifestations of acute cerebrovascular arterial obstructions vary according to the size and location of the lesion. Some variation may also occur with patient age. The most common manifestation of a large cerebral infarct is acute hemiplegia. Infarcts involving the anterior or middle cerebral arteries usually produce an acute hemiplegia that predominates in the upper limb and face. Disturbances of consciousness are usually mild. Infarcts involving the internal capsule and basal ganglia also produce hemiplegia involving the upper and lower limbs and face. Language disorders are common. Infarcts of the internal capsule may produce an ataxic hemiparesis. Parieto-occipital infarcts are uncommon and may produce cortical blindness or homonymous lateral hemianopsia. Occlusions of the posterior fossa circulation

Table 1-10 Etiology of Cerebrovascular Obstruction in Infants and Children

Arterial Obstruction	Venous Obstruction	Capillary Obstruction
Inflammatory disease	Meningitis	Henoch-Schönlein purpura
Henoch-Schönlein purpura	Empyema	Sickle cell disease
Systemic lupus erythematosus	Otitis media	Hemolytic uremic syndrome
Periarteritis nodosa	Leukemia	
	Dehydration	
Infectious disease	Sepsis	
Meningitis	Surgery	
Sinusitis		
Otitis		
Hematologic disease		
Sickle cell disease		
Cardiac disease		
Infective endocarditis		
Right-to-left cardiac shunts		
Trauma		
Blunt or penetrating injury		
Fat embolism		
Cranial irradiation		
Catheterization		
Surgery		
Neoplasm		
Extrinsic compression		
Vascular invasion		
Vascular malformation		
Arteriovenous		
Aneurysm		
Moyamoya		
Primary arterial dysplasia		
Neurofibromatosis		
Fibromuscular dysplasia		
Metabolic diseases		
Hyperlipidemia		
Homocystinuria		

may produce a number of signs and symptoms depending on the location, including pyramidal and cerebellar signs, hemiparesis, cranial nerve palsy, conjugate lateral deviation of the eyes, vertigo, and vomiting.

CT after acute arterial occlusion is usually normal for several hours subsequent to the event. During the first 24 hours, a large infarct may sometimes be demonstrated as an ill-defined

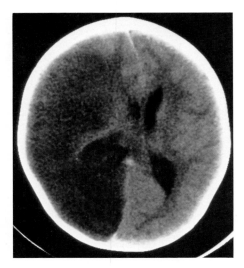

Fig. 1-162 Acute stroke. Unenhanced CT scan of a 2-year-old child 48 hours after the acute onset of left hemiparesis showing extensive low-attenuation abnormality of most of the right cerebral hemisphere as a result of edema. Mass effect due to the stroke causes a shift of the midline structures to the left. This is an acute stroke due to occlusion of the right middle cerebral artery.

during the first week, usually during the latter stages. Contrast enhancement is usually not identifiable in the ischemic area until after 7 days, and this finding is most pronounced between 2 and 3 weeks after the acute event. Eventually, CT may show the changes of encephalomalacia, porencephaly, or focal atrophy.

MRI has greater sensitivity than CT in demonstrating the subtle edema that occurs in the early stages of acute cerebral infarct. This is demonstrated as a region of high signal intensity in the cerebral parenchyma on T_2-weighted images (Fig. 1-163). MRI may also be helpful in demonstrating thrombus or other pathology in the larger intracranial or cervical arteries. The cervical vascular structures may also be evaluated with Doppler sonography.

Radionuclide single-photon emission CT brain imaging with lipophilic neuroimaging agents is quite sensitive for the early diagnosis of an acute cerebral infarct. This technique is of greater sensitivity than CT in the early stages of a stroke. The stroke is seen as a perfusion defect in the cerebral cortex. Follow-up studies may be useful for demonstrating return of perfusion to the affected areas. Hyperemic changes due to collateral circulation or luxury perfusion are sometimes identified as well. Single-photon emission CT brain imaging provides a more physiologic depiction of a stroke than either CT or MRI (Fig. 1-164).[541–543]

area of diminished attenuation. Further decrease in attenuation occurs over the next few days, and the margins become more clearly defined. Mass effect from acute ischemia is usually most marked between 2 and 3 days after the event (Fig. 1-162). Petechial hemorrhage in the ischemic area may occur

Angiography remains the most sensitive technique for the evaluation of the cervicocranial vascular system (Fig. 1-164). Embolic occlusion of an artery is demonstrated as an abrupt cutoff of the vessel lumen; the thrombus may be seen as an intraluminal filling defect. Vascular spasm produces a long

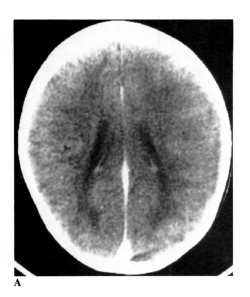

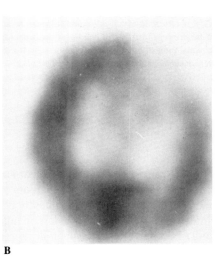

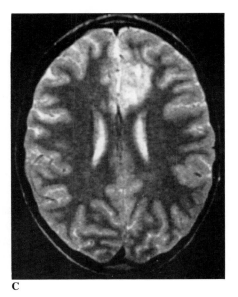

A B C

Fig. 1-163 Arterial obstruction. **(A)** Contrast-enhanced CT scan of an 8-year-old child with sickle cell disease who developed the acute onset of altered mental status several hours before the scan shows a subtle low-attenuation abnormality in the left frontal lobe. **(B)** Axial single-photon emission CT brain image with [123I]iofetamine shows a photopenic region in the left frontal lobe compatible with an acute stroke. **(C)** T_2-weighted MR image shows high-signal abnormality in the left frontal lobe; this is due to vasogenic edema produced by an acute stroke.

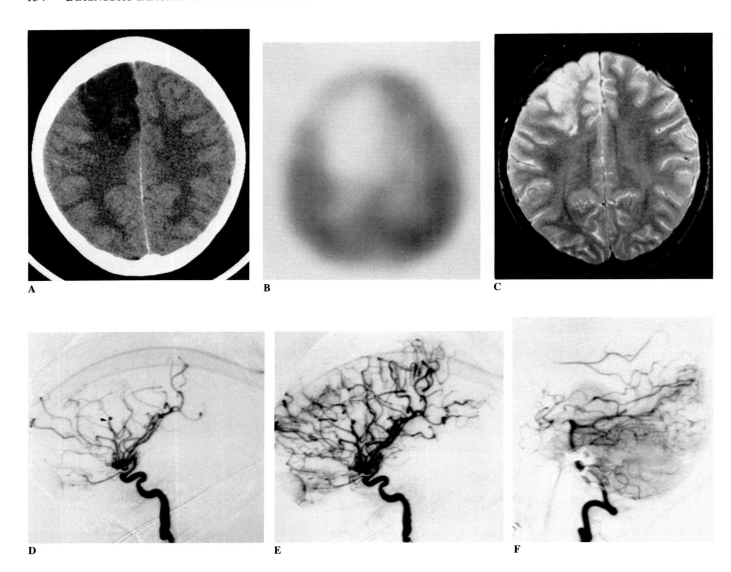

Fig. 1-164 Arterial obstruction. **(A)** Unenhanced axial CT scan of a child with sickle cell disease shows an area of low attenuation in the medial superior aspect of the right frontal lobe. **(B)** Axial single-photon emission CT brain image with [^{123}]iofetamine shows a photopenic appearance in the corresponding region of the right frontal lobe. **(C)** Axial T_2-weighted MR scan shows high signal intensity in this portion of the right frontal lobe as a result of vasogenic edema. **(D)** Lateral right cerebral angiogram shows deficient filling of most of the right anterior cerebral artery territory. There is also an occluded right middle cerebral artery branch (arrow). There is spasm of the intracranial portion of the internal carotid artery. **(E)** Late arterial-phase angiogram shows multiple enlarged collateral vessels arising from the middle cerebral territory. **(F)** Lateral vertebral angiogram shows retrograde filling of collateral vessels that fill from the posterior cerebral artery circulation.

segment of circumferential narrowing that may involve one or more vessels. Extrinsic compression of an artery or vein is demonstrated as a rounded area of compression.

Arteritis and arteriopathy involving the internal carotid artery most often result in progressive narrowing or occlusion just superior to the origin of the ophthalmic artery or distal to the anterior choroidal artery. The occlusion may be complete with either a tapered or an abrupt narrowing (Fig. 1-165). In those cases with incomplete occlusion, there is usually rapid tapering to the stenotic segment with either a localized or a

long-segment stenosis. The margins of the stenotic segment may be smooth or irregular. Multiple narrowings or occlusions are frequently present in the major intracranial branches. With occlusion or high-grade stenosis, the cervical portion of the ipsilateral internal carotid artery is usually small because of decreased blood flow.[544]

Arteritis and arteriopathy involving the cerebral arteries may occur as isolated lesions or in association with internal carotid lesions (Fig. 1-166). The middle cerebral artery is most frequently involved; it is followed in frequency by the

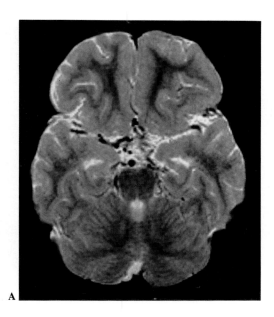

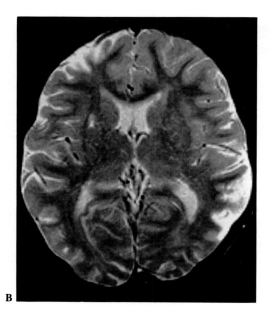

Fig. 1-165 Arteritis in a child with Down syndrome. (**A** and **B**) T₂-weighted axial MR scans show focal areas of atrophy in the right frontal lobe and left parietal lobe due to prior strokes. There is also a small lacunar infarct in the basal ganglia on the right. The more inferior image shows lack of visualization of the internal carotid arteries and left middle cerebral arteries. There are dilated, tortuous collateral vessels visualized in the region of the suprasellar cisterna. (**C**) Lateral cerebral angiogram obtained with a common carotid injection shows complete occlusion of the internal carotid artery. There is filling of cerebral vessels via multiple tortuous collateral arteries that arise from the external carotid system. (**D**) Frontal vertebral angiogram shows occlusion of the right posterior cerebral artery. Numerous tortuous collateral vessels surround the brainstem.

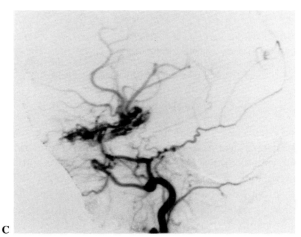

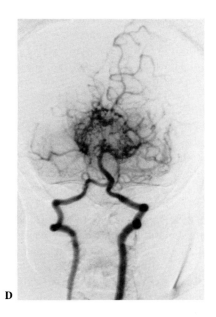

anterior cerebral artery. The posterior cerebral artery is rarely involved. The angiographic findings range from irregular stenoses to abrupt occlusions. Occasionally, the involved arteries have a somewhat beaded appearance.

Moyamoya

Moyamoya is characterized by slowly progressive stenosis of the supraclinoid internal carotid arteries and the proximal main cerebral arteries. The resultant collateral circulation of small branches from the lenticulostriate and thalamoperforating arteries causes an angiographic appearance likened to that of a puff of smoke, from which the name of this condition is derived; the Japanese word *moyamoya* means "hazy" or "unclear."

The etiology of moyamoya is unknown, and the pathophysiology may be multifactorial. Conditions that may be associated with this disease include neurofibromatosis,

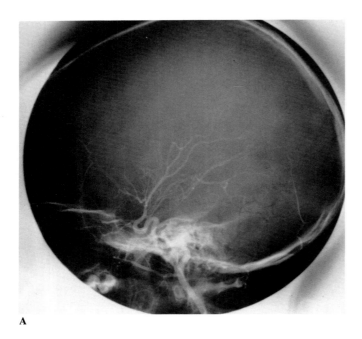

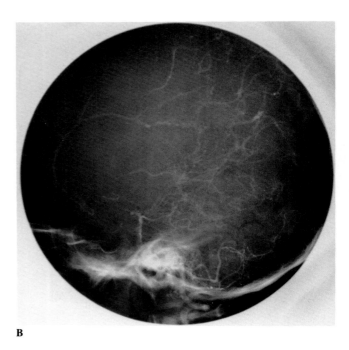

A

B

Fig. 1-166 Arteritis in a child with neurofibromatosis type 1. (A) Lateral cerebral angiogram shows marked tapering of the supraclinoid portion of the internal carotid artery. There is complete occlusion of the anterior cerebral artery and multiple middle cerebral artery branches. The remaining patent middle cerebral artery branches show narrowing of their proximal portions. (B) Late arterial-phase lateral vertebral angiogram shows retrograde filling of the anterior cerebral artery by way of collaterals that fill from the posterior cerebral circulation.

Down syndrome, radiation therapy, and genetic factors. Some investigators have proposed an association with previous nasopharyngeal infections, severe pyrexia, and exanthems. Approximately 70% of reported cases of moyamoya are identified in patients younger than 20 years of age and 50% in children younger than 10 years of age. Pediatric cases are usually manifested clinically by recurrent transient ischemic attacks and progressive neurologic impairment. In young children seizures are common; recurrent headache is common in older children. Moyamoya accounts for 4% to 5% of ischemic strokes in children in North America.[545,546]

The arterial stenoses of moyamoya almost invariably involve the supraclinoid portions of the internal carotid arteries with extension into the proximal portions of the anterior and middle cerebral arteries. The posterior cerebral arteries are occasionally involved, but the vertebral arteries are only rarely affected. Dilatation of the lenticulostriate and thalamoperforating vessels occurs in response to the gradual occlusion of the major feeding vessels. Leptomeningeal anastomoses between cortical branches of the vertebrobasilar and internal carotid systems provide additional collateral circulation. The pathologic changes in the stenotic vessels include marked fibromuscular thickening of the arterial intima, thickening or lamination of the internal elastic lamina, and atrophy and focal necrosis of the media. There is usually relentless progression of the vascular occlusions, which results in progressive clinical deterioration.[547,548]

CT and MRI in cases of moyamoya usually show multiple cerebral infarcts. The infarcts are usually in different stages of evolution. Some infarcts may show contrast enhancement. There may also be enhancement in the basal ganglia as a result of either infarction or opacification of the collateral vessels. In some cases, there is failure of normal visualization of the proximal cerebral vessels and internal carotid arteries in the region of the circle of Willis; this is particularly evident on MRI. Collateral blood vessels of sufficient size may be identified on MRI as multiple curvilinear structures that show flow void at the base of the brain and in the region of the basal ganglia. As the disease progresses, cerebral atrophy and intracranial calcifications may develop.[549,550]

Angiography provides a definitive diagnosis of moyamoya and determines the extent of the disease. Angiography shows stenotic lesions, often multiple, involving the supraclinoid internal carotid arteries, proximal anterior cerebral arteries, and proximal middle cerebral arteries. The findings may be asymmetric or even unilateral, but subsequent studies almost always demonstrate progression to bilateral disease. Eventually, complete occlusions develop. The collateral vessels are demonstrated as innumerable dilated and tortuous lenticulostriate and thalamoperforating arteries. Prominent flow through smaller vessels may produce a generalized blush in the region of the basal ganglia, causing the puff of smoke appearance (Fig. 1-167). Cortical and transdural collateral arterial flow may also be demonstrated.[551]

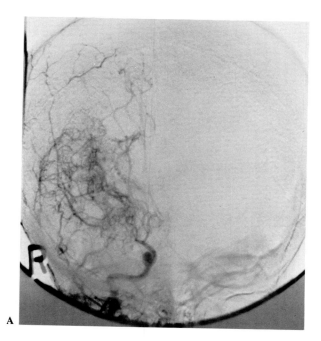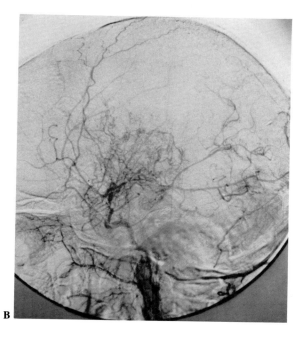

Fig. 1-167 Moyamoya. (**A**) Anteroposterior and (**B**) lateral right cerebral angiograms show occlusion of the supraclinoid portion of the internal carotid artery. There are innumerable dilated and tortuous thalamoperforating and lenticulostriate arteries that produce the puff of smoke appearance of moyamoya.

Venous Thrombosis

Acute thrombosis of superficial or deep veins or of the intracranial venous sinuses may occur as an idiopathic abnormality or in association with various predisposing conditions. In infants and children, intracranial venous thrombosis is most often associated with fluid and electrolyte imbalance, sickle cell disease, head and neck infection, meningitis, disseminated intravascular coagulopathy, and intrinsic hypercoagulable states. Although any venous structure may be involved, venous thrombosis most often occurs in superficial veins or intracranial venous sinuses. Depending on the adequacy of collateral venous drainage, acute venous thrombosis may or may not cause cerebral infarction. Venous infarcts tend to be superficial and hemorrhagic.

Unenhanced CT in the presence of acute cerebral venous thrombosis shows the intraluminal clot as high-attenuation material. Thrombosis of small superficial veins may be obscured by the adjacent calvaria. Coronal images may be helpful in demonstrating thrombus in the superior sagittal sinus. Within several days, the thrombus usually becomes isodense to brain. Contrast-enhanced images show lack of normal enhancement of the thrombosed vein. Thrombus in the superior sagittal sinus is indicated by absence of contrast opacification of the sinus and intense enhancement of the dural walls and dural collateral venous channels around the clot. This is termed the delta sign.

Occasionally, contrast-enhanced CT in the presence of superficial cerebral venous thrombosis shows punctuate and linear enhancing structures in the deep white matter. These are presumed to represent dilated transcerebral medullary veins that serve as collateral channels.

CT may also show evidence of parenchymal abnormalities due to venous infarcts. Venous infarcts do not conform to the territories of a single artery or watershed zone. Small venous infarcts are often superficial and patchy. The involved area produces low attenuation on unenhanced scans as a result of edema and necrosis. The margins tend to be more ill defined than those of an arterial infarct. The gray matter may be slightly hyperdense because of congestive dilatation of the capillaries and the presence of petechial hemorrhage. Contrast-enhanced images often demonstrate prominent gyral enhancement in the area of a venous infarction. This is presumably due to capillary engorgement and breakdown of the blood-brain barrier in the presence of high venous back pressure. Hemorrhage is frequently associated with venous infarcts. This may range from minimal petechial hemorrhage to a large space-occupying hematoma.[552]

MRI provides greater sensitivity and specificity for the demonstration of cerebral venous thrombosis. During the subacute phase, the thrombus produces high signal intensity on T_1-weighted images and moderate intensity on T_2-weighted images. Sagittal images are particularly helpful for evaluation of the superior sagittal sinus. Coexistent venous infarcts produce prolongation of T_1- and T_2-relaxation times. Cerebral angiography is occasionally helpful for further characterization of the extent of venous thrombosis (Fig. 1-168).[553,554]

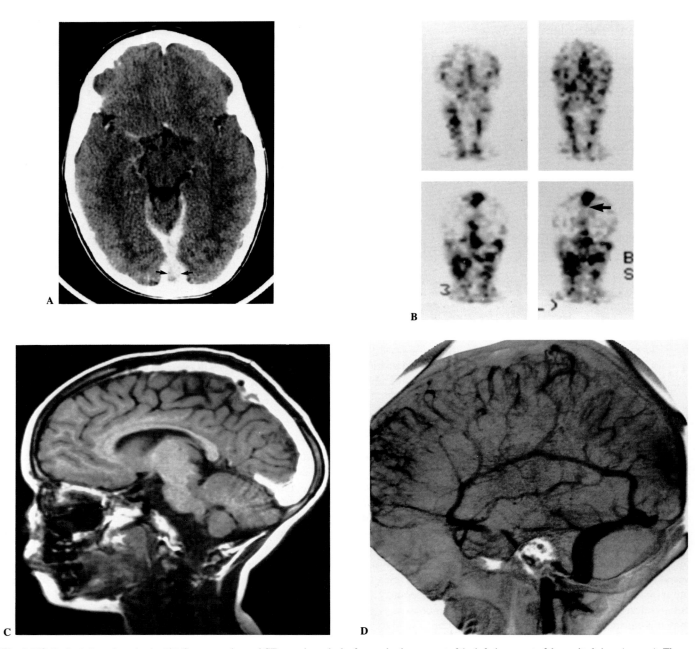

Fig. 1-168 Sagittal sinus thrombosis. (**A**) Contrast-enhanced CT scan shows lack of normal enhancement of the inferior aspect of the sagittal sinus (arrows). There is intense dural enhancement around the margins of the sagittal sinus and along the leaves of the tentorium as a result of small dural collateral veins. (**B**) Radionuclide angiogram shows lack of visualization of a segment of the superior sagittal sinus (arrow). (**C**) Sagittal T_1-weighted MR image shows subacute thrombus that produces high signal; this fills most of the superior sagittal sinus and a portion of the straight sinus. (**D**) Venous phase of a lateral cerebral angiogram shows failure of opacification of the superior sagittal sinus. There are prominent superficial venous collaterals. The sigmoid sinus is opacified. Acute thrombosis of the superior sagittal sinus in this child was due to an intrinsic hypercoagulable state.

REFERENCES

1. Sadler LR, Tarr RW, Jungreis CA, Sekhar L. Sinus pericranii: CT and MR findings. *J Comput Assist Tomogr*. 1990;14:124–127.

2. Witrak BJ, Davis PC, Hoffman JC Jr. Sinus pericranii. A case report. *Pediatr Radiol*. 1986;16:55–56.

3. Tait MV, Gilday DL, Ash JM, et al. Craniosynostosis: correlation of bone scans, radiographs, and surgical findings. *Radiology*. 1979;133:615–621.

4. Cohen MM Jr. Genetic perspectives on craniosynostosis and syndromes with craniosynostosis. *J Neurosurg*. 1977;47:886–898.

5. Coccia PF. Cells that resorb bone. *N Engl J Med*. 1984;310:456–458. Editorial.

6. Stein SA, Witcop C, Hill S, et al. Sclerosteosis: neurogenetic and pathophysiologic analysis of an American kinship. *Neurology*. 1983;33:267–277.

7. Carlson DH, Harris GB. Craniometaphyseal dysplasia. A family with three documented cases. *Radiology.* 1972;103:147–151.

8. Millard DR Jr, Maisels DO, Batstone JH, Yates BW. Craniofacial surgery in craniometaphyseal dysplasia. *Am J Surg.* 1967;113:615–621.

9. Shibuya H, Suzuki S, Okuyama T, Yukawa Y. The radiological appearances of familial metaphyseal dysplasia. *Clin Radiol.* 1982;33:439–444.

10. Kolawole TM, Hawass ND, Patel PJ, Mahdi AH. Osteopetrosis: some unusual radiological features with a short review. *Eur J Radiol.* 1988;8:89–95.

11. Lehman RA, Reeves JD, Wilson WB, Wesenberg RL. Neurological complications of infantile osteopetrosis. *Ann Neurol.* 1977;2:378–384.

12. Bartynski WS, Barnes PD, Wallman JK. Cranial CT of autosomal recessive osteopetrosis. *AJNR.* 1989;10:543–550.

13. Wu XR, Swaiman KF. Reversible hydrocephalus caused by bilateral jugular vein catheterization. *Brain Dev.* 1982;4:397–400.

14. van der Knaap MS, Valk J. Classification of congenital abnormalities of the CNS. *AJNR.* 1988;9:315–326.

15. Bird CR, Hedberg M, Drayer BP, Keller PJ, Flom RA, Hodak JA. MR assessment of myelination in infants and children: usefulness of marker sites. *AJNR.* 1989;10:731–740.

16. Chervenak FA, Isaacson G, Mahoney MJ. Advances in the diagnosis of fetal defects. *N Engl J Med.* 1986;315:305–307.

17. Giorud A. Anencephaly. *Handb Clin Neurol.* 1977;30:173–208.

18. Cox GG, Rosenthal SJ, Holsapple JW. Exencephaly: sonographic findings and radiologic-pathologic correlation. *Radiology.* 1985;155:755–756.

19. Pagon RA, Chandler JW, Collie WR, et al. Hydrocephalus, agyria, retinal dysplasia, encephalocele (HARD ± E) syndrome: an autosomal recessive condition. *Birth Defects.* 1978;14:233–241.

20. Barkovich AJ, Vander Merck P, Edwards MSB, Cogen PH. Congenital nasal masses: CT and MR imaging features in 16 cases. *AJNR.* 1991;12:105–116.

21. Naidich TP, McLone DG, Fulling KH. The Chiari II malformation: part IV. The hindbrain deformity. *Neuroradiology.* 1983;25:179–197.

22. Curnes JT, Oakes WJ, Boyko OB. MR imaging of hindbrain deformity in Chiari II patients with and without symptoms of brainstem compression. *AJNR.* 1989;10:293–302.

23. Wolpert SM, Scott RM, Platenberg C, Runge VM. The clinical significance of hindbrain herniation and deformity as shown on MR images of patients with Chiari II malformation. *AJNR.* 1988;9:1075–1078.

24. Cohen MM Jr, Jirasek JE, Guzman RT, Gorlin RJ, Peterson MQ. Holoprosencephaly and facial dysmorphia: nosology, etiology, and pathogenesis. *Birth Defects.* 1971;7:125–135.

25. Barkovich AJ, Norman D. Absence of the septum pellucidum: a useful sign in the diagnosis of congenital brain malformations. *AJNR.* 1988;9:1107–1114.

26. Matsunaga E, Shiota N. Holoprosencephaly in human embryos: epidemiologic studies of 150 cases. *Teratology.* 1977;16:261–272.

27. Nyberg DA, Mack LA, Bronstein A, Hirsch J, Pagon RA. Holoprosencephaly: prenatal sonographic diagnosis. *AJR.* 1987;149:1051–1058.

28. Barkovich AJ. Apparent atypical callosal dysgenesis: analysis of MR findings in six cases and their relationship to holoprosencephaly. *AJNR.* 1990;11:333–339.

29. O'Dwyer JA, Newton TH, Hoyt WF. Radiologic features of septo-optic dysplasia. *AJNR.* 1980;1:443–448.

30. Sarwar M. The septum pellucidum: normal and abnormal. *AJNR.* 1989;10:989–1005.

31. Aicardi J, Goutieres F. The syndrome of absence of the septum pellucidum with porencephalies and other developmental defects. *Neuropediatrics.* 1981;12:319–329.

32. Atlas SW, Shkolnik A, Naidich TP. Sonographic recognition of agenesis of the corpus callosum. *AJR.* 1985;145:167–173.

33. Larsen PD, Osborn AG. Computed tomographic evaluation of corpus callosum agenesis and associated malformations. *J Comput Tomogr.* 1982;6:225–230.

34. Davidson HD, Abraham R, Steiner RE. Agenesis of the corpus callosum: magnetic resonance imaging. *Radiology.* 1985;155:371–373.

35. Barkovich AJ, Norman D. Anomalies of the corpus callosum: correlation with further anomalies of the brain. *AJNR.* 1988;9:493–501.

36. Kazner E, Stochdorph O, Wende S, Grumme T. Intracranial lipoma. Diagnostic and therapeutic considerations. *J Neurosurg.* 1980;52:234–245.

37. Truwit CL, Barkovich AJ. Pathogenesis of intracranial lipoma: an MR study in 42 patients. *AJR.* 1990;155:855–864. Review.

38. Dean B, Drayer BP, Beresini DC, Bird CR. MR imaging of pericallosal lipoma. *AJNR.* 1988;9:929–931.

39. Abrahams JJ, Trefelner E, Boulware SD. Idiopathic growth hormone deficiency: MR findings in 35 patients. *AJNR.* 1991;12:155–160.

40. Kuroiwa T, Okabe Y, Hasuo K, Yasumori K, Mizushimạ A, Masuda K. MR imaging of pituitary dwarfism. *AJNR.* 1991;12:161–164.

41. Aicardi J, Bauman F. Supratentorial extracerebral cysts in infants and children. *J Neurol Neurosurg Psychiatry.* 1975;38:57–68.

42. Hoffman HJ, Hendrick EB, Humphreys RP, Armstrong EA. Investigation and management of suprasellar arachnoid cysts. *J Neurosurg.* 1982;57:597–602.

43. Robertson SJ, Wolpert SM, Runge VM. MR imaging of middle cranial fossa arachnoid cysts: temporal lobe agenesis syndrome revisited. *AJNR.* 1989;10:1007–1010.

44. Harsh GR IV, Edwards MS, Wilson CB. Intracranial arachnoid cysts in children. *J Neurosurg.* 1986;64:835–842.

45. di Rocco C, Caldarelli M, di Trapani G. Infratentorial arachnoid cysts in children. *Childs Brain.* 1981;8:119–133.

46. Naidich TP, McLone DG, Radkowski MA. Intracranial arachnoid cysts. *Pediatr Neurosci.* 1985–86;12:112–122. Review.

47. Golden JA, Rorke LB, Bruce DA. Dandy-Walker syndrome and associated anomalies. *Pediatr Neurosci.* 1987;13:38–44.

48. Hart MN, Malamud N, Ellis WG. The Dandy-Walker syndrome. A clinicopathological study based on 28 cases. *Neurology.* 1972;22:771–780.

49. Barkovich AJ, Kjos BO, Norman D, Edwards MS. Revised classification of posterior fossa cysts and cystlike malformations based on the results of multiplanar MR imaging. *AJNR.* 1989;10:977–988.

50. Banna M. Syringomyelia in association with posterior fossa cysts. *AJNR.* 1988;9:867–873.

51. Halsey JH Jr, Allen N, Chamberlin HR. The morphogenesis of hydranencephaly. *J Neurol Sci.* 1971;12:187–217.

52. Hoffman HJ, Hendrick EB, Humphreys RP, Armstrong EA. Investigation and management of suprasellar arachnoid cysts. *J Neurosurg.* 1982;57:597–602.

53. Barkovich AJ, Norman D. MR of schizencephaly. *AJR.* 1988;150:1391–1396.

54. Miller GM, Stears JC, Guggenheim MA, Wilkening GN. Schizencephaly: a clinical and CT study. *Neurology.* 1984;34:997–1001.

55. Zimmerman RA, Bilaniuk LT, Grossman RL. Computed tomography in migratory disorders of human brain development. *Neuroradiology.* 1983;25:257–263.

56. Smith AS, Weinstein MA, Quencer RM, et al. Association of heterotopic gray matter with seizures: MR imaging. Work in progress. *Radiology.* 1988;168:195–198.

57. Barkovich AJ, Chuang SH, Norman D. MR of neuronal migration anomalies. *AJR.* 1988;150:179–187.

58. Osborn RE, Byrd SE, Naidich TP, Bohan TP, Friedman H. MR imaging of neuronal migrational disorders. *AJNR.* 1988;9:1101–1106.

59. Rakic P. Neuronal migration and contact guidance in the primate telencephalon. *Postgrad Med J.* 1978;54:25–40.

60. Byrd SE, Bohan TP, Osborn RE, Naidich TP. The CT and MR evaluation of lissencephaly. *AJNR*. 1988;9:923–927.

61. Dobyns WB, McCluggage CW. Computed tomographic appearance of lissencephaly syndromes. *AJNR*. 1985;6:545–550.

62. Barkovich AJ, Chuang SH. Unilateral megalencephaly: correlation of MR imaging and pathologic characteristics. *AJNR*. 1990;11:523–531.

63. Kalifa GL, Chiron C, Sellier N, et al. Hemimegalencephaly: MR imaging in five children. *Radiology*. 1987;165:29–33.

64. McComb JG. Recent research into the nature of cerebrospinal fluid formation and absorption. *J Neurosurg*. 1983;59:369–383.

65. Zee CS, Segall H, Apuzzo G, et al. MR imaging of pineal region neoplasms. *J Comput Assist Tomogr*. 1991;15:56–63.

66. Giuffre R, Palma L, Fontana M. Infantile nontumoral aqueductal stenosis. *J Neurosurg Sci*. 1986;30:41–46.

67. Barkovich AJ, Newton TH. MR of aqueductal stenosis: evidence of a broad spectrum of tectal distortion. *AJNR*. 1989;10:471–476.

68. Scotti G, Musgrave MA, Fitz CR, Harwood-Nash DC. The isolated fourth ventricle in children: CT and clinical review of 16 cases. *AJR*. 1980;135:1233–1238.

69. Markowitz RI, Kleinman CS, Hellenbrand WE, Kopf G, Ment LR. Communicating hydrocephalus secondary to superior vena caval obstruction. Occurrence after Mustard's operation for transposition of the great arteries. *Am J Dis Child*. 1984;138:638–641.

70. Kendall B, Holland I. Benign communicating hydrocephalus in children. *Neuroradiology*. 1981;21:93–96.

71. Mathews VP, Kuharit MA, Edwards MK, D'Amour PG, Azzarelli B, Dreesen RG. Dyke award. Gd-DTPA enhanced MR imaging of experimental bacterial meningitis: evaluation and comparison with CT. *AJR*. 1989;152:131–166.

72. Flodmark O, Becker LE, Harwood-Nash DC, Fitzhardinge PM, Fitz CR, Chuang SH. Correlation between computed tomography and autopsy in premature and full-term neonates that have suffered perinatal asphyxia. *Radiology*. 1980;137:93–103.

73. Bell WO, Charney EB, Bruce DA, Sutton LN, Schut L. Symptomatic Arnold-Chiari malformation: review of experience with 22 cases. *J Neurosurg*. 1987;66:812–816.

74. Hirsch JF, Pierre-Kahn A, Renier D, Sainte-Rose C, Hoppe-Hirsch E. The Dandy-Walker malformation. A review of 40 cases. *J Neurosurg*. 1984;61:515–522.

75. Carolan PL, McLaurin RL, Tobin RB, Tobin JA, Engelhoff JC. Benign extra-axial collections of infancy. *Pediatr Neurosci*. 1986;12:140–144.

76. Nickel RE, Gallenstein JS. Developmental prognosis for infants with benign enlargement of the subarachnoid spaces. *Dev Med Child Neurol*. 1987;29:181–186.

77. National Institutes of Health Consensus Development Conference. Conference statement. Neurofibromatosis. *Arch Neurol*. 1988;45:575–578.

78. Huson SM. The different forms of neurofibromatosis. *Br Med J*. 1987;294:1113–1114. Editorial.

79. Huson SM, Harper PS, Compston DA. von Recklinghausen neurofibromatosis. A clinical and population study in south-east Wales. *Brain*. 1988;111:1355–1381.

80. Sobata E, Ohkuma H, Suzuki S. Cerebrovascular disorders associated with von Recklinghausen's neurofibromatosis: a case report. *Neurosurgery*. 1988;22:544–549. Review.

81. Bognanno JR, Edwards MK, Lee TA, Dunn DW, Roos KL, Klatte EC. Cranial MR imaging in neurofibromatosis. *AJR*. 1988;151:381–388.

82. Kingsley DP, Kendall BE, Fitz CR. Tuberous sclerosis: a clinicoradiological evaluation of 110 cases with particular reference to atypical presentation. *Neuroradiology*. 1986;28:38–46.

83. Bender BL, Yunis EJ. The pathology of tuberous sclerosis. *Pathol Annu*. 1982;17:339–382.

84. Martin N, de Broucker T, Cambier J, Marsault C, Nahum H. MRI evaluation of tuberous sclerosis. *Neuroradiology*. 1987;29:437–443.

85. McMurdo SK Jr, Moore SG, Brant-Zawadzki M, et al. MR imaging of intracranial tuberous sclerosis. *AJR*. 1987;148:791–796.

86. Altman NR, Purser RK, Post MJ. Tuberous sclerosis: characteristics at CT and MR imaging. *Radiology*. 1988;167:527–532.

87. Morimoto K, Mogami H. Sequential CT study of subependymal giant-cell astrocytoma associated with tuberous sclerosis. Case report. *J Neurosurg*. 1986;65:874–877.

88. Tsuchida T, Kamata K, Kawamata M, Okada K, Tanaka R, Oyake Y. Brain tumors in tuberous sclerosis. Report of 4 cases. *Childs Brain*. 1981;8:271–283.

89. Iwasaki S, Nakagawa H, Kichikawa K, Fukusumi A. MR and CT of tuberous sclerosis: linear abnormalities in the cerebral white matter. *AJNR*. 1990;11:1029–1034.

90. Di Trapani G, Di Rocco C, Abbamondi AL, Caldarelli M, Pocchiari M. Light microscopy and ultrastructural studies of Sturge-Weber disease. *Childs Brain*. 1982;9:23–36.

91. Wasenko JJ, Rosenbloom SA, Duchesneau PM, Lanzieri CF, Weinstein MA. The Sturge-Weber syndrome: comparison of MR and CT characteristics. *AJNR*. 1990;11:131–134.

92. Probst FP. Vascular morphology and angiographic flow patterns in Sturge-Weber angiomatosis: facts, thoughts and suggestions. *Neuroradiology*. 1980;20:73–78.

93. Elster AD, Chen MY. MR imaging of Sturge-Weber syndrome: role of gadopentetate dimeglumine and gradient-echo techniques. *AJNR*. 1990;11:685–689.

94. Horton WA, Wong V, Eldridge R. von Hippel–Lindau disease: clinical and pathological manifestations in nine families with 50 affected members. *Arch Intern Med*. 1976;136:769–777.

95. Huson SM, Harper PS, Hourihan MD, Cole G, Weeks Rd, Compston DA. Cerebellar hemangioblastoma and von Hippel–Lindau disease. *Brain*. 1986;109:1297–1310.

96. Gardeur D, Palmieri A, Mashaly R. Cranial computed tomography in the phakomatoses. *Neuroradiology*. 1983;25:293–304.

97. Sato Y, Waziri M, Smith W, et al. von Hippel–Lindau disease: MR imaging. *Radiology*. 1988;166:241–246.

98. Lannering B, Marky I, Nordborg C. Brain tumors in childhood and adolescence in west Sweden 1970–1984. Epidemiology and survival. *Cancer*. 1990;66:604–609.

99. Buetow PC, Smirniotopoulos JG, Done S. Congenital brain tumors: a review of 45 cases. *AJNR*. 1990;11:793–799.

100. Rorke LB, Gilles FH, Davis RL, Becker LE. Revision of the World Health Organization classification of brain tumors for childhood brain tumors. *Cancer*. 1985;56:1869–1886.

101. Duffner PK, Cohen ME, Myers MH, Heise HW. Survival of children with brain tumors: SEER Program, 1973–1980. *Neurology*. 1986;36:597–601.

102. Gjerris F, Klinken L. Long-term prognosis in children with benign cerebellar astrocytoma. *J Neurosurg*. 1978;49:179–184.

103. Naidich TP, Zimmerman RA. Primary brain tumors in children. *Semin Roentgenol*. 1984;19:100–114.

104. Gilles FH, Winston K, Fulchiero A, Leviton A. Histologic features and observational variation in cerebellar gliomas in children. *J Natl Cancer Inst*. 1977;58:175–181.

105. Gol A, McKissock W. The cerebellar astrocytomas: a report on 98 verified cases. *J Neurosurg*. 1959;16:287–296.

106. Ringertz N, Nordenstam H. Cerebellar astrocytoma. *J Neuropathol Exp Neurol*. 1951;10:343–367.

107. Kleinman GM, Schoene WC, Walshe TM III, et al. Malignant transformation in benign cerebellar astrocytoma. *J Neurosurg*. 1978;49:111.

108. Zimmerman RA, Bilaniuk LT, Bruno L, Rosenstock J. Computed tomography of cerebellar astrocytoma. *AJR*. 1978;130:929–933.

109. Barkovich AJ, Edwards MS. Brain tumors of childhood. In: *Contemporary Imaging. Pediatric Neuroimaging*. New York: Raven; 1990;1: 149–203.

110. Al-Mefty O, Jinkins JR, El-Senoussi M, el Shakir M, Fox JL. Medulloblastomas: a review of modern management with a report on 75 cases. *Surg Neurol*. 1985;24:606–624.

111. Farwell JR, Dohrmann GJ, Flannery JT. Medulloblastoma in childhood: an epidemiological study. *J Neurosurg*. 1984;61:657–664.

112. George RE, Laurent JP, McCluggage CW, Cheek WR. Spinal metastasis in primitive neuroectodermal tumors (medulloblastoma) of the posterior fossa: evaluation with CT myelography and correlation with patient age and tumor differentiation. *Pediatr Neurosci*. 1986;12:157–160.

113. McComb JG, Davis RL, Isaacs H Jr. Extraneural metastatic medulloblastoma during childhood. *Neurosurgery*. 1981;9:458–551.

114. Packer RJ, Siegel KR, Sutton LN, Litmann A, Bruce DA, Schut L. Leptomeningeal dissemination of primary central nervous system tumors of childhood. *Ann Neurol*. 1985;18:217–221.

115. Duffner PK, Cohen ME, Heffner RR, Freeman AI. Primitive neuroectodermal tumors of childhood. An approach to therapy. *J Neurosurg*. 1981;55:376–381.

116. Black P. Spinal metastasis: current status and recommended guidelines for management. *Neurosurgery*. 1979;5:726–746.

117. Dohrmann GJ, Farwell JR, Flannery JT. Ependymomas and ependymoblastomas in children. *J Neurosurg*. 1976;45:273–283.

118. Coulon RA, Till K. Intracranial ependymomas in children: a review of 43 cases. *Childs Brain*. 1977;3:154–168.

119. Pierre-Kahn A, Hirsch JF, Roux FX, Renier D, Sainte-Rose C. Intracranial ependymomas in childhood. Survival and functional results of 47 cases. *Childs Brain*. 1983;10:145–156.

120. Swartz JD, Zimmerman RA, Bilaniuk LT. Computed tomography of intracranial ependymomas. *Radiology*. 1982;143:97–101.

121. Spoto GP, Press GA, Hesselink JR, Solomon M. Intracranial ependymoma and subependymoma: MR manifestations. *AJNR*. 1990;11:83–91.

122. Cohen ME, Duffner PK, Heffner RR, Lacey DJ, Brecker M. Prognostic factors in brainstem gliomas. *Neurology*. 1986;36:602–605.

123. Zimmerman RD, Russell EJ, Leeds NE. Axial CT recognition of anteroposterior displacement of fourth ventricle. *AJNR*. 1980;1:65–70.

124. Stroink AR, Hoffman HJ, Hendrick EB, Humphreys RP. Diagnosis and management of pediatric brain stem gliomas. *J Neurosurg*. 1986;65: 745–750.

125. Lee BC, Kneeland JB, Walker RW, Posner JB, Cahill PT, Deck MD. MR imaging of brainstem tumors. *AJNR*. 1985;6:159–163.

126. Michels VV. Investigative studies in von Hippel–Lindau disease. *Neurofibromatosis*. 1988;1:159–163.

127. Lee SR, Sanches J, Mark AS, Dillon WP, Norman D, Newton TH. Posterior fossa hemangioblastomas: MR imaging. *Radiology*. 1989; 171:463–468.

128. Elster AD, Arthur DW. Intracranial hemangioblastomas: CT and MR findings. *J Comput Assist Tomogr*. 1988;12:736–739.

129. Page LK, Lombrosco CT, Matson DD. Childhood epilepsy with late detection of cerebral glioma. *J Neurosurg*. 1969;31:253–261.

130. Palma L, Guidetti B. Cystic pilocytic astrocytomas of the cerebral hemispheres. Surgical experience with 51 cases and long term results. *J Neurosurg*. 1985;62:811–815.

131. Tomita T, McLone DG, Naidich TP. Mural tumors with cysts in the cerebral hemispheres of children. *Neurosurgery*. 1986;19:998–1005.

132. Tans J, de Jongh IE. Computed tomography of supratentorial astrocytoma. *Clin Neurol Neurosurg*. 1978;80:156–168.

133. Waga S, Shimizu T, Sakakura M. Diencephalic syndrome of emaciation (Russell's syndrome). *Surg Neurol*. 1982;17:141–146.

134. Lee YY, Van Tassel P, Bruner JM, Moser RP, Share JC. Juvenile pilocytic astrocytomas: CT and MR characteristics. *AJNR*. 1989;10: 363–370.

135. Savoiardo M, Harwood-Nash DC, Tadmor R, Scotti G, Musgrave MA. Gliomas of the intracranial anterior optic pathways in children. The role of computed tomography, angiography, pneumoencephalography, and radionuclide brain scanning. *Radiology*. 1981;138:601–610.

136. Lin SR, Bryson MM, Gobien RP, Fitz CR, Lee YY. Radiologic findings of hamartomas of the tuber cinereum and hypothalamus. *Radiology*. 1978;127:697–703.

137. Boyko OB, Curnes JT, Oakes WJ, Burger PC. Hamartomas of the tuber cinereum: CT, MR, and pathologic findings. *AJNR*. 1991;12:309–314.

138. Benitez WI, Sartor KJ, Angtuaco EJ. Case report: craniopharyngioma presenting as a nasopharyngeal mass: CT and MR findings. *J Comput Assist Tomogr*. 1988;12:1068–1072.

139. Lipper MH, Kishore PR, Ward JD. Craniopharyngioma: unusual computed tomographic presentation. *Neurosurgery*. 1981;9:76–78.

140. Freeman MP, Kessler RM, Allen JH, Price AC. Craniopharyngioma: CT and MR imaging in nine cases. *J Comput Assist Tomogr*. 1987;11:810–814.

141. Young SC, Zimmerman RA, Nowell MA, et al. Giant cystic craniopharyngiomas. *Neuroradiology*. 1987;29:468–473.

142. O'Sullivan RM, Sheehan M, Poskitt KJ, Graeb DA, Chu AC, Joplin GF. Langerhans cell histiocytosis of hypothalamus and optic chiasm: CT and MR studies. *J Comput Assist Tomogr*. 1991;15:52–55.

143. Tien RD, Newton TH, McDermott MW, Dillon WP, Kucharczyk J. Thickened pituitary stalk on MR images in patients with diabetes insipidus and Langerhans cell histiocytosis. *AJNR*. 1990;11:703–708.

144. Sumner TE, Volberg FM. Cushing's syndrome in infancy due to pituitary adenoma. *Pediatr Radiol*. 1982;12:81–83.

145. Hemminghytt S, Kalkhoff RK, Daniels DL, Williams AL, Grogan JP, Haughton VM. Computed tomographic study of hormone-secreting microadenomas. *Radiology*. 1983;146:65–69.

146. Lee BC, Deck MD. Sellar and juxtasellar lesion detection with MR. *Radiology*. 1985;157:143–147.

147. Pojunas KW, Daniels DL, Williams AL, Haughton VM. MR imaging of prolactin-secreting microadenomas. *AJNR*. 1986;7:209–213.

148. Johannsson JH, Rekate HL, Roessmann U. Gangliogliomas: pathological and clinical correlation. *J Neurosurg*. 1981;54:58–63.

149. Sutton LN, Packer RJ, Rorke LB, Bruce DA, Schut L. Cerebral gangliogliomas during childhood. *Neurosurgery*. 1983;13:124–128.

150. Benitez WI, Glasier CM, Husain M, Angtuaco EJ, Chadduck WM. MR findings in childhood gangliogliomas. *J Comput Assist Tomogr*. 1990; 14:712–716.

151. Castillo M, Davis PC, Takei Y, Hoffman JC Jr. Intracranial ganglioglioma: MR, CT, and clinical findings in 18 patients. *AJR*. 1990;154: 607–612.

152. Armington WG, Osborn AG, Cubberly DA, et al. Supratentorial ependymoma: CT appearance. *Radiology*. 1985;157:367–372.

153. Centeno RS, Lee AA, Winter J, Barba D. Supratentorial ependymomas: neuroimaging and clinicopathological correlation. *J Neurosurg*. 1986;64:209–215.

154. Hart MN, Earle KM. Primitive neuroectodermal tumors of the brain in children. *Cancer*. 1973;32:890–897.

155. Kosnik EJ, Boesel CP, Bay J, Sayers MP. Primitive neuroectodermal tumors of the central nervous system in children. *J Neurosurg*. 1978;48: 741–746.

156. Kingsley DP, Harwood-Nash DC. Radiological features of the neuroectodermal tumors of childhood. *Neuroradiology*. 1984;26:463–467.

157. Davis PC, Wichman RD, Takei Y, Hoffman JC Jr. Primary cerebral neuroblastoma: CT and MR findings in 12 cases. *AJNR*. 1990;11:115–120.

158. Valladares JB, Perry RH, Kalbag RM. Malignant choroid plexus papilloma with extraneural metastasis. Case report. *J Neurosurg*. 1980;52:251–255.

159. Tomita T, McLone DG, Flannery AM. Choroid plexus papillomas of neonates, infants, and children. *Pediatr Neurosci*. 1988;14:23–30.

160. Kendall B, Reider-Grosswasser I, Valentine A. Diagnosis of masses presenting within the ventricles on computed tomography. *Neuroradiology*. 1983;25:11–22.

161. Morrison G, Sobel DF, Kelley WM, Norman D. Intraventricular mass lesions. *Radiology*. 1984;153:435–442.

162. Schellhas KP, Siebert RC, Heithoff KB, Franciosi RA. Congenital choroid plexus papilloma of the third ventricle: diagnosis with real-time sonography and MR imaging. *AJNR*. 1988;9:797–798.

163. Maeder PP, Holtås SL, Basibüyük LN, Salford LG, Tapper UA, Brun A. Colloid cysts of the third ventricle: correlation of MR and CT findings with histology and chemical analysis. *AJNR*. 1990;1:575–581.

164. Edwards MS, Davis RL, Laurent JP. Tumor markers and cytologic features of cerebrospinal fluid. *Cancer*. 1985;56(suppl):1773–1777.

165. Jooma R, Kendall BE. Diagnosis and management of pineal tumors. *J Neurosurg*. 1983;58:654–665.

166. Shokry A, Janzer RC, von Hochstetter AR, Yasargil MG, Hedinger C. Primary intracranial germ-cell tumors. A clinicopathological study of 14 cases. *J Neurosurg*. 1985;62:826–830.

167. Soejima T, Takeshita I, Yamamoto H, Tsukamoto Y, Fukui M, Matsuoka S. Computed tomography of germinomas in basal ganglia and thalamus. *Neuroradiology*. 1987;29:366–370.

168. Kilgore DP, Strother CM, Starshak RJ, Haughton VM. Pineal germinoma: MR imaging. *Radiology*. 1986;158:435–438.

169. Zimmerman RA, Bilaniuk LT, Wood JH, Bruce DA, Schut L. Computed tomography of pineal, parapineal and histologically-related tumors. *Radiology*. 1980;137:669–677.

170. Nakagawa H, Iwasaki S, Kichikawa K, et al. MR imaging of pineocytoma: report of two cases. *AJNR*. 1990;11:195–198.

171. Vonofakos D, Marcu H, Hacker H. Oligodendrogliomas: CT patterns with emphasis on features indicating malignancy. *J Comput Assist Tomogr*. 1979;3:783–788.

172. Lee YY, Tassel PV. Intracranial oligodendrogliomas: imaging findings in 35 untreated cases. *AJNR*. 1988;10:119–127.

173. Horowitz BL, Chari MV, James R, Bryan RN. MR of intracranial epidermoid tumors: correlation of in vivo imaging with in vitro 13C spectroscopy. *AJNR*. 1990;11:299–302.

174. Drolshagan LF. Dense dermoid cyst of the posterior fossa. *AJNR*. 1991;12:317–318.

175. Zimmerman RA, Bilaniuk LT, Dolinskas C. Cranial computed tomography of epidermoid and congenital fatty tumors of maldevelopment origin. *J Comput Assist Tomogr*. 1979;3:40–50.

176. Amendola A, Garfinkle WB, Ostrum BJ, Katz MR, Katz RI. Preoperative diagnosis of a ruptured intracranial dermoid cyst by computerized tomography. Case report. *J Neurosurg*. 1978;48:1035–1037.

177. Goldberg R, Byrd S, Winter J, et al. Varied appearance of trigeminal neuroma on CT. *AJR*. 1980;134:57–60.

178. Pinto RS, Kricheff II. Neuroradiology of intracranial neuromas. *Semin Roentgenol*. 1984;19:44–52.

179. Latack JT, Gabrielsen TO, Knake JE, et al. Facial nerve neuromas: radiologic evaluation. *Radiology*. 1983;149:731–739.

180. Curati WL, Graif M, Kingsley DP, Niendorf HP, Young IR. Acoustic neuromas: Gd-DTPA enhancement in MR imaging. *Radiology*. 1986;158:447–451.

181. Kingsley DP, Brooks GB, Leung AW, Johnson MA. Acoustic neuromas: evaluation by magnetic resonance imaging. *AJNR*. 1985;6:1–5.

182. Camins MB, Takeuchi J. Normotopic plus heterotopic atypical teratomas. *Childs Brain*. 1978;4:151-160.

183. Ganti SR, Hilal SK, Stein BM, Silver AJ, Mawad M, Sane P. CT of pineal region tumors. *AJR*. 1986;146:451–458.

184. Kushnet MW, Goldman RL. Lipoma of the corpus callosum associated with a frontal bone defect. *AJR*. 1978;131:517–518.

185. Deen HG Jr, Scheithauer BW, Ebersold MJ. Clinical and pathological study of meningiomas of the first two decades of life. *J Neurosurg*. 1982;56:317–322.

186. Soffer D, Pittaluga S, Feiner M, Beller AJ. Intracranial meningiomas following low-dose irradiation to the head. *J Neurosurg*. 1983;59:1048–1053.

187. Mamourian AC, Lewandowski AE, Towfighi J. Cystic intraparenchymal meningioma in a child. Case report. *AJNR*. 1991;12:366–367.

188. Aoki S, Sasaki Y, Machida T, Tanioka H. Contrast-enhanced MR images in patients with meningioma: importance of enhancement of the dura adjacent to the tumor. *AJNR*. 1990;11:935–938.

189. Drake JM, Hendrick EB, Becker LE, Chuang SH, Hoffman HJ, Humphreys RP. Intracranial meningiomas in children. *Pediatr Neurosci*. 1986;12:134–139.

190. Sano K, Wakai S, Ochiai C, Takakura K. Characteristics of intracranial meningiomas in childhood. *Childs Brain*. 1981;8:98–106.

191. Hochberg FH, Miller DC. Primary central nervous system lymphoma. *J Neurosurg*. 1988;68:835–853.

192. Levy RM, Rosenbloom S, Perrett LV. Neuroradiologic findings in AIDS: review of 200 cases. *AJNR*. 1986;7:833–839.

193. Ramsey RG, Geremia GK. CNS complications of AIDS: CT and MR findings. *AJR*. 1988;151:449–454.

194. Goldstein JD, Zeifer B, Chao C, et al. CT appearance of primary CNS lymphoma in patients with acquired immunodeficiency syndrome. *J Comput Assist Tomogr*. 1991;15:39–44.

195. Rippe DJ, Boyko OB, Friedman HS, et al. Gd-DTPA–enhanced MR imaging of leptomeningeal spread of primary intracranial CNS tumor in children. *AJNR*. 1990;11:329–332.

196. Han JS, Zee CS, Ahmadi J, Ro HI, Segall HD, Stowe S. Intracranial metastatic Wilms' tumor in children: a report of two cases. *Surg Neurol*. 1983;20:157–159.

197. Armstrong EA, Harwood-Nash DC, Ritz CR, Chuang SH, Pettersson H, Martin DJ. CT of neuroblastomas and gangliogliomas in children. *AJR*. 1982;139:571–576.

198. Handa J, Suzuki F, Nioka H, Koyama T. Clivus chordoma in childhood. *Surg Neurol*. 1987;28:58–62.

199. Meyer JE, Oot RF, Lindfors KK. CT appearance of clival chordomas. *J Comput Assist Tomogr*. 1986;10:34–38.

200. Oot RF, Melville GE, New PF, et al. The role of MR and CT in evaluating clival chordomas and chondrosarcomas. *AJNR*. 1988;9:715–723.

201. Sze G, Uichanco LS, Brant-Zawadzki MN, et al. Chordomas: MR imaging. *Radiology*. 1988;166:187–191.

202. de Divitiis E, Spaziante R, Cirillo S, Stella L, Donzelli R. Primary sellar chondromas. *Surg Neurol*. 1979;11:229–232.

203. Nowell MA, Grossman RI, Hackney DB, Zimmerman RA, Goldberg HI, Bilaniuk LT. MR imaging of white matter disease in children. *AJNR*. 1988;9:503–509.

204. Nagao H, Kida K, Matsuda H, Shishido T, Matsuoka K, Nonaka I. Alexander disease: clinical, electrodiagnostic and radiographic studies. *Neuropediatrics*. 1981;12:22–32.

205. Russo JL, Aron A, Anderson J. Alexander's disease: a report and reappraisal. *Neurology*. 1976;26:607–614.

206. Farrell K, Chuang S, Becker LE. Computed tomography in Alexander's disease. *Ann Neurol*. 1984;15:605–607.

207. Trommer BL, Naidich TP, Dal Canto MC, McLone DG, Larsen MB. Noninvasive CT diagnosis of infantile Alexander disease: pathologic correlation. *J Comput Assist Tomogr*. 1983;7:509–516.

208. Shah M, Ross JS. Infantile Alexander disease: MR appearance of a biopsy-proved case. *AJNR*. 1990;11:1105–1106.

209. Adachi M, Torii J, Schneck L, Volk BW. Electron microscopic and enzyme histochemical studies of the cerebellum in spongy degeneration (van Bogaert and Bertrans type). *Acta Neuropathol.* 1972;20:22–31.

210. Feigin J, Pena CE, Budzilovich G. The infantile spongy degenerations. *Neurology.* 1968;18:153–166.

211. Jellinger K, Seitelberger F. Juvenile form of spongy degeneration of the CNS. *Acta Neuropathol.* 1969;13:276–281.

212. Andriola MR. Computed tomography in the diagnosis of Canavan's disease. *Ann Neurol.* 1982;11:323–324.

213. Rushton AR, Shaywitz BA, Duncan CC, Geehr RB, Manuelidis EE. Computed tomography in the diagnosis of Canavan's disease. *Ann Neurol.* 1981;10:57–60.

214. McAdams HP, Geyer CA, Done SL, Deigh D, Mitchell M, Ghaed VN. CT and MR imaging of Canavan disease. *AJNR.* 1990;1:397–399.

215. Lisson G, Leupold D, Bechinger D, Wallesch C. CT findings in a case of deficiency of 3-hydroxy-3-methylglutaryl CoA lyase. *Neuroradiology.* 1981;22:99–101.

216. Clarke JT, Ozere RL, Krause VW. Early infantile variant of Krabbe globoid cell leucodystrophy with lung involvement. *Arch Dis Child.* 1981;56:640–642.

217. Farrell DF, Swedberg K. Clinical and biochemical heterogeneity of globoid cell leucodystrophy. *Ann Neurol.* 1981;10:364–368.

218. Hagberg B. Krabbe's disease: clinical presentation of neurological variants. *Neuropediatrics.* 1984;15(suppl):11–15.

219. Baram TZ, Goldman AM, Percy AK. Krabbe disease: specific MRI and CT findings. *Neurology.* 1986;36:111–115.

220. Ieshima A, Eda I, Matsui A, Yoshino K, Takashima S, Takeshita K. Computed tomography in Krabbe's disease: comparison with neuropathology. *Neuroradiology.* 1983;25:323–327.

221. Kwan E, Drace J, Enzmann D. Specific CT findings in Krabbe disease. *AJR.* 1984;143:665–670.

222. Haltia T, Palo J, Haltia M, Icen A. Juvenile metachromatic leucodystrophy. Clinical, biochemical and neuropathological studies in nine new cases. *Arch Neurol.* 1980;37:42–46.

223. Naidu S, Hofmann KJ, Moser HW, Maumenee IH, Wenger DA. Galactosylceramide-beta-galactosidase deficiency in association with cherry red spot. *Neuropediatrics.* 1988;19:46–48.

224. Alves D, Pires MM, Guimaraes A, Miranda MD. Four cases of late onset metachromatic leukodystrophy in a family: clinical, biochemical, and neuropathological studies. *J Neurol Neurosurg Psychiatry.* 1986;49:1417–1422.

225. Schipper HI, Seidel D. Computed tomography in late onset metachromatic leukodystrophy. *Neuroradiology.* 1984;26:39–44.

226. Renier WO, Gabriëls FJ, Husbinz TW, et al. Connatal Pelizaeus-Merzbacher disease with congenital stridor in 2 maternal cousins. *Acta Neuropathol.* 1981;54:11–17.

227. Malone MJ. The cerebral lipidoses. *Pediatr Clin North Am.* 1976;23:303–326.

228. Shimomura C, Matsui A, Choh H, Funahashi M, Suzuki Y, Tsuchiya K. Magnetic resonance imaging in Pelizaeus-Merzbacher disease. *Pediatr Neurol.* 1988;4:124–125.

229. Silverstein AM, Hirsh DK, Trobe JD, Gebarski SS. MR imaging of the brain in five members of a family with Pelizaeus-Merzbacher disease. *AJNR.* 1990;11:495–499.

230. Statz A, Boltshauser E, Schinzel A, Spiess H. Computed tomography in Pelizaeus-Merzbacher disease. *Neuroradiology.* 1981;22:103–105.

231. Dabbagh O, Swaiman KF. Cockayne syndrome: MRI correlates of hypomyelination. *Pediatr Neurol.* 1988;4:113–116.

232. Soffer D, Grotsky HW, Rapin I, Suzuki K. Cockayne syndrome: unusual neuropathological findings and review of the literature. *Ann Neurol.* 1979;6:340–348.

233. Watanabe I, McCaman R, Dyken P, Zeman W. Absence of cerebral myelin sheaths in a case of presumed Pelizaeus-Merzbacher disease. Electron microscopic and biochemic studies. *J Neuropathol Exp Neurol.* 1969;28:243–256.

234. Aubourg P, Diebler C. Adrenoleukodystrophy—its diverse CT appearances and an evolutive or phenotypic variant: the leukodystrophy without adrenal insufficiency. *Neuroradiology.* 1982;24:33–42.

235. Hong-Magno ET, Muraki AS, Huttenlocher PR. Atypical CT scans in adrenoleukodystrophy. *J Comput Assist Tomogr.* 1987;11:333–336.

236. Kumar AJ, Rosenbaum AE, Naidu S, et al. Adrenoleukodystrophy: correlating MR imaging with CT. *Radiology.* 1987;165:497–504.

237. Marler JR, O'Neill BP, Forbes GS, Moser HW. Adrenoleukodystrophy (ALD): clinical and CT features of a childhood variant. *Neurology.* 1983;33:1203–1205.

238. Bewermeyer H, Bamborschke S, Ebhardt G, et al. MR imaging in adrenoleukomyeloneuropathy. *J Comput Assist Tomogr.* 1985;9:793–796.

239. Svenningsson A, Runmarker B, Lycke J, Andersen O. Incidence of MS during two fifteen-year periods in the Gothenburg region of Sweden. *Acta Neurol Scand.* 1990;82:161–168,

240. Hauser SL, Bresnan MJ, Reinherz EL, Weiner HL. Childhood multiple sclerosis: clinical features and demonstration of changes in T cell subsets with disease activity. *Ann Neurol.* 1982;11:463–468.

241. Brandt S, Gyldensted C, Offner H, Melchior JC. Multiple sclerosis with onset in a two-year old boy. *Neuropediatrics.* 1981;12:75–82.

242. Sears ES, McCammon A, Bigelow R, Hayman LA. Maximizing the harvest of contrast enhancing lesions in multiple sclerosis. *Neurology.* 1982;32:815–820.

243. Weisberg L. Contrast enhancement visualized by computerized tomography in acute multiple sclerosis. *J Comput Assist Tomogr.* 1981;5:293–300.

244. Sheldon JJ, Siddharthan R, Tobias J, Sheremata WA, Soila K, Viamonte M Jr. MR imaging of multiple sclerosis: comparison with clinical and CT examinations in 74 patients. *AJR.* 1985;145:957–964.

245. Osborn AG, Harnsberger HR, Smoker WR, Boyer RS. Multiple sclerosis in adolescents: CT and MR findings. *AJNR.* 1990;11:489–494.

246. Cadman TE, Rorke LB. Central pontine myelinolysis in childhood and adolescence. *Arch Dis Child.* 1969;44:342–350.

247. Laureno R. Central pontine myelinolysis following rapid correction of hyponatremia. *Ann Neurol.* 1983;13:232–242.

248. Takeda K, Sakuta M, Saeki F. Central pontine myelinolysis diagnosed by magnetic resonance imaging. *Ann Neurol.* 1985;17:310–311.

249. Gerard E, Healy GE, Hesselink JR. MR demonstration of mesencephalic lesions in osmotic demyelination syndrome (central pontine myelinolysis). *Neurology.* 1987;29:582–584.

250. Hazratji SMA, Kim RL, Lee SH, Marasigan AV. Evolution of pontine and extrapontine myelinolysis. *J Comput Assist Tomogr.* 1983;7:356–361.

251. Koci TM, Chiang F, Chow P, et al. Thalamic extrapontine lesions in central pontine myelinolysis. *AJNR.* 1990;11:1229–1233.

252. Peylan-Ramu N, Poplack DG, Pizzo PA, Adornato BT, DiChiro G. Abnormal CT scans of the brain in asymptomatic children with acute lymphocytic leukemia after prophylactic treatment of the central nervous system with radiation and intrathecal chemotherapy. *N Engl J Med.* 1978;298:815–818.

253. Croft PB. Para-infections and post-vaccinal encephalomyelitis. *Postgrad Med J.* 1969;43:392–400.

254. Reik L Jr. Disseminated vasculomyelinopathy: an immune complex disease. *Ann Neurol.* 1980;7:291–296.

255. Tolly TL, Wells RG, Sty JR. MR features of fleeting CNS lesions associated with Epstein-Barr virus infection. *J Comput Assist Tomogr.* 1989;13:665–668.

256. Dietrich RB, Bradley WG, Zagaroza EJ, et al. MR evaluation of early myelination patterns in normal and developmentally delayed infants. *AJNR.* 1988;9:69–76.

257. Barkovich AJ, Kjos BO, Jackson DE Jr, Norman D. Normal maturation of the neonatal and infant brain: MR imaging at 1.5 T. *Radiology*. 1988;166:173–180.

258. Kjos BO, Umansky R, Barkovich AJ. Brain MR imaging in children with developmental retardation of unknown cause: results in 76 cases. *AJNR*. 1990;11:1035–1040.

259. Oepen G, Ostertag C. Diagnostic value of CT in patients with Huntington's chorea and their offspring. *J Neurol*. 1981;225:189–196.

260. Osborne JP, Munson P, Burman D. Huntington's chorea. *Arch Dis Child*. 1972;57:99–103.

261. Simmons JT, Pastakia B, Chase TN, Shults CW. Magnetic resonance imaging in Huntington disease. *AJNR*. 1986;7:25–28.

262. Oliver J, Dewhurst K. Childhood and adolescent forms of Huntington's disease. *J Neurol Neurosurg Psychiatr*. 1969;32:455–459.

263. Nausieda PA, Burton BJ, Koller WC, et al. Sydenham chorea: an update. *Neurology*. 1980;30:331–334.

264. Kienzle GD, Breger RK, Chun RW, Zupanc ML, Sackett JF. Sydenham chorea: MR manifestations in two cases. *AJNR*. 1991;12:73–76.

265. Harik SI, Post JD. Computed tomography in Wilson's disease. *Neurology*. 1981;31:107–110.

266. Kvicala V, Vymazal J, Nevsimalova S. Computed tomography of Wilson disease. *AJNR*. 1983;4:429–430.

267. DeHaan J, Grossman RI, Civitello L, et al. High-field magnetic resonance imaging of Wilson's disease. *J Comput Tomogr*. 1987;11:132–135.

268. DiMauro S, Servidei S, Zeviani M, et al. Cytochrome c oxidase deficiency in Leigh syndrome. *Ann Neurol*. 1987;22:498–506.

269. Richter RB. Infantile subacute necrotizing encephalopathy (Leigh's disease). Its relationship to Wernicke's encephalopathy. *Neurology*. 1968;18:1125–1132.

270. Pincus JH. Subacute necrotizing encephalomyelopathy (Leigh's disease): a consideration of clinical features and etiology. *Dev Med Child Neurol*. 1972;14:87–101.

271. Geyer CA, Sartor KJ, Prensky AJ, Abramson CL, Hodges FJ, Gado MH. Leigh disease (subacute necrotizing encephalomyelopathy): CT and MR in five cases. *J Comput Assist Tomogr*. 1988;12:40–44.

272. Koch TK, Lo WD, Berg BO. Variability of serial CT scans in subacute necrotizing encephalomyelopathy (Leigh disease). *Pediatr Neurol*. 1985;1:48–51.

273. Medina L, Chi TL, DeVivo DC, Hilal SK. MR findings in patients with subacute necrotizing encephalomyelopathy (Leigh syndrome): correlation with biochemical defect. *AJNR*. 1990;11:379–384.

274. Mirowitz SA, Sartor K, Prensky AJ, Gado M, Hodges FJ III. Neurodegenerative diseases of childhood: MR and CT evaluation. *J Comput Assist Tomogr*. 1991;15:210–222.

275. Egger J, Kendall BE. Computed tomography in mitochondrial cytopathy. *Neuroradiology*. 1981;56:741–752.

276. Allard JC, Tilak S, Carter AP. CT and MR of MELAS syndrome. *AJNR*. 1988;9:1234–1238.

277. Swaiman KF, Smith SA, Trock GL, Siddiqui AR. Sea-blue histiocytes, lymphocytic cytosomes, movement disorder and ^{59}Fe-uptake in basal ganglia: Hallervorden-Spatz disease or ceroid storage disease with abnormal isotope scan? *Neurology*. 1983;33:301–305.

278. Dooling EC, Schoene WC, Richardson EP Jr. Hallervorden-Spatz syndrome. *Arch Neurol*. 1974;30:70–83.

279. Boltshauser E, Lang W, Janzer R, et al. Computed tomography in Hallervorden-Spatz disease. *Neuropediatrics*. 1987;18:81–83.

280. Littrup PJ, Gebarski SS. MR imaging of Hallervorden-Spatz disease. *J Comput Assist Tomogr*. 1985;9:491–493.

281. Horowitz AL, Kaplan R, Sarpel G. Carbon monoxide toxicity: MR imaging in the brain. *Radiology*. 1987;162:787–788.

282. Taylor R, Holgate RC. Carbon monoxide poisoning: asymmetric and unilateral changes on CT. *AJNR*. 1988;9:975–977.

283. Heiman-Patterson TD, Bonilla E, Di Mauro S, Foreman J, Schotland DL. Cytochrome-c–oxidase in a floppy infant. *Neurology*. 1982;32:898–901.

284. Langenstein I, Schwendemann G, Kuhne D, Koepp P, Stahnke N, Sternowsky HJ. Neuronal ceroid lipofuscinosis: CCT findings in fourteen patients. *Acta Paediatr Scand*. 1981;70:857–860.

285. Maertens PM, Machen BC, Williams JP, et al. Magnetic resonance imaging of mesial temporal sclerosis: case reports. *J Comput Tomogr*. 1987;11:136–139.

286. Heinz ER, Crain BJ, Radtke RA, et al. MR imaging in patients with temporal lobe seizures: correlation of results with pathologic findings. *AJNR*. 1990;11:827–832.

287. Terplan KL, Krauss RF. Histopathologic brain changes in association with ataxia-telangiectasia. *Neurology*. 1969;19:446–454.

288. Jason JM, Gelfand EW. Diagnostic considerations in ataxia-telangiectasia. *Arch Dis Child*. 1979;54:682–686.

289. Hosking G. Ataxia telangiectasia. *Dev Med Child Neurol*. 1982;24:77–80.

290. Dekaban AS, Constantopoulos G. Mucopolysaccharidosis types I, II, IIIA and V. Pathological and biochemical abnormalities in the neural and mesenchymal elements of the brain. *Acta Neuropathol (Berl)*. 1977;39:1–7.

291. McKusick VA, Neufeld EF. The mucopolysaccharide storage diseases. In: Stanbury JB, ed. *The Metabolic Basis of Inherited Disease*. New York: McGraw-Hill; 1983:751–823.

292. Watts RW, Spellacy E, Kendall BE, du Boulay G, Gibbs DA. Computed tomography studies on patients with mucopolysaccharidoses. *Neuroradiology*. 1981;21:9–23.

293. Nelson J, Grebbell FS. The value of computed tomography in patients with mucopolysaccharidosis. *Neuroradiology*. 1987;29:544–549.

294. Aicardi J, Castelein P. Infantile neuroaxonal dystrophy. *Brain*. 1979;102:727–748.

295. Kilbride HW, Daily DK, Matiu I, Hubbard AM. Neurodevelopmental follow-up of infants with birth weight less than 801 grams with intracranial hemorrhage. *J Perinatol*. 1989;9:376–381.

296. Paneth N, Stark RI. Cerebral palsy and mental retardation in relation to indicators of perinatal asphyxia. An epidemiologic overview. *Am J Obstet Gynecol*. 1983;147:960–966.

297. Nelson KB. What proportion of cerebral palsy is related to birth asphyxia? *J Pediatr*. 1988;112:572–574. Editorial.

298. Enzmann D, Murphy-Irwin K, Stevenson D, Ariagno R, Barton J, Sunshine P. The natural history of subependymal germinal matrix hemorrhage. *Am J Perinatol*. 1985;2:123–133.

299. Schellinger D, Grant EG, Manz HJ, Patronas NJ. Intraparenchymal hemorrhage in preterm neonates: a broadening spectrum. *AJNR*. 1988;9:327–333.

300. Scher MS, Wright FS, Lockman LA, Thompson TR. Intraventricular haemorrhage in the full-term neonate. *Arch Neurol*. 1982;39:769–772.

301. Fawer CL, Calame A, Perentes E, Anderegg A. Periventricular leukomalacia: a correlation study between real-time ultrasound and autopsy findings. Periventricular leukomalacia in the neonate. *Neuroradiology*. 1985;27:292–300.

302. Trounce JQ, Rutter N, Levene MI. Periventricular leucomalacia and intraventricular haemorrhage in the preterm neonate. *Arch Dis Child*. 1986;16:1196–1202.

303. Gilles FH, Murphy SF. Perinatal telencephalic leucoencephalopathy. *J Neurol Neurosurg Psychiatry*. 1969;32:404–413.

304. Leech RW, Alvord EC. Glial fatty metamorphosis. An abnormal response of premyelin glia frequently accompanying periventricular leukomalacia. *Am J Pathol*. 1974;74:603–612.

305. Barmada MA, Moossy J, Shuman RM. Cerebral infarcts with arterial occlusion in neonates. *Ann Neurol*. 1979;6:495–502.

306. Volpe JJ. Brain injury in the premature infant: is it preventable? *Pediatr Res.* 1990;27:S28–S33.

307. Novotny EJ Jr. Hypoxic-ischemic encephalopathy. In: Stevenson DK, Sunshine P, eds. *Fetal and Neonatal Brain Injury.* Philadelphia: Decker; 1989:113–122.

308. Paneth N, Rudelli R, Monte W, et al. White matter necrosis in very low birth weight infants: neuropathologic and ultrasonographic findings in infants surviving six days or longer. *J Pediatr.* 1990;116:975–984.

309. Takashima S, Tanaka K. Development of cerebrovascular architecture and its relationship to periventricular leukomalacia. *Arch Neurol.* 1978;35:11–16.

310. Shankaran S, Slovis TL, Bedard MP, Poland RL. Sonographic classification of intracranial hemorrhage. A prognostic indicator of mortality, morbidity, and short-term neurologic outcome. *J Pediatr.* 1982;100:469–475.

311. Rumack CM, Manco-Johnson ML, Manco-Johnson MJ, Koops BL, Hathaway WE, Appareti K. Timing and course of neonatal intracranial hemorrhage using real-time ultrasound. *Radiology.* 1985;154:101–105.

312. Hecht ST, Filly RA, Callen PW, Wilson-Davis SL. Intracranial hemorrhage: late onset in the preterm neonate. *Radiology.* 1983;149:697–699.

313. Fleischer AC, Hutchison AA, Bundy AL, et al. Serial sonography of posthemorrhagic ventricular dilatation and porencephaly after intracranial hemorrhage in the preterm neonate. *AJR.* 1983;141:451–455.

314. Grant EG, Kerner M, Schellinger D, et al. Evolution of porencephalic cysts from intraparenchymal hemorrhage in neonates: sonographic evidence. *AJR.* 1982;138:467–470.

315. Smith WL, McGuiness G, Cavanaugh D, Courtney S. Ultrasound screening of premature infants: longitudinal follow-up of intracranial hemorrhage. *Radiology.* 1983;147:445–448.

316. Grant EG, Schellinger D, Richardson JD, Coffey ML, Smirniotopoulous JG. Echogenic periventricular halo: normal sonographic finding or neonatal cerebral hemorrhage. *AJR.* 1983;140:793–796.

317. Bowerman RA, Donn SM, DiPietro MA, D'Amato CJ, Hicks SP. Periventricular leukomalacia in the pre-term newborn infant: sonographic and clinical features. *Radiology.* 1984;151:382–388.

318. Grant EG, Schellinger D. Sonography of neonatal periventricular leukomalacia: recent experience with a 7.5-MHz scanner. *AJNR.* 1985;6:781–785.

319. Carson SC, Hertzberg BS, Bowie JD, Burger PC. Value of sonography in the diagnosis of intracranial hemorrhage and periventricular leukomalacia: a postmortem study of 35 cases. *AJNR.* 1990;11:677–683.

320. Flodmark O, Roland EH, Hill A, Whitfield MF. Periventricular leukomalacia: radiologic diagnosis. *Radiology.* 1987;162:119–124.

321. Flodmark O, Lupton B, Li D, et al. MR imaging of periventricular leukomalacia in childhood. *AJNR.* 1989;10:111–118.

322. Baker LL, Stevenson DK, Enzmann DR. End-stage periventricular leukomalacia: MR evaluation. *Radiology.* 1988;168:809–815.

323. McArdle CB, Richardson CJ, Hayden CK, Nicholas DA, Crofford MJ, Amparo EG. Abnormalities of the neonatal brain: MR imaging. Part I. Intracranial hemorrhage. *Radiology.* 1987;163:387–394.

324. Keller MS, DiPietro MA, Teele RL, et al. Periventricular cavitations in the first week of life. *AJNR.* 1987;8:291–295.

325. Barkovich AJ. Metabolic and destructive brain disorders. In: *Contemporary Neuroimaging: Pediatric Neuroimaging.* New York: Raven Press; 1990;1:35–75.

326. Barkovich AJ, Truwit CL. Brain damage from perinatal asphyxia: correlation of MR findings with gestational age. *AJNR.* 1990;11:1087–1096.

327. Roland EH, Hill A, Norman MG, Flodmark O, MacNab AJ. Selective brainstem injury in an asphyxiated newborn. *Ann Neurol.* 1988;23:89–92.

328. Wilson ER, Mirra SS, Schwartz JF. Congenital diencephalic and brain stem damage: neuropathologic study of three cases. *Acta Neuropathol (Berl).* 1982;57:70–74.

329. Billmire ME, Myers PA. Serious head injury in infants: accident or abuse? *Pediatrics.* 1985;75:340–342.

330. Hobbs CJ. Skull fracture and the diagnosis of abuse. *Arch Dis Child.* 1984;59:246–252.

331. Craft AW, Shaw DA, Cartlidge NE. Head injuries in children. *Br Med J.* 1972;4:200–203.

332. Bruce DA, Alavi A, Bilaniuk L, Dolinskas C, Obrist W, Uzzell B. Diffuse cerebral swelling following head injuries in children: the syndrome of "malignant brain edema." *J Neurosurg.* 1981;54:170–178.

333. Sharples PM, Storey A, Aynsley-Green A, Eyre JA. Causes of fatal childhood accidents involving head injury in northern region, 1979–86. *BMJ.* 1990;301:1193–1197.

334. Gentry LR, Godersky JC, Thompson B. MR imaging of head trauma: review of the distribution and radiopathologic features of traumatic lesions. *AJNR.* 1988;9:101–110.

335. Kelly AB, Zimmerman RD, Snow RB, Gandy SE, Heier LA, Deck MD. Head trauma: comparison of MR and CT—experience in 100 patients. *AJNR.* 1988;9:699–708.

336. Hernansanz J, Munoz F, Rodriquez D, Soler C, Principe C. Subdural hematomas of the posterior fossa in normal-weight newborns. A report of two cases. *J Neurosurg.* 1984;61:972–974.

337. Koch TK, Jahnke SE, Edwards MS, Davis SL. Posterior fossa hemorrhage in term newborns. *Pediatr Neurol.* 1985;1:96–99.

338. Hesselink JR, Dowd CF, Healy ME, Hajek P, Baker LL, Luerssen TG. MR imaging of brain contusions: a comparative study with CT. *AJNR.* 1988;9:269–278.

339. Berger MS, Pitts CH, Lovely M, Edwards MS, Bartkowski HM. Outcome from severe head injury in children and adolescents. *J Neurosurg.* 1985;62:194–199.

340. Zimmerman RA, Bilaniuk LT, Genneralli T. Computed tomography of shearing injuries of the cerebral white matter. *Radiology.* 1978;127:393–396.

341. Aoki N. Epidural haematoma in the newborn infants: therapeutic consequences from the correlation between haematoma content and computed tomography features. A review. *Acta Neurochir (Wien).* 1990;106:65–67.

342. Frowein RA, Schiltz F, Stammler U. Early post-traumatic intracranial hematoma. *Neurosurg Rev.* 1989;12(suppl 1):184–187.

343. Wright RL. Traumatic hematomas of the posterior cranial fossa. *J Neurosurg.* 1966;25:402–409.

344. Danzinger A, Price H. The evaluation of head trauma by computed tomography. *J Trauma.* 1979;19:1–5.

345. Aoki N, Masuzawa H. Infantile acute subdural hematoma. Clinical analysis of 26 cases. *J Neurosurg.* 1984;61:273–280.

346. Mealey J Jr. Infantile subdural hematomas. *Pediatr Clin North Am.* 1975;22:433–442.

347. Vielvoye GJ, Peters AC, van Dulken H. Acute infratentorial traumatic subdural hematoma associated with a torn tentorium cerebelli in a one-year-old boy. *Neuroradiology.* 1982;22:259–261.

348. Snow RB, Zimmerman RD, Gandy SE, Deck MD. Comparison of magnetic resonance imaging and computed tomography in the evaluation of head injury. *Neurosurgery.* 1986;18:45–52.

349. Smith WP Jr, Batnitzky S, Rengachary SS. Acute isodense subdural hematomas: a problem in anemic patients. *AJR.* 1981;136:543–546.

350. Bergstrom M, Ericson K, Levander B, Svendsen P. Computed tomography of cranial, subdural and epidural hematomas: variation of attenuation related to time and clinical events such as rebleeding. *J Comput Assist Tomogr.* 1977;1:449–455.

351. Zimmerman RD, Heier LA, Snow RB, Liu DP, Kelly AB, Deck MD. Acute intracranial hemorrhage: intensity changes on sequential MR scans at 0.5 T. *AJNR*. 1988;9:47–57.

352. Gomori JM, Grossman RI, Goldberg HI, Zimmerman RA, Bilaniuk LT. Intracranial hematomas: imaging by high-field MR. *Radiology*. 1985;157:87–93.

353. Dolinskas CA, Zimmerman RA, Bilaniuk LT. A sign of subarachnoid bleeding on cranial computed tomography of pediatric head trauma patients. *Radiology*. 1978;126:409–411.

354. Han JS, Kaufman B, Alfidi RJ, et al. Head trauma evaluated by magnetic resonance and computed tomography: a comparison. *Radiology*. 1984;150:71–77.

355. Pozzati E, Grossi C, Padovani R. Traumatic intracerebellar hematomas. *J Neurosurg*. 1982;56:691–694.

356. Merten DF, Osborne DR. Craniocerebral trauma in the child abuse syndrome. *Pediatr Ann*. 1983;12:882–887.

357. Tsai FY, Zee CS, Apthorp JS, Dixon GH. Computed tomography in child abuse head trauma. *J Comput Tomogr*. 1980;4:277–286.

358. Zimmerman RA, Bilaniuk LT, Bruce D, Schut L, Uzzell B, Goldberg HI. Computed tomography of craniocerebral injury in the abused child. *Radiology*. 1979;130:687–690.

359. Zimmerman RA, Bilaniuk LT, Bruce D, Dolinskas C, Obrist W, Kuhl D. Computed tomography of pediatric head trauma: acute general cerebral swelling. *Radiology*. 1978;126:403–408.

360. Hadley MN, Sonntag VK, Rekate HC, Murphy A. The infant whiplash–shake injury syndrome: a clinical and pathological study. *Neurosurgery*. 1989;141:536–540.

361. Caffey J. The whiplash shaken infant syndrome: manual shaking by the extremities with whiplash-induced intracranial and intraocular bleedings, linked with residual permanent brain damage and mental retardation. *Pediatrics*. 1974;54:396–403.

362. Ommaya AK, Faas F, Yarnell P. Whiplash injury and brain damage: an experimental study. *JAMA*. 1968;204:285–289.

363. Merten DF, Osborne DR, Radkowski MA, Leonidas JC. Craniocerebral trauma in the child abuse syndrome: radiological observations. *Pediatr Radiol*. 1984;14:272–277.

364. Hahn YS, Raimondi AJ, McLone DG, Yamanouchi Y. Traumatic mechanisms of head injury in child abuse. *Childs Brain*. 1983;10:229–241.

365. Till K. Subdural haematoma and effusion in infancy. *Br Med J*. 1968;2:400–402.

366. Duhaime AC, Gennarelli TA, Thibault LE, Bruce DA, Margulies SS, Wiser R. The shaken baby syndrome. A clinical, pathological, and biomechanical study. *J Neurosurg*. 1987;66:409–415.

367. Hamlin H. Subgaleal hematoma caused by hair-pull. *JAMA*. 1968;205:314.

368. James HE, Schut L. The neurosurgeon and the battered child. *Surg Neurol*. 1974;2:415–418.

369. O'Neill JA Jr, Meacham WF, Griffin JP, Sawyers JL. Patterns of injury in the battered child syndrome. *J Trauma*. 1973;13:332–339.

370. Hobbs CJ. Skull fracture and the diagnosis of abuse. *Arch Dis Child*. 1984;59:246–252.

371. Kravitz H, Driessen G, Gomberg R, Korach A. Accidental falls from elevated surfaces in infants from birth to one year of age. *Pediatrics*. 1969;44(suppl):869–876.

372. Helfer RE, Slovis TL, Black M. Injuries resulting when small children fall out of bed. *Pediatrics*. 1977;60:533–535.

373. Kleinman PK. Head trauma. In: *Diagnostic Imaging of Child Abuse*. Baltimore: Williams & Wilkins; 1987:159–199.

374. Martin HP, Beezley P, Conway EF, Kempe CH. The development of abused children. Part I. A review of the literature. Part II. Physical neurologic and intellectual outcome. *Adv Pediatr*. 1974;21:25–73.

375. Cohen RA, Kaufman RA, Myers PA, Towbin RB. Cranial computed tomography in the abused child with head injury. *AJR*. 1986;146:97–102.

376. Ellison PH, Tsai FY, Largent JA. Computed tomography in child abuse and cerebral contusion. *Pediatrics*. 1978;62:151–154.

377. Valmari P. Primary diagnosis in a life-threatening childhood infection. A nationwide study on bacterial meningitis. *Ann Clin Res*. 1985;17:310–315.

378. Dunn DW, Daum RS, Weisberg L, Vargas R. Ischemic cerebrovascular complications of *Haemophilus influenzae* meningitis. The value of computed tomography. *Arch Neurol*. 1982;39:650–652.

379. Skoch MG, Walling AD. Meningitis: describing the community health problem. *Am J Public Health*. 1985;75:550–552.

380. Schlech WF III, Ward JI, Band JD, Hightower A, Fraser DW, Broome CV. Bacterial meningitis in the United States, 1978 through 1981. The National Bacterial Meningitis Surveillance Study. *JAMA*. 1985;253:1749–1754.

381. Berman PH, Banker BQ. Neonatal meningitis. A clinical and pathological study of 29 cases. *Pediatrics*. 1966;38:6–24.

382. Tarr PI, Peter G. Demographic factors in the epidemiology of *Hemophilus influenzae* meningitis in young children. *J Pediatr*. 1978;92:884–888.

383. Syrogiannopoulos GA, Nelson JD, McCracken GH Jr. Subdural collections of fluid in acute bacterial meningitis: a review of 136 cases. *Pediatr Infect Dis*. 1986;5:343–352.

384. Moseley IF, Kendall BE. Radiology of intracranial empyemas, with special reference to computed tomography. *Neuroradiology*. 1984;26:333–345.

385. Naidu S, Glista G, Fine M, Brumlik J, Palacios E. Serial CT scan in *Haemophilus influenzae* meningitis of childhood. *Dev Med Child Neurol*. 1982;24:69–76.

386. Snyder RD, Stovring J. The follow-up CT scan in childhood meningitis. *Neuroradiology*. 1978;16:22–23.

387. Schultz P, Leeds NE. Intraventricular septations complicating neonatal meningitis. *J Neurosurg*. 1973;38:620–626.

388. Naidich TP, McLone DG, Yamanouchi Y. Periventricular white matter cysts in a murine model of Gram-negative ventriculitis. *AJNR*. 1983;4:461–465.

389. Chiras J, Dubs M, Bories J. Venous infarctions. *Neuroradiology*. 1985;27:593–600.

390. Rao KC, Knipp HC, Wagner EJ. Computed tomographic findings in cerebral sinus and venous thrombosis. *Radiology*. 1981;140:391–398.

391. Sze G, Simmons B, Krol G, Walker R, Zimmerman RD, Deck MD. Dural sinus thrombosis: verification with spin-echo techniques. *AJNR*. 1988;9:679–686.

392. Friede RL. Cerebral infarcts complicating neonatal leptomeningitis. Acute and residual lesions. *Acta Neuropathol*. 1973;23:245–253.

393. Renier D, Flandin C, Hirsch E, Hirsch JF. Brain abscesses in neonates. A study of 30 cases. *J Neurosurg*. 1988;69:877–882.

394. Dastur DK. The pathology and pathogenesis of tuberculous encephalopathy and myeloradiculopathy: a comparison with allergic encephalomyelitis. *Childs Nerv Syst*. 1986;2:13–19.

395. Klein NC, Damsker B, Hirschman SZ. Mycobacterial meningitis. Retrospective analysis from 1970 to 1983. *Am J Med*. 1985;79:29–34.

396. Schoeman J, Hewlett R, Donald P. MR of childhood tuberculous meningitis. *Neuroradiology*. 1988;30:473–477.

397. Bachman DS. Computed tomography in a verified case of tuberculous meningitis. *Neurology*. 1980;30:347.

398. Chu NS. Tuberculous meningitis. Computerized tomographic manifestations. *Arch Neurol*. 1980;37:458–460.

399. Chang KH, Han MH, Roh JK, Kim IO, Han MC, Kim CW. Gd-DTPA–enhanced MR imaging of the brain in patients with meningitis: comparison with CT. *AJNR*. 1990;11:69–76.

400. Price HI, Danziger A. Computed tomography in cranial tuberculosis. *AJR*. 1978;130:769–771.

401. Weingarten K, Zimmerman RD, Becker RD, Heier LA, Haimes AB, Deck MD. Subdural and epidural empyemas: MR imaging. *AJR*. 1989;152:615–621.

402. Carter BL, Bankhoff MS, Fisk JD. Computed tomographic detection of sinusitis responsible for intracranial and extracranial infections. *Radiology*. 1983;147:739–742.

403. Enzmann DR, Britt RH, Placone R. Staging of human brain abscess by computed tomography. *Radiology*. 1983;146:703–708.

404. Enzmann DR, Britt RH, Yeager AS. Experimental brain abscess evolution: computed tomographic and neuropathologic correlation. *Radiology*. 1979;133:113–122.

405. Daniels SR, Price JK, Towbin RB, McLaurin R. Nonsurgical cure of brain abscess in a neonate. *Childs Nerve Syst*. 1985;1:346–348.

406. Fischer EG, McLennan JE, Suzuki Y. Cerebral abscess in children. *Am J Dis Child*. 1981;135:746–749.

407. Blaquière RM. The computed tomographic appearances of intra and extracerebral abscesses. *Br J Radiol*. 1983;56:171–181.

408. Britt RH, Enzmann DR, Yeager AJ. Neuropathological and computerized tomographic findings in experimental brain abscess. *J Neurosurg*. 1981;55:590–603.

409. Dobkin JF, Healton EB, Dickinson PC, Brust JC. Nonspecificity of ring enhancement in "medically cured" brain abscess. *Neurology*. 1984;34:139–144.

410. Calabet A, Guibert-Tranier F, Piton J, Billerey J, Elie G, Caille JM. Diagnosis and follow-up of cerebral abscesses by CT scanning. 35 cases. *J Neuroradiol*. 1980;7:57–72.

411. Zimmerman RD, Haimes AB. The role of MR imaging in the diagnosis of infections of the central nervous system. *Curr Clin Top Infect Dis*. 1989;10:82–108.

412. Haimes AB, Zimmerman RD, Morgello S, et al. MR imaging of brain abscesses. *AJNR*. 1989;10:279–291.

413. Whitley RJ, Corey L, Arvin A, et al. Changing presentation of herpes simplex virus infection in neonates. *J Infect Dis*. 1988;158:109–116.

414. Neils EW, Lukin R, Tomsick TA, Tew JM. Magnetic resonance imaging and computerized tomography scanning of herpes simplex encephalitis. Report of two cases. *J Neurosurg*. 1987;67:592–594.

415. Schroth G, Gawehn J, Thron A, Vallbracht A, Voigt K. Early diagnosis of herpes simplex encephalitis by MRI. *Neurology*. 1987;37:179–183.

416. Enzmann DR, Ranson B, Norman D, Talberth E. Computed tomography of herpes simplex encephalitis. *Radiology*. 1978;129:419–425.

417. Zimmerman RD, Russell EJ, Leeds NE, Kaufman D. CT in the early diagnosis of herpes simplex encephalitis. *AJR*. 1980;134:61–66.

418. Zupanc ML, Handler EG, Levine RL, et al. Rasmussen encephalitis: epilepsia partialis continua secondary to chronic encephalitis. *Pediatr Neurol*. 1990;6:397–401.

419. Krawiecki NS, Dyken PR, El Gammal T, DuRant RH, Swift A. Computed tomography of the brain in subacute sclerosing panencephalitis. *Ann Neurol*. 1984;15:489–493.

420. Duda EE, Huttenlocher PR, Patronas NJ. CT of subacute sclerosing panencephalitis. *AJNR*. 1980;1:35–38.

421. Pedersen H, Wulff CH. Computed tomographic findings of early subacute sclerosing panencephalitis. *Neuroradiology*. 1982;23:31–32.

422. Lyons RW, Andriole VT. Fungal infections of the CNS. *Neurol Clin*. 1986;4:159–170.

423. Sabetta JR, Andriole VT. Cryptococcal infection of the central nervous system. *Med Clin North Am*. 1985;69:333–344.

424. Tan CT, Kuan BB. Cryptococcus meningitis, clinical-CT considerations. *Neuroradiology*. 1987;29:43–46.

425. Cornell SH, Jacoby CG. The varied computed tomographic appearance of intracranial cryptococcosis. *Radiology*. 1982;143:703–707.

426. Penar PL, Kim J, Chyatte D, Sabshin JK. Intraventricular cryptococcal granuloma. Report of two cases. *J Neurosurg*. 1988;68:145–148.

427. Popovich MJ, Arthur RH, Helmer E. CT of intracranial cryptococcosis. *AJNR*. 1990;11:139–142.

428. Salaki JS, Louria DB, Chmel H. Fungal and yeast infections of the central nervous system. A clinical review. *Medicine (Baltimore)*. 1984; 63:108–132.

429. Dublin AB, Phillips HE. Computed tomography of disseminated coccidioidomycosis. *Radiology*. 1980;135:361–368.

430. Roe DC, Haynes RE. *Candida albicans* meningitis successfully treated with amphotericin B. *Am J Dis Child*. 1972;124:926–929.

431. Averback P, Wigglesworth FW. Miliary fungal granulomata confined to the brain: mechanism of meningitis. *Childs Brain*. 1978;4:33–37.

432. Katz DA, Dworzack DL, Horowitz EA, Bogard PJ. Encephalitis associated with Rocky Mountain spotted fever. *Arch Pathol Lab Med*. 1985;109:771–773.

433. Salgo MP, Telzak EE, Currie B, et al. A focus of Rocky Mountain fever within New York City. *N Engl J Med*. 1988;318:1345–1348.

434. Horney LF, Walker DH. Meningoencephalitis as a major manifestation of Rocky Mountain spotted fever. *South Med J*. 1988;81:915–918.

435. Bia FJ, Barry M. Parasitic infections of the central nervous system. *Neurol Clin*. 1986;4:171–206.

436. Rodriguez-Carbajal J, Salgado P, Gutierrez-Alvarado R, Escobar-Izquierdo A, Aruffo C, Palacios E. The acute encephalitic phase of neurocysticercosis: computed tomographic manifestations. *AJNR*. 1983;4: 51–55.

437. Sotelo J, Guerrero F, Rubio F. Neurocysticercosis: a new classification based on active and inactive forms. A study of 753 cases. *Arch Intern Med*. 1985;145:442–445.

438. Lopez-Hernandez A, Garaizar C. Childhood cerebral cysticercosis: clinical features and computed tomographic findings in 89 Mexican children. *Can J Neurol Sci*. 1982;9:401–407.

439. Byrd SE, Locke GE, Biggers S, Percy AK. The CT appearance of cerebral cysticercosis in adults and children. *Radiology*. 1982;144:819–823.

440. Suss RA, Maravilla KR, Thompson J. MR imaging of intracranial cysticercosis: comparison with CT and anatomopathologic features. *AJNR*. 1986;7:235–242.

441. Martinez HR, Rangel-Guerra R, Elizondo G. MR imaging in neurocysticercosis: a study of 56 cases. *AJNR*. 1989;10:1011–1019.

442. Carcassonne M, Aubrespy P, Dor V, Choux M. Hydatid cysts in childhood. *Prog Pediatr Surg*. 1973;5:1–35.

443. Kaya U, Ozden B, Turker K, Tarcan B. Intracranial hydatid cysts. Study of 17 cases. *J Neurosurg*. 1975;42:580–584.

444. Hamza R, Touibi S, Jamoussi M, Bardi-Bellagha I, Chtioui R. Intracranial and orbital hydatid cysts. *Neuroradiology*. 1982;22:211–214.

445. Vaquero J, Jimenez C, Martinez R. Growth of hydatid cysts evaluated by CT scanning after presumed cerebral hydatid embolism. Case report. *J Neurosurg*. 1982;57:837–838.

446. Federle MP. A radiologist looks at AIDS. Imaging evaluation based on symptom complexes. *Radiology*. 1988;166:553–562.

447. Stagno S, Pass RF, Alford CA. Perinatal infections and maldevelopment. *Birth Defects*. 1981;17:31–50.

448. Stagno S, Reynolds DW, Huang ES, Thames SD, Smith RJ, Alford CA. Congenital cytomegalovirus infection. *N Engl J Med*. 1977;296: 1254–1258.

449. Stagno S, Pass RF, Cloud G, et al. Primary cytomegalovirus infection in pregnancy. Incidence, transmission to fetus, and clinical outcome. *JAMA*. 1986;256:1904–1908.

450. Hanshaw JB. On deafness, cytomegalovirus, and neonatal screening. *Am J Dis Child*. 1982;136:886–887.

451. Hanshaw JB, Scheiner AP, Moxley AW, Gaev L, Abel V, Scheiner B. School failure and deafness after "silent" congenital cytomegalovirus infection. *N Engl J Med*. 1976;295:468–470.

452. Williamson WD, Desmond MM, LaFevers N, Taber LH, Catlin FI, Weaver TG. Symptomatic congenital cytomegalovirus. Disorders of language, learning, and hearing. *Am J Dis Child*. 1982;136:902–905.

453. Pass RF, Stagno S, Myers GJ, Alford CA. Outcome of symptomatic congenital cytomegalovirus infection: results of long-term longitudinal follow-up. *Pediatrics*. 1980;66:758–762.

454. Tissin GB, Maklad NF, Stewart RR, Bell ME. Cytomegalic inclusion disease: intrauterine sonographic diagnosis using findings involving the brain. *AJNR*. 1991;12:117–122.

455. Marques-Dias MJ, Harmant-van Rijckevorsel G, Landrieu P, Lyon G. Prenatal cytomegalovirus disease and cerebral microgyria: evidence for perfusion failure, not disturbance of histogenesis, as the major cause of cytomegalovirus encephalopathy. *Neuropediatrics*. 1984;15:18–24.

456. Bale JF Jr, Bray PF, Bell WE. Neuroradiographic abnormalities in congenital cytomegalovirus infection. *Pediatr Neurol*. 1985;1:42–47.

457. Stagno S, Pass RF, Reynolds DW, Moore MA, Nahmias AJ, Alford CA. Comparative study of diagnostic procedures for congenital cytomegalovirus infection. *Pediatrics*. 1980;65:251–257.

458. Bray PF, Bale JF, Anderson RE, Kern ER. Progressive neurological disease associated with chronic cytomegalovirus infection. *Ann Neurol*. 1981;9:499–502.

459. Grose C, Itani O, Weiner CP. Prenatal diagnosis of fetal infection: advances from amniocentesis to cordocentesis—congenital toxoplasmosis, rubella, cytomegalovirus, varicella virus, parvovirus and human immunodeficiency virus. *Pediatr Infect Dis J*. 1989;8:459–468.

460. Koppe JG, Rothova A. Congenital toxoplasmosis. A long-term follow-up of 20 years. *Int Ophthalmol*. 1989;13:387–390.

461. Wilson CB, Remington JS, Stagno S, Reynolds DW. Development of adverse sequelae in children born with subclinical congenital *Toxoplasma* infection. *Pediatrics*. 1980;66:767–774.

462. Stagno S, Reynolds DW, Amos CS, et al. Auditory and visual defects resulting from symptomatic and subclinical congenital cytomegaloviral and *Toxoplasma* infections. *Pediatrics*. 1977;59:669–678.

463. Freij BJ, Sever JL. Toxoplasmosis. *Pediatr Rev*. 1991;12:227–236.

464. Bambirra EA, Pittella JE, Rezende M. Toxoplasmosis and hydranencephaly. *N Engl J Med*. 1982;306:1112–1113.

465. Diebler C, Dusser A, Dulac O. Congenital toxoplasmosis. Clinical and neuroradiological evaluation of the cerebral lesions. *Neuroradiology*. 1985;27:125–130.

466. Prober CG, Sullender WM, Yasukawa LL, Au DS, Yeager AS, Arvin AM. Low risk of herpes simplex virus infections in neonates exposed to the virus at the time of vaginal delivery to mothers with recurrent genital herpes simplex virus infections. *N Engl J Med*. 1987;316:240–244.

467. Brown ZA, Vontver LA, Benedetti J, et al. Genital herpes in pregnancy: risk factors associated with recurrences and asymptomatic viral shedding. *Am J Obstet Gynecol*. 1985;153:24–30.

468. Prober CG, Arvin AM. Congenital infections as causes of neurologic sequelae: prevention, diagnosis and treatment. In: Stevenson DK, Sunshine P, eds. *Fetal and Neonatal Brain Injury*. Philadelphia: Decker; 1989:79–91.

469. Boucher FD, Yasukawa LL, Bronzan RN, Hensleigh PA, Arvin AM, Prober CG. A prospective evaluation of primary genital herpes simplex virus type 2 infections acquired during pregnancy. *Pediatr Infect Dis J*. 1990; 9:499–504.

470. Noorbehesht B, Enzmann DR, Sullinder W, Bradley JS, Arvin AM. Neonatal herpes simplex encephalitis: correlation of clinical and CT findings. *Radiology*. 1987;162:813–819.

471. Junck L, Enzmann DR, DeArmond SJ, Okerlund M. Prolonged brain retention of contrast agent in neonatal herpes simplex encephalitis. *Radiology*. 1981;140:123–126.

472. Peckham GS. Clinical and laboratory study of children exposed in utero to maternal rubella. *Arch Dis Child*. 1972;47:571–577.

473. Ueda K, Nishida Y, Oshima K, Shepard TH. Congenital rubella syndrome: correlation of gestational age at time of maternal rubella with type of defect. *J Pediatr*. 1979;94:763–765.

474. Sarwar M, Azar-Kia B, Schechter MM, Valsamis M, Batnitzky S. Aqueductal occlusion in the congenital rubella syndrome. *Neurology*. 1974;24:198–201.

475. Fox GN, Strangarity JW. Varicella-zoster virus infections in pregnancy. *Am Fam Physician*. 1989;39:89–98.

476. Grose C, Itani O. Pathogenesis of congenital infection with three diverse viruses: varicella-zoster virus, human parvovirus, and human immunodeficiency virus. *Semin Perinatol*. 1989;13:278–293.

477. Borzyskowski M, Harris RF, Jones RW. The congenital varicella syndrome. *Eur J Pediatr*. 1981;37:335–338.

478. Shannon KM, Ammann AJ. Acquired immune deficiency in childhood. *J Pediatr*. 1985;106:332–342.

479. Davis SL, Halsted CC, Levy N, Ellis W. Acquired immune deficiency syndrome presenting as progressive infantile encephalopathy. *J Pediatr*. 1987;110:884–888.

480. Epstein LG, Sharer LR, Joshi VV, Fojas MM, Koenigsberger MR, Oleske JM. Progressive encephalopathy in children with acquired immune deficiency syndrome. *Ann Neurol*. 1985;17:488–496.

481. Epstein LG, Sharer LR, Oleske JM, et al. Neurologic manifestations of human immunodeficiency virus infection in children. *Pediatrics*. 1986;78:678–687.

482. Schoenberg BS, Mellinger JF, Schoenberg DG. Cerebrovascular disease in infants and children: a study of incidence, clinical features, and survival. *Neurology*. 1978;28:763–768.

483. Volpe JJ, Perlman JM, Hill A, McMenamin JB. Cerebral blood flow velocity in the human newborn: the value of its determination. *Pediatrics*. 1982;70:147–152.

484. Kirsch JR, Traystman RJ, Rogers MC. Cerebral blood flow measurement techniques in infants and children. *Pediatrics*. 1985;75:887–895.

485. Volpe JJ. Intracranial hemorrhage in the newborn: current understanding and dilemmas. *Neurology*. 1979;29:632–635.

486. MacDonald MM, Koops BL, Johnson ML, et al. Timing and antecedents of intracranial hemorrhage in the newborn. *Pediatrics*. 1984;74:32–36.

487. Perlman JM, Nelson JS, McAlister WH, Volpe JJ. Intracerebellar hemorrhage in a premature newborn: diagnosis by real-time ultrasound and correlation with autopsy findings. *Pediatrics*. 1983;71:159–162.

488. Hill A, Martin DG, Daneman A, Fitz CR. Focal ischemic cerebral injury in the newborn: diagnosis by ultrasound and correlation with computed tomographic scan. *Pediatrics*. 1983;71:790–793.

489. Celli P, Ferrante L, Palma L, Cavedon G. Cerebral arteriovenous malformations in children. Clinical features and outcome of treatment in children and in adults. *Surg Neurol*. 1984;22:43–49.

490. Perret G, Nishioka H. Report on the cooperative study of intracranial aneurysms and subarachnoid hemorrhage: section VI. Arteriovenous malformations. An analysis of 545 cases of cranio-cerebral arteriovenous malformations and fistulae reported to the cooperative study. *J Neurosurg*. 1966;25:467–490.

491. Parkinson D, Bachers G. Arteriovenous malformations. Summary of 100 consecutive supratentorial cases. *J Neurosurg*. 1980;53:285–299.

492. Martin NA, Wilson CB. Medial occipital arteriovenous malformations. Surgical treatment. *J Neurosurg*. 1982;56:798–802.

493. Kumar AJ, Fox AJ, Vinuela F, Rosenbaum AE. Revisited old and new CT findings in unruptured larger arteriovenous malformations of the brain. *J Comput Assist Tomogr*. 1984;8:648–655.

494. LeBlanc R, Ethier R, Little JR. Computerized tomography findings in arteriovenous malformations of the brain. *J Neurosurg.* 1979;51:765–772.

495. LeBlanc R, Levesque M, Comair Y, Ethier R. Magnetic resonance imaging of cerebral arteriovenous malformations. *Neurosurgery.* 1987;21:15–20.

496. Schorner W, Bradac GB, Treisch J, Bender A, Felix R. Magnetic resonance imaging (MRI) in the diagnosis of cerebral arteriovenous angiomas. *Neuroradiology.* 1986;28:313–318.

497. Smith HJ, Strother CM, Kikuchi Y, et al. MR imaging in the management of supratentorial intracranial AVMs. *AJNR.* 1988;9:225–235.

498. Nüssel, Wegmüller, Huber P. Comparison of magnetic resonance angiography, magnetic resonance imaging and conventional angiography in cerebral arteriovenous malformation. *Neuroradiology.* 1991;33:56–61.

499. McCormick WF. The pathology of vascular ("arteriovenous") malformations. *J Neurosurg.* 1966;24:807–816.

500. Pozzati E, Padovani R, Morrone B, Finizio F, Gaist G. Cerebral cavernous angiomas in children. *J Neurosurg.* 1980;53:826–832.

501. Voigt K, Yasargil MG. Cerebral cavernous haemangiomas or cavernomas. Incidence, pathology localization, diagnosis, clinical features and treatment. Review of the literature and report of an unusual case. *Neurochirurgia (Stuttg).* 1976;19:59–68.

502. Savoiardo M, Strada L, Passerini A. Intracranial cavernous hemangioma: neuroradiologic review of 36 operated cases. *Am J Neuroradiol.* 1983;4:945–950.

503. Bartlett JE, Kishore PR. Intracranial cavernous angioma. *Am J Roentgenol.* 1977;128:653–656.

504. Numagushi Y, Fukui M, Miyake G, Kishikawa T, Ikeda J. Angiographic manifestations of intracerebral cavernous hemangioma. *Neuroradiology.* 1977;14:113–116.

505. Lemme-Plaghos L, Kucharczyk W, Brandt-Zawadzki M, et al. MRI of angiographically occult vascular malformations. *AJR.* 1986;146:1223–1228.

506. Rigamonti D, Hadley MN, Drayer BP, et al. Cerebral cavernous malformation: incidence and familial occurrence. *N Engl J Med.* 1988;319:343–347.

507. Sarwar M, McCormick WF. Intracerebral venous angioma. Case report and review. *Arch Neurol.* 1978;35:323–325.

508. Saito Y, Kobayashi N. Cerebral venous angiomas: clinical evaluation and possible etiology. *Radiology.* 1981;139:87–94.

509. Rothfus WE, Albright AL, Casey KF, Latchaw RE, Roppolo HM. Cerebellar venous angioma: "benign" entity? *AJNR.* 1984;5:61–66.

510. Fierstien SB, Pribram HW, Hieshima G. Angiography and computed tomography in the evaluation of cerebral venous malformations. *Neuroradiology.* 1979;17:137–148.

511. Olson E, Gilmor RL, Richmond B. Cerebral venous angiomas. *Radiology.* 1984;151:97–104.

512. Lasjaunias P, ter Brugge K, Lopez-Ibor L, et al. The role of dural anomalies in vein of Galen aneurysms: report of six cases and review of the literature. *AJNR.* 1987;8:185–192.

513. Gold AP, Ransohoff JR, Carter S. Vein of Galen malformation. *Acta Neurol Scand.* 1964;40(suppl 11):5–31.

514. Norman M, Becker LE. Cerebral damage in neonates resulting from arteriovenous malformations of the vein of Galen. *J Neurol Neurosurg Psychiatr.* 1985;37:252–258.

515. Silverman BK, Brekz T, Craig J, et al. Congestive failure in the newborn caused by cerebral AV fistula. *Am J Dis Child.* 1959;89:539–543.

516. Hoffman HJ, Chuang S, Hendrick EB, Humphreys RP. Aneurysms of the vein of Galen. Experience at the Hospital for Sick Children, Toronto. *J Neurosurg.* 1982;57:316–322.

517. Seidenwurm D, Berenstein A, Hyman A, Kowalski H. Vein of Galen malformation: correlation of clinical presentation, arteriography, and MR imaging. *AJNR.* 1991;12:347–354.

518. Cubberley DA, Jaffe RB, Nixon GW. Sonographic demonstration of galenic arteriovenous malformations in the neonate. *AJNR.* 1982;3:435–439.

519. Martelli A, Scotti G, Harwood-Nash DC, Fitz CR, Chuang SH. Aneurysms of the vein of Galen in children: CT and angiographic correlations. *Neuroradiology.* 1980;20:123–133.

520. Albright AL, Latchaw RE, Price RA. Posterior dural arteriovenous malformations in infancy. *Neurosurgery.* 1983;13:129–135.

521. Ito J, Imamura H, Kobayashi K, Tsuchida T, Sato S. Dural arteriovenous malformations of the base of the anterior cranial fossa. *Neuroradiology.* 1983;24:149–154.

522. Lasjaunias PL, Chiu M, ter Brugge K, Tolia A, Hurth M, Bernstein M. Neurological manifestations of intracranial dural arteriovenous malformations. *J Neurosurg.* 1986;64:724–730.

523. Houser OW, Baker HL Jr, Rhoton AL Jr, Okazaki H. Intracranial dural arteriovenous malformations. *Radiology.* 1972;105:55–64.

524. Newton TH, Weidner W, Greitz T. Dural arteriovenous malformations in the posterior fossa. *Radiology.* 1968;90:27–35.

525. Miyasaka K, Takei H, Nomura M, et al. Computerized tomography findings in dural arteriovenous malformations. Report of three cases. *J Neurosurg.* 1980;53:698–702.

526. Newton TH, Hoyt WF. Dural arteriovenous shunts in the region of the cavernous sinus. *Neuroradiology.* 1970;1:71–81.

527. Pang D, Kerber C, Biglan AW, Ahn HS. External carotid–cavernous sinus fistula in infancy: case report and review of the literature. *Neurosurgery.* 1981;8:212–218.

528. Halbach VV, Higashida RT, Hieshima GB. Treatment of vertebral arteriovenous fistulas. *AJNR.* 1988;9:741–749.

529. Reizine D, Laouiti M, Guimaraens L, Riche MC, Merland JJ. Vertebral arteriovenous fistulas. Clinical presentation, angiographical appearance and endovascular treatment. A review of 25 cases. *Ann Radiol (Paris).* 1985;28:425–438.

530. Heiskanen O, Vilkki J. Intracranial arterial aneurysms in children and adolescents. *Acta Neurochir (Wien).* 1981;59:55–63.

531. Locksley HB. Report on the Cooperative Study of Intracranial Aneurysms and Subarachnoid Hemorrhage. Section V, part 1: natural history of subarachnoid hemorrhage, intracranial aneurysms and arteriovenous malformations. Based on 6,368 cases in the Cooperative Study. *J Neurosurg.* 1966;25:219–239.

532. Ostergaard JR, Voldby B. Intracranial arterial aneurysms in children and adolescents. *J Neurosurg.* 1983;58:832–837.

533. Patel AN, Richardson AE. Ruptured intracranial aneurysms in the first two decades of life. A study of 58 patients. *J Neurosurg.* 1971;35:571–576.

534. Thrush AL, Marano GD. Infantile intracranial aneurysm: report of a case and review of the literature. *AJNR.* 1988;9:903–906.

535. Bohmfalk GL, Story JL, Wissinger JP, Brown WE Jr. Bacterial intracranial aneurysm. *J Neurosurg.* 1978;48:369–382.

536. Roach MR, Drake CG. Ruptured cerebral aneurysms caused by microorganisms. *N Engl J Med.* 1965;273:240–244.

537. Rout D, Sharma A, Mohan PK, Rao VR. Bacterial aneurysms of the intracavernous carotid artery. *J Neurosurg.* 1984;60:1236–1242.

538. Heidelberger KP, Layton WM Jr, Fisher RG. Multiple cerebral mycotic aneurysms complicating posttraumatic *Pseudomonas* meningitis. Case report. *J Neurosurg.* 1968;29:631–635.

539. Frazee JG, Cahan LD, Winter J. Bacterial intracranial aneurysms. *J Neurosurg.* 1980;53:633–641.

540. Tomita T, McLone DG, Naidich TP. Mycotic aneurysm of the intracavernous portion of the carotid artery in childhood. *J Neurosurg.* 1981;54:681–684.

541. Park CH, Madsen MT, McLellan T, Schwartzman RJ. Iofetamine HCl I-123 brain scanning in stroke: a comparison with transmission CT. *RadioGraphics.* 1988;8:305–326.

542. Toshiaki H, Tanaka T, Ikekubo K, Komatsu T, Torizuka K. SPECT with *N*-isopropyl-*p*-iodoamphetamine in occlusive cerebrovascular diseases. *Clin Nucl Med*. 1986;11:855–859.

543. Hayashida K, Nishimura T, Imakita S, et al. Change of accumulation and filling pattern in evolution of cerebral infarction with I-123 IMP brain SPECT. *Neuroradiology*. 1991;33:9–14.

544. Hilal SK, Soloman GE, Gold AP, Carter S. Primary cerebral arterial occlusive disease in children. II. Neurocutaneous syndromes. *Radiology*. 1971;99:87–94.

545. Harwood-Nash DC, Fitz CR. *Neuroradiology in Infants and Children*. St Louis: Mosby; 1976;3:902–964.

546. Rajakulasingam K, Cerullo LJ, Raimondi AJ. Childhood moya-moya syndrome. Postradiation pathogenesis. *Childs Brain*. 1979;5:467–475.

547. Haltia M, Iivanainen M, Majuri H, Puranen M. Spontaneous occlusion of the circle of Willis (moyamoya syndrome). *Clin Neuropathol*. 1982;1:11–22.

548. Suzuki J, Takaku A. Cerebrovascular "moyamoya" disease. Disease showing abnormal netlike vessels in base of brain. *Arch Neurol*. 1969;20:288–299.

549. Takahashi M, Miyauchi T, Kowada M. Computed tomography of moyamoya disease: demonstration of occluded arteries and collateral vessels as important diagnostic signs. *Radiology*. 1980;134:671–676.

550. Takeuchi S, Kobayashi K, Tsuchida T, Imamura H, Tanaka R, Ito J. Computed tomography in moyamoya disease. *J Comput Assist Tomogr*. 1982;6:24–32.

551. Suzuki J, Kodama N. Moyamoya disease—a review. *Stroke*. 1983;14:104–109.

552. Rao KC, Knipp HC, Wagner EJ. Computed tomographic findings in cerebral sinus and venous thrombosis. *Radiology*. 1981;140:391–398.

553. Gabrielsen TO, Seeger JF, Knake JE, Stilwill EW. Radiology of cerebral vein occlusion without dural sinus occlusion. *Radiology*. 1981;140:403–408.

554. Rippe DJ, Boyko OB, Spritzer CE, et al. Demonstration of dural sinus occlusion by the use of MR angiography. *AJNR*. 1990;11:199–201.

Chapter 2

The Spine

DEVELOPMENTAL ABNORMALITIES

Embryogenesis of the Spine and Spinal Cord

The interpretation of imaging studies of the spine and intraspinal structures in infants and children requires a thorough understanding of the normal development of these structures and the important developmental variations that can occur in this process. The embryologic development of the spine is complex. There are three distinct stages: membranous (also termed precartilaginous) development, chondrification, and ossification. Ossification is divided into primary and secondary stages.[1]

During week 3 of embryogenesis, the paraxial mesoderm (which lies lateral to the notochord and beneath the neural plate) thickens to form a pair of longitudinal strips. By day 20, this tissue becomes segmented into paired blocks of tissue called somites. The first somites appear in the midportion of the embryo just caudal to the cranial end of the notochord. With further differentiation, the ventromedial portion of each somite forms a sclerotome. The sclerotomal cells form the primordia of the cartilage, bones, and ligaments of the vertebrae and ribs.

The dorsolateral portion of the somite is called the dermomyotome. The cells in the medial portion of the dermomyotome differentiate into myoblasts that give rise to the paraspinal muscles. The laterally situated cells migrate beneath the ectoderm to form the dermis and subcutaneous tissues.

The membranous stage of spinal development is characterized by migration of sclerotomal cells to form the membranous anlagen of the vertebrae and ribs. At approximately day 25 of gestation, the notochord separates from the ectoderm and endoderm. At this stage two zones exist: a ventral subchordal zone between the notochord and the endoderm, and a dorsal epichordal zone between the notochord and the neural tube. As this separation occurs, sclerotomal cells migrate medially into both the subchordal and epichordal zones, thereby surrounding the notochord and neural tube (Fig. 2-1). These cells unite to form a dense longitudinal column of mesenchyme that is termed the perichordal sheath.

This process begins in the cervical region and progresses caudally. The perichordal sheath retains a segmental configuration, with each sclerotome level consisting of densely packed cells caudally and loosely arranged cells cranially that surround the intersegmental arteries. These layers of cells are the precursors of the vertebral bodies and the intervertebral discs. As the superficial ectoderm separates from the closed neural tube, sclerotomal cells complete their migration around the dorsal aspect of the neural tube; they eventually form the membranous neural arches of the vertebrae. These cells also form the precursors of the meninges and paraspinous muscles. Cells derived from the ventrolateral aspects of the sclerotomes give rise to the membranous costal processes of the vertebrae and the membranous ribs.

Beginning on approximately day 24, a major resegmentation occurs in the membranous vertebral bodies. The cells of the caudal half of each sclerotome proliferate more rapidly than those in the cranial half. Clefts develop at the midportion of each sclerotome, thereby dividing the dense caudal half from the less dense cephalic half. The sclerotomes then separate along these clefts and reunite in a complex fashion, such

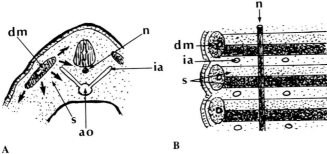

Fig. 2-1 Embryologic development of the spine. **(A)** Partial cross-section through the midportion of a 4-week embryo shows the dermomyotome (dm) lying dorsal and lateral to the intersegmental artery (ia) that arises from the aorta (ao). The mesenchymal cells of the sclerotome (s) spread dorsally, ventrally, and anteriorly to surround the neural tube and the notochord (n). **(B)** Diagrammatic coronal image of the embryo at the same stage of gestation shows the condensation of the sclerotome around the notochord. The sclerotome consists of a cranial area of loosely packed cells and a caudal area of closely packed cells. The dermomyotome lies at the lateral aspect of the sclerotome.

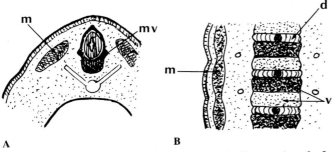

Fig. 2-2 Embryologic development of the spine. **(A)** Cross-section of a 5-week embryo shows condensation of the sclerotomal cells about the notochord and the neural tube to form the precartilaginous mesenchymal vertebra (mv). Cells from the myotome (m) give rise to the paraspinal muscles. **(B)** Diagrammatic coronal section of the same stage of gestation shows that the vertebral body (v) forms from the cranial and caudal halves of two successive sclerotomal masses. The intersegmental arteries now cross the bodies of the vertebrae, and the spinal nerves lie between the vertebrae. The notochord is undergoing degeneration except in the region of the intervertebral disc (d), where it ultimately forms the nucleus pulposus.

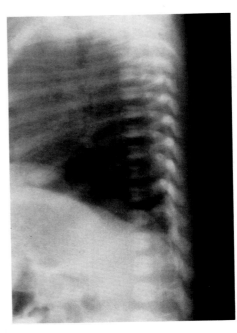

Fig. 2-3 Lateral radiograph of the thoracic spine of a neonate showing the site of fusion of the two sclerotomes as a radiolucent band through the center of the vertebral bodies. Note the notchlike deformity of the anterior surface of the vertebral bodies. This is a normal finding in the neonatal period.

that the dense caudal portion of one sclerotome unites with the less dense cells of the next most caudal sclerotome; this results in formation of new precartilaginous primitive vertebral bodies (Fig. 2-2). This process also results in entrapment of the intersegmental arteries in the central portions of the new vertebral bodies. In infants, the site of fusion of the sclerotomes is often visible on lateral radiographs of the spine as a lucent band across the midportions of the vertebral bodies (Fig. 2-3).

Some of the cells from the denser half of the sclerotome contribute to the formation of the annulus fibrosus of the intervertebral disc and the enchondral growth plates of the centra of the vertebrae. This fusion proceeds bilaterally and symmetrically at each segment, such that cleavage and fusion of the sclerotomes on each side form the ipsilateral half of each vertebral body. This process begins in the lower cervical and upper thoracic region and proceeds both cranially and caudally.

During resegmentation and fusion of the membranous vertebral bodies, the notochord also undergoes significant changes. Initially, the notochord has a uniform caliber throughout its length. During formation of the membranous vertebrae, the cells of the notochord that lie in the region of the future centrum become compressed and degenerate, and the cells that lie in the region of the future intervertebral disc proliferate and undergo mucoid degeneration. This portion of the notochord is thereby converted into the nucleus pulposus of the intervertebral disc. Additional notochordal tissue persists as the apical ligaments of the dens and as occasional remnants in the skull base, sacrum, and vertebral bodies.

The chondrification stage of vertebral development begins with the appearance of centers of chondrification in the mesenchyme of the membranous vertebral column on approximately day 39. The process of chondrification begins at the cervicothoracic junction and extends both cranially and caudally. Chondrification is initiated earlier in the centrum than in the neural arches. In the centrum, two centers of chondrification appear, one on either side of the midline. A chondrification center also develops in each half of the neural arch lateral to the neural tube. Each of these centers later fuses with its mate to form the chondral neural arch and spinous process. Two additional centers of chondrification appear at the junction of

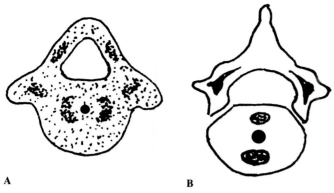

Fig. 2-4 Chondrification. **(A)** The chondrification centers that appear in the mesenchymal vertebra at gestation week 6 consist of two ringlike condensations of cartilage on either side of the notochord. In addition, there are two chondrification centers in each side of the neural arch. **(B)** Primary centers of ossification appear in the cartilaginous vertebra at gestation week 7. There are two centers in the vertebral body, one anterior and one posterior to the degenerating notochord. A roughly triangular primary ossification center appears in the posterior elements on either side.

the neural arch with the centrum; these centers extend laterally into the transverse processes. Therefore, three pairs of chondrification centers develop in each vertebra (Fig. 2-4A).

The process of ossification overlaps that of chondrification. The primary ossification stage begins at gestation week 8 or 9. Each vertebral arch develops two primary ossification centers, one on each side. Ossification of the arches begins in the cervical and thoracic regions and extends caudally. Fusion of the laminae into complete bony arches begins in the lumbar region and progresses cranially, however.

Ossification of the vertebral bodies begins in the lower thoracic and upper lumbar region and extends both cranially and caudally. Initially, each vertebral body centrum develops two primary ossification centers, one anterior to and one posterior to the vestigial mucoid streak of the notochord (Fig. 2-4B). These centers rapidly fuse into a single ossification center that progressively enlarges. The residual unossified cartilage cephalad and caudal to the ossification center in the centrum then forms two cartilaginous plates that lie adjacent to the intervertebral discs. A C-shaped cartilaginous ring develops at the ventral and lateral aspects of the interspace between the centrum and the disc, forming the annular (ring) epiphyses. At about the time of puberty, secondary ossification centers develop at the tips of the transverse processes, at the tips of the spinous processes, and in the annular epiphyses. Complete fusion of these secondary centers occurs by approximately 25 years of age.

The eventual fusion of the vertebral arch and the centrum occurs anterior to the pedicles at the site of the neurocentral synchondroses. Consequently, the vertebral body is composed of bone derived from the ossification centers of the arch as well as those of the centrum. Fusion of the arch and centrum occurs between years 3 and 6.

Continuing development of the spine after birth results in several radiographic findings. The vertebral bodies in the neonate tend to be rectangular in the thoracic area and oval in the lumbar region (Fig. 2-5). Also, a bone-within-bone appearance is common during the first 2 months of life. Anterior and posterior vascular channels are prominent in the newborn and young infant. The anterior channels gradually disappear in infancy, whereas the posterior channels are sometimes still visible in the adult. At birth, the synchondrosis between the ossified halves of the posterior arch is readily identified as a radiolucent line in the midline on frontal radiographs. The costovertebral synchondroses (between the ribs and the neural arches) and the neurocentral junctions (between the centra and arches) are also visible.

Between the ages of 8 and 10 years, formation of secondary ossification centers begins in the annular epiphyses at the superior and inferior margins of the vertebral body. Each is formed from several nuclei that vary in number from 2 to 20. Before fusion, the multicentric nature of ossification of the annular epiphyses is demonstrated on frontal radiographs as an irregularity that is most prominent in the midthoracic and midlumbar regions. On lateral radiographs, the cartilaginous epiphysis appears as a steplike defect in the vertebral body. The defect is deep along the anterior surface and more shallow posteriorly. As ossification occurs, irregular foci of calcification appear in the bony defect, forming wedge-shaped fragments. These irregularities should not be confused with fractures or other pathologic entities. Fusion of the ring epiphyses with the vertebral bodies occurs between 20 and 25 years of age.

The development of the atlas (C-1) and axis (C-2) differs significantly from that of the remainder of the vertebral column. During the mesenchymal stage of development, the atlas arises from the fourth occipital and first cervical sclerotomes.

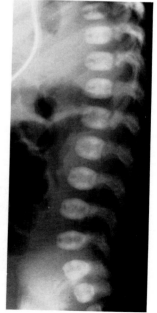

Fig. 2-5 Lateral radiograph of the lower thoracic and lumbar spine of a neonate showing the lower thoracic vertebral bodies to be roughly rectangular. The site of fusion of the two sclerotomes is visible as a radiolucent band. In the lumbar region the vertebral bodies are oval. A radiolucent line is seen posterior to the vertebral body at the junction of the centrum and the neural arch.

Ossification of the atlas occurs from three primary centers, one for each lateral mass (appearing at the end of month 2 of gestation) and one for the anterior arch (appearing in the first year). The posterior arch of the atlas is ossified by extension from the lateral masses.

The dens, which actually represents the body of the atlas, develops primarily from the caudal half of the fourth occipital sclerotome and the cranial half of the first cervical sclerotome. The apex of the dens develops from the cranial portion of the fourth occipital sclerotome. The body and neural arch of the axis arise from the first and second cervical sclerotomes. The dens ossifies from three primary centers. Two laterally placed centers appear at about month 6 of gestation and unite before birth. The tip of the dens has a separate ossification center that appears during the second year of life and fuses at about 12 years of age.

In infants, the dens is a separate bone that remains separated from the body of the axis by a disc-shaped cartilaginous plate that persists for about 6 years. Ossification begins at the periphery of the plate and progresses toward the center; a portion may remain cartilaginous until early adulthood. Failure of complete ossification of this plate results in the appearance of the dens as a separate bone, the os odontoideum.

The neurocentral synchondroses between the vertebral bodies and posterior arches begin to fuse in the cervical region at about 3 years of age. This fusion progresses inferiorly to the lumbar region and is complete by about 6 years of age. Conversely, the posterior neural arches fuse in the lumbar region during the first year of life, with the fusion progressing cephalad. The cervical laminae are the last to fuse. This occurs during the third year.

In summary, most of the vertebrae ossify from eight major ossification centers, three primary and five secondary. The secondary ossification centers include one for the spinous process, two for the transverse processes, and two for the ring epiphyses. Each lumbar vertebra has two additional secondary ossification centers for the mamillary processes.

The embryogenesis of the spinal cord and meninges is closely related to the events involved in formation of the spine. There is a broad spectrum of errors in embryogenesis that lead to the different types of dysraphic lesions and other anomalies of the cord, meninges, and vertebrae. Spinal cord embryogenesis can be divided into three general stages: neurulation, canalization, and retrogressive differentiation.

During gestation week 3, pluripotent ectodermal cells proliferate along the surface of the embryo to form a plate termed the primitive streak. The cranial end of the primitive streak develops a nodular group of rapidly proliferating cells that is termed the primitive node (Hensen node). A small depression develops in the primitive node (the primitive pit or the neuropore) that is contiguous with a groove in the primitive streak. At approximately day 16 of embryonic life, cells migrate from the primitive node in a cephalad direction to form the notochordal process, which eventually develops into the notochord. As described above, the notochord is intimately involved in the formation of the vertebral column.

The notochord induces a thickening of the dorsal ectoderm that results in the formation of the neural plate. By the end of week 3 of gestation, the lateral portions of the neural plate become thickened and elevated, thereby forming the neural folds. The thinner midline portion of the plate forms the neural groove. The neural folds progressively bend dorsally along the entire length of the neural groove, fusing eventually in the midline to form the neural tube.

The process of closure of the neural tube is termed neurulation. This fusion of the neural folds begins in the upper cervical region and proceeds in both cephalad and caudal directions. As fusion occurs, a continuous ectodermal covering is formed over the neural structures. The most cephalad segment of the neural tube is termed the anterior neuropore; this closes at approximately gestation day 24 at the lamina terminalis. The caudal end of the neural tube is termed the posterior neuropore; this closes in the region of the future lumbar spine at approximately day 26 or 27.

There is further contribution to the caudal growth of the neural tube by cells from the tail bud. The tail bud is a focus of proliferating mesodermal cells that lies ventral and caudal to the caudal aspect of the neural tube. Cells from the tail bud are continuously added to the caudal ends of the notochord and neural tube. The resulting solid cord of cells develops small cavities that coalesce to form a central lumen, which ultimately becomes contiguous with the lumen of the neural tube. The embryogenesis of the spinal cord, therefore, involves both neural plate neurulation and medullary cord neurulation. This process of rostral extension of the neural tube from medullary cord structures is termed canalization. The transition zone between these two portions of the cord is the location of most dysraphic lesions.[2]

The third stage of formation of the spinal cord is termed retrogressive differentiation. This begins at approximately gestation day 38, when the caudal medullary cord and the central lumen of the caudal neural tube decrease in size. This process results in formation of the distal portion of the conus medullaris, the filum terminale, and the ventriculus terminalis (a focal dilatation of the central canal that is contained in the conus medullaris).

Developmental Abnormalities of the Spinal Column

The spine forms from chondrification and subsequent ossification of growth centers for the centra and posterior arches. Abnormal development or fusion of these growth centers and persistence of portions of the notochord are responsible for most of the major vertebral malformations. Various osseous spinal abnormalities also occur in conjunction with developmental anomalies of the meninges and cord structures.

Most congenital malformations of the vertebral bodies are due to alterations in the processes of chondrification and ossification. Fusion anomalies may involve the vertebral body, the neural arch, or both. Anomalies of the vertebral bodies may occur with or without associated intraspinal or other organ maldevelopment. Dysraphic states typically include complex anomalies of the vertebral arches.

Anomalies of Vertebral Segmentation

Block Vertebra. The term *block vertebra* refers to partial or complete fusion of two or more vertebrae. Because the fusion in cases of congenital block vertebra occurs during embryonic development, growth is inhibited; the involved vertebrae are decreased in sagittal diameter. There is usually a thin remnant of disc material at the site of fusion.

Fusion that involves only two vertebral segments is usually asymptomatic. Symptoms of variable severity are often present in those unusual cases in which numerous vertebrae are incorporated into a single block vertebra. These may include deformity and limitation of motion. Block vertebrae occur most commonly in the cervical and thoracic regions, usually in the upper thoracic and lower cervical areas. In most cases, the anomaly is isolated; block vertebrae also occur in patients with other skeletal abnormalities, however, such as dysraphism or Klippel-Feil syndrome.

The involved vertebral bodies as seen on lateral radiographs are variably increased in height compared to adjacent normal vertebrae. The sagittal diameter of the vertebral bodies is usually decreased. Bony trabeculae are visible coursing through the fused segments. A line of condensation or a linear radiolucency is seen in the midportion of the fused vertebrae at the site of the absent or rudimentary intervertebral disc. Frequently, the interspaces above and below the block vertebra are somewhat narrowed (Fig. 2-6).

Fusion also may involve the posterior elements, sometimes causing obliteration of the neural foramina at the level of the fusion. The apophyseal joints usually also are fused if the posterior elements are involved.

Klippel-Feil Syndrome. The clinical definition of Klippel-Feil syndrome is the triad of short neck, limited neck mobility, and a low posterior hairline. This entity was originally described in 1912. The radiographic indication of this syndrome is fusion of two or more cervical vertebrae. Klippel-Feil syndrome is of unknown etiology and occurs in 1 in 40,000 to 1 in 50,000 births. The mean age at the time of diagnosis is approximately 2 to 3 years.

There are three subtypes of the syndrome. In type I, there is extensive fusion of numerous cervical and upper thoracic vertebrae. In type II, there is fusion of one or two pairs of cervical vertebrae; this is the most common type. The C2–3 interspace is most frequently involved, and the C5–6 interspace is the second most common site. The type II anomaly is usually asymptomatic. Type III combines anomalies of types I and II with either thoracic or lumbar vertebral fusions. Additional anomalies of the cervical spine may be present in Klippel-Feil syndrome. These include spina bifida, hemivertebra, vertebral body clefts, spinal stenosis, enlarged or obliterated neural foramina, occipital assimilation, deformity of the odontoid process, and basilar invagination.[3]

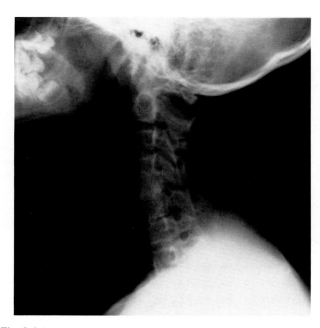

Fig. 2-6 Lateral radiograph of the cervical spine shows lack of segmentation of C-4 through C-7. Several of the intervertebral discs are rudimentary, and others are completely obliterated. The vertebral bodies are decreased in anteroposterior diameter but are increased in height. Note the slight narrowing of the interspace between C-7 and T-1. These findings are typical of block vertebrae.

Patients with Klippel-Feil syndrome frequently have other anomalies, including abnormalities of the genitourinary, central nervous, musculoskeletal, dermatologic, cardiovascular, respiratory, or gastrointestinal system. Approximately 60% of these children have significant anomalies of the genitourinary tract, such as renal agenesis, ectopia or dysgenesis of the kidney, hypospadias, cryptorchidism, vaginal agenesis, and bicornuate uterus.

Anomalies of the external, middle, and inner ear are common in Klippel-Feil syndrome, with 25% to 30% of these children having some hearing impairment. Various neurologic disabilities also occur, some of which are related to spinal stenosis or vertebral artery compression in the involved portions of the cervical spine. Rarely, a motor disorder called synkinesia is exhibited, consisting of involuntary mirror motion of the hands. This is thought to be the result of incomplete decussation of the pyramidal tracts. Progressive scoliosis occurs in about half the children with Klippel-Feil syndrome. In about 25% of patients there is high position of a scapula (Sprengel deformity). Conversely, about 40% of patients who present with Sprengel deformity are shown to have Klippel-Feil syndrome. An omovertebral bone (an anomalous bone that connects the scapula with the cervical spine) is identified in many of these cases.

Radiographs in cases of Klippel-Feil syndrome show a short neck with segmentation anomalies of the cervical spine. Most often, there are two or more cervical block vertebrae. In severe cases, there is extensive fusion of all or most of the cervical

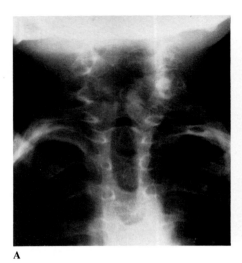
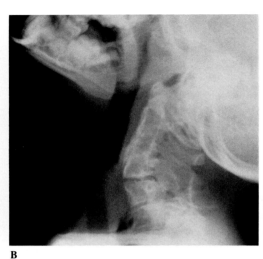

A   **B**

Fig. 2-7 Klippel-Feil syndrome. (**A**) Anteroposterior and (**B**) lateral radiographs of the cervical spine show extensive fusion anomalies of the cervical vertebrae, involving both the vertebral bodies and the posterior elements. This is typical of the type I Klippel-Feil anomaly.

vertebrae (Fig. 2-7). There may be associated curvature anomalies of the cervical spine. Anomalies of the upper thoracic vertebrae and the upper ribs sometimes occur in association with Klippel-Feil syndrome.

In infants, Klippel-Feil syndrome may be difficult to detect radiographically because the sites of fusion are mostly cartilaginous at this age. Fusion of one or more spinous processes in the cervical spine is often the earliest indicator of Klippel-Feil syndrome. Subsequent evaluation as the child ages will show progression to fusion of several cervical vertebrae.[4]

Klippel-Feil deformity is well demonstrated on magnetic resonance imaging (MRI). The block vertebrae are demonstrated as narrowed, fused vertebral bodies, sometimes with partial interspace formation. This is best shown on sagittal images. MRI is particularly useful for demonstrating associated abnormalities of the intracranial and intraspinal structures.

Hemivertebra. Most hemivertebrae are the result of failure of normal development of one or more chondrification or ossification centers during embryogenesis of the spine. As described above, the vertebral centra are predominantly formed from two side-by-side chondrification centers and two primary ossification centers, one anterior and one posterior. In most cases, the patterns of hemivertebra formation are readily explained by alterations in these developmental processes. A hemivertebra also can be produced by the formation of a supernumerary ossification center.

Hemivertebrae are most common in the thoracolumbar spine. A hemivertebra may or may not have a pedicle and may or may not fuse with the adjacent vertebra. The abnormality may occur at single or multiple levels. Multiple hemivertebrae can be ipsilateral or can alternate. Some hemivertebrae are incidental findings, and others cause progressive scoliosis. Thoracic lateral hemivertebrae are usually associated with rib anomalies, such as aplasia, hypoplasia, fusion, or supernumerary rib.

The rare failure of development of the ventral half of the vertebra produces a dorsal (posterior) hemivertebra that is usually associated with progressive angular kyphosis (gibbous deformity). Posterior slippage of a dorsal hemivertebra due to underdevelopment of the posterior arch can cause impingement on the spinal cord or nerve roots, sometimes leading to paraplegia, respiratory compromise, or other neurologic problems (Fig. 2-8).

Hemivertebrae are characterized as balanced or unbalanced according to the relationship to the adjacent vertebrae. With balanced multiple hemivertebrae, there are alternating hemi-

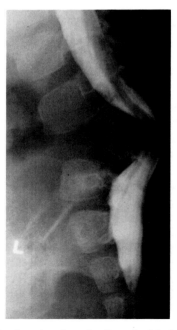

Fig. 2-8 Dorsal hemivertebra. Lateral radiograph of the lower lumbar spine shows a dorsal hemivertebra between L-5 and the sacrum. The hemivertebra is displaced posteriorly, indents the contrast-opacified subarachnoid space, and impinges on the nerve roots. This is the typical appearance of a dorsal hemivertebra.

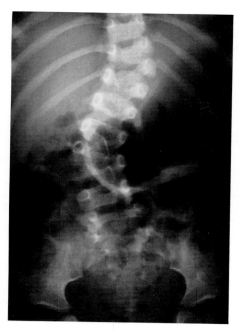

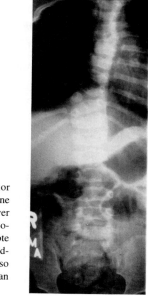

Fig. 2-10 Hemivertebra. Anteroposterior radiograph of the thoracic and lumbar spine shows a hemivertebra on the right in the lower thoracic spine. This causes an angular scoliosis with the hemivertebra at the apex. Note also the segmentation anomalies in the mid-thoracic spine. The left pedicle of L-3 is also absent. This anomaly is an example of an unbalanced hemivertebra.

Fig. 2-9 Hemivertebra. Anteroposterior radiograph of the lumbar spine shows a hemivertebra at the thoracolumbar junction on the left. In addition, there is a hemivertebra on the right in the midlumbar region. This is an example of so-called balanced hemivertebrae. Note that each hemivertebra causes scoliotic deformity, with the hemivertebra being located at the apex of the scoliotic curve, and that the curves are opposite each other, which lessens the overall deformity.

the population. Typically, a vertebra at the margin of a segment of the spine (junctional vertebra) is incorporated into a higher or lower segment; an actual deviation from the normal total number of vertebrae is rare.

Numeric variability is most frequent in the sacrococcygeal region. A common anomaly in this portion of the spine is the addition of one vertebra to the sacrum and the loss of one vertebra from the coccyx. Variation in the lumbosacral and thoracolumbar regions is also common. This results in either an increase or a decrease in the number of lumbar vertebrae, with a corresponding increase or decrease in the number of thoracic or sacral vertebrae.

vertebrae in a pattern that cancels the deforming effects (Fig. 2-9). A balanced single hemivertebra refers to ipsilateral undergrowth and contralateral overgrowth of the adjacent vertebral bodies, such that significant deformity is lacking. With unbalanced hemivertebrae, significant scoliosis (often angular) is present (Fig. 2-10). All types of hemivertebra cause some degree of spinal deformity. Serial examination of these children is important to ensure early detection of a progressive scoliosis, kyphosis, or kyphoscoliosis.[5]

Butterfly Vertebra. A butterfly vertebra is the result of a lack of fusion of the lateral chondrification centers of the vertebral centrum, thereby producing a sagittal cleft (Fig. 2-11). This anomaly is also known as a double-wedge vertebra. With weight bearing, there is usually progressive lateral displacement of the two halves. The anomalous vertebral body ultimately assumes the configuration of two triangles in apposition. The two halves of the butterfly vertebra can be asymmetric. If the asymmetry is significant, a butterfly vertebra can result in scoliosis.

Alterations in the Number of Vertebrae

The vertebral column is made up of 7 cervical, 12 thoracic, 5 lumbar, 5 sacral, and 4 coccygeal vertebrae. The number of cervical vertebrae is constant, but there is variability in the number of thoracic or lumbar vertebrae in more than 10% of

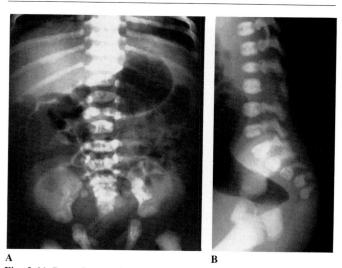

A   B

Fig. 2-11 Butterfly vertebra. (**A**) Anteroposterior and (**B**) lateral radiographs of the lumbar spine of a neonate with the VACTERL association of anomalies show a butterfly vertebra at L-2. The two components of the vertebral centrum are separated by an unossified central portion. In addition, the pedicles of L-3 are absent.

A transitional vertebra is a junctional vertebra that has characteristics common to both the segment above and the segment below. This anomaly most often occurs at the lumbosacral junction. A transitional vertebra is usually of no clinical significance.

The extreme forms of transitional vertebrae are sacralization of L-5 and lumbarization of S-1. In the normal spine vertebra 24 is the last lumbar vertebra, and vertebra 25 is the first sacral vertebra. Sacralization refers to changes in vertebra 24 (the presacral vertebra) that produce the appearance of a sacral vertebra. Sacralization is characterized by unilateral or bilateral enlargement of the transverse processes or partial or complete fusion of a transverse process or vertebral body of the presacral vertebra with the sacrum. With sacralization there are only four vertebrae that have lumbar characteristics. Lumbarization indicates changes in the first sacral vertebra (vertebra 25) such that it has the characteristics of a lumbar vertebra. With lumbarization, there is unilateral or bilateral lack of formation of the lateral masses of the first sacral vertebra. The vertebral body may either be assimilated or become the last presacral vertebra. This is much less common than sacralization.

A transitional lumbosacral vertebra has features intermediate between those of complete sacralization and lumbarization. One or both transverse processes are enlarged and may articulate with or fuse to the sacrum or the iliac bones. The body of the transitional vertebra is usually square and is separated from the next most inferior vertebral body by a rudimentary disc.

Anomalies of the Neural Arches

The neural arch ossifies from two primary centers that normally fuse during the first year of life. Fusion begins in the lumbar region and progresses to the cervical region. Fusion defects of the neural arches that can be detected radiographically can be due to a true developmental defect or failure of ossification of an arch that is present in membranous or chondral form. A midline cleft due to an ossification defect in the fifth lumbar vertebra or first sacral vertebra is a frequent finding in childhood and is of no clinical significance. Although uncommon, midline clefts also can occur in any other portion of the spine as well. They are most common in the lower thoracic or upper lumbar region.

In addition to the midline cleft, a number of other neural arch defects can occur. These include any combination of defects of the laminae, pedicles, and spinous processes. Although the spinous process often remains unossified if there are bilateral defects in the laminae, there are instances when the ossification center of the spinous process fuses unilaterally with a single lamina or joins the spinous process of the next higher or lower vertebra. Bilateral congenital defects in the laminae can be associated with spondylolisthesis.

Congenital absence of a pedicle is a rare anomaly that occurs in the lumbar spine and, less frequently, in the cervical spine. This anomaly is extremely rare in the thoracic area.[6]

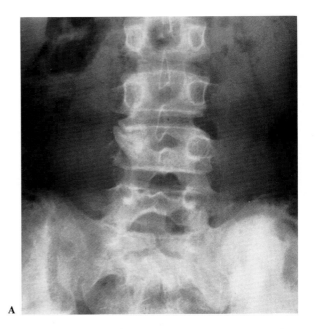

A

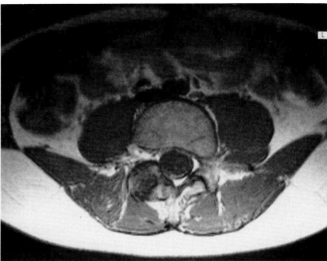

B

Fig. 2-12 Neural arch anomalies. (**A**) Anteroposterior radiograph of the lower lumbar spine shows absence of the right pedicle of L-4. The right L3–4 facet joint has abnormal angulation and spur formation as a result of abnormal motion. (**B**) Axial T_1-weighted MR image shows absence of the right pedicle of L-4. Note the abnormal right apophyseal joint.

Unilateral congenital absence of a pedicle does not usually cause significant symptoms and often is an incidental radiographic finding. There may be significant instability of the spine in the rare cases of bilateral absence of the pedicles (Figs. 2-11 and 2-12).

Congenital absence of the pedicle is thought to be due to a defect in cartilaginous development. The chondrification center that develops in each side of the neural arch gives rise to a pedicle, the superior and inferior articular processes, the transverse process, and the lamina with its spinous process. Consequently, congenital absence of the pedicle is usually associated with other anomalies of the neural arch and vertebral appendages.

Both absence and severe hypoplasia of the pedicle can occur with neurofibromatosis as a manifestation of the mesodermal dysplasia. A more consistent finding in neurofibromatosis, however, is scoliosis. Deficiencies in the pedicles of the lumbar vertebrae have been reported in association with renal aplasia and other renal anomalies.

Unilateral congenital absence of a pedicle typically causes stress changes in the contralateral pedicle and neural arch that lead to hypertrophy with or without sclerosis (Fig. 2-13). This is a useful radiographic observation to aid in distinguishing absence of the pedicle from acquired destruction due to neoplastic disease or trauma. The severity of this finding is related to age. Acquired absence of a pedicle is uncommon in children.

Some degree of underdevelopment of the neural arch, most often the superior facet, usually accompanies congenital absence of a pedicle. Likewise, the spinous process is abnormal. A small transverse process on the ipsilateral side is abnormally angulated (up or down); this is best identified on the lateral projection. Absence of a pedicle usually causes enlargement of the ipsilateral intervertebral foramen. Hypoplasia and aplasia of a pedicle are associated with hypoplasia of the ipsilateral superior facet.

Absence of the pedicle can result in a photopenic region on bone scintigraphy. Computed tomography (CT), especially with oblique reconstructions, is useful for defining the defect. CT or MRI readily detects the absence of the pedicle and the hypoplasia of the superior articular facet and confirms the hypertrophy of the contralateral lamina and pedicle.

Anomalies of the Transverse Processes

The most common anomaly of the transverse process is development of unilateral or bilateral supernumerary ribs at C-7 (cervical rib). This anomaly occurs in about 0.5% of otherwise normal individuals. Four varieties of cervical ribs are described: a complete rib that articulates anteriorly with the manubrium, an incomplete rib with a bulbous free anterior end, a rib that consists partly of bone and partly of fibrous tissue, and a fibrous branch that cannot be identified on standard radiography. The anomaly is unilateral in about 50% of cases.

Most cervical ribs are asymptomatic. Rarely, there is symptomatic compression of adjacent nerves or vessels. The subclavian artery and brachial plexus pass through a narrow triangle that is bounded anteriorly by the scalenus anterior muscle, posteriorly by the scalenus medius muscle, and inferiorly by the first rib. Elevation of the inferior border of the triangle as a result of the interposition of a cervical rib can cause a variable degree of compression of the subclavian artery and the first thoracic nerve. This can result in neck pain, ischemia of the fingers, or paralysis in the distribution of the first thoracic or lower cervical nerves (thoracic outlet or scalene syndrome).

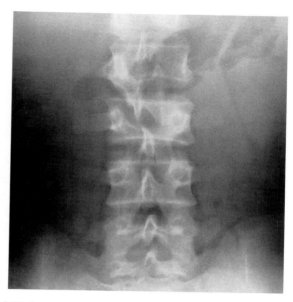

Fig. 2-13 Anteroposterior radiograph of the lumbar spine showing absence of the left pedicle of L-2. Note the stress changes in the contralateral pedicle of the same vertebra as well as abnormal orientation of the contralateral apophyseal joint. The left apophyseal joint is markedly hypoplastic.

Anomalies of the Craniovertebral Region

Basilar Invagination. Basilar invagination is an anomaly in which there is superior displacement of the margins of the foramen magnum into the posterior fossa of the skull or an abnormally cephalad location of the first cervical vertebra and odontoid process. This anomaly occurs in congenital and acquired forms. The congenital type is more common. This may exist as an isolated anomaly or occur in association with occipitalization of the atlas, hypoplasia of the atlas, Klippel-Feil syndrome, achondroplasia, or cleidocranial dysplasia.[7] The acquired variety is much less common and is seen in conditions such as rickets, osteogenesis imperfecta, hypothyroidism, rheumatoid arthritis, Paget disease, vertebral neoplasm, and vertebral osteomyelitis.

Most patients with basilar invagination are asymptomatic. With severe basilar invagination, the odontoid protrudes into the foramen magnum and may encroach on the brainstem or basilar artery.[3] Neurologic symptoms usually are not specific and may include cervical or occipital pain, cranial nerve palsy (due to compression of the upper cervical cord or brainstem), or signs and symptoms of syringomyelia or syringobulbia.

The diagnosis of basilar invagination is usually made by conventional radiography. Myelography, CT myelography, or MRI may be useful in showing the relationship of the bony abnormality to adjacent neural structures. MRI is especially useful in detecting coexisting syringomyelia, ventricular dilatation, or compression of the brainstem (Fig. 2-14).[8–10]

A number of radiologic measurements have been devised to aid in the diagnosis of basilar invagination. These include the

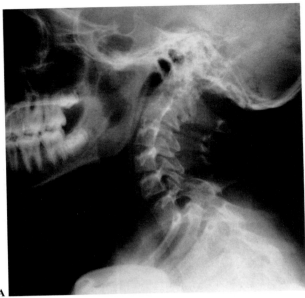
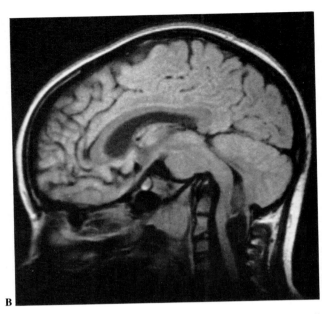

Fig. 2-14 Basilar invagination. (**A**) Lateral radiograph of the cervical spine shows that the upper cervical vertebrae are invaginated into the base of the skull. The clivus is oriented nearly horizontally. Note that there is an increase in the sagittal diameter of the cervical spinal canal. (**B**) Proton density–weighted sagittal MR image shows extensive basilar invagination, with the pons and the medulla being distorted by the invaginated cervical vertebrae. An oval cystlike structure extends inferiorly from the cerebellum posterior to the cervical spinal cord.

Chamberlain line, McGregor line, Bull angle, and McRae line. The Chamberlain line extends from the dorsal margin of the hard palate to the dorsal lip of the foramen magnum as viewed on a true lateral skull radiograph. Projection of the odontoid process 6.6 mm or more above this line is the two–standard deviation value for this measurement. The McGregor line is drawn from the superior surface of the posterior aspect of the hard palate to the most caudal plane of the occipital curve in the occipital bone as seen on a lateral skull radiograph. The tip of the odontoid should project no more than 5 mm above this line. Normal values for this measurement based on patient age are available.[11] The Bull angle is formed between the Chamberlain line and a line connecting the central plane of the anterior and posterior portions of the atlas. An angle of greater than 13° is considered indicative of basilar invagination. This method, however, is of limited usefulness because of its variation with flexion and extension of the head.

A major shortcoming with the use of the Chamberlain line and McGregor line for the determination of basilar invagination is that these lines are drawn from the hard palate, a structure that is not directly related to the anatomy of the skull base. The position and plane of the hard palate are somewhat variable and are altered by developmental changes in the facial bones. A low palate may give the false impression of basilar invagination, whereas a high palate may cause the correct diagnosis to be missed. Further complicating the diagnosis of this anomaly is the fact that the odontoid process can extend to a high position without true basilar invagination. This may occur with a congenitally elongated odontoid or with occipitalization of the atlas.

The McRae line is drawn from the anterior lip of the foramen magnum (the basion) to the posterior lip of the foramen magnum (the opisthion) on a lateral radiograph of the skull. This line measures the anteroposterior dimension of the foramen magnum. The squamous portions of the occipital bone on each side of the foramen magnum are visualized as curved, thin, dense plates of bone that are convex inferiorly. These bones normally lie below the McRae line. Basilar invagination is present if the occipital squamae at the foramen magnum are oriented in a convex upward manner or if they extend above the McRae line.

Platybasia. Platybasia is an anthropologic term that refers to an abnormal obtuseness of the basal angle of the skull (ie, flattening of the skull base). Although basilar invagination and platybasia may coexist, the two terms are not synonymous. The basal angle of the skull is the angle between a line drawn from the nasion (nasal frontal suture) to the center of the pituitary fossa and the line from the center of the pituitary fossa to the anterior rim of the foramen magnum. The normal basal angle varies between 103° and 131°. Platybasia exists if the basal angle is equal to or exceeds 145°.[12]

Occipitalization of the Atlas. Occipitalization of the atlas is rare but is the most common developmental abnormality of the craniocervical junction. Occipitalization refers to partial or complete fusion of the atlas (C-1) with the occipital bone. If the fusion is complete, this is referred to as assimilation of the atlas.

Occipitalization of the atlas can be an isolated and asymptomatic anomaly, but it is associated more often with other cra-

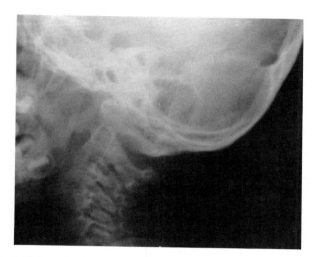

Fig. 2-15 Lateral radiograph of the cervical spine showing fusion of the posterior elements of C-1 to the occiput. The posterior elements appear as a bony ridge inferior to the occipital bone. The arch of C-1 is slightly hypoplastic and lies above the tip of the odontoid process. This is an example of occipitalization of the atlas.

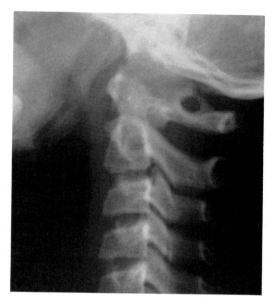

Fig. 2-16 Lateral radiograph of the cervical spine showing a complete foramen for the vertebral artery at C-1. This is an example of the arcuate foramen or ponticulus posticus.

niovertebral anomalies. These include atlantoaxial subluxation, cervical vertebral fusions, basal invagination, herniation of the cerebellar tonsils, and dural bands. Associated fusion of C2–3 occurs in about 70% of cases of this anomaly.[7] Most patients with occipitalization of the atlas develop symptoms of spinal cord compression that can be attributed to one or more of these abnormalities.[13]

Fusion of the atlas with the occiput may occur anteriorly, posteriorly, or both. Typically, radiographs show fusion of the anterior arch of the atlas with the anterior lip of the foramen magnum. The fused posterior arch is usually identified as a bony ridge at the posterior margin of the foramen magnum (Fig. 2-15). The lateral masses of the atlas may fuse with the occiput either unilaterally or bilaterally and frequently asymmetrically. Complete occipitalization or assimilation of the atlas refers to complete fusion of all components of the atlas with the base of the skull.[12]

Occipitalization of the atlas may be difficult to evaluate radiographically in infants and young children. The anterior arch of C-1 is not ossified at birth in about 80% of children, and a portion of the posterior arch of C-1 normally is not ossified at this age as well.

Arcuate Foramen. The arcuate foramen (ponticulus posticus) is the most frequent anomaly of the atlas. This refers to ossification of the atlanto-occipital ligament as it arches over the groove for the vertebral artery. This bony bridge can be partial or complete, unilateral or bilateral. It is seen on a lateral radiograph of the cervical spine as a ringlike projection of bone from the posterior elements of C-1 (Fig. 2-16). The arcuate foramen is an asymptomatic variant of normal.

Ossification Anomalies of the Atlas. The atlas develops from three primary ossification centers: one for the anterior arch and one for each lateral mass. The posterior elements

ossify from the posterior portions of the lateral ossification centers. The two sides of the posterior arch usually unite between years 3 and 5, either directly or with an interposed separate ossicle. Occasionally union does not occur until 10 to 12 years. Failure of complete midline fusion of the posterior arch of the atlas occurs in about 2% of the general population. This anomaly is entirely asymptomatic.

Failure of fusion of the posterior elements of the atlas is usually best demonstrated on frontal or oblique radiographs but may also be seen on the lateral view (Fig. 2-17). The

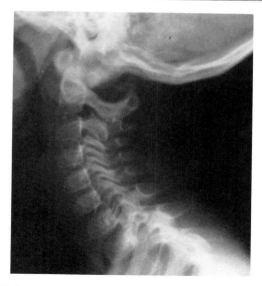

Fig. 2-17 Lateral radiograph of the cervical spine showing a normal-appearing anterior arch of C-1. The posterior elements are extremely hypoplastic, with only a small portion of the laminae and spinous process being ossified.

laminae usually have a rounded appearance near the midline and do not meet. Occasionally, a separate ossicle is seen in the midline between the separated laminae.[14]

There are two types of anomalies of ossification of the anterior arch of the atlas: accessory ossicles and ossification defects. At birth, the anterior arch of the atlas consists of a ring of fibrocartilage that undergoes ossification near the end of the first year. There are two contiguous nuclei that fuse to form a single ossification center. Occasionally, an extra inferior ossification center persists to form an accessory ossicle of variable size. An ossification defect of the anterior arch of the atlas is an unusual anomaly. It is recognized radiographically by the absence of a bony ring anterior to the dens.

Occipital Vertebra. The occipital vertebra, or proatlas, is the most cephalad of the primitive vertebrae. Normally, it fuses with other primitive vertebrae to form the basilar process of the occipital bone. Failure of normal fusion leads to the development of a small area of abnormal bone along the outer surface of the skull along the anterior portion of the foramen magnum. It may be an isolated entity or occur in combination with other abnormalities.

The most frequent radiographic manifestation of an occipital vertebra is the so-called third condyle; this is a midline bony structure that is adjacent to, but distinct from, the anterior portion of the foramen magnum.[15] This condyle may be a single tuberosity with an anterior articular facet, or it may occur as an articular depression in the foramen magnum. This anomaly is best visualized on a lateral radiograph.[16]

Asymmetry of the Lateral Masses of the Atlas. This is an unusual but clinically significant anomaly. Torticollis or significant limitation of neck motion is the usual result. The deformity is usually partially compensated by reverse asymmetry of the lateral masses of the axis.

Ossification Anomalies of the Dens. Ossification anomalies of the dens are clinically important because they can simulate traumatic or pathologic lesions on radiographs. The most common anomalies are the ossiculum terminale, os odontoideum, and hypoplasia or aplasia of the dens.

During embryologic development, the body of the odontoid process becomes separated from the centrum of C-1 and fuses caudally with C-2.[17] The odontoid process is cartilaginous during the neonatal period; ossification does not occur until later in infancy and childhood. By 2 to 3 years of age, the odontoid process is fairly well ossified; there is a persistent V-shaped vertical cleft at its tip, however. Also, a lucent cartilaginous line, which is present in all children younger than 4 years, separates the odontoid process from the main body of the axis. Complete fusion of the odontoid with the body of C-2 occurs around the age of 10 to 12 years. Failure of fusion of the odontoid process and its base results in a persistent radiolucent cartilage plate and a platelike sclerotic depression in the superior facet of the axis. The unfused dens is termed an os odontoideum. The atlantoaxial joint is stable with this anomaly, and no symptoms occur.

In some cases, the os odontoideum has the configuration of a small oval or round ossicle that is separated from and cephalad to a hypoplastic odontoid process. The ossicle may lie in the normal position at the tip of the odontoid process, or it may lie near the basion, either separate from or fused to it. This anomaly is also asymptomatic.

Some cases of os odontoideum may be due to an unrecognized fracture of the dens during infancy. This can be followed by nonunion, vascular compromise of the bone above the fracture, and partial or complete failure of further development of this avascularized segment. In these cases, the dens is small as a result of diminished growth and bone resorption and is usually separated from the main body of C-2 by a significant gap. In these situations, the atlantoaxial joint is often unstable, and there may be a risk of neurologic complications (Fig. 2-18).[18]

Early in childhood, a separate ossification center develops in the V-shaped cleft at the tip of the odontoid process. This can be identified in approximately 25% of children between the ages of 5 and 11 years. By the age of 12, this ossification center is normally fused to the tip of the odontoid process. Occasionally fusion does not occur, and a separate ossicle (the ossiculum terminale) persists (Fig. 2-19). This finding is a variation of normal that is not associated with symptoms.

Developmental Abnormalities of the Spinal Cord and Meninges

Spinal Dysraphism

The term *dysraphism* is derived from the Greek *raphe*, meaning "seam," and the prefix *dys*, meaning "bad." Spinal dysraphism refers to all types of incomplete midline closure of mesenchymal, osseous, or nervous tissue. Spinal dysraphism therefore includes incomplete fusion of the neural tube, meninges, vertebral column, or skin; failure of normal separation of the three germ cell layers (eg, a deep dermal dimple); abnormal growth of ectopic cell rests (dermoid or epidermoid cyst); and abnormal growth of otherwise normal tissue (intraspinal or intramedullary lipoma or hamartoma). Dysraphism often includes incomplete closure of the posterior bony elements of the spine; this is termed spina bifida.

Clinically, spinal dysraphism can be divided into spina bifida cystica and occult spinal dysraphism. Spina bifida cystica (spina bifida aperta) includes all dysraphic states in which there is an externally obvious closure defect of the spinal canal. Included in this category are myelomeningocele, myelocele (myeloschisis), myelocystocele, and some cases of meningocele. Myelomeningocele is a herniation of neural tissue and meninges through a closure defect, and a meningocele is a herniation of meninges only. Myelocele is the externalization of neural tissue without a meningeal covering. Myelocystocele, or syringomyelocele, is a rare anomaly in which there is dilatation of the spinal canal in a herniated sac.

Occult spinal dysraphism includes abnormalities that develop beneath an intact dermis and epidermis, there being no exposed neural tissue.[19] Included in this category are

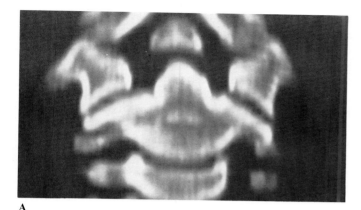

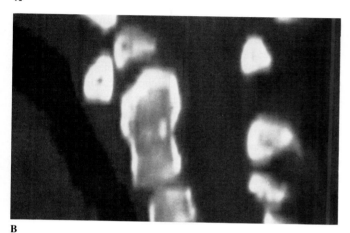

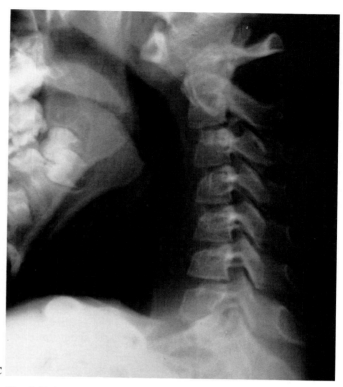

Fig. 2-18 Os odontoideum. **(A)** Coronal and **(B)** sagittal reformatted CT images of the upper cervical spine show a triangular ossicle above the tip of a blunted and rounded odontoid. This is an example of an acquired os odontoideum from prior trauma. **(C)** Lateral radiograph of the cervical spine with flexion shows forward motion of the arch of C-1 and this triangular os odontoideum with respect to the blunted odontoid process. Atlantoaxial instability is a common complication of an acquired os odontoideum.

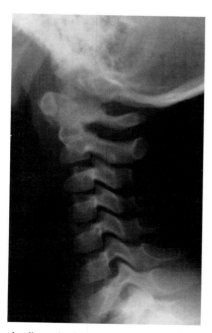

Fig. 2-19 Lateral radiograph of the cervical spine showing a triangular ossicle above the tip of the odontoid process. This is the typical appearance of an ossiculum terminale.

tethered cord syndrome, intraspinal lipoma, dermoid cyst, epidermoid cyst, dorsal dermal sinus, diastematomyelia, neurenteric cyst, split notochord syndrome, and some cases of meningocele. The simplest form of occult spinal dysraphism is spina bifida occulta, in which there is a small, clinically undetectable defect in the posterior elements of one or more vertebrae. Most of these conditions are not truly occult because they tend to be associated with a cutaneous abnormality, such as a hairy tuft, nevus, or sinus, that suggests the presence of an underlying developmental abnormality. Also, a subcutaneous lipoma or meningocele may be palpable. MRI is the diagnostic tool of choice to evaluate the intraspinal structures in these patients.[20]

Myelomeningocele and Myelocele

Myelomeningocele (from the Greek *myelo*, indicating the spinal cord, and *kele*, meaning "hernia") and myelocele (myeloschisis) are common types of spina bifida cystica. These disorders are thought to be due to lack of closure of a portion of the neural tube during embryonic development. At the affected site the neural tube remains open, and the neural folds are in continuity with the skin. The exposed segment of cord is termed the neural placode. The dura is deficient posterior to the placode. The pia and arachnoid line the ventral aspect of the placode and dura, thereby forming an arachnoid sac that communicates with the subarachnoid space. The spinal cord is tethered at a more caudal location than normal. The dorsal and ventral nerve roots arise from the ventral surface of the placode. With a myelomeningocele, expansion of the ventral subarachnoid space causes posterior displacement of the placode. With a myelocele, the placode lies at the same level as the surrounding skin surface.

Because the neural folds remain in continuity with the cutaneous ectoderm at the site of a myelocele or myelomeningocele, the mesenchyme cannot migrate into its normal posterior position to form the posterior elements of the vertebrae. Therefore, spina bifida occurs in the region of the neural abnormality. The pedicles and laminae are externally rotated, and the spinal canal is enlarged in the region of the spina bifida. Anomalies of the vertebral bodies are infrequent.

Myelomeningocele and myelocele are probably the most common clinically significant congenital anomalies of the central nervous system, having a prevalence of about 1 in 1000 live births in the United States. There are several clinical factors that alter the rate of occurrence of these disorders; the mechanisms of these associations are, however, unknown or poorly understood. The condition is twice as common in pregnancies in which the mother is older than 35 years of age. The subsequent sibling of a child born with a myelomeningocele carries a 15-fold increased risk of this anomaly. A child of a parent with spina bifida carries 15 times the baseline risk for this disorder. There is a significantly increased risk of anencephaly in infants with myelomeningocele. The presence of occult spinal dysraphism in a parent or sibling does not signify an increased risk for either myelomeningocele or anencephaly.[21]

Essentially all children with myelomeningocele or myelocele have Chiari II malformation. Of these children, 85% have some degree of hydrocephalus. Occult spinal dysraphism, however, is rarely if ever associated with Chiari II malformation. The reason for this difference between the two dysraphic states has not been established.[22]

Chiari malformation consists of a spectrum of hindbrain malformations in which there are various degrees of caudal protrusion of the hindbrain through the foramen magnum. There are two distinct types, termed type I and type II. The two types differ markedly with respect to both the anatomic characteristics of the anomaly and the implications regarding other central nervous system malformations. Type I consists of elongation of the cerebellar tonsils and medial inferior lobes of the cerebellum. This type of malformation is not associated with spinal dysraphism.[23]

With type II Chiari malformation, there is caudal displacement of tissue derived from the inferior cerebellar vermis into the cervical canal with concomitant caudal displacement of the medulla, pons, and fourth ventricle. The type II malformation is almost always associated with hydrocephalus of variable severity. Essentially all cases of type II Chiari malformation occur in patients with myelomeningocele. Other neural malformations that are associated with the Chiari type II anomaly include microgyria, heterotopic cortical tissue, enlargement of the massa intermedia, fenestration of the falx, fusion of the quadrigeminal plate (tectal beaking), forking of the aqueduct, hydromyelia, and meningeal gliosis. There is evidence that the association among these various malformations is due to different regional responses to a common insult.[24]

Signs and symptoms of hydrocephalus are often absent in newborns with myelomeningocele and Chiari II malformation. A normal or small head size at birth has no prognostic significance. Head circumference measurements are not always reliable for predicting the development of hydrocephalus. The early diagnosis of hydrocephalus in these infants frequently requires direct imaging, usually with sonography.

Spina bifida is the dominant osseous spinal abnormality in children with myelocele or myelomeningocele. There is external rotation of the spinal laminae and widening of the interpedicular distances at the level of the lesion. In addition to spina bifida, other vertebral anomalies are commonly identified at levels above, within, or below the lesion. These associated vertebral anomalies tend to occur in two main regions. (1) There is a propensity for vertebral arch fusion anomalies at the cranial end of the spina bifida. Vertebral body fusion anomalies, hemivertebrae, and vertebral body aplasia also may occur in this area. (2) Hemivertebrae often occur at the cervicothoracic junction. Other dysraphic lesions also may occur in other regions of the spine but are less common. Rib anomalies, such as agenesis, defective development, and synostosis, are frequent, particularly in the T-5 through T-8 region.

Spinal deformities are important factors in the long-term management of children with myelocele and myelomeningocele. Clinically significant scoliosis occurs in more than half these patients. The scoliosis is generally thought to be due to a paralytic collapsing spine, although the exact mechanism is not well understood. Unopposed contraction of the iliopsoas muscle has been suggested as a contributing factor, but this does not account for the frequent thoracic location of the scoliosis. A disturbance of innervation of the paraspinal muscles is also unlikely because the spinal curvature is usually located above the myelocele. Further, at birth the spinal neurons above the spinal defect are histologically normal. Some investigators have implicated congenital dislocation of the hips as a causative factor, but a similar incidence of hip dislocation is found in myelocele patients with or without scoliosis.

Children who are not severely incapacitated by myelocele or myelomeningocele at birth may later develop spasticity and increased weakness of the extremities, sometimes associated with developmental scoliosis. In these cases, the possibility of hydromyelia needs to be considered. Hydromyelia in these patients is thought to be due to passage of cerebrospinal fluid from a dilated ventricular system into the central canal of the spinal cord. Hydromyelia can, however, occur in patients with myelomeningocele who have normal-size ventricles. In developmental hydromyelia, communication with the ventricles probably serves to compensate for hydrocephalus. Clinical signs of increased intracranial pressure are uncommon in these patients. Ventricular shunting in patients with developmental hydromyelia, even those who do not show ventricular dilatation, often results in significant improvement of the neurologic deficits and arrests the progression of developmental scoliosis.[25]

The initial imaging study in the evaluation of children with meningocele or myelomeningocele should be standard radiographs to detect the nature, degree, and extent of bony defects. Marked thinning of the calvaria in a patchy distribution is visible on skull radiographs in many infants with myelomeningocele. This is commonly termed lacunar skull (lückenschädel). The lacunae are most evident in early infancy; they gradually become less recognizable and completely disappear by about 6 months of age. The lacunar skull is not the result of hydrocephalus or increased intracranial pressure; it is presumed to represent a developmental dysplasia of the membranous calvaria. It may be seen in patients with small heads; the distribution of lacunae does not conform to brain convolutions.

Spine radiographs show severe spina bifida at the level of the myelocele or myelomeningocele with absence of the spinous processes and separation and eversion of the pedicles and laminae (Fig. 2-20). As a general rule, if the spina bifida involves T-12 through L-1, the entire lumbar and sacral regions will be involved; if T-12 and L-1 are intact, the spina bifida will be localized to the involved portion of the lumbar, sacral, or (uncommonly) thoracic spine. The radiographs also may

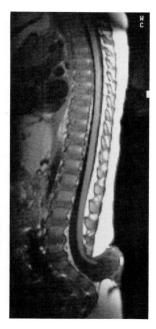

Fig. 2-21 Sagittal T_1-weighted MR image of an infant with a myelomeningocele showing the spinal cord to be tethered to the S-1 level and to curve posteriorly. It terminates in a saclike structure. Neural tissue can be seen in the superior-posterior aspect of the myelomeningocele. Note the disruption of the normal subcutaneous fat.

demonstrate a number of other vertebral anomalies adjacent to, or remote from, the area of the spina bifida.

Sonography is frequently useful for evaluating infants after surgical repair of a myelocele or myelomeningocele. The osseous defect provides a window for evaluation of the intraspinal structures. In most cases, the spinal cord and nerve roots can be imaged effectively on sonography. CT is most useful for demonstrating the spinal osseous anomalies and for evaluating the intracranial structures.[26]

MRI is the most effective imaging technique for the evaluation of the intraspinal structures in patients with myelocele or myelomeningocele.[27,28] If performed before repair of the lesion, MRI shows a myelocele or myelomeningocele as a posterior or midline mass, usually in the lumbar region. Most of the lesion produces signal of cerebrospinal fluid intensity. The placode is demonstrated as irregular tissue along the posterior aspect of the cystic component that has signal intensity approximately equal to that of the spinal cord. The cutaneous tissues posterior to the placode are deficient. Tethering of the spinal cord is also demonstrated (Fig. 2-21).

The changes associated with Chiari type II malformation in the upper cervical region can be demonstrated on MRI, myelography, or CT myelography. These studies show the upper portion of the cervical spinal cord and medulla to be displaced inferiorly. The upper cervical nerve roots ascend toward their neural foramina. The medulla is displaced inferiorly, and there is often a posterior kink at the cervicomedullary junction. Inferior herniation of the cerebellar vermis produces a thin tongue of tissue that extends posterior to the medulla (Fig. 2-22). This most often extends inferiorly to C-2 through C-4 but may extend as low as the upper thoracic spine (Fig. 2-23).

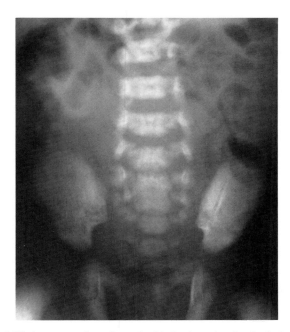

Fig. 2-20 Anteroposterior radiograph of the lumbar spine showing lack of the spinous processes of the lower lumbar spine and sacrum. The pedicles and laminae are everted, and the interpedicular distances are widened. The appearance is typical of the severe spina bifida that occurs with myelomeningocele.

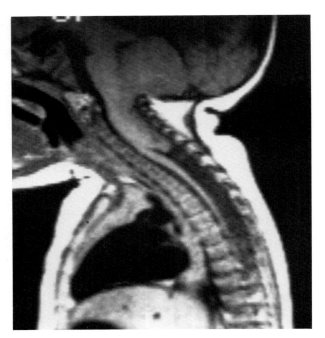

Fig. 2-22 Sagittal T$_1$-weighted MR image of a child with a myelomeningocele showing marked caudal descent of the hindbrain, with cerebellar tissue extending to the level of C-7. This is severe Chiari type II malformation.

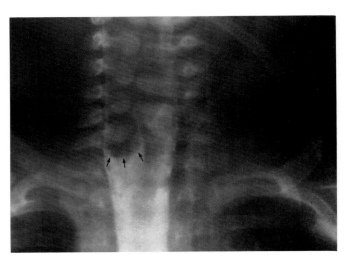

Fig. 2-23 Myelography with water-soluble contrast material in a child with myelomeningocele showing cerebellar tissue as a crescentic filling defect (arrows) posterolateral to the spinal cord at the C7–T1 level.

Hydromyelia is best detected on MRI. There is fusiform enlargement of the involved portion of the cord. The central canal is dilated, and the contents have signal characteristics identical to those of cerebrospinal fluid (Fig. 2-24). Hydromyelia most often is seen in the lower cervical or upper thoracic segments of the spinal cord. Even so, the entire central canal or one or more short segments of any portion of the cord may be involved. Hydromyelia does not occur distal to the placode.

Associated abnormalities seen in these children are also effectively evaluated with MRI. A lipoma, dermoid, or epidermoid may occur in association with a myelocele or myelomeningocele. These are demonstrated as an intraspinal mass of variable signal intensity. A lipoma or dermoid usually produces high signal on T$_1$-weighted images. An epidermoid

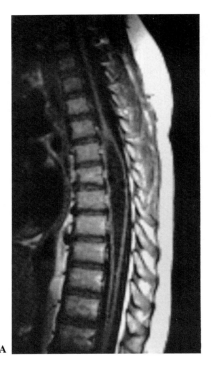

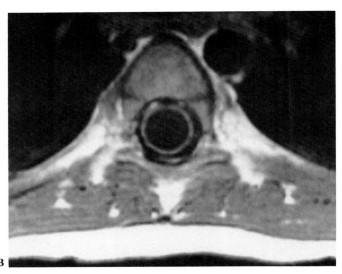

Fig. 2-24 Hydromyelia. **(A)** Sagittal T$_1$-weighted MR image of the thoracic spine in a patient who had repair of myelomeningocele shows fusiform enlargement of the central portion of the spinal canal. The signal characteristics are identical to those of cerebrospinal fluid. **(B)** Axial T$_1$-weighted MR image through the midportion of the thoracic cord reveals marked thinning of the substance of the cord by the central hydromyelia.

is often approximately isointense to cerebrospinal fluid on T_1-weighted sequences.

Approximately 30% to 40% of patients with myelomeningocele have an associated diastematomyelia (ie, a sagittal division of a portion of the spinal cord). The spinal cord may be divided above, below, or at the same level as the myelomeningocele.[29] If the two hemicords are equal in size, they are positioned next to each other in the coronal plane. If they are asymmetric, the smaller segment most often lies ventral to the larger hemicord. In about 5% of cases of myelomeningocele, there is duplication of the central canal in the region of the defect without a true splitting of the cord.

Hemimyelocele refers to a specific type of myelomeningocele with diastematomyelia; it occurs in 5% to 10% of patients with myelomeningocele. The most common form of hemimyelocele is characterized by diastematomyelia, with one of the two hemicords being contained in a small myelomeningocele (usually lying on one side of the midline); the other hemicord either is normal or has a much smaller meningocele at a lower level. The hemicords are usually contained in separate dural sacs. The septum that separates the cords may be bony or fibrous. Less commonly, the two hemicords lie in a single dural sac that is deficient at the level of the divided cord.

From an imaging standpoint, hemimyelocele is best evaluated on MRI. The cord divides into two hemicords at the level of the bony defect. The associated myelomeningocele is demonstrated as a cerebrospinal fluid–containing cystic structure. A spur that courses between the hemicords may or may not be present.

Meningocele

Meningocele is a herniation of arachnoid and dura through an osseous spinal defect that is covered by skin. The great majority of meningoceles occur dorsally, although lateral and anterior types are occasionally identified. The great majority of meningoceles occur in the lumbosacral region; cervical and thoracic meningoceles are uncommon. The sac contains no neural tissue, and there is no association with hydrocephalus, Chiari malformation, or syringohydromyelia. The conus medullaris is usually in a normal position.

Conventional radiographs are useful in cases of dorsal meningocele to determine the character and extent of the osseous defects. The bony abnormalities range from a small defect of the posterior elements of a single vertebra to a long-segment spina bifida. The contents of the sac can be evaluated with sonography or CT to determine whether any neural structures or other tissues are present (Fig. 2-25). MRI is also helpful to ensure that the mass is a meningocele and not a myelomeningocele, lipoma, cystic tumor, or other developmental cystic abnormality. A lipoma is recognized on MRI by the high signal intensity produced on T_1-weighted images.

Anterior sacral meningocele is herniation of a cerebrospinal fluid–containing meningeal sac through an abnormal sacral foramen or other anterior defect in the sacrum. The sacrum is

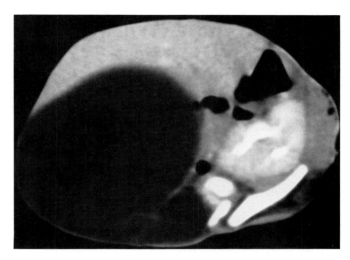

Fig. 2-25 Contrast-enhanced CT of the midlumbar region revealing a large dorsal and lateral meningocele. The right lamina of the vertebra is absent. In this patient, similar bony changes extended from the lower thoracic region to involve the entire lumbar spine and sacrum.

anomalous, with hypoplasia of one side of the sacrum being the most common malformation. This is identified radiographically as a sickle- or comma-shaped malformation. There is an equal sex distribution and rare familial cases. This lesion occasionally occurs in patients with neurofibromatosis or Marfan syndrome.

Anterior sacral meningocele frequently presents during childhood with constipation, urinary dysfunction, or neurologic symptoms. Some cases remain asymptomatic or present during adulthood with low back pain and sciatica or symptoms of local pressure on the pelvic organs. In women, many cases of anterior sacral meningocele are discovered during a pelvic examination or after a difficult labor. Other complications of anterior sacral meningocele include ureteric obstruction, recurrent meningitis, and spontaneous rupture.[30]

Anterior sacral meningocele is shown as a midline pelvic mass on sonography, CT, barium enema, cystography, or MRI. The mass has the imaging characteristics of cerebrospinal fluid. The lesion may be unilocular or multiloculated. In some cases, nerve roots course through the lumen or the wall of the meningocele. Communication with the spinal subarachnoid space can be documented with MRI, myelography, or CT myelography.

Myelocystocele

Myelocystocele is a rare, occult spinal dysraphism in which a segment of a hydromyelic spinal cord and the covering arachnoid layer are herniated through a posterior spina bifida. The resulting cyst is in continuity with the dilated central canal of the spinal cord. There is often an associated meningocele that does not communicate directly with the lumen of the myelocystocele. The most common type is the terminal myelocystocele, in which the spinal cord inserts in the posterior wall of a meningocele; a separate ependymal-lined cyst that communicates with the central canal is also present. Myelocystocele most often occurs in the lumbosacral spine; rarely, the cervical or thoracic segments can be involved. Terminal myelocystoceles frequently occur in association with sacral dysgenesis and anomalies of the gastrointestinal and genitourinary tracts, especially exstrophy of the cloaca.

Myelography or CT myelography shows a myelocystocele as a mass that does not communicate directly with the subarachnoid space. A coexistent meningocele, when present, is readily opacified with intrathecal contrast material. Delayed opacification of the myelocystocele may occur as contrast material gains access to the dilated central canal of the spinal cord.

Myelocystocele is demonstrated on sonography or MRI as a thin-walled cyst. The communication of the myelocystocele with the hydromyelic spinal cord may or may not be demonstrable. When a meningocele is also present, the spinal cord is seen to traverse the meningocele. The myelocystocele is most often located posterior and inferior to the meningocele and is usually the larger of the two cysts (Fig. 2-26).[31]

Dorsal Dermal Sinus

A dorsal dermal sinus is an epithelium-lined tract that extends inward from the dorsal skin surface to the region of the spine. This developmental anomaly is the result of a region of incomplete separation of cutaneous ectoderm from neural ectoderm. Because the embryonic spinal cord ascends in relation to the spine and skin, the dermal sinus usually follows a long oblique course extending from inferior to superior. During embryonic development, the neural folds first fuse into the primitive neural tube in the cervical region, with fusion progressing superiorly and inferiorly from this point. This developmental sequence is thought to account for the propensity for dermal sinuses to occur in the lumbosacral region; most are located in the region of closure of the caudal neuropore.[32]

Some dermal sinuses extend from the skin surface into the subcutaneous tissue but end blindly. In most cases, however, the tract extends intraspinally. The sinus tract may reach the dura without passing through it, causing a tenting of the dura at this site. If the sinus passes through the dura, it may communicate with the subarachnoid space or may traverse the subarachnoid space to terminate in the conus medullaris, filum terminale, or dorsal aspect of the cord. It may also end in a dermoid or epidermoid cyst. About half the dermal sinuses pass into an intraspinal dermoid or epidermoid cyst, presumably as a result of incorporation of surface ectodermal cells into the neural tube during closure of the caudal neuropore. Conversely, about 25% of dermoid and epidermoid cysts are associated with a dermal sinus tract. Dermal sinuses that have

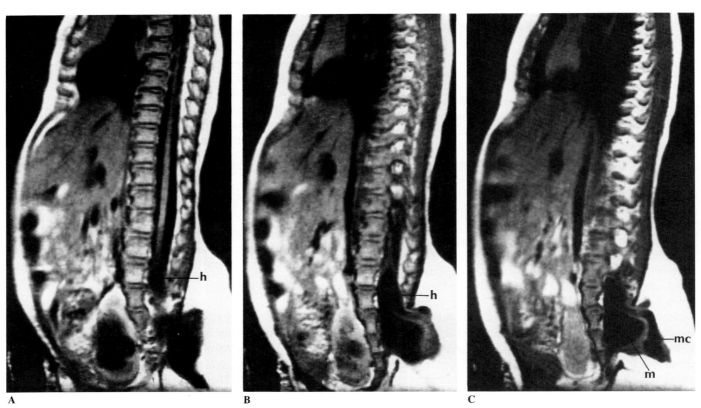

Fig. 2-26 Myelocystocele. Sagittal T_1-weighted MR images in the midline (**A**) and left parasagittal regions (**B** and **C**) show the spinal cord to be tethered at the L5–S1 level. The distal spinal cord is hydromyelic (h) and communicates through a defect posteriorly to terminate in a myelocystocele (mc). The myelocystocele lies posterior and slightly inferior to a meningocele (m). Also note a pelvic kidney anterior to the sacrum.

a midline orifice tend to be associated with a midline dermoid or epidermoid; those that have a paramedian orifice are usually associated with an epidermoid cyst that is located laterally in the subarachnoid, subdural, or epidural spaces. The length and course of the dermal sinuses vary.[33]

Midline posterior vertebral anomalies are often associated with congenital dermal sinuses. There may be a groove on the upper surface of the spinous process and lamina, a hypoplastic spinous process, a single bifid spinous process, multilevel spina bifida, or a laminar defect. In some cases, the sinus tract extends in the space between two adjacent spinous processes, but no bony abnormalities are found.

Clinically, a dermal sinus is identified as a midline (or, less commonly, a paramedian) dimple or pinpoint ostium in the skin of the back. Frequently there is a hypopigmented patch, a surrounding hairy nevus, or a capillary angioma in the region of the ostium. The lesion is asymptomatic in some cases. Symptoms may be caused by infection or compression of intraspinal structures by an associated dermoid or epidermoid cyst. Passage of organisms through the tract may result in meningitis or abscess formation in the skin, paraspinal soft tissues, epidural space, subdural space, or subarachnoid space.[34]

The course of a dermal sinus tract may be demonstrated on sonography, CT, or MRI. The most important consideration from an imaging standpoint is the detection of associated intraspinal pathology. Epidermoid cysts are usually best identified on CT myelography. An epidermoid cyst is demonstrated as a thin-walled structure that has signal characteristics of cerebrospinal fluid on MRI and as a nonopacified cystic structure on CT myelography. Dermoid cysts typically show the CT and MR characteristics of fat. Nerve roots adjacent to the dermoid or epidermoid cyst are frequently adherent to the capsule of the cyst. The cord may be expanded by an intramedullary dermoid or epidermoid cyst; an extramedullary lesion can displace the cord and adjacent nerve roots. The imaging studies also frequently demonstrate a posterior vertebral defect of variable size in the region of the dermal sinus (Fig. 2-27).[35,36]

Lipoma

Spinal lipoma is a developmental tumor that almost always is accompanied by spina bifida aperta. The lesion occurs as a partially encapsulated mass of fat and connective tissue that is connected to the leptomeninges or spinal cord. Spinal lipomas are generally divided into four types: intradural lipoma (less than 5%), epidural lipoma (rare), lipomyelomeningocele and lipomyelocele (80% to 85%), and fibrolipoma of the filum terminale (10% to 15%). Intradural lipomas, lipomyelomeningoceles, and lipomyeloceles account for approximately 35% of skin-covered lumbosacral masses.[37] A spinal lipoma is present in between 40% and 75% of cases of spina bifida aperta.[38]

An intradural lipoma is contained in an intact dural sac. This lesion accounts for less than 1% of primary intraspinal neo-

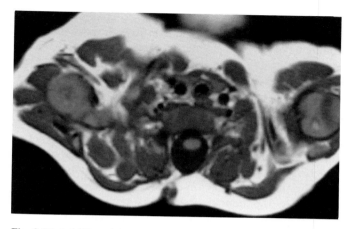

Fig. 2-27 Axial T_1-weighted MR image of the C-7 vertebra showing absence of the posterior elements. In this patient, this extended over six contiguous vertebral segments. The subarachnoid space is enlarged posteriorly. A dermal sinus is seen extending posteriorly from the dilated subarachnoid space to terminate in a dimpled area of low signal in the subcutaneous fat just below the midline. This an example of a dorsal dermal sinus.

plasms. The clinical manifestations of intradural lipoma often exhibit a slow, progressive course. Intradural lipomas in the cervical and thoracic areas typically present with an ascending paraparesis, spasticity, and sensory loss. Compression of the posterior columns may produce ataxia. Pain and temperature sensations are usually less affected than with intramedullary spinal cord tumors. Lumbosacral intradural lipomas often present with dysfunction of the rectal and bladder sphincters and flaccid paralysis of the lower extremities. The skin overlying the lesion is usually normal.

An intradural lipoma can occur at any level of the spine. The most common locations are the cervical and thoracic regions, with about 12% being found in the cervical spine, 24% in the cervicothoracic spine, and 30% in the thoracic spine. About 75% are positioned in the dorsal aspect of the cord. Syringohydromyelia is a rare coexistent abnormality.[39]

Intradural lipoma is a subpial-juxtamedullary lesion. The dorsal aspect of the spinal cord fails to fuse at the level of the tumor; the lipoma fills the space between the central canal and the dorsal pia. In almost all cases, a portion of the tumor is exophytic; the exophytic component, with its overlying pia, projects into the subarachnoid space, usually dorsal to the cord. A fibrous layer separates the lipoma from the cells of the cord; although the cord is deformed, true microscopic infiltration by the lipoma does not occur.

In some cases of intradural lipoma, the bony spinal canal is normal. In most cases, however, there is focal enlargement of the spinal canal, and occasionally there is enlargement of adjacent neural foramina. A focal area of spina bifida may be present at the level of the lipoma.

Rarely, an intraspinal lipoma that is unassociated with spina bifida can occur in the epidural space. In this case, the mass usually lies dorsal to the cord. Most epidural lipomas are unencapsulated and are not attached to the dura. The most common location is the thoracic region. The histologic features of these lesions often differ from those of the more common types of spinal lipomas. Epidural lipomas may contain embryonic fat cells and may have the histologic characteristics of a fibrolipoma or angiolipoma.[40]

Lipomyelocele and lipomyelomeningocele refer to myeloceles and myelomeningoceles that are associated with a lipomatous subcutaneous connective tissue mass. With both these anomalies, there is a lipoma that is attached to the dorsal surface of the neural placode; the skin overlying the lipoma is intact. Therefore, these are types of occult spinal dysraphism.

As occurs with simple myelocele, the subarachnoid space ventral to the neural placode is normal in cases of lipomyelocele. The placode lies in the spinal canal. The lipoma of a lipomyelocele extends extraspinally from the surface of the placode through the area of spina bifida to become continuous with the extraspinal subcutaneous fat. The configuration of the intraspinal portion of the lipoma causes a variable degree of distortion of the shape of the neural placode.

With lipomyelomeningocele, the subarachnoid space ventral to the neural placode is expanded, causing dorsal displacement of the placode, the subarachnoid space, the dura, and the adjacent lipoma. The dura is deficient in the region of the spinal dysraphism and is attached to the lateral aspect of the neural placode posterior to the site of origin of the dorsal nerve roots. The dorsal surface of the placode is, in turn, attached to the lipoma, and, as with lipomyelocele, the lipoma is continuous with the subcutaneous fat. The extent of the intraspinal component of the lipoma is variable. It may occur superiorly along the dorsal aspect of the neural placode, in the central canal of the spinal cord, or in the epidural space. In some patients, the intraspinal component of the lipoma is asymmetric and causes rotation and posterior herniation of a portion of the placode, nerve roots, and the subarachnoid space.[41]

The clinical presentation of lipomyelomeningocele and lipomyelocele usually occurs before the age of 6 months. The findings include a lumbosacral mass, sensory loss, bladder dysfunction, motor loss, and orthopedic deformities of the lower limb. These anomalies are more common in girls.

Fibrolipoma of the filum terminale is included in the spectrum of spinal lipomatous malformations. This lesion may involve any portion of the filum terminale. Many are small and asymptomatic. This lesion frequently occurs in association with myelomeningocele.

The precise mechanisms involved in the pathogenesis of spinal lipomas are unknown. Potential sources of the fat cells from which a spinal lipoma may develop include normal fat cells in the pia and arachnoid, remnants of ectodermal cells in the spinal canal, and perivascular mesenchymal cells. Intradural lipoma, lipomyelomeningocele, and lipomyelocele are thought to result from premature separation of the cutaneous ectoderm from the neuroectoderm during the process of neurulation (ie, focal premature disjunction). The premature separation presumably allows perineural mesenchyme to enter the central canal of the as yet unfused neural tube. The presence of this abnormal tissue prevents normal closure of the neural

folds at this site. The mesenchyme in the neural tube is induced to form a lipoma. Lipomas of the filum terminale appear to result from abnormal development of the tail bud (caudal cell mass), in which there is an anomaly in the sequence of canalization and retrogressive differentiation.

Radiographs in cases of spinal lipoma are useful to demonstrate the bony abnormalities. Intradural lipomas may or may not be associated with spina bifida. When present, the dorsal spinal defect is usually small. Both intradural and epidural spinal lipomas are often associated with an area of focal enlargement of the spinal canal. This is usually best appreciated as an area of widening of the interpedicular distance, sometimes with thinning of the margins of one or more pedicles.

In cases of lipomyelomeningocele or lipomyelocele, radiographs demonstrate gross spina bifida and enlargement of the spinal canal. Butterfly vertebrae and segmental anomalies of one or more vertebral bodies are demonstrated in approximately 40% of these patients. Sacral anomalies are also common.[42]

The pathologic anatomy of a spinal lipoma and the intraspinal structures can be demonstrated on CT myelography or MRI. On CT, the lipoma produces negative attenuation values that are characteristic of fat. MRI is the single best method for imaging spinal lipomas. The characteristic high signal intensity of this fatty neoplasm on T_1-weighted images allows clear differentiation from surrounding structures.

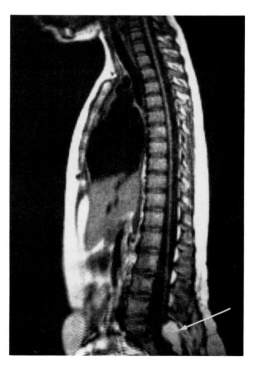

Fig. 2-28 Sagittal T_1-weighted MR image showing a tethered spinal cord that terminates in a fatty mass (arrow) at the S1–3 level. This is an example of a lipomyelocele. The overlying skin has been repaired.

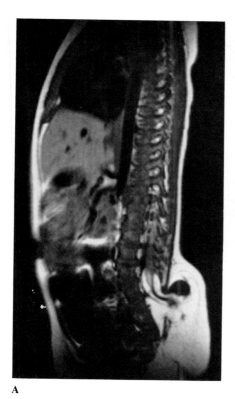

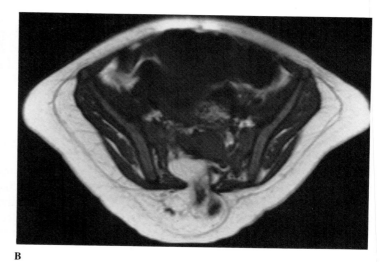

Fig. 2-29 Lipomyelomeningocele. (**A**) Parasagittal T_1-weighted MR image shows a tethered cord that terminates in a fatty mass that has both intraspinal and extra-spinal components. The fat extends intradurally to surround the tethered spinal cord. A small meningocele is present at the superior margin of the bony defect. (**B**) Axial T_1-weighted MR image shows the intradural fat to blend imperceptibly with the sub-cutaneous fat. The meningocele lies to the left of the midline. The overlying skin has been repaired. There is dysraphism of the posterior elements.

An intradural lipoma is imaged as a fatty mass along the surface of the spinal cord or in the region of the cauda equina. Typically, the lesion lies along the dorsal aspect of the cord and grows for a variable distance superiorly and inferiorly in the spinal canal. The spinal cord is deformed at the site of the lesion. An epidural lipoma also lies in the spinal canal and causes some degree of deformation of the adjacent spinal cord; the lesion is separated from the spinal cord by the dura.

Cross-sectional imaging of lipomyelocele and lipomyelo-meningocele demonstrates a mass with the characteristics of fatty tissue in association with a tethered cord and spina bifida (Fig. 2-28). Portions of the lipoma blend with the subcutaneous fat. With a lipomyelocele, the subarachnoid space ventral to the neural placode is of normal size. The neural placode may be deformed by intraspinal extension of the lipoma. With a lipomyelomeningocele the subarachnoid space is expanded, and the neural placode and subarachnoid space are displaced posteriorly. The growth pattern of the lipoma causes a variable degree of distortion and deformity of these structures. In some cases of lipomyelomeningocele or lipomyelocele, the lipoma grows superiorly in the central canal or the adjacent subarachnoid or epidural spaces (Fig. 2-29).

A fibrolipoma of the filum terminale is imaged as an area of enlargement of the filum that has the CT and MR characteristics of fat (Fig. 2-30). These lesions vary from small, asymptomatic masses to larger masses that cause displacement of nerve roots and enlargement of the spinal canal. Evidence of tethering of the spinal cord may or may not be identified.

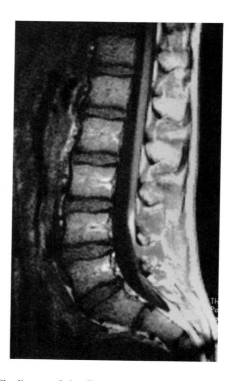

Fig. 2-30 Fibrolipoma of the filum terminale. Sagittal T_1-weighted MR image of an adolescent with incontinence showing tethering of the spinal cord. The spinal cord terminates in an elongated area of high signal, representing a lipoma of the filum terminale. The nerve roots can be seen exiting below the lipoma.

Dermoid and Epidermoid Cysts

Intraspinal dermoid and epidermoid cysts are developmental tumors that frequently occur in association with spina bifida. A dermoid cyst is lined with squamous epithelium that contains elements of skin appendages such as hair, sweat glands, and sebaceous glands. An epidermoid cyst is lined by a membrane that is composed of epidermal elements of the skin only. They are thought to arise from congenital dermal or epidermal cell rests. These congenital tumors account for approximately 10% of spinal cord tumors in children. Twenty percent are associated with dermal sinuses.

Most intraspinal dermoids present in late adolescence, and most epidermoids tend to present in early to middle adulthood. Intraspinal dermoids and epidermoids may produce a slowly progressive myelopathy. A chemical meningitis can occur if the cyst ruptures. Epidermoids are more common in boys; there is no sex predilection with dermoids.

About 80% of dermoids occur in the lumbosacral region of the spinal cord or in the area of the cauda equina. Epidermoids have a more uniform incidence distribution throughout the spinal column, although involvement of the more caudal areas is slightly more common. Sixty percent of dermoids and epidermoids are extramedullary, and the remainder are intramedullary.[43]

On myelography, a dermoid or epidermoid is demonstrated as a nonspecific intraspinal mass (Fig. 2-31). Those dermoids that are primarily composed of fat produce low attenuation on CT or high signal intensity on T_1-weighted MR images. There is some degree of variability in the content of individual dermoids. There are uncommon lesions that have a high water content and little fat; these may not show the characteristic CT and MR appearances. The contents of an epidermoid cyst are typically similar to cerebrospinal fluid on both CT and MR images. Epidermoid cysts are often best demonstrated on CT myelography. It may be difficult to detect the thin wall of an epidermoid cyst on MRI. Spinal dermoid and epidermoid cysts may lie either within or outside the dural sac.

Hamartoma

A hamartoma is a malformation that consists of a mixture of normal tissues found in an abnormal location. These lesions are composed of mesodermal elements such as muscle, fat, cartilage, and bone. Spinal hamartomas are dorsal skin-covered lesions that occur in the midline of the midthoracic, thoracolumbar, and lumbar regions. Associated cutaneous angiomas may be present. Radiographs show spina bifida in more than 50% of these patients and widening of the spinal canal in about 80%. The characteristics of the mass on CT and MRI are determined by the tissue composition.[44]

Tethered Cord Syndrome

During development of the fetal spine, the cord extends the entire length of the embryo, and the spinal nerves are oriented horizontally to pass through the vertebral foramina. With subsequent development of the embryo, the vertebral column and dura lengthen more rapidly than the spinal cord, and the caudal portion of the cord undergoes simultaneous retrogressive differentiation. This causes the conus medullaris to ascend to the level of L-2 at birth.[45] Normal ascent of the cord fails to occur if the conus becomes entrapped at a low level during development by an abnormally thickened or short filum or as a result of a number of spinal anomalies, such as lipoma, sagittal septum (diastematomyelia), myelomeningocele, myeloschisis, or myelocystocele. This abnormal low position of the spinal cord is termed a tethered cord.

If the tethering causes severe stretching of the conus, neurologic disturbances usually become apparent early in infancy. A lesser degree of traction may cause minor nonprogressive neurologic deficits that only become clinically manifest later during childhood. Initial clinical presentation in adulthood is uncommon. The symptoms are due to longitudinal traction or compression of the cord, with ischemia possibly being involved as well.

During childhood, patients with tethered cord may present with orthopedic, neurologic, urologic, or cutaneous abnormalities. Common initial findings include foot deformity, leg length inequality, lower limb atrophy, abnormal lower extremity reflexes, gait disturbance, delay in toilet training, enuresis, recurrent urinary tract infection, or a birthmark or hair patch in the lower back. The adult patient, however, typically presents with pain in the perineal region, diffuse pain over both legs, or, occasionally, shocklike sensations in the legs. Affected adults also may present with progressive leg weakness, walking difficulties, atrophy of one leg, progres-

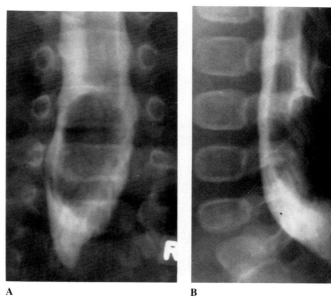

A   **B**

Fig. 2-31 Extramedullary epidermoid cyst. (**A**) Posteroanterior and (**B**) lateral radiographs of the lumbar spine with intrathecal contrast material demonstrate tethering of the spinal cord at the L5–S1 level. The spinal cord terminates in an irregular mass posteriorly. Spina bifida is present in the region of the mass.

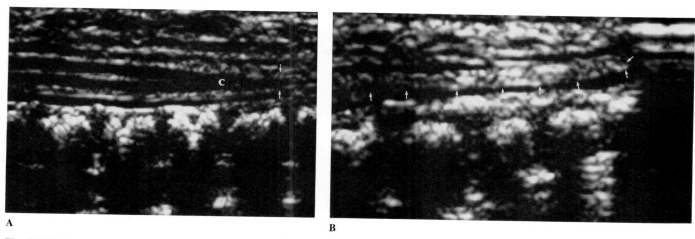

Fig. 2-32 Tethered cord syndrome. **(A)** Longitudinal sonogram of the lower lumbar region shows abnormal inferior extension of the spinal cord (c). The cord merges inferiorly with a thickened filum terminale (arrows). **(B)** An image at the level of the sacrum shows tethering of the caudal portion of the spinal cord to the short, thick filum (arrows). The filum becomes contiguous with the dorsal aspect of the dura inferiorly. A small dimple was visible at this point in the overlying skin.

sive scoliosis, or bladder or bowel dysfunction. Cutaneous stigmata of dysraphism are nearly always present in children with tethered cord, whereas these findings are present in less than 50% of patients who first present as adults. Some degree of spina bifida is nearly always present. The development of symptoms in adults is sometimes precipitated by trauma, stretching exercises, childbirth, or degenerative disease of the spine.[46–48]

Radiographs of the spine in patients with tethered cord syndrome can show various bony abnormalities that are associated with dysraphism. These findings range from a small focus of spina bifida to total absence of the neural arches at several contiguous levels. Scoliosis occurs in about 20% of cases. In infants and young children, these spinal abnormalities are often subtle and difficult to detect. Direct measurement of the interpedicular distances is sometimes helpful; a difference of 3 or 4 mm between consecutive lumbar vertebrae should raise the suspicion of intraspinal pathology.

In neonates and infants, before complete ossification of the posterior neural elements sonography can demonstrate the level of the conus medullaris and detect a number of intraspinal lesions (Fig. 2-32).[49] Myelography, CT, CT myelography, and MRI are also valuable for evaluating the intraspinal structures in infants and children. With a tethered cord, imaging studies show the conus medullaris to be located below the level of the L2–3 disc space. The conus may be tethered to the dura in the upper sacrum by a short filum, no demonstrable filum, or a thickened filum (greater than 2 mm in thickness). The filum is usually closely applied to the dura posteriorly (Fig. 2-33). A fibrolipoma is sometimes present; this is identified as a region of high signal intensity in the filum on T_1-weighted MR images.

The nerve roots normally exit the cord at an angle of 15° or less with respect to the long axis of the cord. In cases of a tethered cord, the nerve roots course more laterally than nor-

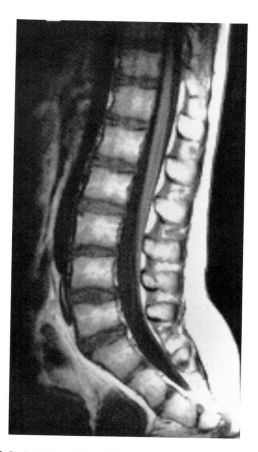

Fig. 2-33 Sagittal T_1-weighted MR image of an adolescent with urinary incontinence and fecal soiling showing the spinal cord to be tethered in the lower lumbar region. The filum terminale is slightly thickened and lies posteriorly. The thecal sac extends to the S-3 level. Note that the lumbar spinous processes are normal. This is an example of a tethered cord with only localized spina bifida of the lower sacrum.

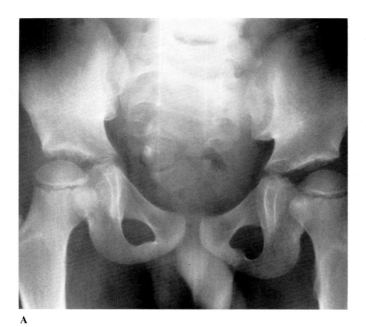

A

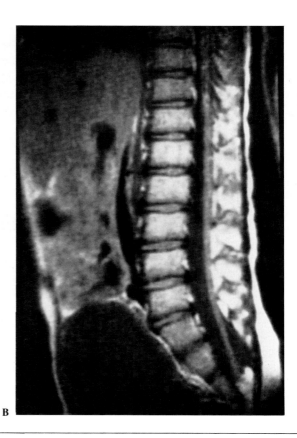

Fig. 2-34 Tethered cord syndrome. (**A**) Anteroposterior radiograph of the pelvis shows a cleft in the midline of the lower sacrum with hypoplasia of its left lateral aspect. (**B**) Sagittal T_1-weighted MR image shows the spinal cord to be tethered at the S-3 level. The spinal cord terminates in a small irregular area of high signal, representing a lipoma. A markedly distended neurogenic bladder is also seen.

B

mal and may actually ascend at an angle greater than 90° to reach the neural foramina. Dural ectasia often occurs in association with a low-lying conus. Imaging studies are valuable for defining the spinal anomalies that frequently are associated with tethering of the cord. These include intraspinal lipoma, myelomeningocele, myelocele, myelocystocele, and diastematomyelia (Fig. 2-34).[46,47]

Diastematomyelia

The word *diastematomyelia* is derived from the Greek words *diastema,* meaning ''cleft,'' and *myelos,* meaning ''spinal cord.'' Diastematomyelia is a congenital anomaly in which a portion of the spinal cord is divided sagittally into two segments. At the level of the defect, there are two frequently asymmetric hemicords. Each hemicord contains a central canal and a single dorsal and ventral horn that give rise to ipsilateral nerve roots. Each hemicord is surrounded by a layer of pia. Overlying bone or soft tissue anomalies are usually present.[50]

The length of the segment of split in the spinal cord in diastematomyelia is variable, usually ranging from two to four vertebral segments. Most often, the two hemicords reunite distally.[51] In 60% to 70% of cases there is a single dural sheath, and the cord is not split around a dividing fibrous or osteocartilaginous septum. If separate dural sheaths and subarachnoid spaces are present, a fibrous or osteocartilaginous

septum often splits the spinal canal and lies between the two hemicords.[52] The septum may be bony, cartilaginous, or fibrous. The spur, when ossified, is a diagnostic sign of diastematomyelia and represents the actual site of the split cord; this is visualized radiographically in about 20% of the cases. The spur is thought to develop from a separate ossification center and does not arise from the vertebral body.

Despite the division of the spinal cord, there are only two pairs of nerve roots in cases of diastematomyelia. Each pair consists of a motor and a sensory root on the lateral surface of the split cord. In contradistinction, in diplomyelia (or duplication of the spinal cord) there are four pairs of nerve roots. One pair is attached to the lateral and one pair to the medial surface of each hemicord. True diplomyelia is exceedingly rare.

Diastematomyelia can occur at any level but is most common from the lower thoracic spine to the sacrum. The upper thoracic and cervical regions are rarely involved.[52] Potential associated anomalies include thickening of the filum terminale, tethered cord, intradural lipoma, epidermoid or dermoid cyst, aberrant dorsal nerve roots that often tether the cord, and syringohydromyelia. Abnormal caudal extension of the conus medullaris occurs in more than 75% of cases. Diastematomyelia is usually associated with focal segmentation anomalies of the vertebral bodies, such as hemivertebrae, sagittal split vertebrae, or widening of the interpedicular distance.[53,54]

The clinical manifestations of diastematomyelia are similar to those of other types of occult spinal dysraphism. Girls are

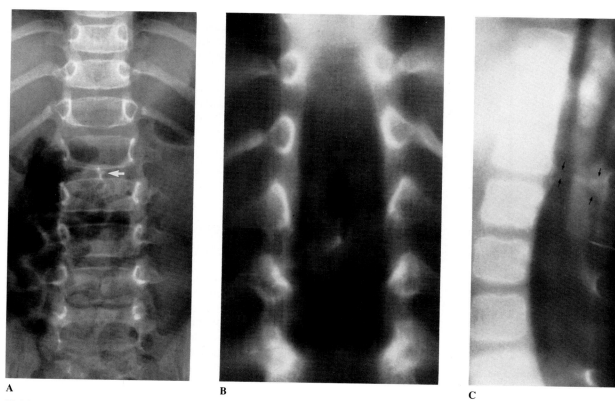

Fig. 2-35 Diastematomyelia. (**A**) Anteroposterior radiograph of the lumbar spine shows a crescentic spicule of bone (arrow) that projects at the L1–2 interspace. Note that the pedicles of the lumbar vertebrae are widely spaced and thinned. (**B**) Anteroposterior and (**C**) lateral linear tomograms obtained during air myelography show the spicule of bone to course from the posterior aspect of the interspace through the split in the spinal cord to end in the spinous process. The spinal cord terminates at the L-3 level. The subarachnoid space is enlarged.

more commonly affected than boys. Affected children may exhibit an abnormal gait, leg length discrepancy, dorsal midline cutaneous abnormalities (nevi, hypertrichosis, lipomas, skin dimples, or hemangiomas), unilateral or bilateral leg weakness, muscle atrophy, or urinary or fecal incontinence. On rare occasions, symptoms may not develop until adolescence or adulthood. The rare patient with diastematomyelia who presents as an adult often has experienced a secondary pathologic process, such as spondylosis or vascular disease, that leads to clinically significant findings in a previously asymptomatic patient. Diastematomyelia occurs in 5% of cases of congenital scoliosis and must be excluded in this clinical setting. Scoliosis, on the other hand, occurs in approximately 75% of patients with diastematomyelia and is more frequent when the anomaly involves the more cephalad portions of the spine.

The evaluation of diastematomyelia should begin with radiographs of the spine. Vertebral anomalies are present in virtually all cases. Although a bony spur is a valuable finding when present, it cannot be demonstrated in many cases of diastematomyelia. Other radiographic findings include spina bifida occulta, widening of the interpedicular distances, and segmentation anomalies (Fig. 2-35). In many cases, there is thickening and fusion of two or more laminae. Spina bifida in

association with fusion of one or more laminae in a diagonal direction with respect to the contralateral laminae (intersegmental laminar fusion) is a relatively specific finding for diastematomyelia. The neural arch at the level of the septum is usually completely ossified, and the spinous process is prominent. Anomalies of the vertebral bodies are commonly identified; these may include hemivertebrae, block vertebrae, butterfly vertebrae, and disc space narrowing. There may be a decrease in the anteroposterior diameters of the vertebral bodies adjacent to the intraspinal pathology.[55]

Myelography, CT, or MRI allows detection of the cord defect and, when present, the intervening septum (Fig. 2-36). These studies are also helpful for the detection of other associated anomalies, such as hydromyelia, tethered cord, or lipoma of the filum terminale.[56] CT provides valuable structural details concerning the size, shape, nature, and extent of the septum. CT is particularly useful in those cases in which inversion of the lamina indents or splits the cord.

With MRI, the morbid anatomy of diastematomyelia is best demonstrated in the coronal and axial projections. If there is severe scoliosis and kyphosis, coronal, oblique, and axial projections may be required. Hydromyelia is seen in about 50% of cases. Areas of high signal intensity on T_1-weighted images suggest the presence of a lipoma; this may be located at

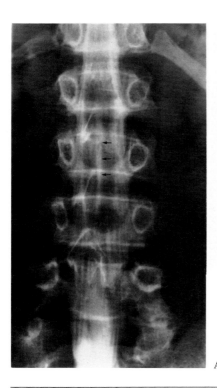

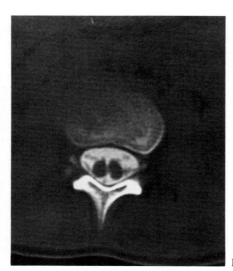

A

Fig. 2-36 Diastematomyelia without a tethering spicule. (**A**) Anteroposterior lumbar myelogram shows abnormal enlargement of the caudal end of the spinal cord. A collection of contrast material is seen extending longitudinally in the midline (arrows). No spinal anomalies are evident. (**B**) CT scan at the L-3 level shows two asymmetric hemicords, the left being larger than the right. A single set of dorsal and ventral nerve roots is seen exiting each hemicord.

B

the lesion, the conus, or the filum terminale.[57] MRI is relatively insensitive for identifying the fibrous or osteocartilaginous septum that sometimes is present. If there is a true bony spicule in the spinal canal, moderate signal from the fatty marrow in the spicule may be seen on MR scans (Fig. 2-37).[58]

Neurenteric Cyst

Neurenteric cyst is a congenital cystic lesion of developmental origin in which there is a connection of an extraspinal mass with the intraspinal structures through an anterior vertebral defect. The connection with the spinal canal may be in the form of a fibrous tract or a true fistula. The lesion may occur as a posterior mediastinal mass, an abdominal mass, or an intraspinal cyst. There are often associated anomalies of the spinal cord, such as a tethered cord or an intradural cyst containing gastrointestinal mucosa. In addition to the defect in the anterior surface of one or more adjacent vertebrae that is usually present in cases of neurenteric cyst, various other vertebral anomalies also may occur, such as scoliosis, hemivertebra, or spina bifida. These vertebral anomalies are usually located cephalad to the neurenteric cyst that is found in the cervical or thoracic regions.[59,60]

The precise mechanism or origin of a neurenteric cyst is unknown. One theory holds that the lesion is caused by incomplete or delayed closure of the primitive neurenteric canal (the canal of Kovalevsky), which is an evanescent communication between the notochord and the endoderm. An alternate hypothesis is that a neurenteric cyst is due to focal adherence of the endoderm of the yolk sac to the notochord. As

the notochord migrates dorsally during development of the spine, a diverticulum of endoderm is carried along. This endodermal tissue may give rise to a diverticulum, a cyst, or a duplication of the alimentary tract. This aberrant tissue also interferes with formation of the vertebral centrum to cause anterior vertebral clefts.

The clinical presentation of neurenteric cyst varies according to the size and location of the lesion and the nature of the intraspinal involvement. In many cases, an otherwise asymptomatic posterior mediastinal mass is identified on a chest radiograph. In some cases, a posterior mediastinal or abdominal neurenteric cyst produces symptoms that are due to effects on adjacent structures. Meningitis may occur if there is a fistulous communication with the intestinal tract. This is a common mode of presentation in the newborn period. Intraspinal extension can cause various neurologic symptoms, such as radicular pain or paraplegia. Some patients are, however, neurologically normal. Most neurenteric cysts are discovered in childhood. There is an increased incidence in boys.

On imaging studies, the characteristic feature of a neurenteric cyst is the association of anterior spina bifida with one or more of the following: a soft tissue mass in the posterior mediastinum, most commonly to the right of the midline; an abdominal mass due to a giant intestinal diverticulum or duplication; or an intraspinal cyst. The cervical and thoracic areas are the most frequent locations.

Radiographs in cases of a neurenteric cyst typically demonstrate a vertebral cleft (anterior spina bifida) or clustered segmentation anomalies. A paraspinal mass may be identified inferior to the vertebral anomalies. Scoliosis may be present. Rarely, the spine is radiographically normal.

When radiographs show vertebral anomalies in association with a paraspinal mass, evaluation of the intraspinal structures is essential. This may be achieved with myelography, CT myelography, or MRI. A spectrum of intraspinal abnormalities may be demonstrated in cases of neurenteric cyst. In

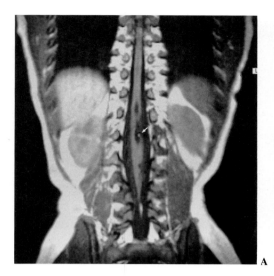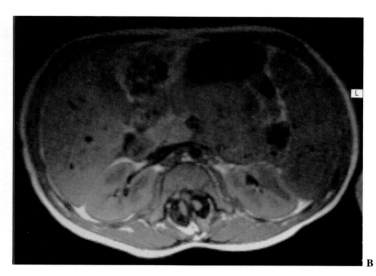

Fig. 2-37 Diastematomyelia with an intervening bony spicule. (**A**) Coronal T$_1$-weighted MR scan shows an area of hydromyelia in the midlumbar region. A focal area of high signal representing the marrow in the bony spicule is seen in the center of the spinal cord. The cortex produces a rim of low signal surrounding the marrow. Also note a linear area of bright signal in the filum terminale, which is due to a small lipoma. The spinal cord is tethered at L-4. (**B**) Axial T$_1$-weighted MR image at the level of the septum shows the bony spicule to extend obliquely from right to left. There is spina bifida. The two hemicords are asymmetric, with the right hemicord being slightly larger and somewhat flattened.

some cases the intraspinal structures are normal, or there is tenting of the dura at the site of a fibrous tract that extends through an anterior vertebral defect to communicate with a paraspinal neurenteric cyst. Alternatively, an intraspinal cyst may be present, either in association with a paraspinal mass or as an isolated lesion. The intraspinal cyst may occur in any location, but most are intradural extramedullary lesions. The intraspinal lesion may communicate with a paraspinal mass by either a fibrous tract or a fistula. The spinal cord is usually narrowed and displaced by the intraspinal mass (Fig. 2-38). Rarely, an intraspinal neurenteric cyst passes through the cleft of a diastematomyelia.

Split Notochord Syndrome

The split notochord syndrome refers to a spectrum of anomalies that is believed to be due to a splitting or deviation of the notochord during fetal development. This causes a cleft in the vertebral column in association with an enteric malformation.[61,62] The most severe form of this syndrome is a complete dorsal enteric fistula, in which there is a persistent communication between the gastrointestinal tract and the skin surface in the midline posteriorly. Any portion of a dorsal enteric fistula may become obliterated or persist, thereby resulting in an isolated diverticulum, duplication, cyst, fibrous cord, or sinus at any point along the tract of the fistula. The cysts that may occur in the split notochord syndrome can be enterogenic (ie, containing gastrointestinal mucosa) or neurenteric.

The embryogenesis of these anomalies is complex. As the notochord grows cephalad toward the prechordal plate, it must separate both from the dorsal ectoderm (the future skin) and from the ventral endoderm (the future intestinal tract). If there

is a point at which the ectoderm fails to separate, the notochord must either split or deviate around the adhesion. The mesoderm that normally envelopes the notochord to form the vertebrae is also displaced by the anomaly, causing a split or deviated spinal column. In some cases, there is a persistent connection between the dorsal surface of the gut and the skin surface in the midline of the back. With growth and variable degrees of migration, the adhesion may become quite long and connect structures that are segmentally related but topographically distant.[63] Because the notochord may split or deviate, the connection of the cysts to the vertebral bodies can be in the midline or in a paramedian location.

The clinical presentation of split notochord syndrome varies according to the character and severity of the anomaly. When a patent dorsal enteric fistula is present, the abnormality is usually clinically apparent at birth. Bowel contents may be noted to pass intermittently from the opening of the fistula. In some cases, there is a palpable dorsal cystic mass that may or may not have an opening through the skin. Enterogenic cysts in the mediastinum or abdomen may or may not produce symptoms. An intraspinal cyst produces neurologic symptoms, such as radicular pain or paralysis, if there is compression of the spinal cord or nerve roots.

Imaging studies in children with split notochord syndrome typically demonstrate vertebral anomalies of variable severity, such as anterior spina bifida, posterior spina bifida, hemivertebrae, segmentation anomalies, partial fusions, and scoliosis. Enlargement of the spinal canal may be identified at the site of an intraspinal cyst. MRI or CT myelography should be performed in these children to demonstrate cord involvement and the presence or absence of intraspinal or paraspinal cysts. On T$_1$-weighted MR scans, an intraspinal cyst may produce signal

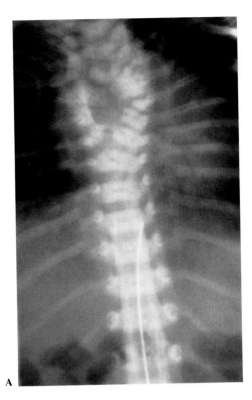

A

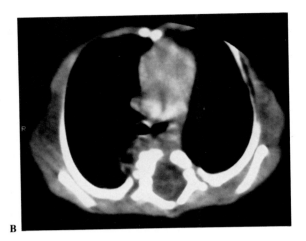

B

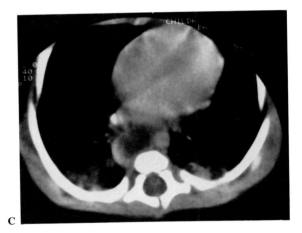

C

Fig. 2-38 Neurenteric cyst. **(A)** Anteroposterior radiograph of the thoracolumbar spine of a neonate who presented with meningitis shows numerous anomalous vertebrae in the midthoracic region and a central defect in the midportion. The spinal canal is widened from side to side. Contrast material is seen in the lumbar subarachnoid space. **(B)** Contrast-enhanced CT scan shows a defect in the vertebral centrum anteriorly. The spinal canal is filled with irregular high-attenuation material. Similar density is seen anterior and slightly to the right of the defect. **(C)** CT scan at a slightly lower level shows a mass in the right side of the mediastinum that is largely cystic. The mass lies to the right of the aorta and posterior to the pulmonary veins. **(D)** Sagittal T_2-weighted MR scan shows an irregular, high–signal intensity mass (arrows) that fills the anterior portion of the enlarged subarachnoid space. The spinal cord is displaced posteriorly. An area of high signal extends through the defect in the vertebral bodies to enter the right side of the mediastinum. This is typical of a neurenteric cyst. This cyst was lined with esophageal mucosa.

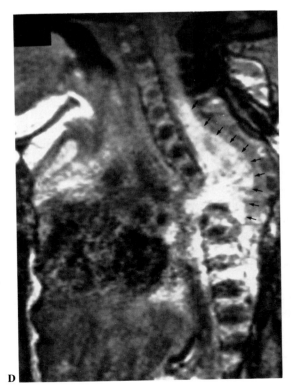

D

identical to that of cerebrospinal fluid or may have slightly greater signal intensity than that of cerebrospinal fluid, depending on the content of the lesion.

Caudal Regression Syndrome

Caudal regression syndrome refers to a spectrum of abnormalities that include fusion of the lower extremities (sirenomelia), absence of the caudal portion of the spine (lumbosacral agenesis), anal atresia, abnormal external genitalia, renal anomalies, and pulmonary hypoplasia.[64] About 16% of infants with caudal regression syndrome are offspring of diabetic mothers; this anomaly occurs in approximately 1% of the offspring of diabetic mothers.[65] Exposure during pregnancy to toxic organic solvents has been implicated in some cases. This anomaly is probably related to disturbed formation of the caudal cell mass of the tail bud, causing defective development of the caudal portions of the spinal cord, notochord, and spine. The prevalence of caudal regression syndrome is about 1 in 7500 births.[64,66]

The symptoms and clinical presentation of caudal regression syndrome vary greatly according to the severity of the anomaly. In those patients who have bony anomalies but no significant associated neurologic defects, the lesion may be clinically silent or may cause obstructed labor during childbirth. The spectrum of orthopedic abnormalities in children with caudal regression syndrome includes foot deformities, distal muscle weakness, hip dislocation, hypoplasia of the lower extremities, and fusion of the lower extremities. Most patients have a neurogenic bladder. Neurologic examination typically demonstrates more severe motor deficits than sensory losses. Sphincter dysfunction and lower extremity motor deficits are common. Meningocele or other forms of spina bifida occur in some cases. Anal atresia and severe genitourinary anomalies are frequently present in children with the more severe forms of caudal regression.

The radiographic appearance of the lumbosacral spine in children with caudal regression syndrome may be classified into four main types. Type 1 refers to partial unilateral sacral agenesis. In type 2, there are partial bilateral defects in the sacrum. The iliac bones articulate with the first sacral vertebra. The distal segments of the sacrum and coccyx are absent. Type 3 refers to total sacral agenesis. With this type, the iliac bones articulate with the lowest segment of the lumbar spine. Type 4, the most severe form of lumbosacral dysgenesis, has complete absence of the coccyx, sacrum, and one or more lumbar vertebrae. The iliac bones are fused posteriorly, and the lowest remaining vertebra rests above the iliac bones. Two or more of the caudalmost vertebral bodies are frequently fused (Fig. 2-39). Also, there is often narrowing of the dural sac inferior to the last intact vertebra.[67]

MRI or CT myelography is helpful in cases of caudal regression for accurately demonstrating the osseous abnormalities and for detecting abnormalities of the spinal cord and nerve roots. Evaluation of the level and shape of the conus will determine the presence of a tethered cord. Sagittal MR images show a characteristic blunt, wedge-shape appearance of the conus in those cases that are not tethered. The distal cord has a tapered appearance when the cord is tethered. A tethering lipoma or lipomyelomeningocele may be present. Axial CT or MR images need to be obtained immediately adjacent to the level of regression to demonstrate spinal stenosis or dural stenosis.

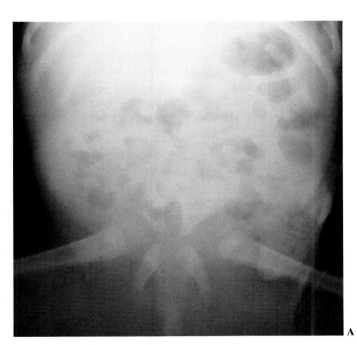

A

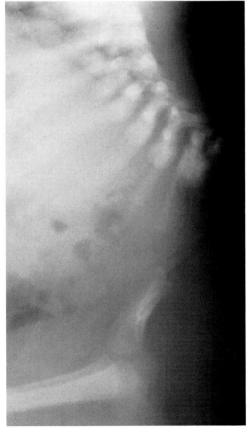

B

Fig. 2-39 Type 4 caudal regression. **(A)** Anteroposterior and **(B)** lateral radiographs of the abdomen of an infant of a diabetic mother show absence of nearly all the lumbar vertebrae and complete absence of the sacrum. The iliac bones are fused. The two most caudal vertebral bodies are fused.

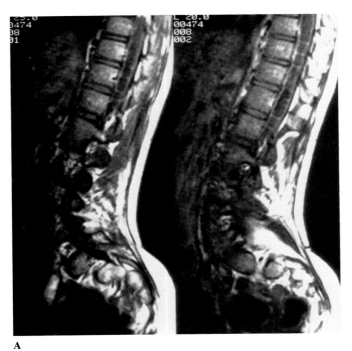
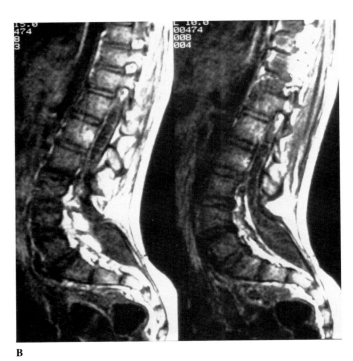

A   B

Fig. 2-40 (**A** and **B**) Parasagittal T_1-weighted MR images of the lumbar area showing extensive syringohydromyelia involving the entire spinal cord. The spinal cord is tethered and terminates at the S-4 level. The syringohydromyelia extends to the caudal end of the spinal cord. Note the areas of septation in the spinal cord, producing a beaded appearance. There is spina bifida extending from L-5 through the sacrum.

Syringohydromyelia

Syringohydromyelia refers to an abnormal fluid-filled cavity in the spinal cord. The term *hydromyelia* refers to dilatation of the central canal of the spinal cord, and *syringomyelia* refers to fluid-filled cavities in the substance of the cord that may or may not communicate with the central canal. Because both abnormalities often coexist, the term *syringohydromyelia* is customarily applied.

Syringohydromyelia is usually a congenital disorder in children, although acquired forms related to trauma, neoplasm, or infection also can occur. Congenital syringohydromyelia, often extensive, is relatively common in association with Chiari malformations. There are various theories as to the etiology of syringohydromyelia in these cases; most postulate chronic increased pressure in the central canal of the spinal cord. Hydromyelia, usually localized, occurs in about 50% of cases of diastematomyelia.

The clinical presentation of congenital syringohydromyelia usually begins in late childhood, adolescence, or early adulthood. The severity and progression of symptoms are quite variable. Common manifestations include segmental weakness and muscle atrophy of the hands and arms and loss of deep tendon reflexes. There may be loss of pain and temperature sense, with preservation of the sense of touch over the neck, shoulders, and arms. There is often significant pain in the affected extremities. The symptoms are often more severe in, or are confined to, the lower extremities. Unilateral symptoms may occur.[68,69]

Myelography or CT myelography in cases of syringohydromyelia demonstrates nonspecific enlargement of one or more portions of the spinal cord. MRI is the most useful diagnostic method for the evaluation of this abnormality. One or more cerebrospinal fluid–intensity fluid collections are identified in the spinal cord. These collections usually extend over a fairly long segment of the cord and cause a variable degree of enlargement of the cord. There may be septations in the cavity, producing a beaded appearance (Fig. 2-40). In some cases, the abnormality extends into the brainstem (syringobulbia).[70]

SPINAL DEFORMITIES

Spondylolysis

A bony defect in the pars interarticularis is termed spondylolysis. Spondylolysis may be unilateral or bilateral. This abnormality occurs in approximately 5% of the population. It may or may not be accompanied by significant symptoms. Bilateral defects in the pars interarticularis are often associated with subluxation of the involved vertebra (ie, spondylolisthesis).

Ninety percent of pars defects occur at L-5, 8% at L-4, and 1% to 2% at L-3. Occasionally, more than one vertebra is involved. Spondylolysis is unilateral in about 30% of cases. Two-thirds of adult patients with bilateral defects have some degree of spondylolisthesis. When present, partial sacralization of L-5 tends to stabilize the vertebra, making it less likely to develop spondylolisthesis.

The etiology of spondylolysis is somewhat speculative. Currently, the most popular theory is that spondylolysis is a type of fatigue fracture that fails to heal, occurring as a result of repeated minor trauma rather than a single acute traumatic event. The timing and precise mechanism of the fracture are uncertain. It is not known, for instance, whether flexion or extension injuries are most important; nor is it known at what age the defect appears in individual patients. Some have suggested that the pars interarticularis is subjected to increased stress during the toddler period, when the child begins to walk and is prone to many falls. It has been postulated that landing on the buttocks with the legs outstretched and the lumbar spine hyperextended may lead to this abnormality. The validity of this theory is contraindicated, however, by the fact that spondylolysis is seldom identified in children younger than 5 years of age. Rather, early cases of spondylolysis are most often seen between the ages of 5 and 7, which is coincidental with the age at which children begin school and are required to sit for prolonged periods with lordotic posture. This age period is also one of increased physical exertion during play and recess periods.[71]

The effect of stress cannot be considered without reference to the strength of the bone that it affects. The pars interarticularis in most individuals is a thick, bony strut; there are probably individuals, however, in whom the pars interarticularis is relatively hypoplastic and prone to fracture at any age. Inherent weakness of a pars as a result of hereditary factors may play a role in the pathogenesis. Some families have been shown to have a high incidence of spondylolysis. The pre-existing condition of the pars and the severity of stress are probably two equally important factors in the etiology.[72]

The radiographic evaluation of spondylolysis should include frontal, lateral, and oblique views. Stress-induced osseous changes in the pars interarticularis can occur as microfractures that cannot be detected on standard radiography during the early stages of disease. The earliest radiographic finding is sclerosis due to reactive bone formation; this is not visible in all cases, however. Continued microfractures result in bone fatigue, and eventually cortical bone fracture occurs. Spondylolysis is usually shown most clearly on oblique radiographs. With this projection, the pars defect is seen as a radiolucent band, often with sclerotic margins (Fig. 2-41). The radiolucent band often can be identified on lateral radiographs as well, where it is seen just caudal to the pedicle. The lateral radiograph is also important for demonstrating the presence or absence of spondylolisthesis that can occur with bilateral defects. A pars defect is often poorly visualized on frontal radiographs, although it is sometimes seen as a radiolucent band inferior to the pedicle. At times, an elongated but intact pars interarticularis occurs. This most often represents a healed stress fracture.

With a unilateral pars defect, sclerosis, thickening, and enlargement of the contralateral lamina and pedicle are fre-

quently observed. This is termed Wilkinson syndrome. These findings are probably produced by stress changes related to weakening of the posterior elements of the vertebra caused by the defect.[73]

Spondylolysis is demonstrated on axial CT scans as a defect in the pars interarticularis that has irregular, jagged margins. Occasionally, bilateral pars interarticularis defects are mistaken for facet joints on axial images. Pars defects are, however, located 10 to 15 mm above the intervertebral disc space, whereas the facet joints are located at or immediately adjacent to the disc space. Also, pars defects have irregular, jagged margins, whereas facet joints have smooth, corticated margins (Fig. 2-42). In some cases, callous or granulation tissue is identified adjacent to a pars defect. This can cause compression of the thecal sac or a nerve root, although this complication is more common in adults. With unilateral spondylolysis, sclerosis and hypertrophy are often demonstrated in the contralateral neural arch and pedicle.[72,74]

With MRI, spondylolysis is best shown on sagittal or oblique T_1-weighted images. As with CT, the defect also can be demonstrated on axial images. The most important function of MRI in cases of spondylolysis is to demonstrate encroachment on the thecal sac, nerve root compression, or coexistent

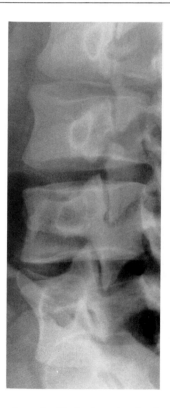

Fig. 2-41 Oblique radiograph of the lumbar spine showing a defect in the pars interarticularis between L-3 and L-4. The defect is broad and has sclerotic margins. There is also a defect in the pars interarticularis between L-2 and L-3. This defect is less broad but is well defined and has sclerotic margins. This is an example of spondylolysis at two levels.

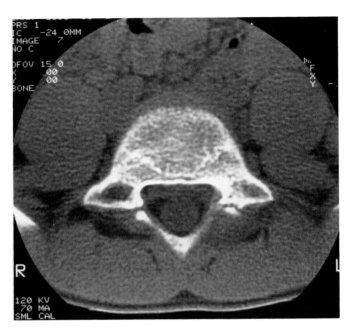

Fig. 2-42 Unenhanced CT scan of the L-5 vertebral body showing an irregular defect in the pars interarticularis on the left. There is a similar but somewhat more sclerotic defect on the right. There is minimal sclerosis of the left pedicle of L-5, arising as a stress phenomenon due to the defects.

disc disease. Spondylolysis is diagnosed on sagittal MR images by a loss of marrow signal in the pars interarticularis between the superior and inferior facets. If there is a wide space at the site of the spondylolysis, interposed epidermal fat may produce increased signal on T_1-weighted sequences.

The scintigraphic appearance of spondylolysis is somewhat variable. In most cases, delayed images from bone scintigraphy show mild to moderate increased uptake in the region of the pars defect. In some cases, however, bone scintigraphy is normal despite the presence of a radiographically demonstrable pars defect. This variable appearance is explained by the fact that scintigraphy does not demonstrate the defect itself but rather the sclerotic reactive changes that occur in response to the defect. In cases of unilateral pars defect, scintigraphy often shows increased uptake in the contralateral lamina and pedicle as a result of the stress changes (Wilkinson syndrome). This can be differentiated from the increased uptake that occurs as the result of an osteoid osteoma by observing that blood pool (tissue phase) images are normal with stress changes due to a pars defect but show intense uptake in the presence of an osteoid osteoma (Fig. 2-43).[75]

Spondylolisthesis

Spondylolisthesis means subluxation or slippage of one vertebra on another (Greek *spondylos*, "vertebra"; *olisthesis*, "slippage"; and *lysis*, "dissolution"). There are three major types of spondylolisthesis: dysplastic, spondylitic, and degenerative. In children, the degenerative type is rare.[76]

Dysplastic spondylolisthesis usually occurs at the level of L-5 and is due to an associated developmental abnormality. There is deficient development of the neural arch of L-5 and hypoplasia or dysplasia of the superior articular facets of S-1. This developmental abnormality results in structural weakness of the vertebra. The stress transmitted through the more supe-

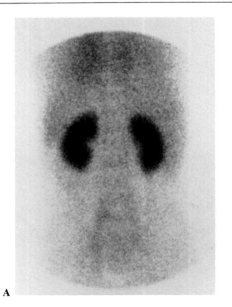

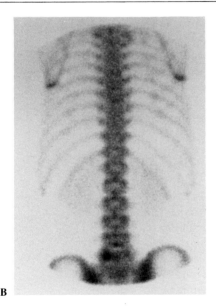

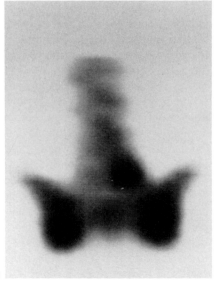

A   B   C

Fig. 2-43 Spondylolysis. **(A)** Blood pool image from bone scintigraphy of the lumbar spine is normal. **(B)** Posterior delayed image shows a focal intense area of tracer uptake on the left at L-5. **(C)** Coronal single photon emission computed tomography (SPECT) image shows the focal area of increased activity to lie in the posterior elements of L-5. In this patient, radiographs demonstrated a contralateral defect in the pars interarticularis. The increased uptake is a stress phenomenon due to the unilateral pars defect (Wilkinson syndrome). A normal blood pool image excludes an osteoid osteoma.

rior lumbar vertebrae gradually causes anterior and inferior displacement of L-5 over S-1. The spinous process of L-5 is carried forward and impinges on the first sacral neural arch, eventually causing an indentation. Unlike the spondylolisthesis that occurs with spondylolysis, the slippage that occurs in the dysplastic type is due to progressive elongation of the neural arch in the sagittal direction, predominantly involving the interarticular portion of the arch. The pars interarticularis becomes elongated and thinned and occasionally fractures. The dysplastic type of spondylolisthesis is most often identified in children or young adults and is twice as common in girls. Unilateral involvement is much less common than bilateral disease.

Spondylitic spondylolisthesis is the most common type of spondylolisthesis in all age groups. The peak age at diagnosis is, however, in young adults. The presence of bilateral pars interarticularis defects allows forward slippage of the vertebral body, the pedicles, transverse processes, and superior articular facets. The inferior facets remain in a normal position, articulating with the superior facets of the adjacent inferior vertebral body. In children spondylolytic spondylolisthesis is more common in boys.

The severity of spondylolisthesis is usually categorized according to the degree of displacement of the vertebral body relative to the anterior margin of the adjacent inferior vertebral body. Grade I spondylolisthesis indicates that one-third or less of the vertebral body is displaced anteriorly. Slippage of between one-third and two-thirds of the vertebral body width indicates a grade II slip. A grade III slip is present when two-thirds to the entire vertebral body is displaced anteriorly. Grade IV spondylolisthesis occurs when the entire vertebral body lies anterior to the more inferior vertebral body.

A well-positioned lateral radiograph allows accurate determination of the degree of spondylolisthesis (Figs. 2-44 and 2-45). Oblique radiographs demonstrate bilateral pars interarticularis defects or dysplastic elongation and thinning of the pars. In the presence of spondylolisthesis, oblique radiographs also may show widening of the facet joints. A clue to the presence of spondylolisthesis on frontal radiographs is isolated lateral deviation of the spinous process of the involved vertebra. Severe spondylolisthesis at L5-S1 produces the "upside-down Napoleon hat sign" on frontal radiographs as a result of superimposition of the L-5 vertebral body on S-1.[77,78]

Axial CT at the level of spondylolisthesis may show pseudoherniation of the disc, with disc material being visualized posterior to the L-5 vertebral body. A more inferior image, however, will show that the superior endplate of the next most inferior vertebral body correlates with the position of the disc material. Also, the epidural fat, thecal sac, and nerve roots show no evidence of compression in the absence of disc herniation. CT demonstrates unilateral or bilateral neural foraminal stenosis in about 25% of symptomatic patients with spondylitic spondylolisthesis. CT is also quite useful for demonstrating the elongation and narrowing of the pars interarticularis that occur with dysplastic spondylolisthesis.[74,79]

Sagittal MR images are well suited for demonstrating the severity of spondylolisthesis and for detecting untoward effects on the intraspinal structures. Although not present in most cases of spondylolisthesis, disc herniation is an impor-

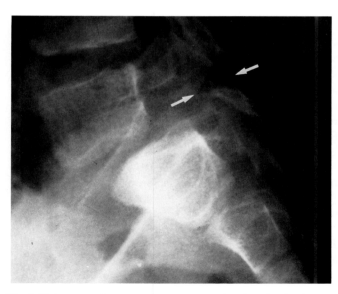

Fig. 2-44 Lateral radiograph of the lumbosacral junction showing forward offset of the body of L-5 on S-1. This is a grade I spondylolisthesis. The intervertebral disc is narrowed. Note that there are bilateral defects in the pars interarticularis between L-5 and S-1 (arrows).

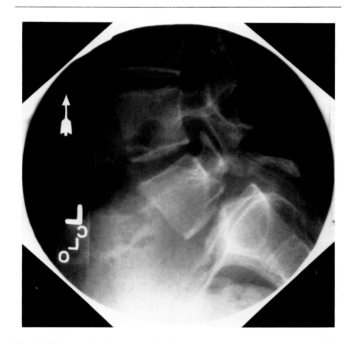

Fig. 2-45 Lateral radiograph of the lumbosacral region showing slight forward offset of the body of L-5 on S-1. This is a grade I spondylolisthesis. The intervertebral disc space is narrowed. Note that the partes interarticularis between L-5 and S-1 are elongated. The inferior facet joints are hypoplastic. This is an example of the dysplastic type of spondylolisthesis.

tant complication that is well demonstrated on MRI. Disc herniation is actually more likely to occur at the next most superior level. MRI is also well suited for depicting encroachment on the neural foramina.

Scoliosis

General Considerations

The term *scoliosis* means curvature and is the Anglicization of the Greek word *skoliosis*. Spinal scoliosis is usually a complex deformity that includes a lateral curvature and vertebral rotation often associated with kyphosis.

Both structural and nonstructural forms of scoliosis occur. Structural scoliosis is a fixed deformity that persists regardless of the position of the patient. Limitation and asymmetry of normal lateral bending occur with structural scoliosis, and there usually is a rotational deformity as well. Nonstructural scoliosis is a flexible deformity that can be made to vary with changes in body position. The curve with nonstructural scoliosis tends to be relatively mild and is most commonly located in the thoracolumbar or lumbar spine. Spinal motion is symmetric, and there is no significant rotational deformity with this type.[80]

There are two main types of nonstructural scoliosis: postural and compensatory. Postural scoliosis typically develops during the last half of the first decade of life. The spinal curvature is mild and disappears with recumbency or forward bending. Compensatory scoliosis occurs in response to pathologic tilt of the pelvis, leg length inequality, muscular spasm, or spinal deformity at another level. Nonstructural scoliosis often is not progressive.

Structural scoliosis is categorized into three major types according to etiology. Idiopathic scoliosis is the most common type. Neuropathic and myopathic scoliosis occur in association with myelomeningocele, syringohydromyelia, spinal cord tumors, neurofibromatosis, cerebral palsy, and poliomyelitis, and also in association with muscular diseases, such as muscular dystrophy and Werdnig-Hoffmann disease. Osteopathic scoliosis results from one or more specific structural abnormalities of the spine, such as congenital vertebral anomalies, traumatic compression, osteomyelitis, tumor, or skeletal dysplasia.[80]

Idiopathic Scoliosis. As stated above, idiopathic scoliosis is the most common type of structural scoliosis. This type occurs in the absence of any significant congenital spinal abnormality, musculoskeletal disease, or neurologic disease.[81] On the basis of age, idiopathic scoliosis is divided into three major groups: infantile (birth to 3 years of age), juvenile (4 to 9 years of age), and adolescent (10 years of age to the end of the period of skeletal growth). The etiologies, none of which has been conclusively proved, include imbalance in the proprioceptive system, peripheral neuropathy, myopathy, muscle imbalance, and metabolic abnormality.

Infantile idiopathic scoliosis is more common in Europe than in North America. There is a male preponderance. The curve patterns with this type of scoliosis tend to be specific. The thoracic curve is almost always convex to the left, and the lumbar curve is convex to the right. This is the opposite of the pattern that occurs with adolescent idiopathic scoliosis. Infantile idiopathic scoliosis resolves spontaneously in about 75% of cases.[82] The potential for spontaneous resolution is greatest in those infants with relatively mild curves, usually less than 30°. In those patients with progressive scoliosis, there is usually an increase in the spinal curvature of about 5° per year up to about 100°.[28]

Juvenile idiopathic scoliosis occurs in children between 4 and 9 years of age. The incidence is greater in girls. In boys, the peak incidence of this type of scoliosis is in the 4- to 6-year age range. Girls are most often affected between the ages of 7 and 9 years. A right thoracic curve is most common. In patients diagnosed before the age of 10 years, there is an 85% chance that the scoliosis will progress by 5° or more. The curve will progress by 10° or more in 75% of these patients. The risk of progression of 10° or more in scoliosis diagnosed at an older age is only 30%. In general, patients who have an initial curve that is greater than 30° or who are prepubertal are at a greater risk for curve progression.[83–85]

Adolescent idiopathic scoliosis is by far the most common form of scoliosis. In most cases, there is a right thoracic curve that extends from T-4, T-5, or T-6 to T-11, T-12, or L-1 (Fig. 2-46). A left thoracic curve is uncommon. This type is thought to be caused by disproportionate growth between the vertebral column and the intraspinal neural structures.[86] Those cases that occur at an earlier age and those that involve the more superior aspects of the spine tend to be more clinically apparent.

The reported incidence of adolescent idiopathic scoliosis varies somewhat because of differing criteria relating to the severity and pattern of the spinal curvature, the age at presentation, and other clinical features.[87] This type probably accounts for two-thirds or more of children with clinically significant scoliosis. The female-to-male ratio is approximately 10:1. The incidence of idiopathic scoliosis among first-degree relatives of affected patients is 15 to 20 times greater than that of the general population. There is some evidence that the hereditary factor is a sex-linked trait that has incomplete penetrance and variable expression.[88]

Although 20% to 25% of children with adolescent idiopathic scoliosis experience significant progression of the curve, the course of the disorder in individual patients is unpredictable. Mild curves between 15° and 20° may be unnoticed and, when detected, usually require no treatment. Progression of the deformity is usually most marked during the years of rapid skeletal growth. Nevertheless, about 70% of cases in which the curve is greater than 30° have progressive scoliosis after growth of the spine has ceased.[88]

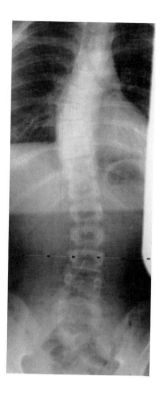

Fig. 2-46 Anteroposterior radiograph of the thoracolumbar spine of a 14-year-old girl showing an S-shaped scoliosis convex to the right in the mid-thoracic region and convex to the left at the thoracolumbar junction. This is typical of the idiopathic scoliosis of adolescence.

Osteopathic Scoliosis. Congenital scoliosis refers to scoliosis that is present from birth. Most cases are due to developmental abnormalities of the spine and, therefore, represent types of osteopathic scoliosis. Developmental vertebral abnormalities that often lead to scoliosis include failure of formation (hemivertebra or wedge vertebra), failure of segmentation (intervertebral bars, block vertebrae, and the like), and dysraphism (abnormal bone or neural development).[89] In approximately 15% of patients with congenital scoliosis, there is a coexistent intraspinal lesion; the most common of these is diastematomyelia.[90] Scoliosis is present in about 80% of patients with diastematomyelia.[91]

Congenital scoliosis is most commonly located in the thoracic spine. In most cases, there is a progressive increase in the curvature with increasing age.[92] Progression of the deformity is most marked in the thoracic and thoracolumbar regions. The most rapid progression of the curvature typically occurs during the preadolescent growth spurt. This progression continues as long as growth continues. During childhood and adolescence, about 15% of patients with congenital scoliosis have no progression; 50% have moderate progression of between 10° and 30°, and 35% demonstrate severe progression of greater than 30°.[92] The severity of progression of congenital scoliosis

increases with the degree of curvature and the number of abnormal vertebrae in the curve. On average, the curve in patients with congenital scoliosis progresses at about 5° per year.[80]

Of the various congenital anomalies that cause scoliosis, a unilateral bar is the most serious. This anomaly is due to unilateral failure of segmentation. The bar may involve two or more adjacent vertebrae.[89] The vertebral bodies, the posterior elements, or both may be involved. The presence of a bar typically is associated with progressive scoliosis because of a lack of growth ipsilateral to the lesion and normal or exaggerated growth on the contralateral side.

Another congenital abnormality that leads to pronounced scoliosis is multiple contiguous hemivertebrae on the same side of the spine. A solitary hemivertebra usually produces mild to moderate deformity, but there are occasional instances in which severe angular scoliosis occurs. Growth of the hemivertebra causes the spine to lengthen excessively on the convex side. In addition, the angular deformity produces pressure on the concave side that retards the rate of growth of the epiphyseal plate on that side, thereby contributing to the progression of the scoliosis.

Approximately 18% of patients with congenital scoliosis (excluding those with myelomeningocele) have coexisting urologic abnormalities. The most common of these include unilateral renal agenesis, renal duplication, renal ectopia, and obstructive uropathy.[93] The incidence of scoliosis among patients with congenital heart disease is between 3.3% and 19%, compared to an incidence of between 0.03% and 6% in the general population. More than a third of these patients are older than 13 years of age. Scoliosis is three times more common among patients with cyanotic compared to non-cyanotic heart disease.[94]

Neuropathic and Myopathic Scoliosis. Scoliosis frequently complicates neuromuscular and muscular disorders such as myelomeningocele, muscular dystrophy, syringomyelia, spinal cord tumor, neurofibromatosis, cerebral palsy, Friedreich ataxia, and poliomyelitis. These are termed neuropathic and myopathic scolioses. In the absence of associated vertebral anomalies, the mechanism of scoliosis in these disorders is generally attributed to asymmetric muscular action or imbalance, with the stronger muscles being on the concave side of the curve. This produces a C-shaped curve rather than the S shape seen in most cases of idiopathic scoliosis (Fig. 2-47).

Scoliosis occurs in about 15% of children with neurofibromatosis. In the absence of specific vertebral anomalies, the scoliosis is thought to be due to a congenital mesodermal defect. Right thoracic curves predominate in neurofibromatosis, although there is an increased incidence of left thoracic curves in neurofibromatosis compared to idiopathic scoliosis. In some cases there is a short, sharply angular curve, usually in the lower thoracic region. Other dystrophic spinal changes that may occur with neurofibromatosis include apical

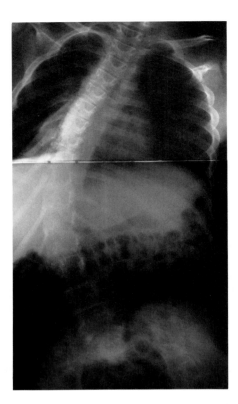

Fig. 2-47 Anteroposterior radiograph of the thoracolumbar spine of a young man with muscular dystrophy showing a single C-shaped scoliosis of the thoracolumbar spine that is convex to the right. This single scoliotic curve is typical of scoliosis that complicates neuromuscular and muscular disorders. Also note atelectasis of the right lower lobe, which is due to compression of the bronchus by the scoliotic deformity.

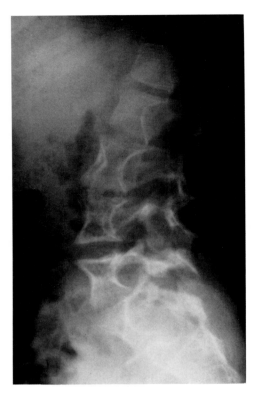

Fig. 2-48 Lateral radiograph of the lumbar spine of an adolescent with neurofibromatosis showing extensive scalloping of the posterior aspects of all the lumbar vertebrae. In addition, there is scalloping of the anterior aspects of L-3, L-4, and L-5. Note the enlargement of the neural foramina. The sagittal diameter of the spinal canal is also enlarged. The posterior scalloping that occurs in neurofibromatosis reflects dural ectasia in most cases.

wedging and rotation, vertebral scalloping (both anterior and posterior), foraminal enlargement, and spindling of the transverse processes and pedicles (Fig. 2-48).[95] Skeletal dysplasias that are sometimes associated with significant scoliosis include spondyloepiphyseal dysplasia congenita, diastrophic dysplasia, and chondrodystrophic calcificans congenita.

Scoliosis frequently occurs in patients with syringomyelia, with reported incidences being up to 80%. In some patients, the spinal curvature is due to asymmetric weakness of the trunk muscles or imbalance of muscular tone. In others, the scoliosis does not appear to correlate with the neurologic deficit. In a third group of patients, the development of scoliosis precedes the onset of neurologic symptoms. The mechanism of the spinal deformity in these latter two groups remains unclear.

There is considerable variation in the pattern of scoliosis that occurs in patients with syringomyelia. Most often there is a double curve, with the thoracic deformity usually being the more severe. These curves usually remain relatively mild and seldom require surgical correction. Forcible straightening of the spine in patients with untreated scoliosis due to syringomyelia may cause hemorrhage in the spinal cord.

Pathologic Mechanisms of Scoliosis

The various types of scolioses, whether idiopathic or due to an underlying disorder, cause similar structural alterations in the spine that progress during growth and usually stabilize when growth is complete.[96] These alterations are due to continued adaptation of the spine to the deformity during the growth period. There are changes in enchondral bone formation, appositional bone growth, and bone resorption. These changes are most pronounced during the preadolescent growth spurt.

Scoliosis causes a persistent and increasing stress on the concave side of the curve. With time, the chondrocyte columns along the concave aspect become compressed, leading to diminished enchondral bone formation in this location. On the convex side of the curve, the bone is under decreased stress, resulting in increased chondrogenesis and bone formation. These two factors—suppressed growth on the concave aspect and increased growth on the convex side—eventually lead to lateral vertebral body wedging.

With progressive lateral wedging deformity, the periosteum along the concave side is drawn away from the vertebral body, creating stress on the underlying Sharpey fibers. As the stress progresses, there is increased vascularity and osteoblastic activity, leading to cortical thickening at this location. Along the convex side, the periosteum of the bone is stretched and often avulsed. This avulsion is associated with resorption of the cortical bone along the convex aspect of the involved vertebral bodies. The intervertebral disc is also compressed along the concave aspect and distracted on the convex side. The disc is eventually forced to migrate in the direction of the convexity of the curve.

Lateral curvature in one area of the spine is almost always accompanied by a compensatory curve or curves in the opposite direction. The result of the compensatory curve is positioning of the head vertical to the middle of the sacrum. The area of the vertebral column in which the structural curvature has occurred forms the primary curve and is the diseased area that needs to be corrected. There may be a single primary curve with a compensatory curve or double primary curves. A long C curve or a collapsing spine is associated with paralytic diseases.

Measurement of Scoliosis

The two methods most often used for measuring the degree of scoliosis (and kyphosis) are the Cobb method and the Ferguson method. With the Cobb method, a line is drawn parallel to the superior surface of the most cephalad vertebra of the scoliotic curve. This is the vertebra whose superior surface demonstrates the greatest slant toward the concavity of the curve. A second line is drawn parallel to the inferior surface of the most caudal vertebra in the curve. This is the vertebra whose inferior surface slants maximally toward the concavity of the curve. Lines are then drawn perpendicular to both these lines. The angle formed at the intersection of these perpendicular lines is the angle or degree of scoliotic curvature. All the intervertebral disc spaces in this measured curve should exhibit widening on the convex side of the curve.[97]

In the Ferguson method, the apex of the curvature is defined as the vertebra that exhibits the greatest amount of rotation. The center of this vertebral body is found by the intersection of lines that connect the superior corner of one side of the vertebra with the inferior corner of the opposite side. If the vertebra has become wedge shaped, the wedge is altered to the shape of a rectangle to aid in identifying the center. The proximal and distal vertebrae to be measured are those that demonstrate the least amount of rotation, that is to say those that have the spinous process near or at the midline. The center of these vertebrae is determined in the same fashion as for the vertebra at the apex. Lines are then drawn to connect the centers of the end vertebrae with the center of the vertebra at the apex of the curve. The angle of the curvature is the divergence of these lines from 180°.[98,99]

The Cobb method magnifies the degree of curvature as the curve progresses. In addition, there is a better percentage of correction with the Cobb method after surgery than with the Ferguson method.[100] The Cobb method cannot be used reli-ably to measure curves that are less than 50°.[64] The Ferguson method is more accurate and is a more direct method of measuring the curve because it does not rely on the angle of the surface of the last vertebra of the curve. The Ferguson method is more difficult to use with curves that are greater than 50°.

Vertebral body rotation cannot be measured accurately. Nevertheless, an estimate can be made by measuring the degree of displacement of the spinous process from the midline or by evaluating the displacement and configuration of the pedicles of the involved vertebral body.[101] The pedicle method consists of measuring the degree of displacement of the pedicle on the convex border of the vertebral body as it moves toward the concave aspect of the vertebra. This is calculated as the percentage of the lateral dimension of the vertebral body. The pedicle method is easier to perform with various degrees of rotation because the pedicles are less distorted than the spinous process. The values obtained by the spinous process method of measurement often underestimate the degree of rotation compared to the pedicle method.

Kyphosis

Kyphosis refers to abnormally increased convexity in the curvature of the spine as viewed from the side. A kyphotic curve of the thoracic spine that measures greater than 15° by the Cobb method is considered clinically significant.[101] The lumbar curve is normally lordotic, so that any loss of the lordosis is considered a relative kyphosis. Both congenital and acquired forms of kyphosis occur. The most commonly affected area is the thoracolumbar region. As with scoliosis, the degree of kyphosis progresses most rapidly during the preadolescent growth spurt.

Congenital kyphosis is the result of a developmental abnormality of the vertebrae, such as an anterior or posterior hemivertebra or an anterior bar. All patients with an anterior unsegmented bar will develop progressive kyphosis. These patients also often have associated congenital abnormalities, most commonly involving the genitourinary system.

Of the acquired forms of kyphosis, adolescent or juvenile kyphosis, also known as Scheuermann disease, is the most common. Scheuermann disease, or round-back deformity, is reported in 5% of otherwise healthy adolescents. It must be differentiated from postural kyphosis. In Scheuermann disease, the cartilage of the vertebral growth plate is abnormal, leading to weakening of the vertebral endplate and subsequent formation of Schmorl nodes, which protrude into the vertebral body. The growth and ossification of the vertebra are impaired in these locations, leading to anterior wedging and subsequent kyphosis. These abnormalities are most frequently seen in the thoracic spine at the T6–10 levels.

Kyphosis also may occur in association with neuromuscular diseases, skeletal dysplasias, trauma, inflammatory diseases, the arthritides, and tumors. Kyphosis is common in patients with Marfan syndrome. In children with neurofibromatosis, kyphosis occurs less commonly than scoliosis but, when present, is often severe.

VERTEBRAL ABNORMALITIES WITH SKELETAL DYSPLASIAS, METABOLIC DISORDERS, AND SYSTEMIC DISEASES

Achondroplasia

The defective enchondral bone formation of achondroplasia affects all bones that are preformed in cartilage, particularly at those sites that normally have the most active growth. Although the changes of achondroplasia are most marked in the extremities, spinal involvement is an important aspect of this disorder. Clinically a lumbar gibbus is common in infancy, but after the first year of life this almost always disappears and is replaced by a straight middle and upper back with a prominent lumbar lordosis. Older patients may develop neurologic abnormalities as a result of spinal stenosis in the cervical or lumbar areas.[102]

In normal individuals, the vertebrae grow in all directions. This growth is most pronounced in the lumbar spine. The normal lumbar vertebrae gradually increase in size from L-1 to L-5. Because the effects of the cartilage defect in achondroplasia are accentuated at sites of greater growth, the failure of enchondral bone formation is most pronounced in the lumbar spine, particularly at L-5. This causes the spinal canal to taper from L-1 to L-5. The smaller size of the vertebral bodies causes the interpedicular distances to become progressively narrowed.[103] Likewise, there is inadequate longitudinal growth of the pedicles, so that they achieve only approximately half their normal length.[104] Premature fusion between the pedicles and the ossification centers of the vertebral body further contributes to blunted growth of the pedicles. These features, combined with the narrow interpedicular distances, result in spinal stenosis that is usually most severe in the lumbosacral region.

Radiographs of infants and young children with achondroplasia show wedge-shaped or hypoplastic vertebral bodies, these being most marked in the thoracolumbar and upper lumbar regions. The vertebrae are often bullet shaped during infancy. There is slight concavity of the posterior surfaces of the vertebral bodies (posterior scalloping) that becomes more pronounced as adult life is reached. This posterior vertebral scalloping is caused by pulsations of the thecal sac in the narrow spinal canal. The vertebral bodies appear small and cuboid shaped when viewed in the lateral projection. Frequently, there is irregularity of the anterior margins of the T-12 and L-1 vertebral bodies.

A mild kyphosis may develop at the thoracolumbar junction before the infant begins to stand. This kyphosis is thought to be due to muscle hypotonia; the deformity resolves once the child begins to walk and muscular strength improves.[105] Angular kyphosis in older children with achondroplasia is usually associated with hypoplasia of the anterior portion of a vertebral body, usually at the upper lumbar level. Kyphosis occurs in about one-third to one-half of cases of achondroplasia and is severe in about one-third. In addition there is exaggeration of lumbar lordosis, with an increase in this deformity as the child begins to walk. This is noted in approximately 70% of patients with achondroplasia (Fig. 2-49).[102]

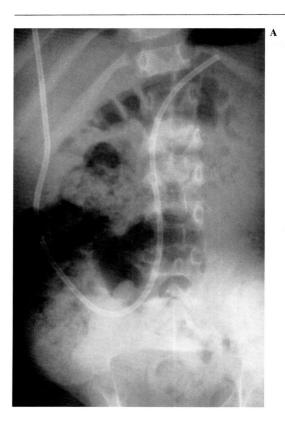
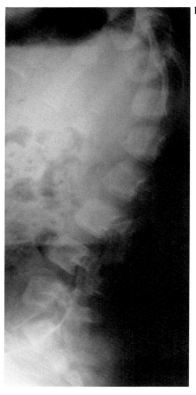

Fig. 2-49 Achondroplasia. (**A**) Anteroposterior and (**B**) lateral radiographs of the lumbar spine of a toddler with achondroplasia show an exaggerated thoracolumbar kyphosis and increased lumbar lordosis. The vertebral bodies are small and cuboid in configuration. The pedicles are foreshortened, and there is posterior scalloping of the vertebral bodies. The interpedicular distances narrow from superior to inferior. A diversionary shunt catheter is in place for treatment of hydrocephalus, a common complication of achondroplasia.

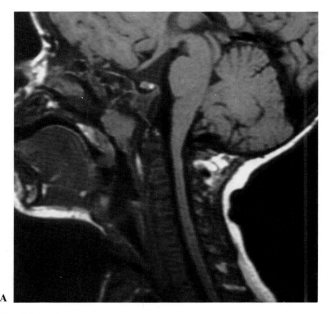

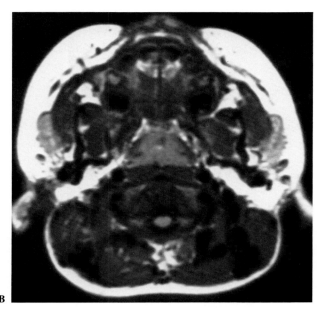

Fig. 2-50 Achondroplasia. (**A**) Sagittal and (**B**) axial T_1-weighted MR scans of the craniocervical junction show compression of the medulla at the small foramen magnum. The cranial base is also foreshortened. Stenosis of other cranial foramina, especially the jugular foramen, is common in achondroplasia.

As described above, spinal stenosis is common in achondroplasia. When it occurs at the craniocervical junction, it is most often due to a small and misshapen foramen magnum, which causes compression of the medulla and upper cervical spinal cord (Fig. 2-50). Significant spinal stenosis also can occur in the lumbosacral region. In this location, radiographs show the spinal canal to be narrowed in both dimensions as a result of the diminished interpedicular distance and the shortening of the pedicles.[106]

Symptoms of lumbosacral spinal stenosis usually become most evident in adult patients; symptoms are uncommon before the age of 15 years. In adults, bulging of the annulus fibrosus, protrusion of disc material, osteophyte formation, progressive lumbar lordosis, and thoracolumbar kyphosis all contribute to the development of neurologic symptoms because there is compromise of an already narrowed spinal canal. The intervertebral discs are somewhat hyperplastic, and multiple protruding discs are common. Nearly half the patients with achondroplasia develop clinically significant spinal complications at some time during their lives.

A number of parameters have been identified that are helpful in predicting which patients with achondroplasia are at particular risk for developing severe neurologic symptoms as adults. These parameters include accentuated thoracolumbar kyphosis, prominent lumbar lordosis, and an interpedicular distance less than 20 mm at L-1 and less than 16 mm at L-5.[107]

Mucopolysaccharidoses

The mucopolysaccharidoses are a group of inherited disorders caused by enzyme deficiencies that result in incomplete degradation of acid mucopolysaccharides (glycosaminoglycans). The clinical manifestations of these disorders are due to accumulation of these mucopolysaccharides in various organs. Because the mucopolysaccharides are major components of the intercellular substance of connective tissues, bony changes are characteristic of these disorders. The skeletal deformities produce a radiographic pattern that is termed dysostosis multiplex. Significant spinal abnormalities occur in several of the mucopolysaccharidoses.

Radiographs of the spine in patients with Hurler syndrome, the prototype example of dysostosis multiplex, show ovoidshaped vertebral bodies in the lower thoracic and upper lumbar regions. The heights of the vertebral bodies are normal or slightly increased. Beaklike projections develop on the anteroinferior vertebral body margins. This is usually most marked at the second lumbar vertebra (Fig. 2-51). The beaklike deformity is probably caused by anteroinferior herniation of disc tissue, which prevents normal ossification of the vertebral margin.[108] The deformity causes a gibbus at the thoracolumbar junction that usually develops after the first year of life.

The interpedicular distances are normal in Hurler syndrome. There may be posterior scalloping of the vertebral bodies as a result of dural ectasia produced by connective tissue abnormalities or osseous dysplasia.[109] In addition, dural thickening resulting from infiltration with mucopolysaccharides is common.

Patients with Hunter syndrome have similar, but less marked, radiographic changes compared to those with Hurler syndrome. They usually do not have a thoracolumbar gibbus deformity, although most have a mild kyphosis. The radiographic features of Sanfilippo syndrome are somewhat variable but usually are similar to those of Hurler and Hunter syndromes.

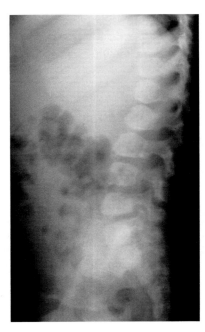

Fig. 2-51 Lateral radiograph of the lumbar spine of an infant with Hurler syndrome showing ovoid vertebral bodies. There is inferior beaking at the L-1 and L-2 levels.

The spinal manifestations of Morquio syndrome are distinct from those of the other varieties of mucopolysaccharidoses. In early childhood, the vertebrae show mild flattening (platyspondyly) and are oval in shape. There is defective ossification of the anterior portions of the thoracolumbar and upper lumbar vertebrae that produces inferior beaking. In older children with Morquio syndrome, the thoracic vertebral bodies exhibit slow growth in height. There is a central tongue (central beak) that protrudes anteriorly from the oval-shaped thoracic and lumbar vertebrae except at the thoracolumbar junction, where inferior beaking persists. Irregularity of the vertebral endplates is also usually present. As the child grows the intervertebral discs become widened, and platyspondyly becomes more pronounced. Platyspondyly is a helpful finding in the differentiation of Morquio syndrome from the other mucopolysaccharidoses. The odontoid process is mildly hypoplastic in early childhood and is severely hypoplastic or absent in older children.[110] The hypoplasia of the odontoid process results in atlantoaxial instability of variable severity.

Diastrophic Dysplasia

Diastrophic dysplasia is a rare autosomal recessive abnormality that produces short stature, micromelia, clubfoot deformity, and a characteristic abducted and proximally positioned thumb (hitchhiker thumb). Scoliosis and lumbar lordosis are commonly noted in these patients and usually develop at around 8 to 10 years of age. Kyphosis in the cervical region is common; if it is severe, there may be significant cord

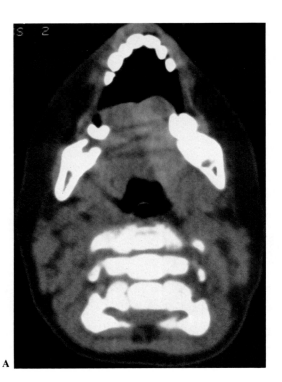

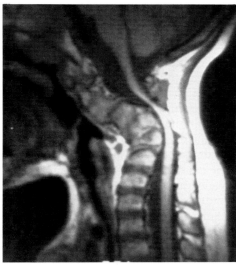

Fig. 2-52 Dystrophic dysplasia. (**A**) Unenhanced CT scan of the upper cervical spine shows occult spina bifida. In addition, the diameter of the cervical canal is markedly narrowed in the sagittal plane but is broadened from side to side. (**B**) Sagittal T_1-weighted MR image shows a marked kyphosis in the midcervical region that compresses the spinal cord at the apex of the kyphosis. A cervical kyphosis is common in diastrophic dysplasia.

compression. In most cases, there are no significant underlying vertebral abnormalities. The vertebral bodies are usually of normal height and width. The pedicles are normal or show slight shortening. Spina bifida occulta is commonly present, usually involving the lower cervical spine. This ranges from a small cleft in the spinous process to a large defect in the vertebral arch (Fig. 2-52).

Spondyloepiphyseal Dysplasia

Spondyloepiphyseal dysplasia congenita is a hereditary bone dysplasia that occurs in two forms. The more severe congenital form is seen primarily in infants. The milder tarda form occurs primarily in adolescents. Spondyloepiphyseal dysplasia tarda may be detected during childhood because of truncal shortness.

Radiographically, there is universal platyspondyly. The vertebral bodies are flattened but increased in their anteroposterior diameter. The intervertebral disc spaces are increased in height. There is a mild epiphyseal dysplasia with small irregular epiphyses. The growth plates tend to fuse prematurely. This disorder leads to premature osteoarthritis in young adults (Fig. 2-53).

Down Syndrome (Trisomy 21)

Radiographs of children with Down syndrome (trisomy 21) frequently show some degree of increase in height of the vertebral bodies. The lumbar vertebrae may be somewhat narrow in their anteroposterior diameters. Posterior scalloping and accentuated anterior vertebral concavity are common. The pedicles may be elongated.[111]

A

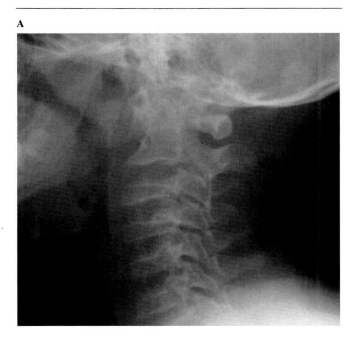

Fig. 2-53 Spondyloepiphyseal dysplasia tarda. (**A**) Lateral radiograph of the cervical spine shows severe platyspondyly. The vertebral bodies are increased in their anteroposterior diameter, and the intervertebral disc spaces are widened. Note the hypoplasia of the odontoid process. (**B**) Anteroposterior and (**C**) lateral radiographs of the lumbar spine show severe platyspondyly. The endplates are slightly irregular. The vertebral bodies are increased in their sagittal and transverse diameters. (**D**) Posteroanterior radiograph of the right hand shows premature closure of the growth plates of the phalanges and metacarpals. There is mild distortion of the epiphyses and metaphyses as a result of the epiphyseal dysplasia that occurs in spondyloepiphyseal dysplasia tarda.

B **C** **D**

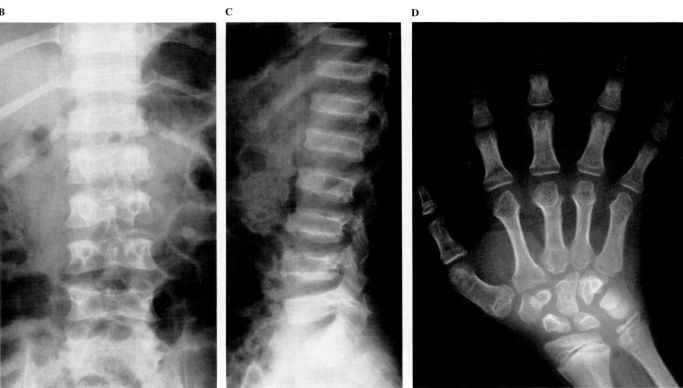

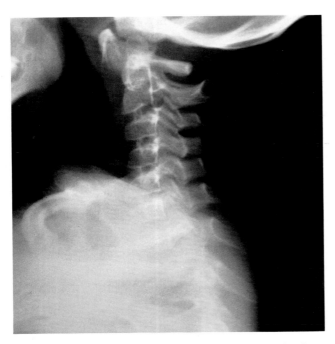

Fig. 2-54 Lateral radiograph of the cervical spine with flexion showing anterior displacement of the arch of C-1 with respect to the odontoid. This atlantoaxial instability is due to the abnormalities of the transverse ligament that occur in trisomy 21.

Abnormalities of the odontoid process that can occur in Down syndrome include os odontoideum, ossiculum terminale, and dysplasia or hypoplasia of the odontoid. One or more of these abnormalities is present in approximately 6% of children with Down syndrome.[112] These children also have abnormalities of the transverse ligament resulting from laxity, malformation, or aplasia. The abnormalities of the odontoid process and of the transverse ligament place children with Down syndrome at increased risk for atlantoaxial subluxation, which occurs in 10% to 30% of patients with this disorder (Fig. 2-54).[113]

Osteogenesis Imperfecta

Osteogenesis imperfecta is classified into autosomal recessive, potentially lethal congenital forms, and autosomal dominant tarda forms. Although the age of onset and severity differ with these two forms, the clinical features of both include short-limbed dwarfism, ligamentous laxity, blue sclerae, increased fragility of the bones, discoloration of the teeth, and thin skin. There is failure of normal periosteal and endosteal bone formation that leads to osteopenia and frequent fractures. Spinal involvement consists of vertebral body collapse with concave endplates (Fig. 2-55). Scoliosis and kyphosis are often present. There is scalloping of the dorsal aspects of the vertebral bodies.

Rickets

The radiologic manifestations of rickets in the spine of children are similar to those associated with osteomalacia in adults. There is loss of the secondary trabeculae as well as generalized osteopenia. The vertebral bodies demonstrate biconcavity and widened disc spaces. In severe cases of rickets, there may be platyspondyly and anterior beaking. After therapy, the density and height of the vertebrae may be restored. Scoliosis often develops in older children with rickets. In severe cases, basilar invagination has been reported.[114]

Juvenile Rheumatoid Arthritis

Involvement of the cervical spine is relatively common in children with juvenile rheumatoid arthritis. An early radiographic abnormality is limitation of motion on flexion and extension views. Atlantoaxial subluxation and subluxation at other levels (especially C-2 through C-4) are common. In

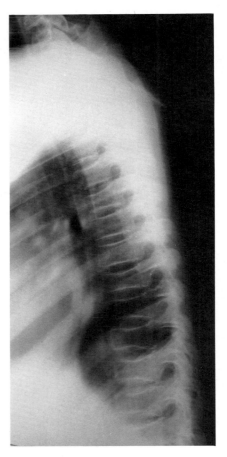

Fig. 2-55 Lateral radiograph of the thoracic spine showing numerous compression fractures. The vertebral bodies appear mildly osteoporotic. Note a biconcave appearance of the endplates of several of these vertebral bodies. This appearance is common in osteogenesis imperfecta tarda.

children, a separation between the anterior arch of C-1 and the base of the odontoid of greater than 5 mm on a lateral radiograph indicates subluxation. Frequently, there are later manifestations of inflammatory changes in the apophyseal joints, such as joint space narrowing and erosions. Apophyseal ankylosis in the upper half of the cervical spine is fairly common in longstanding juvenile rheumatoid arthritis. Fusion of the apophyseal joints results in diminished growth of the vertebral bodies, which become narrow in their anteroposterior diameter and decreased in height. There is also a decrease in height of the intervertebral discs in the involved segment of the spine (Fig. 2-56). Significant abnormalities of the thoracic or lumbar portions of the spine are infrequent. Vertebral collapse related to generalized skeletal demineralization, especially as a complication of steroid therapy, can occur in any portion of the spine.[115]

Anemias

Spinal changes are common with chronic anemias. Sickle cell disease and thalassemia produce significant hyperplasia of the marrow in the spine. Spinal abnormalities in children with sickle cell disease and the mixed hemoglobinopathies also can be produced by ischemia and infarction.

Hyperplastic marrow in chronic anemias causes diminution in the size and number of the horizontal trabeculae in the vertebrae. This produces the radiographic appearance of osteopenia. Forces transmitted through the demineralized vertebrae cause reactive new bone formation in the vertical trabeculae, radiographically producing a coarsened pattern. These findings are usually most prominent in cases of thalassemia, but they also occur to some extent in children with sickle cell disease.[116]

The demineralization that occurs with marrow hyperplasia in the vertebrae results in a propensity for vertebral compression fractures. This may produce flattening of multiple vertebrae, usually in the lumbar and lower thoracic regions. Depression of the weakened vertebral body endplates by disc material frequently produces concave compressions. These smooth, concave compression deformities are distinct from the H-shaped central cupping deformities that result from vertebral endplate ischemia.

Radiographs frequently demonstrate widening of the anterior vertebral vascular channels in children with sickle cell disease, thalassemia, and other severe chronic anemias. These vascular channels are normally visible in young children but are frequently enlarged or persist abnormally into late childhood and adulthood in these patients.

A unique central cupping deformity of the vertebra occurs in 40% to 50% of patients with sickle cell disease, in lesser numbers of patients with sickle cell–thalassemia and sickle cell–hemoglobin C disease, and rarely in patients with thalassemia. This abnormality is thought to be due to localized inhibition of bone growth in the central portions of the vertebra as a result of recurrent episodes of red cell sickling in the

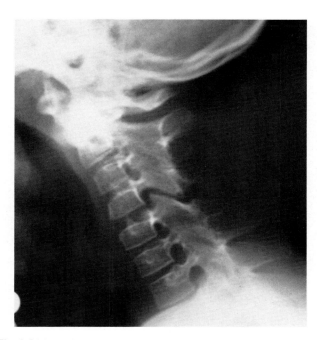

Fig. 2-56 Lateral radiograph of the cervical spine showing a slight forward positioning of the arch of the atlas with respect to the odontoid. In this patient, the forward positioning increased further with flexion. There is ankylosis of the apophyseal joints from C2–5 and from C-5 through C-7. There is diminished growth of the vertebral bodies in the upper cervical and midcervical regions. These findings are common in longstanding juvenile rheumatoid arthritis.

nutrient vessels that supply the central portions of the vertebral endplates. Normal growth of the peripheral aspects of the endplates results in the progressive central cupping deformity, or H-shaped vertebrae. When this finding is present, multiple vertebral bodies are usually involved (Fig. 2-57).[117]

TRAUMA

Cervical Spine Trauma

Radiographic Signs of Injury

Major spinal injuries are much less common in infants and children than in adolescents and adults. Less than 5% of all cervical spine injuries occur in children, despite the fact that the mechanical features of a young child's spine make it more susceptible to injury during rapid deceleration. Cervical spine injuries in infants tend to involve the more superior aspects because the pivot point of cervical spine motion C2–3 is high in this age group. Significant neurologic deficits may occur with spinal injury in children in the absence of an overt fracture because the developing spine has more elasticity than the spinal cord, which is fixed by the nerve roots. Most injuries are of the flexion type; these are followed in frequency by hyperextension and rotation injuries.

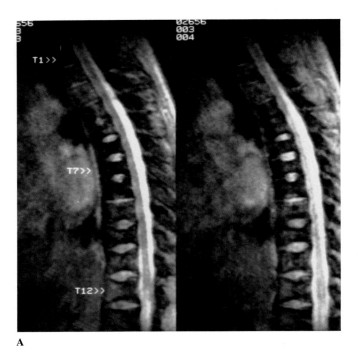
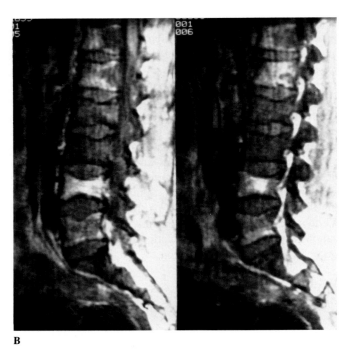

A   B

Fig. 2-57 Sickle cell disease. Sagittal T_2-weighted MR images of (**A**) the thoracic spine and (**B**) the lumbar spine in this adolescent show scattered areas of very low signal in many vertebral bodies and bright signal in others. The low signal may be due to hemosiderin deposits or vertebral sclerosis from prior bone infarction. The areas of bright signal correspond to edema of the marrow spaces. Note also the central cupping deformity of the T-7 and T-8 vertebral bodies. There are biconcave compressions of many of the lumbar vertebrae.

The paramount role of radiology in cases of spinal injury is to determine whether a fracture is present and whether or not the injury is stable. A systematic evaluation, especially of the cervical spine, is essential. The lateral view is the most informative projection and should be subjected to a number of assessments before a frontal view is obtained. In general, it is most useful to view the entire curvature of the included portions of the spine and then to assess specific structures. Specifically, attention should be directed to the prevertebral soft tissues, predental space, odontoid process, vertebral bodies, disc spaces, apophyseal joints, neural arches, and spinous processes. The included portion of the skull also should be inspected for fractures or other abnormalities.[118–120]

The cervical spine assumes a lordotic curve in the neutral position, as is seen on the lateral radiograph, and is straight on the frontal view. Any deviation from this appearance usually reflects muscle spasm or injury of the osseous or ligamentous structures. Spasm usually straightens the spine, as is seen on the lateral view, and can lead to an element of anterior kyphotic angulation of C-2 on C-3. Localized kyphosis at other levels usually indicates ligamentous injury due to hyperflexion. Muscle spasm may produce scoliosis on the frontal view.

Prevertebral soft tissue widening is a nonspecific but important finding in cervical spine injuries.[121,122] It can be due to edema or hemorrhage. Prevertebral soft tissue widening does not occur with all cervical injuries, however, and is frequently absent with minimal compression fractures or with un-

displaced fractures of the dens. There is wide variability in the thickness of the normal prevertebral space among children and in the same child with changes in position of the neck. Nevertheless, an overall rule can be applied: Below the level of the glottis, the width of the normal soft tissue in the prevertebral space is less than twice the anteroposterior diameter of the adjacent vertebral body. This measurement can serve as a standard, regardless of patient age.

The most frequent cause of a misdiagnosis of thickening of the prevertebral soft tissues is lack of adequate extension of the spine. Pathologic prevertebral soft tissue thickening usually produces anterior displacement and indentation of the airway. When there is questionable soft tissue thickening along the lower cervical spine, it may be useful to evaluate the prevertebral fat stripe for anterior displacement. Displacement of this fat stripe is presumptive evidence of vertebral injury. The prevertebral fat stripe, however, is not always identifiable in infants and young children. Therefore, visualization of the stripe in a normal or displaced position is useful, but absence of the stripe is not diagnostic of injury.

An increase in the size of the predental space (from the anterior arch of C-1 to the dens) is suggestive of ligamentous or osseous injuries in this region. As with the prevertebral soft tissue space, however, normal variation occurs, and the variation is more pronounced in infants and children. In adults a distance of greater than 2.5 mm is usually considered abnormal, but in children distances of 4 to 5 mm are seen normally.[123] It should be understood that the predental space often changes somewhat with extension and flexion of the neck. Variations of up to 2 mm can occur. Consequently, the radiographic evaluation of the predental space must take into account the normal variations that occur in children.

Abnormal alignment of the vertebral bodies as viewed on lateral radiographs may cause diagnostic difficulty. Most often, displacement of one vertebral body on another is a significant finding and indicates an underlying instability. Most of these cases involve anterior displacement of a vertebral body with respect to the next most inferior vertebra. This is usually due to a flexion injury, but on occasion it will occur with rotary or extension injuries.

Anterior vertebral body displacement in the upper cervical spine of children must be viewed cautiously because normal physiologic displacement is common. Physiologic displacement may involve the upper four vertebral bodies or C-2 on C-3 only. In cases in which multiple vertebral bodies are involved, the findings are clearly physiologic; when isolated anterior displacement of C-2 on C-3 occurs, however, interpretation may be troublesome. Swischuk[124] developed the posterior cervical (spinolaminar) measurement as a method for differentiating physiologic from pathologic subluxation of C-2 on C-3. A line is drawn from the anterior aspect of the cortex of the spinous process of C-1 to the same point on C-3. One assesses the relationship of this line to the anterior cortex of the spinous process of C-2 (Fig. 2-58). If the line misses the anterior cortex of the C-2 spinous process by 2 mm or more, a true dislocation should be present. This finding is most often associated with a hangman fracture. There are occasional cases in which the posterior cervical line falls within the normal range despite the presence of significant ligamentous injury and instability of C-2 and C-3. A normal posterior cervical line excludes a hangman fracture but does not absolutely rule out ligamentous injury.[125]

It is important that the posterior cervical line be applied only when the lateral radiograph actually shows anterior displacement of C-2 on C-3. With the spine in neutral position, the posterior cervical line misses the posterior arch of C-2 by 2 mm or more in the normal patient. This is because the position of the posterior arch of C-2 normally lies posterior to the arches of C-3 and C-1. It is only when C-2 appears to be displaced forward on C-3 that a distance of 2 mm or more becomes significant.[124]

Posterior displacement of one cervical vertebral body on another is uncommon but can occur during the acute phase of an extension injury. Such displacement, however, is usually transient because neutral positioning of the neck or hyperflexion during a whiplash injury tends to re-establish normal alignment. Lateral vertebral body displacement is usually associated with a fracture dislocation.

Alterations in height of one or more disc spaces occasionally occur with trauma. Disc space narrowing or widening is best appreciated on lateral radiographs. In normal patients, the cervical intervertebral disc spaces are of equal height. Any discrepancy raises the possibility of a longitudinal ligament injury and suggests that instability is probably present. Disc

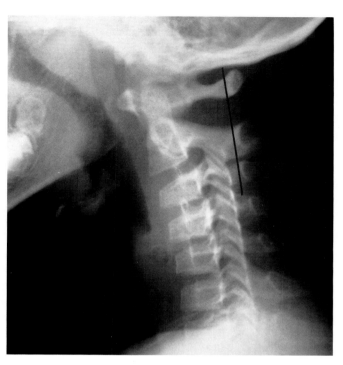

Fig. 2-58 Lateral radiograph of the cervical spine in a young child who was involved in a motor vehicle accident. The radiograph was obtained in the cross-table lateral projection. There is slight forward offset of the body of C-2 on C-3. The spinolaminar line is normal, however, indicating that this offset is physiologic and not due to a pathologic subluxation.

space narrowing can occur with flexion and rotation injuries, but widening of a disc space almost always indicates that an extension injury has occurred.

Abnormalities of the apophyseal joints may be detected on a lateral radiograph of the cervical spine. If there is an abrupt discrepancy in the alignment of the apophyseal joints at any one level, a rotary subluxation with a locked facet is usually the etiology. Apophyseal joint dislocation is almost always due to a flexion injury. In these cases, the joints, in addition to being anteriorly dislocated, may appear unduly widened or narrowed.

Widening of the joints of Luschka is another uncommon abnormal finding in cases of cervical spine trauma. On frontal radiographs obtained with lateral bending, the contralateral joints of Luschka normally uniformly increase in width. A prominent widening at one or two levels raises the possibility of a significant ligamentous injury.

Disruption of the posterior spinal ligaments with hyperflexion injuries produces an increase in the interspinous distance. This may be identified on both lateral and frontal radiographs and indicates an unstable injury. It is important to recognize, however, that the distance between the spinous tips of C-1 and C-2 often appears somewhat widened in normal individuals.[126]

Lateral deviation of the spinous process is best identified on the frontal view. The deviation may be due to a vertebral arch fracture or a unilateral locked facet. When a unilateral locked facet is present, the spinous process above the locked facet is displaced toward the side of locking.

Location of Injuries

Spinal injuries are uncommon in infants and children. About 50% of spinal injuries in children involve the cervical spine, and more than one-third occur at multiple levels. Trauma to the cervical spine may produce isolated or complex fractures of the vertebral arch and the vertebral bodies or even more complex fracture-dislocations. Cervical spine injuries in older children and adolescents are more common in the lower (C-3 through C-7) than the upper portions. In infants, there is a predilection for injury to the upper portions of the cervical spine.[120,127] The vertebral bodies are the most common site of cervical spine injury in children. Most occur in the lower three cervical vertebrae, with more than half occurring at the C-6 and C-7 levels.

Fractures of the vertebral arch are uncommon in children. Most occur in the articular pillars, especially at the C-6 level.[128] Fractures of the articular pillars are often difficult to diagnose radiographically, and CT is especially helpful in these cases. These injuries should be suspected whenever there is significant prevertebral soft tissue swelling.

Fractures of elements of the vertebral arch other than the pillars are less common. Most fractures of the laminae occur at the C-5 and C-6 levels, and most fractures of the spinous processes occur at the C-6 and C-7 levels.[128] Most fractures of the pedicles occur at the C-2 level. Fractures of the transverse processes are rare and difficult to identify. They usually involve the C-7 level and at this level are commonly associated with injuries of the brachial plexus.

Burst (Jefferson) and focal arch fractures are the most common fractures of C-1. A C-1 Jefferson fracture is not common in childhood. Fractures of the atlas constitute about 5% of all cervical spine fractures. Both flexion and extension injuries can produce fractures at the base of the dens; fractures of the dens account for 5% to 10% of cervical spine fractures. The upper cervical spine also can be involved with atlantoaxial dislocation or atlanto-occipital dislocation. Children who sustain upper cervical spine trauma frequently have associated severe head trauma.

Fracture-dislocations are serious injuries that may be caused by severe hyperextension or hyperflexion trauma, usually in motor vehicle accidents or falls. Fractures of the face or mandible correlate with extension injuries.[129] Neurologic signs and symptoms of cord compression often develop but may be absent initially with some traumatic lesions.[130] It must be emphasized that approximately one-third of patients with cervical spinal cord injury have clinical signs of injury between the C-6 and T-1 levels, areas that are difficult to evaluate with conventional radiography.[131]

Mechanisms and Types of Cervical Injuries

Injuries to the cervical spine range from minimal ligamentous injury to complete fracture-dislocation with or without spinal cord injury. There are five major mechanisms responsible for cervical spine injuries: flexion, extension, lateral flexion, rotation, and axial compression. In some cases, more than one of these mechanisms is involved in the pathogenesis of the injury.

With flexion, the vertebra is subjected to compressive forces anteriorly and distraction forces posteriorly. This type of injury often results in anterior vertebral body compression, usually with a corner (tear-drop) fracture. Most often, the fracture involves the anteroinferior corner of the vertebral body (Fig. 2-59). These fractures are thought to result from buckling of the anterior longitudinal ligament during hyperflexion. In addition, accompanying ligamentous injury can lead to disc disruption and disc space narrowing. In young children, the equivalent of a tear-drop fracture consists of displacement of a fragment of the vertebral ring epiphysis. The identification of a corner fracture indicates that a hyperflexion injury has occurred and should stimulate a more careful search for possible associated traumatic lesions.[132,133]

Prevertebral soft tissue swelling can occur with flexion injuries, but it is not invariably present. This finding is not usually present with minimal anterior compression fractures; with more severe injuries, especially in the presence of a tear-drop fracture, soft tissue swelling becomes prominent

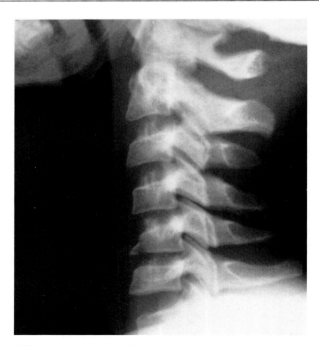

Fig. 2-59 Lateral radiograph of the cervical spine of a child who sustained a flexion injury in a motor vehicle accident. Note a tear-drop fracture at the inferior aspect of C-5. This is the most common fracture that occurs with flexion injuries of the cervical vertebrae. Also note the increased density of the C-6 vertebral body, which is due to compression fracture of C-6. There is widening of the C6–7 interspace.

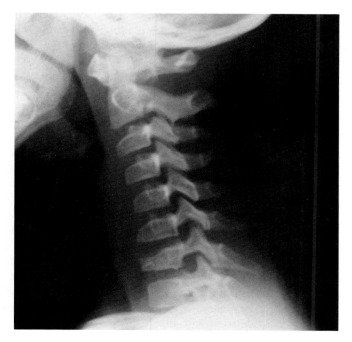

Fig. 2-60 Lateral radiograph of the cervical spine of a young child who sustained a flexion injury in a motor vehicle accident showing a compression fracture of the C-7 vertebral body. There is increased density throughout the vertebral body because of compression of the bony trabeculae. There is loss in height anteriorly. Note also the prevertebral soft tissue swelling.

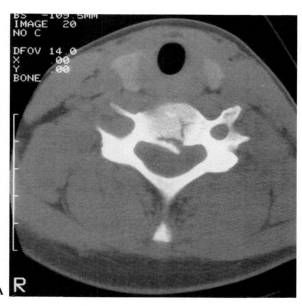

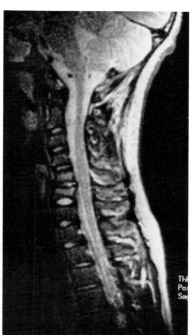

Fig. 2-61 Trauma. (**A**) Unenhanced CT scan of a 12-year-old boy who sustained a flexion injury of the neck reveals a comminuted fracture of the C-6 vertebral body. A small fragment of bone has been retropulsed and abuts the anterior surface of the spinal cord. This patient also had a tear-drop fracture of the inferior surface of the C-5 vertebral body. (**B**) Sagittal T$_2$-weighted MR scan shows a portion of the superior aspect of the C-6 vertebral body to be retropulsed and to lie against the anterior surface of the spinal cord. The signal emanating from the spinal cord is normal. Note the increased signal in the C-5 and C-6 vertebral bodies; this is due to edema of the marrow spaces.

(Fig. 2-60). In injuries in which significant vertebral body compression occurs, a vertical fracture is usually present. On the lateral radiograph, a portion of the compressed vertebral body is displaced posteriorly. CT and MRI show this injury more precisely and are particularly helpful for detecting intraspinal encroachment of fracture components (Fig. 2-61).[134]

The posterior distraction forces associated with hyperflexion injury may lead to ligamentous disruption at the apophyseal joints and between the neural arches and the spinous processes. Involvement of the apophyseal joints may be indicated by either widening or narrowing of the involved segment and variable degrees of anterior subluxation. Dis-

placement of more than 3 mm and anterior angulation of more than 15° are considered abnormal. Ligamentous injury also can result in separation of the spinous processes and widening of the interspinous distance. Occasionally, an avulsion fracture of the posterior elements is identified.

Atlanto-occipital dislocation is a rare and usually fatal flexion injury. It is most often caused by severe motor vehicle accidents. Death is usually produced by transection of the medulla and upper spinal cord; some patients survive this injury, however, and may even present without neurologic impairment.[135] This lesion is more common among children than adults,[136] probably because of the relatively large size of the head of a child with respect to the spine. Radiographically, atlanto-occipital alignment is best evaluated by utilizing the ratio of the distance between the basion and the posterior arch of C-1 to the distance between the anterior arch of the atlas and the opisthion.[137] A ratio greater than 1 as seen on the lateral radiograph indicates anterior dislocation of the occiput on the atlas. This ratio is not affected by patient age. It may not aid in the detection of longitudinal atlanto-occipital dislocation,[135] however, or of the less common posterior type of atlanto-occipital dislocation.[137]

Flexion injuries of the atlas and axis most commonly result in fractures of the base of the dens with anterior displacement of the odontoid process. Widening of the predental space is present if there is an associated atlantoaxial dislocation. In infants and young children, fractures of the base of the dens usually occur through the synchondrosis. This synchondrosis remains open until the latter part of childhood, and the normal radiolucency produced by this structure should not be misinterpreted as a fracture. Slight posterior tilting of the dens is a normal finding; anterior tilting is always abnormal and is usually the result of a significant injury. A nondisplaced fracture of the dens may not be detectable radiographically in infants and young children. The clinical findings include pain and loss of normal motion. Within a few weeks, resorption of bone at the synchondrosis occurs, causing it to appear widened and irregular. In some cases, a fracture of the dens results in eventual resorption of the majority of the bone. This may be followed by compensatory overgrowth of the normal ossiculum terminale, producing the so-called acquired os odontoideum.

Pathologic widening of the predental space occurs with disruption of the transverse ligament that bridges C-1 and the dens. Traumatic disruption of the transverse ligament is uncommon, however, even with fractures of the dens. This is due to the fact that the dens and C-1 tend to move as a unit, so that severe stress usually is not applied to the transverse ligament. In fact, atlantoaxial instability in conditions such as rheumatoid arthritis, Down syndrome, or hypoplasia of the dens is a more common cause of widening of the predental space than traumatic disruption of the transverse ligament. Those patients who have a pre-existing abnormality in this region are prone to atlantoaxial movement and dislocation without fracture. In addition to transverse ligament disruption there are other injuries, such as rotary subluxation of C-1 on C-2 and Jefferson fractures of C-1, that may produce widening of the predental space.

Extension injuries subject the vertebrae to compressive forces posteriorly and distracting forces anteriorly. Vertebral body fractures are not common with this mechanism of injury, but fractures of the articular facets, pillars, and posterior elements occur. Vertebral body fracture with extension injury usually occurs as an avulsion tear-drop fracture. As with the flexion tear-drop fracture, this finding indicates significant ligamentous injury and instability. As opposed to the flexion tear-drop fracture, however, in which there is infraction of the anteroinferior portion of the vertebral body, the extension tear-drop fracture most often involves the anterosuperior corner of the vertebral body. The disc space is usually widened. This fracture results from an avulsive force transmitted through the anterior longitudinal ligament during hyperextension. Prevertebral soft tissue thickening usually accompanies an extension tear-drop fracture.

Hyperextension injuries also can cause various fractures of the posterior components of the vertebrae. When these fractures are unilateral and not associated with any other injuries, the spine is usually stable. Significant instability frequently accompanies bilateral fractures, however, or fractures through the neural arch or pedicles. This injury is termed a hangman fracture when it occurs at C-2 (Fig. 2-62). In many cases, extension injuries of the posterior elements can be difficult to detect radiographically, and supplemental imaging with CT is required.

Extension injuries are among the most common causes of fractures of the posterior arch of C-1, fractures of the dens, and the classic hangman fracture of C-2. Fractures of the posterior arch of C-1 can be bilateral or unilateral. They can be isolated or occur in association with other fractures of C-1 or C-2. These fractures are usually identified as thin radiolucent defects through the posterior arch of C-1 (Fig. 2-63). They must be differentiated from congenital defects of the arch, which are seen as broad defects that may be associated with triangular tapered or irregularly shaped ossifications in the posterior arch of C-1. Occasionally, an extension injury can produce a transverse fracture through the anterior arch of C-1. These fractures are often occult radiographically but are readily demonstrated on CT.

Fractures of the dens caused by extension injuries are usually associated with a variable degree of posterior angulation or displacement. With the hangman fracture of C-2, initial hyperextension causes bilateral fractures through the neural arch or pedicles (or both). With subsequent return to the neutral position or with flexion from whiplash, motion through the fracture site and disc space produces anterior displacement of the body of C-2, the dens, and all of C-1. In some cases the fracture is clearly visible, whereas in others the findings are subtle. Use of the posterior cervical line, as described earlier, may be helpful in some cases.

Lateral flexion injuries of the cervical spine can produce vertebral compression injuries, fractures of the transverse or uncinate processes, and contralateral avulsion of the brachial plexus. Lateral flexion injuries can cause unilateral widening of the joints of Luschka. If such widening is seen at every level, it is probably physiologic. If, however, there is marked disparity at one or two levels, an underlying ligamentous injury is likely. In the upper cervical spine, lateral flexion injury can produce fractures of the dens.[138]

Rotation injuries of the cervical spine usually occur in association with either flexion or extension injuries, most frequently the former. In the lower cervical spine, flexion-rotation injuries result in a unilateral locked facet. Extension-rotation injuries produce fractures of the articular facets, pillars, and posterior elements.

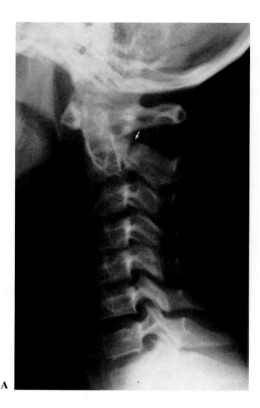

A

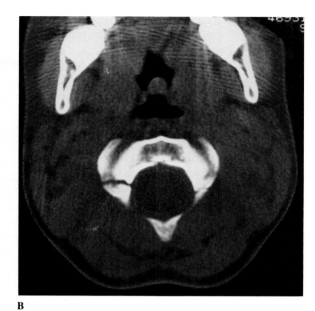

B

Fig. 2-62 Hangman fracture. (**A**) Lateral radiograph of the cervical spine of a young child who had a hyperextension injury shows bilateral fractures of the pedicles of C-2 (arrow). The posterior elements are displaced inferiorly with respect to the body. (**B**) CT confirms transverse fractures of the pedicles of C-2.

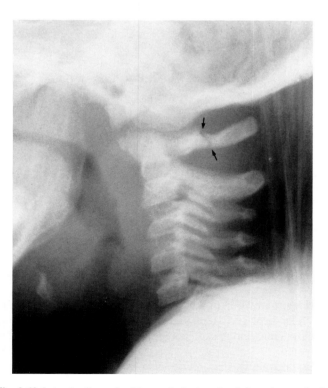

Fig. 2-63 Lateral radiograph of the cervical spine of an infant who sustained an extension injury of the cervical spine showing a fracture of the posterior arch of C-1 (arrows). This is seen as a thin radiolucent line through the lamina of C-1.

Unilateral locked facet can be identified on lateral radiographs as anterior displacement of the involved vertebral body with respect to the next most inferior vertebra or as an abrupt change in the alignment of the apophyseal joints at the level of the injury.[139] Anterior displacement of a vertebral body is usually associated with narrowing of the disc space. In many cases, there is ipsilateral displacement of the upper vertebral body and localized widening of the joints of Luschka. Associated fractures through the articular facets, pillars, or posterior elements also can occur. On the frontal view, a locked facet is suggested when the spinous process of the rotated vertebra and the vertebra above it are shifted off the midline. Locked facet and associated fractures are best demonstrated on oblique radiographs or CT scans.

Rotation injuries of the atlas and axis include rotary dislocation, rotary subluxation, and rotary fixation. Rotary dislocation and subluxation are probably manifestations of different degrees of the same pathophysiologic event. Rotary subluxation usually is reversible with conservative therapy, whereas rotary dislocation requires surgical management.

Rotary subluxation of C-1 and C-2 often occurs with the typical wry neck or torticollis of childhood. Clinically, these patients present with the acute onset of a stiff neck, often with a history of minor trauma. Lateral cervical spine radiographs may be relatively normal or may show malalignment of C-1 and C-2. There is no evidence of true atlantoaxial dislocation, however, and the predental space is normal. On the frontal view, a characteristic alteration in the alignment of the spinous process of C-2 with respect to the tip of the mandible occurs. Normally, when the head is positioned to one side, the spinous processes of the vertebral bodies rotate to the opposite side. With torticollis, the rotated anterior facet of C-1 becomes locked on the underlying facet of C-2, and as a result C-2 cannot rotate in a normal manner. Therefore, the spinous process of C-2 remains on the same side rather than rotating to the side opposite to which the mandible is rotated.

Frontal radiographs of rotary dislocation of C-1 and C-2 show abnormalities similar to those that occur with subluxation. On the lateral view, locking of C-1 and C-2 is more pronounced and fixed. Widening of the predental space and anterior displacement of the rotated articular mass of C-1 also occur (Fig. 2-64).

In rotary fixation, there is offsetting of the involved lateral mass of C-1 that persists no matter which way the head is positioned. The fixed nature of this injury is thought to be the result of invagination of the ligaments into the involved joint. As opposed to the findings with rotary dislocation, there is no widening of the predental space on lateral radiographs. CT is ideal for evaluating this abnormality.

Axial compression injuries of the cervical spine usually result in a bursting type fracture of the vertebra. In the upper cervical spine, a characteristic bursting fracture is the Jefferson fracture of C-1. Typically, this fracture involves the anterior and posterior arches of C-1 and is bilateral. The vector of force in this injury is axial compression applied to the vertex of the skull while the head is in the erect position.[140] This force causes the atlas to become compressed between the occipital condyles of the skull and the superior articular facets of C-2. Because of the obliquity of the articular surfaces of the lateral masses of C-1, the compression force in this injury causes the lateral masses to become laterally displaced.[141] In young children, the fracture may occur through the synchondroses. Frequently, there are associated avulsion fractures arising from the lateral masses. These small avulsion fracture fragments are difficult to detect on conventional radiographs, but they may be well visualized on CT. The Jefferson burst fracture and the focal anterior and posterior arch fractures are the most common fractures of the atlas.[142]

On the normal open-mouth view of the upper cervical spine, the lateral masses of C-1 line up with the articular surfaces of C-2. With a Jefferson fracture, bilateral or, occasionally, unilateral displacement of the lateral masses of C-1 occurs, such that the lateral masses of C-1 overhang the lateral masses of C-2. This displacement is usually greater than 3 mm. If the displacement is greater than 7 mm, there is probably also an injury of the transverse ligament. Jefferson fractures are optimally demonstrated on CT.[143,144]

The detection of anterior and posterior arch fractures of C-1 is often difficult on standard radiographs. This type of injury should be suspected if there is significant prevertebral soft tissue swelling.[145,146] Posterior arch fractures are best seen on the lateral radiograph. A less common finding on the lateral radiograph is the interposition of the basion between the anterior arch of C-1 and the odontoid process; this reflects abnor-

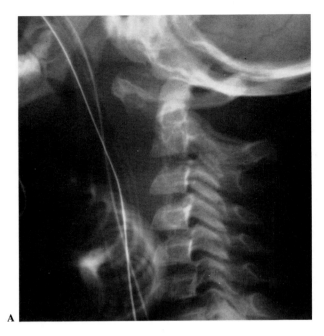

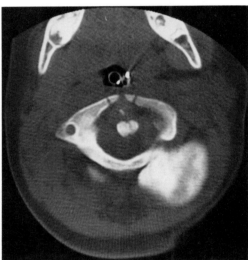

Fig. 2-64 Rotary dislocation of C-1 on C-2. **(A)** Lateral radiograph of the cervical spine of a child who sustained a severe rotational injury of the upper cervical spine shows anterior displacement of C-1 with respect to the odontoid process. Soft tissue swelling is seen in the prevertebral space. **(B)** CT scan shows rotation of C-1 to the right with respect to the tip of the odontoid process. A small avulsion fracture is seen anterior to the dens; this probably arose from the tip of the dens.

mal approximation of the occiput to the axis as a result of the laterally displaced lateral masses of C-1.[147] When any of these radiographic findings are noted, further evaluation with CT is required.

Axial compression injuries also may occur in the body and dens of C-2 and in the lower cervical vertebrae. These injuries produce vertical and oblique fractures and expansion of the vertebral body in all directions. These injuries also are best demonstrated on CT.

Cord and Nerve Root Injuries

Avulsion injuries of the brachial plexus are produced by excessive lateral flexion and rotation of the cervical spine or extensive posterior stretching of the arm. Brachial plexus injury causes paralysis of the affected limb. With a C5–7 nerve root injury, a Duchenne-Erb paralysis of the shoulder and upper arm results. A Klumpke paralysis of the hand results from C8–T1 injuries. Horner syndrome may also occur with C8–T1 injuries. The diagnosis of a brachial plexus injury is usually made clinically.

With an avulsion injury of a cervical nerve root, a cuff of arachnoid and dura mater is torn along with the nerve. Traction and shrinkage of the nerve root stump cause a cavity that eventually becomes sealed off by reactive tissue. The resulting pseudomeningocele at the site of the nerve root avulsion can be demonstrated on myelography as a rounded abnormal extension of contrast material along the expected courses of one or more nerve roots (Fig. 2-65). These abnormalities can also be demonstrated on MRI.

The central cord syndrome refers to injury of the cervical spinal cord in the absence of a displaced fracture or dislocation. There is usually a history of a hyperextension injury of the cervical spine. Clinically, there usually is a clearly defined cord level, and significant neurologic deficits are present. Radiographs do not show a fracture or dislocation in most cases. Nevertheless, this injury should be considered unstable and the neck properly immobilized. The mechanism of this injury involves impingement of the cord between the anterior and posterior walls of the spinal canal as a result of buckling of the ligamentum flavum as the neck is rapidly hyperextended. If significant rotational forces are combined with hyperexten-

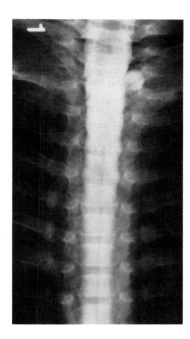

Fig. 2-65 Anteroposterior myelogram showing a rounded collection of contrast material on the left at the C-7 level. This is a pseudomeningocele that is the result of avulsion of the nerve root.

sion, the cord damage may be unilateral; the clinical manifestations in these cases may be those of the Brown-Séquard syndrome. MRI is the most useful imaging technique for the demonstration of injuries of the spinal cord (Fig. 2-66).[148]

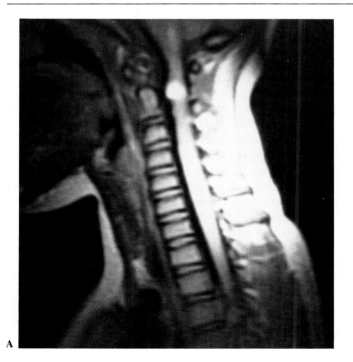

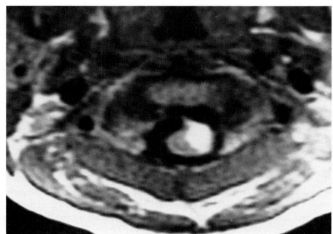

Fig. 2-66 Traumatic spinal cord injury. (**A**) Sagittal T_1-weighted MR image of a child who sustained a rotation-hyperextension injury of the neck shows a rounded area of high signal in the cervical spinal cord at the C-2 level representing subacute hemorrhage. (**B**) Axial T_1-weighted MR scan of C-2 shows that the hemorrhage occupies the left half of the spinal cord. This injury resulted in the Brown-Séquard syndrome.

A   B

Thoracic and Lumbar Spine Trauma

The same general mechanisms of injury that occur in trauma to the cervical spine are involved in trauma to the thoracic and lumbar portions of the spine. The developing spine has greater flexibility because of its ligamentous laxity, underdevelopment of the paraspinal muscles, incompletely ossified bone structures, and shallow orientation of the facets. The mechanisms of injury include flexion, extension, lateral flexion, rotation, and axial compression.

Most thoracic and lumbar spine injuries are due to flexion-compression trauma. Flexion injuries of the thoracolumbar spine typically result in anterior vertebral body compression (Fig. 2-67). The compression forces are accentuated by the normal kyphosis of the thoracic spine. Pure axial compression acting on an abnormal kyphotic curve can produce a similar injury.

Flexion-compression injury usually brings the greatest stress to bear on the anterior aspects of the vertebral body, the anterior longitudinal ligament, and the anterior annulus fibrosus. The posterior aspect of the vertebral body and the posterior annulus fibrosus may or may not be involved. The posterior vertebral structures are often spared, but if the flexion-compression force is of sufficient magnitude there is tension (distraction) posteriorly that results in subluxation, dislocation, or fracture-dislocation of the articular processes or spinous processes. The more severe the injury, the greater the likelihood that posterior ligaments will be disrupted; this is identified as widening of the interspinous distance.

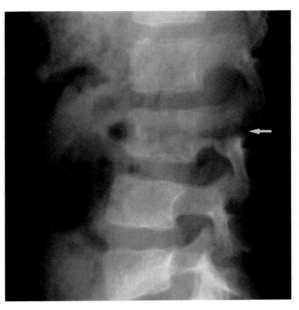

Fig. 2-68 Lateral radiograph of the lumbar spine revealing a splitting fracture of the L-3 vertebral body that extends through the pedicles (arrow). This Chance fracture was the result of severe hyperflexion in a motor vehicle accident. The child was in an infant seat secured with a lap belt.

Anterior compression fractures of the thoracic and lumbar spine occur at all ages, but the incidence increases in older adults as osteoporosis develops. Children with osteoporosis due to an underlying condition, such as steroid therapy or osteogenesis imperfecta, are at increased risk for these fractures. Anterior compression fractures of the thoracolumbar spine may occur in patients who jump or fall from heights. They usually occur at the thoracolumbar junction, although the C7–T1 area is another common site.[149] Flexion-compression fractures are sometimes identified in physically abused children.[150]

In the lower lumbar spine, compression forces are directed more toward the center of the vertebral body because of the normal lumbar lordosis. Consequently, a compression fracture in this portion of the spine sometimes occurs as a central depression in the vertebral body.

In addition to compression fractures, tear-drop fractures can occur in the thoracic and lumbar portions of the spine. In the lumbar spine, tear-drop fractures are often referred to as limbus fractures. If the injury is severe enough, patients with these fractures may demonstrate anterior subluxation of the apophyseal joints. If there is anterior subluxation or separation of the spinous process, the fracture is considered unstable.

Chance fractures result from severe hyperflexion injuries of the lumbar spine. Typically, this is from a sudden deceleration while a person is wearing a lap-type seat belt. The resultant distraction forces cause failure of the posterior and middle columns of the vertebral body. Compressive forces are concomitantly applied to the anterior column. There may be disruption of the posterior ligaments and the facet joints with

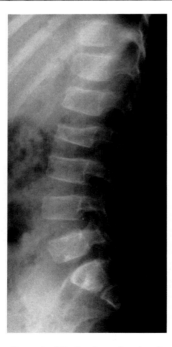

Fig. 2-67 Lateral radiograph of the lumbar spine showing anterior compression of the L-2 vertebral body. There is also minimal loss in height of the L-1, L-3, and L-4 vertebral bodies. Fractures of this variety are the result of flexion-compression forces.

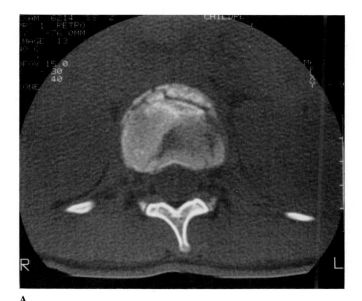

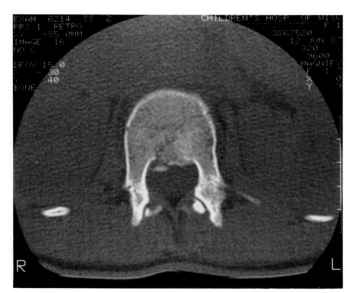

A

B

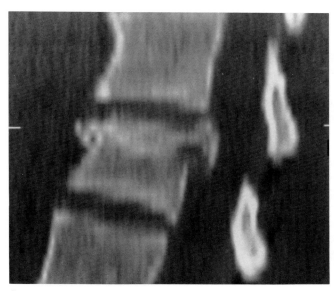

C

Fig. 2-69 Burst fracture. **(A)** Unenhanced CT scan of the superior surface of L-1 shows numerous fracture lines in the anterior portion of the vertebral body. Several of these fracture lines extend posteriorly. **(B)** Unenhanced CT at the level of the pedicles of L-1 shows that several fragments of the vertebral body are retropulsed into the spinal canal. **(C)** Sagittal reformatted image shows the degree of compression of the anterior portion of the vertebral body. The bursting of the superior surface of the vertebra is apparent. Note the large retropulsed fragment.

---

this injury. If the ligaments remain intact, however, a fracture will occur in the transverse plane through the posterior elements with extension into the posterosuperior aspect of the vertebral body (Fig. 2-68). The anterior longitudinal ligament normally remains intact. If this ligament tears, the superior vertebra may sublux anteriorly on the more inferior vertebra. When this occurs the lesion is unstable, and neurologic compromise that is proportional to the degree of subluxation may result.

In a burst fracture, the anterior and middle columns of the vertebral body fail under axial compression forces.[151] The nucleus pulposus of the intervertebral disc is driven into the adjacent inferior vertebral body, which then explodes or bursts.[152] This leads to severe comminution of the vertebral body and fracture of one (usually the superior) or both vertebral endplates. The posterior wall of the vertebral body is tilted, and the fragment is displaced (retropulsed) posteriorly into the spinal canal. There may be spreading of the pedicles, a vertical fracture of the lamina, and splaying of the facet joints. The posterior spinous ligaments usually remain intact.

Radiographs in cases of burst fracture show loss of vertebral body height anteriorly with normal or increased height of the posterior vertebral margin. The fracture in the superior half of the vertebral body is comminuted, and there is usually a sagittally oriented fracture in the inferior half.[153] The retropulsed fragment from the posterosuperior aspect of the vertebral body may rotate significantly, causing the cartilaginous endplate to come to lie anteriorly. Optimal visualization of these fragments is provided by CT (Fig. 2-69). The retropulsed fragment may be displaced several millimeters in the cranial or caudal direction. Most often, the retropulsed fragments become separated from the vertebral body. The interpedicular distance may be widened. Rarely, there is a fracture from the posteroinferior corner of the vertebral body that is rotated clockwise, suggesting that it remains attached to the annulus fibrosus.[154]

Burst fractures are considered unstable, even though they occur without neurologic deficit in more than 50% of cases. The weight-bearing function of the middle column of the vertebral body is significantly compromised. Because of this, further axial loading of the spine may cause the middle column to be forced posteriorly, resulting in further encroachment into the spinal canal. This can be an ominous sign of impending neurologic deficit after the acute injury.[155] Stability is further compromised when there is significant associated interspinous ligament laxity or disruption.

Extension injuries of the thoracolumbar spine are uncommon. In some cases, the only result is nondisplaced fractures of the neural arch and spinous process. Occasionally, a hangman-type fracture mechanism occurs, causing anterior dislocation of the superior vertebral body. This is the pathophysiologic event in so-called traumatic spondylolisthesis.

Another injury that can occur when extension forces are applied to the thoracolumbar spine is the limbus or corner fracture of the vertebral body. This is analogous to the extension tear-drop fracture in the cervical spine. Corner fractures also can be produced by flexion injuries, but some degree of vertebral body compression is often identified in these cases. The hyperextension corner fracture is caused by avulsive forces transmitted through ligamentous attachments and is associated with underlying ligamentous injury and instability. There may be disc space widening and actual posterior displacement of the involved vertebral body.

As in the cervical spine, lateral flexion injuries can result in lateral compression fractures of the vertebral bodies of the thoracolumbar spine. This mechanism also can produce fractures of the transverse processes. These injuries are usually not serious, provided that lateral flexion is the only force involved. Fractures of the transverse process must be differentiated from rudimentary lumbar ribs or bipartite transverse processes.

Rotation injuries involve either rotation-flexion or rotation-extension forces. The upper thoracic spine is especially prone to these injuries. Considerable spinal cord damage may occur because the subarachnoid space is especially narrow in this region.

SPINAL NEOPLASMS

Spinal neoplasms may arise from the cord, nerve roots, meninges, epidural connective tissues, or spinal osseous structures. On the basis of the site of origin, spinal tumors are usually divided into three general categories: intramedullary, intradural extramedullary, and extradural (Table 2-1). Of these, extradural tumors are the most common and account for 40% to 60% of all neoplasms that affect the spine in children. Intradural extramedullary tumors account for 30% to 40%, and purely intramedullary neoplasms constitute 20% to 30%.[156]

Extradural tumors of neural origin account for approximately 20% of spinal neoplasms. Most of these are neuroblastomas arising from the sympathetic nervous system. Tumors arising from the nerve roots and peripheral nerves, such as schwannoma and neurofibroma, may occur in extradural or intradural extramedullary locations (or both). These lesions occur with an increased incidence in children with neurofibromatosis. Tumors arising from the osseous structures of the spine present in the extradural space.

Table 2-1 Spinal Neoplasms in Infants and Children

Intramedullary tumors
 Astrocytoma
 Ependymoma
 Oligodendroglioma
 Ganglioglioma

Intradural extramedullary tumors
 Developmental tumors
  Dermoid cyst
  Epidermoid cyst
  Lipoma
  Teratoma
 Spinal nerve tumors
  Schwannoma
  Neurofibroma
 Meningeal tumors
  Meningioma
 Vascular lesions
  Hemangioma
  Arteriovenous malformation
 Metastatic tumors

Extradural tumors
 Osseous tumors
  Osteoblastoma
  Osteoid osteoma
  Osteosarcoma
  Ewing tumor
  Langerhans cell histiocytosis
 Neural tumors
  Neuroblastoma
  Ganglioneuroblastoma
  Ganglioneuroma
  Neurofibroma
 Lymphoma and leukemia
 Metastatic tumors

The most common spinal tumors in infants are the various congenital (dysplastic) tumors, such as dermoid, epidermoid, lipoma, and teratoma. Most of these occur in the intradural extramedullary space and are often associated with dysraphic malformations. Overall, the most common congenital tumor in neonates in sacrococcygeal teratoma. This lesion may invade the intraspinal spaces but is primarily located in the extradural paraspinal region. There are rare cases of primary intraspinal teratoma.

The most important intramedullary tumors in children are astrocytoma and ependymoma. Intramedullary tumors of the spinal cord constitute 6% to 10% of childhood central nervous system tumors and represent approximately one-third of all spinal neoplasms in children. Astrocytoma accounts for about 60% of intramedullary spinal cord tumors in children, and ependymoma accounts for about 30%. This is the reverse of the prevalence pattern in adults.

Intramedullary neoplasms of the spinal cord in children are frequently slow growing and tend to produce subtle, slowly progressive clinical signs and symptoms. The clinical diagnosis is frequently difficult early in the course of the disease. Symptoms often develop insidiously and may be present for months or years before diagnosis. Weakness, the most common presenting complaint, occurs in about 80% of these children. The weakness can range from a minimal localized abnormality to quadriparesis.

Pain or other sensory changes occur in 60% to 70% of affected children, with back pain being the most common (occurring in about 70%). Back pain is usually dull and aching and tends to be localized to a bone segment adjacent to the tumor. The second most common type of pain is nerve root in origin. Some children manifest a vague burning type of pain associated with paresthesia. Occasionally, the pain is referred to the abdomen. Other potential clinical findings include gait disturbance (40% to 50%), sphincter dysfunction (20%), and signs and symptoms of increased intracranial pressure (12%).[157–161]

Extradural tumors tend to produce bony pain or radicular symptomatology. Nerve root tumors may cause diminished or absent deep tendon reflexes in the distribution of the affected nerves. Congenital intradural tumors, such as lipoma, epidermoid, and dermoid, are usually associated with bony spinal or other external malformations. These children may exhibit sphincter disturbances and gait abnormalities. Pain does not occur until late in the course of the disorder.

Although a spinal neoplasm can occur at any level in the spine, many of these lesions exhibit predilections for specific regions. Astrocytoma most often occurs in the upper portions of the spinal cord, particularly the cervical and cervicothoracic regions. Ependymoma predominates in the lumbosacral region and in the conus medullaris. Lipoma, dermoid, and epidermoid are usually located in the lower portion of the spinal canal. Teratoma occurs in the lumbar and sacrococcygeal regions. Neuroblastoma is most often found in the thoracolumbar and lumbar regions.

Astrocytoma

The most common intramedullary spinal cord neoplasm in children is astrocytoma. This neoplasm is of glial origin. There is a slight male predominance. The average age of presentation is usually after 6 years. The cervical and thoracic portions of the cord are the most frequent locations. The tumor causes diffuse enlargement of the involved portion of the cord and predominantly spreads in a longitudinal manner. At least 50% to 60% of spinal cord astrocytomas extend from the lower brainstem to the conus medullaris; this is termed holocord astrocytoma. About two-thirds of spinal astrocytomas are solid; one-third have significant cystic components. Even tumors that are largely solid usually have a small cyst at either end. Most spinal cord astrocytomas in children are relatively benign (ie, grade 1 or 2 lesions). Malignant forms of spinal astrocytoma are much less common in children than in adults.[160–162]

The signs and symptoms of spinal cord astrocytoma are quite variable. Potential findings include gait disturbance, pain, stiffness, torticollis, scoliosis, paralysis, hyporeflexia,

positive Babinski sign, sphincter dysfunction, and sensory deficits. Torticollis and scoliosis are often the initial manifestations of a mass in the cervical portion of the spinal cord. Thoracic tumors often present initially with gait disturbances. Neoplasms located in the lumbar portion of the cord may produce gait disturbance, scoliosis, or sphincter dysfunction.[163]

Two distinct clinical syndromes are associated with total cord involvement with astrocytoma.[162] The first of these is characterized primarily by weakness of one arm that may be accompanied by neck pain as the initial manifestation. Bowel and bladder functions are preserved. Physical examination reveals mild spastic weakness of the legs. In this group of patients the solid portion of the tumor is in the cervical region, and the caudal portion is cystic.

The second clinical syndrome associated with holocord astrocytoma is characterized by progressive spastic paraplegia sometimes accompanied by thoracic pain and scoliosis. In these patients, the solid portion of the tumor lies in the thoracic or lumbar region. When solid tumor extends into the conus medullaris, deep tendon reflexes in the lower extremities may be diminished or absent, and bladder and bowel functions are impaired.

Radiographs in cases of spinal cord astrocytoma may show widening of the spinal canal. In the cervical region, this is best detected by an increase in the sagittal diameter of the canal. In addition, the posterior surface of the vertebral bodies may be scalloped. In the thoracic and lumbar regions, the pedicles may be eroded and the spinal canal enlarged. Scoliosis occurs in some cases. Rarely, intraspinal calcifications are visible.

Myelography reveals diffuse expansion of the involved segment of the cord (Fig. 2-70). Occasionally, there is a complete block to the flow of contrast material. CT myelography demonstrates more clearly the region of neoplastic cord enlargement. Low-attenuation, nonenhancing cystic components may be identified in or adjacent to the lesion.[164]

MRI is the imaging modality of choice for the evaluation of spinal astrocytoma. Expansion of the cord at the level of the lesion is demonstrated.[165–169] The solid components of the tumor produce moderate to low signal intensity on T_1-weighted images and moderate to high intensity on T_2-weighted images. Cystic components produce low signal, approximately isointense to cerebrospinal fluid, on T_1-weighted images and very high signal on T_2-weighted images. The solid components of the neoplasm usually show prominent enhancement after intravenous administration of gadopentate dimeglumine.

Ependymoma

Ependymoma is a primary glial tumor that arises from the ependymal cells in the spinal canal or filum terminale. Spinal ependymomas are usually slow growing and of low malignancy. Histologically, ependymomas may be of the myxopapillary, cellular, epithelial, or mixed type. In the filum

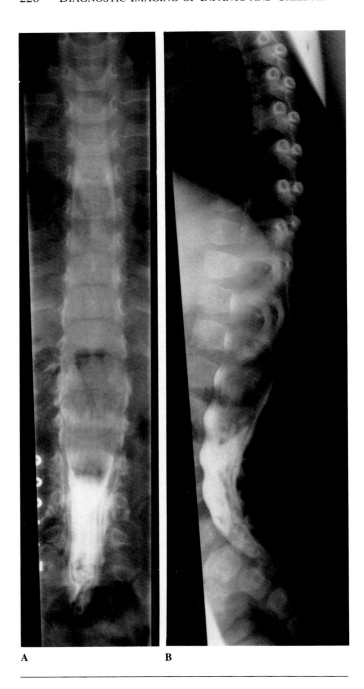

A   B

Fig. 2-70 Astrocytoma. **(A)** Anteroposterior and **(B)** lateral myelograms of the thoracolumbar spine show extensive expansion of the spinal cord from the midthoracic region to the conus. The pedicles are widely separated and eroded, and there is minimal posterior scalloping of the vertebral bodies. There are serpiginous defects at the caudal end of the thecal sac and at the cephalad end of the tumor; these are due to enlarged blood vessels. This appearance is typical of an infiltrating astrocytoma of the spinal cord.

the cauda equina, forming a tumor nodule attached to the nerve roots. Ependymoma is the second most frequent tumor of the filum terminale after lipoma. In children, the prevalence of ependymoma is twice as high in boys as in girls.

The clinical features of spinal ependymoma vary somewhat according to the location of the tumor. The initial manifestations may include scoliosis, pain in the legs or back, paresthesias, or weakness in one or both lower extremities. The pain may worsen in the recumbent position. The diagnosis may be delayed for years when the only clinical manifestation is scoliosis. Eventually all children with ependymoma develop gait disturbances, and it is this symptom that often leads to diagnostic imaging.

Children with ependymoma in the cervical region present with a stiff neck, torticollis, and neck pain that is worse at night. Lesions of the thoracic cord often produce pain localized to the level of the tumor. Ependymomas of the filum terminale may cause chronic low back pain, coccygodynia, or diffuse pain that radiates to the pelvis or lower extremities. Tumors of the filum terminale can rupture, causing subarachnoid hemorrhage, meningismus, fever, and cerebrospinal fluid pleocytosis that mimics bacterial meningitis.[170]

Spastic paraplegia is the usual finding on physical examination of children with ependymoma. Tumors in the cervical region may cause weakness of one arm as well. Tumors of the cauda equina produce flaccid weakness and atrophy of the leg muscles associated with loss of tendon reflexes. The cerbrospinal fluid is often xanthochromic, and the protein content is elevated.

Radiographs of patients with intraspinal ependymoma are usually normal, although there may be widening of the interpedicular distance and posterior vertebral scalloping with lesions of long duration. Myelography demonstrates a smooth or slightly lobulated tumor that is most frequently located in the conus medullaris or filum terminale. The intramedullary nature of the mass may not be appreciable with lesions arising from the tip of the conus or the filum. The absence of spinal dysraphism favors the diagnosis of ependymoma rather than teratoma, dermoid, epidermoid, or lipoma.[165–167]

An intramedullary ependymoma is demonstrated on MRI as an area of focal cord enlargement or a mass in the filum terminale. On T_1-weighted images, homogeneous or heterogeneous areas of low signal intensity may be present; these can be due to tumor, cystic degeneration in the tumor, or cysts

terminale and conus medullaris, the myxopapillary variant occurs most frequently.

Spinal ependymoma can occur at any age. About 25% of all ependymomas present in patients younger than 20 years of age, and 20% appear in patients younger than 15 years of age. Any portion of the spine may be involved, but the filum terminale and conus medullaris are the most common sites. Others arise, in decreasing order of frequency, in the lumbar, thoracic, and cervical portions of the cord. Occasionally, an ependymoma originates from ectopic ependymal cells along

adjacent to the tumor. On T_2-weighted images, the neoplasm produces high signal intensity compared to normal cord. With small lesions, the tumor is usually fairly well circumscribed. Tumor margins may be somewhat obscured by adjacent edema, however. Areas of signal void in and around the neoplasm may be identified; these are due to hemosiderin from prior hemorrhage. T_1-weighted MR images after intravenous administration of gadopentate dimeglumine typically show significant enhancement of the neoplasm (Fig. 2-71). This method provides the most accurate delineation of tumor margins and helps distinguish tumor from edema or associated cysts.[166,167,171]

Oligodendroglioma

Primary spinal cord oligodendroglioma is the rarest of all spinal gliomas. This lesion accounts for less than 1% of all spinal tumors. It occurs in all age groups, and boys and girls are equally affected. The most common location is the thoracic cord, which is followed in frequency by the cervical and lumbar segments. The signs and symptoms of spinal oligodendroglioma are similar to those of other intramedullary tumors. Back pain is the initial manifestation in most patients. Other findings include motor deficits, paresthesias, para-

paresis, sensory deficits, sphincter disturbances, and hyperreflexia below the lesion. Decreased reflexes may occur if the tumor involves nerve roots.[172,173]

At the time of clinical presentation, findings suggestive of an intraspinal mass on plain radiographs appear in a minority of cases of primary spinal oligodendroglioma. Kyphoscoliosis is occasionally present. With large lesions, enlargement of the spinal canal and erosion of pedicles may be identified. MRI clearly demonstrates the intramedullary location of the tumor and defines the extent of cord involvement. As with astrocytoma and ependymoma, cystic areas may be identified in or adjacent to an oligodendroglioma.

Nerve Root Tumors

There are four major histologic types of tumors derived from nerve sheaths. A schwannoma (neurilemoma) is a benign encapsulated tumor composed of Schwann cells. A neurofibroma consists of a mixture of Schwann cells and fibroblasts. This tumor may occur in either localized or diffuse forms and is usually associated with neurofibromatosis type 1. An anaplastic neurilemoma is quite rare. A malignant neurofibroma (neurofibrosarcoma) results from malignant degeneration of a neurofibroma.

Nerve sheath tumors account for approximately 10% of spinal tumors in children. These lesions are approximately twice as common in adults as in children. They may occur anywhere along the spine, but about two-thirds are located in the cervical and lumbar regions. These lesions rarely may occur as intramedullary tumors; the great majority are extramedullary, however, being intradural, extradural, or both. Spinal nerve root tumors frequently extend through an intervertebral foramen, producing a dumbbell-shaped mass that is both intradural and extradural.[174]

In general, the symptoms produced by a spinal nerve root tumor are more intense, occur earlier, and are more frequent in children than in adults. The findings include radicular pain, muscle weakness or paresis, sensory deficits, and local muscular atrophy. The clinical findings typically follow the distribution of a specific nerve root.

The radiographic findings of a spinal nerve root tumor vary according to the size and location of the lesion. Radiographs and CT scans in those cases that have a large intraspinal component may show focal enlargement of the spinal canal, erosion of the pedicles, scalloping of the posterior margins of the vertebral bodies, and thinning of the laminae. It is important to note that posterior vertebral body scalloping occurs frequently in patients with neurofibromatosis without an underlying space-occupying lesion. Extraspinal extension of the lesion frequently causes widening of one or more intervertebral neural foramina (Fig. 2-72). In the thorax the intercostal spaces may be widened, and the posteromedial aspects of the ribs may be eroded. Myelography can be utilized to demonstrate the intraspinal component of a spinal nerve root tumor.

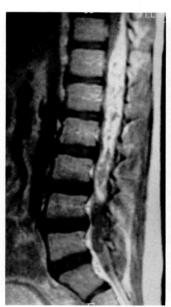
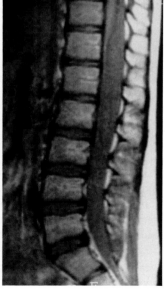

A   B

Fig. 2-71 Ependymoma. (**A**) T_1-weighted sagittal MR image shows a somewhat lobulated mass that is poorly distinguished from the adjacent cerebrospinal fluid. The vertebral bodies appear normal. (**B**) T_1-weighted sagittal MR image with intravenous gadopentate dimeglumine shows intense enhancement of the neoplasm that extends caudally from the conus medullaris to L-4. This appearance is typical of a myxopapillary ependymoma of the spinal cord.

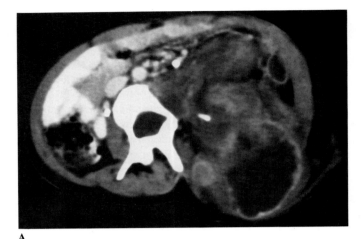

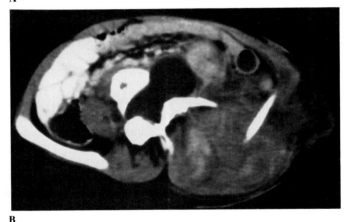

Fig. 2-72 Neurofibromatosis type 1 with neurofibrosarcoma. (**A**) Contrast-enhanced CT scan of the lower lumbar spine shows extensive rotatory scoliosis of the spine. A large inhomogeneous mass extends posteriorly and laterally from the left side of the spine. (**B**) Contrast-enhanced CT at a slightly lower level shows marked dural ectasia and a large lateral meningocele. The neurofibrosarcoma has eroded posteriorly and presents in the flank and buttocks. Dural ectasia and lateral meningoceles are common in neurofibromatosis type 1. The irregular enhancement and areas of necrosis as well as the poor definition of the soft tissue tumor are signs of malignant degeneration.

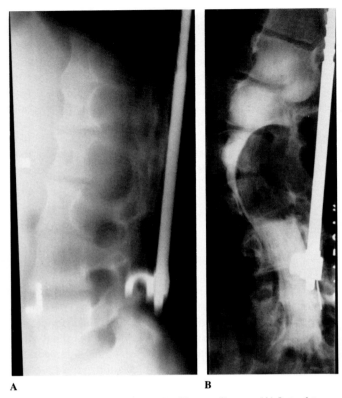

Fig. 2-73 Neurofibromatosis type 1 with neurofibroma. (**A**) Lateral tomogram of the lumbar spine reveals extensive posterior scalloping of the vertebral bodies. Many of the neural foramina are markedly enlarged. Orthopedic spinal instrumentation is in place. (**B**) Anteroposterior myelogram of the lumbar spine reveals most of the posterior scalloping to be due to dural ectasia. A large dumbbell neurofibroma is seen at the L2–3 level.

This technique is particularly useful in those patients with metallic orthopedic spinal hardware that precludes the use of MRI (Fig. 2-73).

On T$_1$-weighted MR images, spinal nerve sheath tumors usually show slightly greater signal intensity than muscle. The lesion shows intense enhancement with gadopentate dimeglumine (Fig. 2-74). Most of the lesion produces relatively high signal intensity on T$_2$-weighted images. Central areas of low signal intensity are frequently identified on T$_2$-weighted images. These appear to correspond histologically to areas of Schwann cell proliferation, whereas the high-signal portions of the tumor are probably due to the high water content of the endoneural myxoid matrix. Malignant neurofibroma (neurofibrosarcoma) usually lacks these well-defined central areas of low signal. Heterogeneous, irregular central areas of high signal intensity are sometimes seen in

malignant lesions; these are due to necrosis. These general patterns, however, do not allow definitive distinction between malignant and benign lesions.[175]

Intraspinal Teratoma

Intraspinal teratoma is an uncommon tumor, accounting for approximately 1% of all intraspinal neoplasms. Unlike other congenital tumors, such as lipoma, dermoid cyst, and epidermoid cyst, intraspinal teratoma is most often not associated with other congenital spinal anomalies. The clinical presentation of this congenital neoplasm can occur at any age. About one third of cases are identified in children younger than age 6 years and one quarter between the ages of 6 and 19 years. The clinical presentation is usually intermittent back pain and signs of cord compression.[176]

Intraspinal teratoma may occur at any level of the spinal canal, but there is a predilection for involvement of the dorsal aspect of the thoracolumbar cord. The lesion may be intramedullary, intradural extramedullary, or both. Most often, the teratoma is adherent to the cord with a poorly defined interface of tumor connective tissue and spinal cord–reactive gliosis. As

Fig. 2-74 Axial T_1-weighted MR image of the cervical spine with intravenous gadopentate dimeglumine showing a large, intensely enhancing, right paraspinal neoplasm that extends into the right neural foramen. This was a large plexiform neurofibroma in a patient with neurofibromatosis.

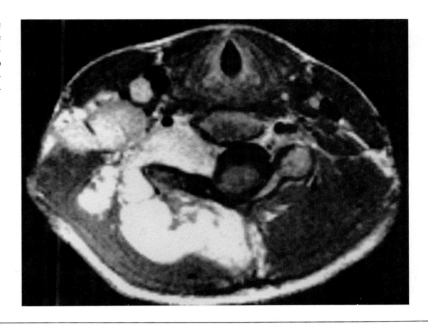

with teratomas elsewhere, the composition of the lesion may be quite variable. Intraspinal teratomas may be solid, partially cystic, or completely cystic. Bone or cartilage may be present.

Radiographs in cases of intraspinal teratoma may show focal enlargement of the spinal canal with thinning of the pedicles and laminae, posterior vertebral body scalloping, and widening of the interpedicular distance. Scoliosis is sometimes present. Most often, the osseous structures of the spine are developmentally normal. There are rare instances of spina bifida, block vertebrae, Klippel-Feil syndrome, or diastematomyelia.

Intraspinal teratoma is demonstrated as a markedly heterogeneous lesion on MRI. Cystic components produce low signal on T_1-weighted images and high signal on T_2-weighted images. Fat, proteinaceous material, or cellular debris in one or more cysts may significantly alter the signal characteristics, however. The solid components of the tumor usually produce signal intensity similar to that of the spinal cord on T_1-weighted images and are somewhat hyperintense on T_2-weighted images. Signal voids in the lesion are due to calcification or ossification.

Arachnoid Cysts

Arachnoid cysts are benign diverticula of the leptomeninges that are lined by arachnoid and have collagen tissue in the wall. They may occur in an intradural, extradural, or perineurial location. They may arise anywhere along the spinal canal, either posterior or anterior to the spinal cord or in both locations.[177]

These cysts are congenital in origin. They can cause symptoms at any age; signs and symptoms depend on the location of the cyst. Those located in the cervical region can cause quad-

riparesis and respiratory difficulties. Those located in the thoracic or lumbar region can produce paraparesis. Spasticity, paresthesias, disturbances of the bowel or bladder, and local pain are common symptoms of arachnoid cysts in any location.

Plain radiographs of the spine are usually normal and specifically do not show widening of the canal or erosion of the pedicles. Extradural arachnoid cysts may increase the interpedicular distance, but intradural lesions do not. Myelography frequently reveals a complete block at the level of the cyst. MRI shows the cyst as a well-demarcated area that has long T_1 and T_2 relaxation times.[178]

Arteriovenous Malformation

Intraspinal arteriovenous malformation may present at any age. The lesions may occur anywhere along the spinal cord. In children, about one half occur in the thoracolumbar region, 28% in the cervical cord, and 21% in the thoracic cord.[179,180]

In many cases, the clinical presentation of intraspinal arteriovenous malformation is acute. The sudden onset of symptoms may occur in association with intense physical activity or the Valsalva maneuver. The clinical findings include back pain, lower extremity motor abnormalities, and sphincter dysfunction. In young children, there may be delayed motor development of the legs, progressive spasticity, and weakness of the lower extremities. Subarachnoid hemorrhage may occur as an acute event. Approximately one-third of cases of spinal cord arteriovenous malformation are associated with a deep or cutaneous angiodysplasia. These angiodysplasias include port wine angiomas, Osler-Weber-Rendu disease, Klippel-Trenaunay syndrome, and Cobb syndrome.

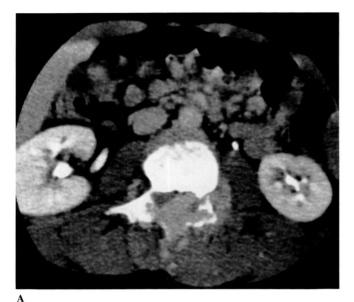

A

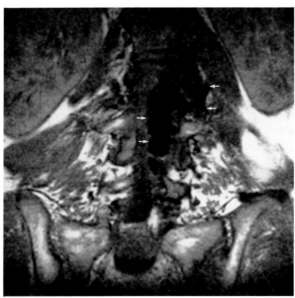

B

Fig. 2-75 Intraspinal arteriovenous malformation. **(A)** Contrast-enhanced CT scan shows an intensely enhancing area posterior to the vertebral body, the left pedicle and lamina of the vertebra that extends laterally beneath the left psoas muscle. The thecal sac is markedly displaced to the right. **(B)** Coronal T_1-weighted MR image shows numerous signal voids (arrows) in the spinal subarachnoid space, which extend to the left, at the L-2 level. This is the level of the eroded pedicle seen on CT. These signal voids were due to large draining veins from the intraspinal arteriovenous malformation.

The radiographs of the spine may show bony abnormalities if the arteriovenous malformation is large. Potential findings include vertebral body scalloping, erosion of the pedicles, focal widening of the vertebral canal, and kyphoscoliosis. Enlarged feeding arteries and draining veins may be identified on myelography as tortuous filling defects on the surface of the cord. An intramedullary arteriovenous malformation causes focal enlargement of the spinal cord.

The typical MR appearance of the juvenile type of intraspinal arteriovenous malformation is multiple, serpiginous areas of signal void in an intramedullary nidus. These signal voids are due to rapid blood flow through the abnormal vasculature. These are seen on both T_1- and T_2-weighted imaging sequences. Large draining veins are often identified as tortuous signal voids extending in both cranial and caudal directions (Fig. 2-75). On T_2-weighted images, there may be areas of high signal interspersed between regions of low signal in the mass resulting from clot in the cord tissue or old hemorrhage. Prior hemorrhage may produce areas of high signal intensity on T_2-weighted images surrounded by a low-signal rim. Depending on the presence of methemoglobin, areas of prior hemorrhage may produce areas of high signal intensity on T_1-weighted images. Most intraspinal arteriovenous malformations show significant contrast enhancement with intravenous administration of gadopentate dimeglumine as a result of abnormal permeability of the local blood-cord barrier or because of enhancement of blood in enlarged draining veins.[181]

Spinal Metastasis

Metastatic disease can involve the vertebrae, meninges, spinal cord (rare), and nerve roots. Between 10% and 25% of spinal neoplasms in children are metastatic in origin. Osseous metastases to the spine in children are predominantly due to neuroblastoma, rhabdomyosarcoma, osteosarcoma, lymphoma, Ewing sarcoma, chondrosarcoma, teratocarcinoma, and the clear cell variant of Wilms tumor. Symptoms in these cases may be produced by pathologic fractures and spinal cord compression. The metastatic lesions also can extend into the epidural space of the spinal canal (Fig. 2-76).

Most intradural metastases are extramedullary; only rare cases of intramedullary lesions have been reported. There are three main types of intradural extramedullary metastases: subarachnoid metastases, intradural extra-arachnoid metastases, and secondary invasion of the intradural spaces from an epidural lesion. The most common are subarachnoid (drop) metastases from an intracranial neoplasm. The most common intracranial lesion associated with subarachnoid metastases is medulloblastoma. Other intracranial neoplasms that may metastasize by this mechanism include ependymoma, pineal neoplasms, astrocytoma, choroid plexus carcinoma, and retinoblastoma. Spinal subarachnoid metastases with these lesions may be present at the time of diagnosis or develop as part of the recurrence of the tumor. The metastatic lesions most often are located in the lumbosacral or lower thoracic region, although any portion of the spinal canal may be affected. This predilection for involvement of the more caudal portions of the thecal sac is probably related to the direction of cerebrospinal fluid flow as well as to the effects of gravity.

Radiographs are usually normal in cases of spinal subarachnoid metastases. Myelography shows multiple intradural

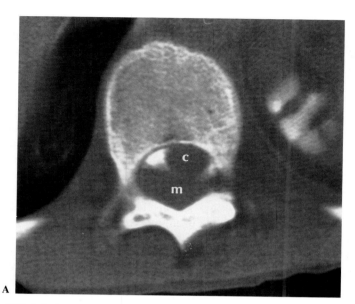
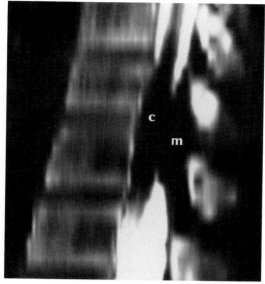

Fig. 2-76 Spinal metastasis. (**A**) CT myelogram of the lower thoracic spine shows the spinal cord (c) and subarachnoid space to be displaced anteriorly. There is a soft tissue mass (m) in the posterior epidural space. (**B**) Sagittal reformatted CT image shows obliteration of the posterior epidural space from T-11 to T-12. This was due to metastatic involvement of the posterior elements of T-12. The primary lesion was a malignant thymoma.

extramedullary nodules that vary in size (Fig. 2-77). These may be located anywhere in the subarachnoid space but are most often seen in the theca terminalis and along the exits of the spinal nerves. Nodules adherent to the surface of the spinal cord also may be identified. CT myelography may be helpful for identifying small nodules and for more accurately defining the effects on the cord and nerve roots.

MRI is also quite sensitive for the detection of spinal subarachnoid metastases. These lesions are usually best detected on T_1-weighted images after the intravenous administration of gadopentate dimeglumine. The metastatic lesions usually show prominent enhancement. MRI is also well suited for showing compression of the spinal cord or nerve roots by metastatic lesions (Fig. 2-78).[165–167]

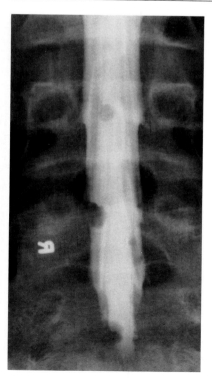

Fig. 2-77 Anteroposterior myelogram of the lumbar spine showing numerous nodules of tumor throughout the subarachnoid space. The nodules are largest in the cul de sac. These are drop metastases from a medulloblastoma.

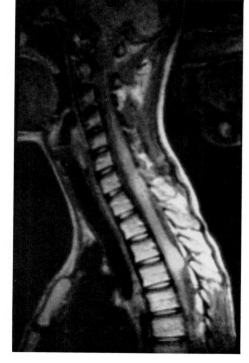

Fig. 2-78 Sagittal proton-density MR image of a patient with medulloblastoma showing two large drop metastases on the surface of the spinal cord. The largest lesion is at the T-4 level. A smaller lesion is at the C7–T1 level.

Paraspinal Tumors

The bony spinal canal is surrounded by a large group of muscles. In the abdomen, the psoas muscles lie lateral to the vertebral bodies and the pedicles, and the paraspinal muscles lie on either side of the spinous processes and laminae. Soft tissue tumors, especially rhabdomyosarcoma, can arise in these muscle groups. Because of the close proximity of these muscle groups, these tumors may extend into the spinal canal through the neural foramina. Similarly, fibrosarcoma can arise in the connective tissue planes and may involve the spinal axis by extension through neural foramina.

The vast majority of masses in the psoas muscles and, to a lesser extent, the paraspinal muscles are due to invasion by other malignant disease, especially lymphoma, Wilms tumor, or Ewing tumor. The psoas muscle also may become involved from extension of osteomyelitis of the vertebral bodies as a result of infection with either pyogenic organisms or *Mycobacterium tuberculosis*. Inflammatory disease in the retroperitoneum, such as appendicitis occurring in a retrocecal appendix, inflammatory bowel disease, and septic arthritis from the sacroiliac joint, also may involve the psoas muscles.

Radiographs of the spine and abdomen in cases of primary tumors of the paraspinal musculature are usually normal or may show a vague soft tissue mass. MRI is the imaging modality of choice for demonstrating the exact extent of these lesions. The involved muscle is enlarged. Scattered areas of increased signal may be seen on T_1-weighted images, reflecting subacute hemorrhage. Otherwise, the mass produces signal equal to that of adjacent muscle. T_2-weighted images demonstrate increased signal from the mass and clearly dem-

onstrate the extent of the lesion, including involvement of the intraspinal contents (Fig. 2-79). Enhancement with intravenous gadopentate dimeglumine further improves distinction of the lesion from adjacent structures.

Neuroblastoma

Neuroblastoma and the other neural crest tumors usually arise from the adrenal gland or from the cervical, thoracic, or abdominal sympathetic ganglia. Although they may occur anywhere from the base of the skull to the pelvis, they are found most commonly in the abdomen and thorax. Most of these sites of origin are in close proximity to the spine. Invasion of the spine is an important complication of neural crest tumors.

There is a pathologic spectrum of neural crest tumors that ranges from the frankly malignant neuroblastoma, to ganglioneuroblastoma (which is intermediate in its aggressive behavior), to ganglioneuroma (which is benign). Neuroblastoma tends to occur in infants and young children; ganglioneuromas most often present in older children and young adults.

Intraspinal extension of a paravertebral neural crest tumor may occur without neurologic symptoms or bone erosion. Intraspinal extension usually occurs via a neural foramen, and the mass remains confined to the extradural space. Neurologic signs and symptoms develop when there is compression of the spinal cord. Paraplegia may be the initial clinical manifestation of a neurogenic tumor that has extended into the epidural space from a paravertebral location. In infants, the initial findings may include irritability, constipation, and pain with limb motion. Spinal involvement in older children may be

A   **B**

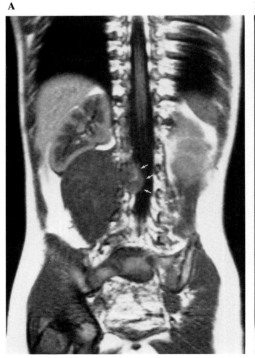
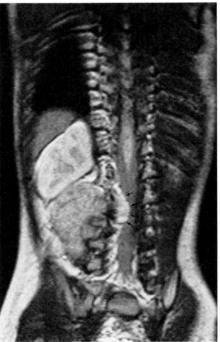

Fig. 2-79 Rhabdomyosarcoma arising from the right psoas muscle. (**A**) Coronal T_1-weighted MR scan shows the right paraspinal mass arising from the psoas muscle. The mass produces signal approximately equal to that of normal skeletal muscle. There is intraspinal extension of the lesion at the L1–2 level on the right (arrows). The mass also causes elevation of the right kidney. (**B**) Coronal T_2-weighted image shows the mass to be of high signal intensity compared to skeletal muscle. The intraspinal component is well demonstrated (arrows).

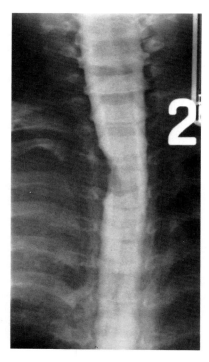

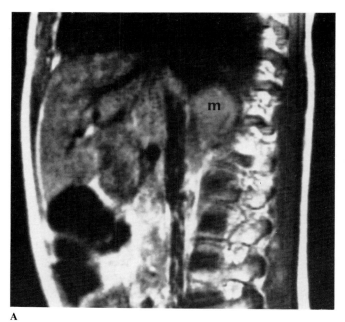

A

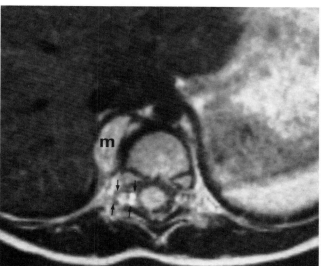

B

Fig. 2-80 Anteroposterior myelogram of the lower cervical and upper thoracic spine showing an epidural mass on the right at the T3–4 level. Note the large mass in the right upper mediastinum that contains flocculent areas of calcification. The right pedicles of T-3 and T-4 are eroded, as is the posterior portion of the right third rib. This is a paraspinal neuroblastoma.

Fig. 2-81 Paraspinal neuroblastoma. **(A)** Parasagittal T_1-weighted MR image shows a small mass (m) posterior to the inferior vena cava. **(B)** Axial T_2-weighted MR image shows the mass (m) to lie in the right paraspinal region. The mass is of bright signal on this image. Note the extension of tumor through the T12–L1 neural foramen (arrow) and effacement of the subarachnoid space on the right lateral aspect of the spinal cord.

manifested by motor signs, back pain, or sphincter dysfunction. Mild weakness may progress to complete paraplegia over a period of hours or days. Physical examination generally reveals a flaccid paraplegia, distention of the urinary bladder, and depressed deep tendon reflexes in the lower extremities. Because of the variability in the clinical presentation of spinal involvement, thorough imaging evaluation of the spine should be performed in all children who have a paraspinal tumor.

Radiographs usually show a paraspinal mass with or without bony erosion and destruction. Enlargement of one or more neural foramina is a strongly suggestive sign of intraspinal extension. If the intraspinal component is large, there may be focal widening of the spinal canal, thinning of the pedicles and laminae, and posterior vertebral body scalloping. With lesions in the thorax, the posterior ribs are usually eroded and thinned. Osseous metastatic disease may be present at the time of presentation.

Intraspinal extension is shown on myelography as an extradural mass (Fig. 2-80). If there is a complete block, an irregular serrated margin is demonstrated on myelography. CT myelography shows displacement of the cord and the subarachnoid space away from the extradural tumor. The tumor is usually calcified.[182]

Neural crest tumors usually produce moderate to low signal intensity on T_1-weighted images and high signal on T_2-weighted images. There is usually prominent enhancement

with intravenous gadopentate dimeglumine. Areas of calcification that are of sufficient size cause focal signal voids. Intraspinal extension is usually demonstrated as passage of a portion of the tumor through one or more neural foramina (Fig. 2-81). The involved foramina may be enlarged. The intraspinal component of the tumor is usually confined to the epidural space, with images showing elevation and displacement of the dura. T_2-weighted images may show high-signal edematous changes in the spinal cord if there is significant compression by the tumor.[165–167]

Vertebral Neoplasms

Neoplastic involvement of the osseous components of the spine can occur by three general mechanisms. The lesion may be a primary tumor (osteoblastoma, osteoid osteoma, aneurysmal bone cyst, osteosarcoma, Ewing sarcoma, fibrosarcoma, osteochondroma, chondrosarcoma, or chordoma); it may involve the spine from contiguous spread from an adjacent tumor (neuroblastoma, ganglioneuroma, germ cell tumor, or sarcoma); or it may be the result of a metastatic lesion from a remote primary tumor or systemic malignancy (neuroblastoma, leukemia, lymphoma, rhabdomyosarcoma, malignant germ cell tumor, Ewing sarcoma, or Wilms tumor). The imaging evaluation of these lesions should include radiographs as well as myelography, CT myelography, or MRI for the detection of intraspinal extension. Intraspinal involvement is usually confined to the epidural space (Figs. 2-82 and 2-83).[165–167,183]

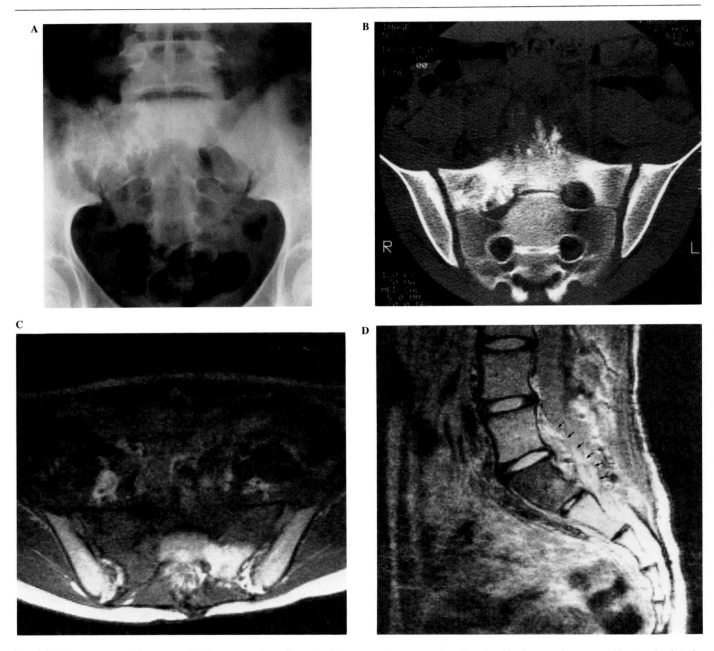

Fig. 2-82 Osteosarcoma of the sacrum. (**A**) Anteroposterior radiograph of the sacrum shows extensive sclerosis of the first sacral segment with extension into the right ala of the sacrum. (**B**) Unenhanced CT confirms the sclerosis of the first sacral segment. Note the extension of malignant new bone anteriorly from the sacrum and into the right S-1 neural foramen. (**C**) Axial T_1-weighted MR scan shows very low signal emanating from most of the S-1 vertebral body as a result of neoplastic replacement of the normal marrow. (**D**) Sagittal photon-density MR scan shows striking low signal from the S-1 vertebral body. Note the high-signal tumor extending into the epidural space posteriorly (arrows).

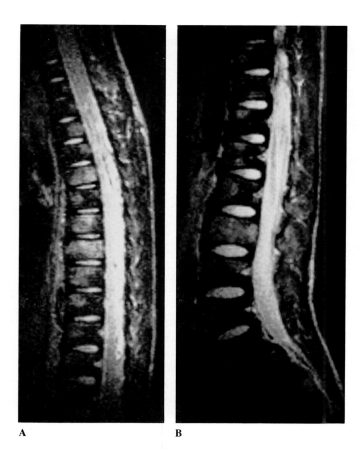

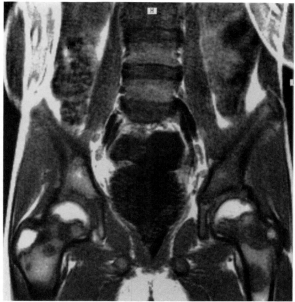

Fig. 2-83 Intraspinal involvement in vertebral neoplasm. Sagittal T_2-weighted MR scans of (**A**) the thoracic and (**B**) the lumbar spine show numerous irregular areas of bright signal in many vertebral bodies. The greatest involvement occurs in the L-3 vertebral body. The epidural space is normal. (**C**) Coronal T_1-weighted MR image of the pelvis shows numerous areas of low signal in the medullary spaces of the proximal femurs and the iliac bones. Only a small area of normal bright signal is seen in the right iliac bone. These changes were due to involvement of the hemopoietic marrow with Hodgkin disease.

Leukemia

Leukemia is the most common malignancy in childhood and involves the hemopoietic marrow. Because the axial skeleton is rich in red marrow, it is frequently affected in leukemia. The incidence and appearance of the radiographic changes of leukemia are highly variable and depend on the type of leukemia and the age of the patient.

A number of radiographic findings have been described in the axial skeleton in children with leukemia, including generalized osteopenia, vertebral body collapse, focal osteolytic lesions, osteosclerosis, and subchondral radiolucent bands. Generalized osteopenia is due to trabecular destruction by the leukemic process itself, resorption caused by marrow hyperplasia, or steroid therapy. Approximately 3% of patients with leukemia demonstrate vertebral body collapse at the time of clinical presentation.[184] This may be in the form of anterior wedging or biconcavity of the vertebral endplates.[185] Severe vertebral collapse and vertebra plana are uncommon findings in leukemia, however.

The focal osteolytic lesions that occur in patients with leukemia are difficult to detect. These lesions may be produced by focal bone destruction related to leukemic infiltration or by infarction due to vascular occlusion.[186] Osteosclerosis may be patchy, focal, or diffuse.[187]

Faint, thin radiolucent bands are occasionally identified in the subchondral portions of the vertebral bodies of children with leukemia. Because the subchondral region of the vertebral body is a metaphyseal equivalent, these bands correspond to similar radiolucencies seen in the metaphyses of the long bones. The bands parallel the vertebral margins and can be seen in both the superior and the inferior vertebral endplates.[188]

Occasionally, central nervous system leukemia may cause deposits of leukemic cells on the spinal cord and nerve roots. This most commonly occurs in the lumbar region, where it causes nerve root enlargement. Leukemia also may cause an extradural mass that compresses the thecal sac as a result of a focal chloroma.[189]

Osteoid Osteoma

Osteoid osteoma is a benign bone tumor that contains osteoid in a stroma of loose vascular connective tissue. This osteoid nidus may contain variable amounts of calcification. Surrounding the osteoid nidus is a zone of sclerotic, but otherwise normal, bone. Osteoid osteoma accounts for approximately 2% of all primary bone tumors of the axial skeleton other than myeloma. Approximately 10% of osteoid osteomas occur in the spine and sacrum, with the great majority occurring in patients younger than 25 years of age. The peak age is between 10 and 12 years. Fifty-nine percent of these lesions occur in the lumbar spine, 27% in the cervical spine, 12% in the thoracic spine, and 2% in the sacrum.[190,191]

Children with osteoid osteoma of the spine often present with backache that is worse at night and is relieved by aspirin.

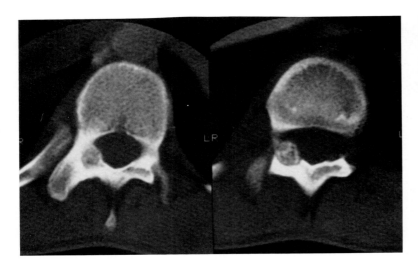

Fig. 2-84 Unenhanced CT scans showing a nidus of an osteoid osteoma in the right lamina of T-12. The nidus projects into the right side of the epidural space and is surrounded by dense reactive bone in the pedicle and in the lamina. The nidus contains several small, flocculent areas of calcification. This is the typical appearance of osteoid osteoma when it occurs in the spine.

The characteristic intense nature of the pain is related both to the vascular nature of the lesion, which causes increased local edema, and to the presence of nerve fibers in the nidus.[192] A localized scoliosis is usually present as a result of paravertebral muscular spasm and localized vertebral or paravertebral tenderness. The osteoid osteoma typically is located on the concave side of the scoliotic curve.[193] Neurologic abnormalities are found in more than 20% of cases.[194] A child who presents with painful scoliosis should always be evaluated for a possible vertebral lesion, such as osteoid osteoma, osteoblastoma, histiocytosis, osteomyelitis, and the like.

The radiographic features of osteoid osteoma of the spine are similar to those of such lesions in other regions of the skeletal system. Osteoid osteoma almost always arises in the vertebral arch.[195] Approximately 50% of vertebral lesions develop in the laminae or pedicles, and 20% occur in the articular processes. There is usually an associated mild scoliotic curve, with the convexity of the curve being oriented away from the side of the lesion.

The nidus of osteoid osteoma is 1 cm in size or smaller and is almost always radiolucent. The radiolucent nidus may not be visible on plain radiographs because of its small size and the surrounding sclerosis, but it is well demonstrated on thin-section CT images.[196] Areas of calcification in the nidus are sometimes identified on CT (Fig. 2-84). Bone scintigraphy shows marked uptake of tracer in the lesion on both blood pool and delayed images. In many cases, the nidus is demonstrated as a small focus of intense uptake that is surrounded by a larger area of moderate uptake in reactive sclerotic bone. Scintigraphy is extremely helpful in confirming the diagnosis or clarifying subtle radiographic findings.[75]

Osteoblastoma

Osteoblastoma refers to a vascular osteoid and bone-forming tumor containing numerous osteoblasts that have a benign histologic appearance. It occurs preferentially in the spine. This lesion constitutes less than 1% of all bone tumors. More than 40% of the reported cases are found in the spine. Like osteoid osteoma, osteoblastoma is associated with scoliosis in many cases; nearly 90% of lesions located in the thoracic or lumbar spine are associated with scoliosis. Osteoblastoma has also been reported in the long bones, the ribs, the calvaria, the facial bones, and the small bones of the hands and feet. Osteoblastoma that occurs in the spine usually involves the spinous and transverse processes. In some cases, the lesion is confined to the vertebral body. The average age at diagnosis is 17 years. Two-thirds of the patients are younger than 30 years of age.[197]

Histologically, osteoblastoma and osteoid osteoma are quite similar. They differ by site, size, and degree of sclerosis. The main characteristics of osteoblastoma are its larger size, its predilection for the spinous and transverse processes of the spine, and its lack of reactive bone formation. The last is the main feature that differentiates osteoblastoma radiographically from osteoid osteoma.

Painful scoliosis due to spasm of the paravertebral musculature is the most common presenting sign of this tumor.[198] Neurologic symptoms resulting from compression of the spinal cord or nerve roots, usually accompanied by adjacent muscle spasm, have been observed in approximately 50% of cases. Radicular pain also occurs in nearly half the patients.[194]

Plain radiographs show a well-circumscribed radiolucent rim that varies in size from 2 to 10 cm. The lesion frequently contains areas at different stages of new bone formation that may be accompanied by a soft tissue component and by a small amount of cortical new bone formation at the periphery. Like osteoid osteoma, osteoblastoma in the thoracic or lumbar region is located in the concavity of the scoliotic curve at or near its apex.

Bone scintigraphy shows a pattern that is similar, if not identical, to that of osteoid osteoma. The size of the lesion, however, is larger with osteoblastoma than osteoid osteoma. Imaging features include marked uptake of tracer in the lesion

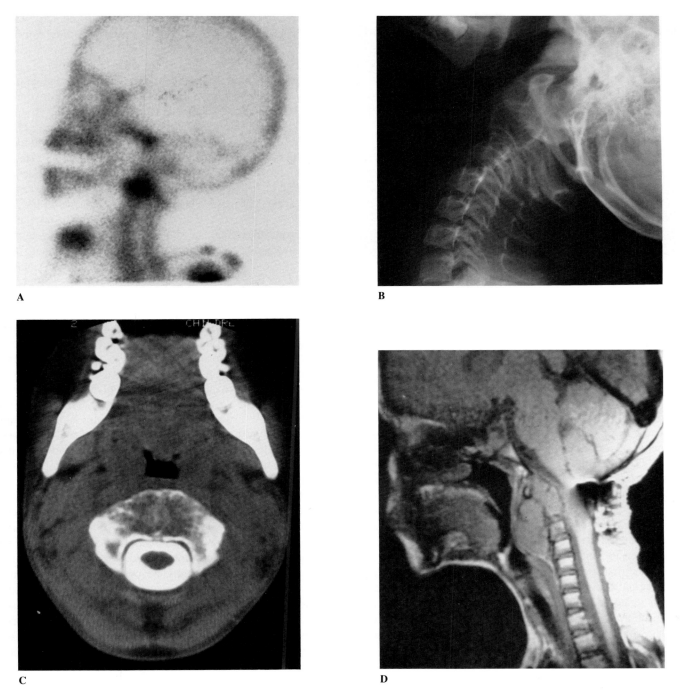

Fig. 2-85 Osteoblastoma. **(A)** Delayed image from bone scintigraphy shows increased tracer uptake in the body of C-2. **(B)** Lateral radiograph of the cervical spine shows expansion and low density of the body and dens of C-2. **(C)** CT myelogram shows expansion and irregular lucency of C-2. There is no intraspinal extension. **(D)** Sagittal T_1-weighted MR scan obtained several months later, after biopsy and posterior fusion, shows a large prevertebral soft tissue mass extending from C-2. The signal void seen posteriorly is due to a fixation wire. This lesion was an aggressive osteoblastoma.

on both blood pool and delayed images. Unlike the situation with osteoid osteoma, a central nidus is rarely demonstrable in an osteoblastoma. Normal bone scintigraphy in a patient with painful scoliosis virtually excludes osteoid osteoma or osteoblastoma as the etiology.[199]

CT or MRI provides information concerning the exact location of the tumor in the spine as well as the status of the surrounding tissues. Osteoblastoma can expand or destroy the cortex and compress adjacent nerve roots or the spinal cord (Figs. 2-85 and 2-86).

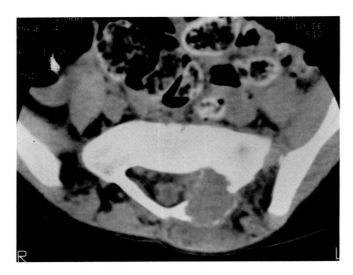

Fig. 2-86 Unenhanced CT of the upper sacrum showing expansion and partial destruction of the left lamina. There is a soft tissue mass that extends into the epidural space and the posterior paraspinal region. Osteoblastoma typically arises in the posterior elements.

Sacrococcygeal Teratoma

Sacrococcygeal teratoma is the most common solid tumor in the neonatal period, having an overall incidence of between 1 in 35,000 and 1 in 40,000 births. There is a striking female preponderance; between 70% and 85% of affected infants are girls. An increased incidence of congenital anomalies has been documented in children with sacrococcygeal teratoma (12% to 18%). These associated anomalies have been reported in all organ systems and range from minor to life threatening.[200–202]

Between 50% and 70% of sacrococcygeal teratomas present during the first few days of life. Large lesions may interfere with vaginal delivery. It is not uncommon for a large sacrococcygeal teratoma to be detected on prenatal sonography.[203] Initial clinical detection of sacrococcygeal teratoma beyond the age of 2 years occurs in 6% or less of cases; initial detection in adulthood is distinctly rare.

The sacrococcygeal region is the most common location of a teratoma; sacrococcygeal teratoma accounts for 40% to 70% of all teratomas. Other locations include the gonads, mediastinum, neck, retroperitoneum, and intracranial structures. As a general rule, teratomas develop in midline or paraxial locations.

By definition, a teratoma is a tumor composed of tissues that are derived from all three germinal layers. These neoplasms are composed of tissues of variable degrees of maturation and organization, with cells of embryonal, fetal, and adult character being contained in a single tumor. Differentiation of ectodermal elements can produce teeth, squamous epithelium, and neural tissue; mesodermal elements can produce bone, cartilage, and muscle; and endodermal elements can produce gastrointestinal and respiratory epithelium and mucous glands. Although most of these tumors are benign, malignancy may develop from cells of any of the three germinal layers. The benign and malignant forms of these tumors can be grouped under the designation of germ cell tumors.

There are three general theories concerning the etiology of teratomas. One theory holds that teratomas arise from embryonic totipotent cells that originate in Hensen node. It is suggested that some of these cells do not migrate normally, escape normal hormonal developmental constraints, and ultimately exhibit uninhibited growth. The most caudal extent of Hensen node is the region of the coccyx; this is thought to be a factor in the high incidence of teratomas in the sacrococcygeal region.

A second proposed theory is that a teratoma arises from primitive germ cells that originate in the yolk sac during embryonic development. These cells progressively migrate from the yolk sac to the hindgut wall, the urogenital ridge, and, eventually, the gonad. Arrest of migration of some of these cells in an abnormal location may result in pathogenetic development of these cells and result in the formation of a teratoma.

A third theory attributes teratomas to an abnormal segmentation of the blastomere. This theory suggests that some teratomas may represent an incomplete attempt at twinning. This theory is supported by an increased family history of twinning in patients with sacrococcygeal teratomas.

Most sacrococcygeal teratomas are benign. Benign teratomas are further classified histologically into mature and immature types. Areas of poorly differentiated embryonic tissues are found in the immature type. There is some evidence that immature teratomas have a greater risk of becoming malignant compared to the mature type.

The malignant neoplasms that are related to teratomas are of germ cell derivation and are termed malignant germ cell tumors. About 15% to 30% of sacrococcygeal germ cell tumors are malignant. Malignant types of teratoma are extremely rare in the newborn period. The incidence of malignancy increases significantly beyond the age of 2 months. Most pediatric malignant germ cell tumors are classified histologically as endodermal sinus or yolk sac tumors. Anaplastic carcinoma or malignancies arising from differentiated cell lines in the teratoma, such as neuroblastoma, are rare.[204]

Sacrococcygeal teratomas arise from and are attached to the anterior portion of the coccyx. Most often, the tumor grows posteriorly and inferiorly to produce an external mass. Growth in an anterior and superior direction results in intrapelvic or intra-abdominal components. A classification system for the gross morphology of sacrococcygeal teratomas has been developed by the Surgical Section of the American Academy of Pediatrics.[205] According to this system, a type I teratoma is predominantly external and has little or no presacral component. A type II tumor is dumbbell shaped and has both significant external and intrapelvic components. A type III tumor has a small external component; most of the lesion lies in the intrapelvic and intra-abdominal spaces. A type IV tumor occupies the presacral and intra-abdominal spaces and has no significant external component. The incidence of malignancy varies significantly with type (Table 2-2).

Table 2-2 Sacrococcygeal Teratoma

Type	Incidence (%)	Incidence of Malignancy (%)
I	47–58	5–8
II	23–35	7–32
III	8–15	21–34
IV	8–10	38–42

Malignant sacrococcygeal germ cell tumors are more common in boys. The incidence of malignancy increases with increasing patient age. The composition of the tumor is also a factor. Purely cystic sacrococcygeal teratomas are usually benign, whereas there is a high incidence of malignancy in purely solid lesions. Teratomas that are of mixed cystic and solid composition are usually benign. Calcification occurs in most benign lesions but only rarely in malignant germ cell tumors.[206]

There is a specific malformation complex (Currarino syndrome) of which sacrococcygeal teratoma may be a component.[207] This complex is a triad characterized by three main features: (1) a congenital anorectal stenosis or other low anorectal malformation; (2) a curvilinear anterior sacral defect; and (3) a presacral mass that may be a meningocele, a teratoma, an enteric cyst, or a combination of these. The malformation complex is frequently familial, although expression of the abnormality varies among family members.

Current imaging techniques allow accurate classification of a sacrococcygeal teratoma according to the staging system of the American Academy of Pediatrics.[208] In this respect, diagnostic imaging aids in surgical planning and also provides important prognostic information. Radiographic signs that are suggestive of benign histology include large cystic components, dense calcification, and a predominantly external location of the mass. Radiographic signs that are suggestive of malignancy include predominantly solid composition, infiltration of adjacent structures, predominantly intrapelvic location, necrosis, lymphadenopathy, and lack of calcification.

Calcification is radiographically visible in at least 50% of sacrococcygeal teratomas. Cystography, excretory urography, and barium gastrointestinal tract studies are occasionally useful for the evaluation of displacement or invasion of adjacent pelvic and abdominal structures. Because intrapelvic extension of sacrococcygeal teratomas occurs between the sacrum and the rectum, the rectum is displaced anteriorly and compressed. Although sacrococcygeal teratomas arise from the coccyx, radiographic abnormalities of the sacrum and coccyx usually are not seen (Fig. 2-87). In rare cases, myelography is helpful for the evaluation of possible intraspinal extension of the neoplasm. A malignant sacrococcygeal teratoma may invade the caudal foramen to involve sacral neural foramina.

Sonography is a rapid and simple technique to characterize and define the intrapelvic extent of a sacrococcygeal teratoma. The sonographic appearance of the mass varies greatly according to the tumor composition. Cystic teratomas are usually multiloculated, although there may be one or two dominant cysts. Debris or fluid-fluid levels may be identified in the cysts. Also, the echogenicity often varies somewhat among individual cysts in the same mass. Calcifications are suggested by areas of acoustic shadowing. Predominantly solid teratomas are frequently heterogeneous sonographically; areas of altered echogenicity may be present, representing necrosis or hemorrhage (Fig. 2-88). Hydronephrosis may result from infiltration or compression of the lower urinary tract.

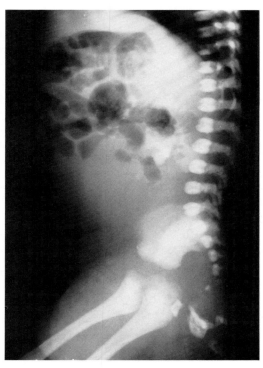

Fig. 2-87 Lateral radiograph of the lumbar spine of a neonate who had a visible external mass showing areas of calcification and ossification inferior to the tip of the sacrum. A large intra-abdominal component is suggested by superior displacement of bowel. The spine appears normal. The character and location of the areas of calcification are typical of sacrococcygeal teratoma.

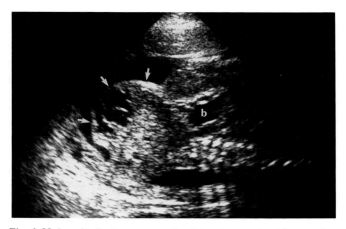

Fig. 2-88 Longitudinal sonogram of a fetus at approximately gestation week 30 showing a complex mass (arrows) anterior and inferior to the sacrum. The mass has sonolucent areas, representing cysts, and other areas of bright echoes, suggesting calcification. There is no gross intra-abdominal extension. The bladder (b) is in a normal position. Many cases of sacrococcygeal teratoma are identified prenatally.

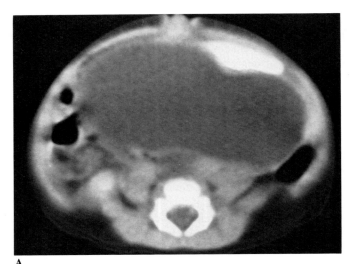

A

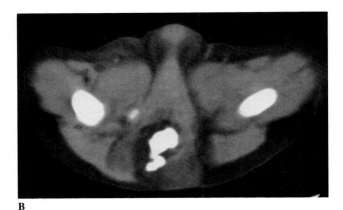

B

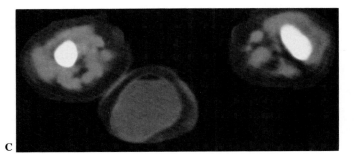

C

Fig. 2-89 Sacrococcygeal teratoma. (**A**) Contrast-enhanced CT scan of the lower abdomen shows a large bilobed cyst posterior to the urinary bladder. (**B**) Image through the floor of the pelvis shows a mass containing dense calcification and fat just beneath the tip of the coccyx. The lesion lies slightly to the right of the midline. (**C**) A more caudal image shows a fat-fluid level in the external component of this large sacrococcygeal teratoma. The predominantly cystic composition and the areas of calcification and fat favor a benign histology.

CT is also an excellent method for characterizing sacrococcygeal teratomas and is the most sensitive imaging modality for the detection of calcification. Areas of fat, fluid, hemorrhage, and necrosis are well demonstrated. As with sonography, the CT attenuation characteristics frequently vary among individual cysts, and fluid-fluid levels are sometimes seen. The size of the intrapelvic component and the presence of infiltration or displacement of pelvic structures are usually well demonstrated on CT (Fig. 2-89). Viewing of bone window images is important for the detection of spinal destruction or invasion.

MRI clearly shows the intimate association of the neoplasm with the coccyx on sagittal images (Fig. 2-90). Sagittal imaging is also particularly well suited for the depiction of the degree of intrapelvic extension and the accurate classification of tumor morphology according to the American Academy of Pediatrics system. MRI allows detection of intraspinal extension and obviates the need for intrathecal contrast media. It is not as sensitive as CT for the detection of calcifications, but calcifications that are of sufficient size produce a signal void. Areas of fat, subacute hemorrhage, or proteinaceous fluid produce high signal intensity on both T_1- and T_2-weighted images. Simple cysts are imaged as low signal on T_1-weighted images and high signal on T_2-weighted images.[165,167,209]

The familial malformation complex that includes a presacral teratoma (Currarino syndrome) can be suggested radiographically by the presence of an anterior sacral defect. The radiographic appearance has been described as a scimitar-shaped, crescentic, or sickle-shaped deformity of the sacrum.

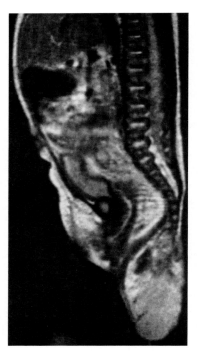

Fig. 2-90 Proton-density sagittal MR scan showing a complex mass arising from the tip of the coccyx. The mass is entirely extrapelvic. Areas of low signal in the mass are due to calcifications. There are also intermediate-signal cystic components and areas of fat signal. This is a benign type I sacrococcygeal teratoma.

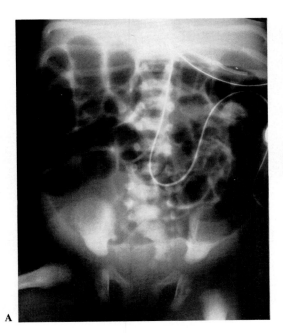

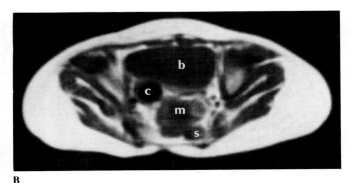

B

Fig. 2-91 Currarino syndrome. **(A)** Anteroposterior radiograph of the abdomen of a neonate with rectal atresia shows hypoplasia of the right side of the sacrum, causing a sicklelike deformity. The bowel proximal to the atretic rectum is distended. **(B)** T_1-weighted MR scan shows a small mass (m) anterior to the sacrum (s), which lies to the left of the midline. The mass lies posterior to the bladder (b) and to the left of the distal colon (c). The mass was a small sacrococcygeal teratoma.

The associated teratoma lies immediately adjacent to the osseous sacral defect. These teratomas are of the presacral variety (type IV). Despite the intrapelvic location of these tumors, the teratomas associated with this syndrome are almost invariably benign, in contradistinction to the relatively high incidence of malignancy with other totally intrapelvic sacrococcygeal teratomas. Anorectal stenosis or atresia also is found in these children (Fig. 2-91).

INFECTION

Osteomyelitis

Involvement of the spine with osteomyelitis in infants and children is much less common than involvement of the long bones. Although infection of the spine usually occurs from hematogenous spread of microorganisms, it may also develop after lumbar puncture, spinal surgery, penetrating trauma, paravertebral abscess formation, or urinary tract infection. The spine is the most common site of bone and joint infection among patients on renal dialysis, even though the incidence of this complication is low.[210]

Although three-quarters of all cases of osteomyelitis occur in children, vertebral osteomyelitis is rare in this age group.[211] Osteomyelitis of the vertebra is more common in the 10- to 15-year age group and among adults 20 to 60 years of age. Spinal osteomyelitis accounts for approximately 2% to 4% of all cases of osteomyelitis.[212] Osteomyelitis of the spine almost invariably involves the vertebral bodies but also may involve the posterior elements. Localized disease of the posterior elements without involvement of the vertebral body is rare.

The location of osteomyelitis in all age groups is determined by the marrow distribution and the vascular supply of the bone marrow. In the young child, all bone marrow is red marrow. As the child ages, marrow conversion occurs and is complete by 20 to 25 years of age. In adults, the axial skeleton has a greater proportion of the total supply of red marrow. The regional marrow blood supply is directly related to the amount of red marrow. These factors, at least in part, account for the greater relative frequency of spinal osteomyelitis in adults compared to children.[213]

In decreasing order of frequency, vertebral osteomyelitis occurs in the lumbar, thoracic, and cervical regions. The subchondral area of the vertebral body, a metaphyseal equivalent, is typically the initial site of infection. Hematogenous spread of infection to the spine is usually by the arterial route, although venous spread via paraspinal and intraspinal venous plexi has been implicated in some cases. There is a rich intraosseous arterial supply to the subchondral areas that have numerous anastomoses in infants and young children. These areas of anastomosis involute with increasing age during childhood and adolescence, leaving the arterial branches to the vertebral bodies as end arteries.[214,215]

The mechanism postulated for the development of vertebral osteomyelitis implicates a septic microembolus traveling in the arterial system that becomes lodged in the metaphyseal arteries in the subchondral portion of a vertebral body. The septic microembolus forms a small wedge-shaped septic infarct in the bone. Among infants and young children, the extensive intraosseous anastomoses in the subchondral areas prevent the formation of the large infarctions that may occur among older patients. Bone infarction is essential in the development of osteomyelitis of the vertebral body.

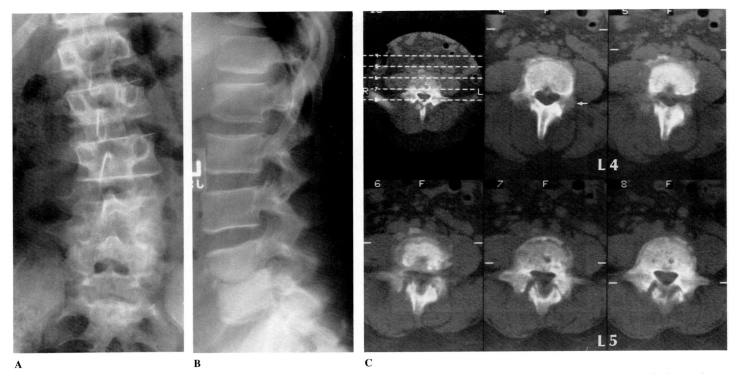

A   B   C

Fig. 2-92 Osteomyelitis. (**A**) Anteroposterior and (**B**) lateral radiographs of the lumbar spine of an adolescent with fever and low back pain show marked narrowing of the L4–5 interspace with irregularity and blurring of the adjacent vertebral margins. The L-4 vertebral body is also displaced slightly forward and to the left. (**C**) Unenhanced CT scans show permeative destruction of the vertebral bodies. The apophyseal joints are also irregular and narrowed. A small soft tissue mass (arrow) is seen posterior to the L-4 pedicle on the left. Vertebral osteomyelitis in adolescents is frequently accompanied by significant bone destruction. In this patient, ankylosis of these vertebral bodies eventually occurred.

The clinical and radiographic changes that are seen in infants and children with vertebral osteomyelitis are usually mild compared to those that occur in adults. The rate and severity of progression of infection in the spine depend on the virulence of the organism and the response of the host.

Numerous organisms have been cultured from vertebral osteomyelitis. The most common offending organism in children and adults is *Staphylococcus aureus*. Other gram-positive organisms, such as *Streptococcus pneumoniae* and other streptococci, and gram-negative organisms, such as *Escherichia coli* and species of *Pseudomonas, Salmonella,* and *Klebsiella,* are much less common. β-Hemolytic streptococcal infection usually affects infants from a few weeks to 2 months of age.[216] *Staphylococcus aureus* is still the most common offending organism in this age group.[217]

Pyogenic osteomyelitis of the vertebral body tends to be an aggressive infection, although some organisms and infections that are partially treated may have a more indolent course. Radiographs are usually normal early in the course of the illness because the infection begins in the subchondral zone of the vertebral body. The first radiographic finding in spinal infection is usually narrowing of the intervertebral disc space. This is believed to be due to the release of proteolytic enzymes that destroy the disc.[218] This process usually begins within days or weeks of the onset of infection. The margins of the vertebral endplate become indistinct, and destruction of the subchondral bone becomes more evident within 1 to 2 weeks of the onset of the infection. These osseous changes are most prominent in the anterior two-thirds of the vertebral body.

As the infection progresses, the vertebral body endplates eventually show bony destruction, cortical permeation, and blurring of the disc space margins (Fig. 2-92). The affected vertebra may show a decrease in height. Extension of the inflammatory process into the soft tissues frequently produces a paravertebral or epidural mass. With healing, the involved vertebra usually shows extensive sclerosis. Eventually, fusion of the involved vertebra with the adjacent vertebra may occur. Calcification in a paraspinal mass is more frequently identified in tuberculous osteomyelitis.

Occasionally, vertebral infection may involve a pedicle or neural arch. The response of the bone to the infection may be sclerotic or lytic, depending on the pathologic process produced. If there is sclerosis of a pedicle, the differential diagnosis includes osteoid osteoma, osteoblastoma, and stress changes contralateral to a defect in the pars interarticularis defect (Wilkinson syndrome).

Radionuclide bone imaging is frequently helpful in the evaluation of spinal osteomyelitis.[219] Scintigraphy shows prominent tracer uptake in a single vertebral body or two adjoining vertebral bodies. If the infection has formed a paravertebral abscess, there may be extended uptake of tracer in the paravertebral region.

MRI is also helpful in assessing spinal infections. This technique is particularly useful for detection of epidural extension and paraspinal abscess formation. On T_1-weighted images, the normal marrow signal is decreased. T_2-weighted images show increased signal in the involved portion of the vertebra, representing edema. Extraosseous extension of infection also produces high signal intensity on T_2-weighted images.[220–222]

Discitis

Discitis is a term that has been applied to symptomatic narrowing of the intervertebral disc space in children. It is a syndrome of uncertain etiology, although many investigators hold that it is the result of an infectious process. The L4–5 interspace is the most common site of involvement; this level accounts for about 40% of cases. The L5–S1 interspace is the next most frequently involved site. Involvement of the thoracolumbar region also may occur.[223]

The mean age of onset of discitis is about 5 years, although the range extends from infancy to adolescence. The symptoms include refusal to walk or complaints of vague pain in the buttocks, thigh, or knee. There is often point tenderness over the spine as well. Many of these symptoms are often partially relieved when the patient assumes a supine position. There is often a mild leukocytosis and elevation of the erythrocyte sedimentation rate.[224–226]

Microorganisms can gain access to the intervertebral disc in several ways. Some investigators hold that hematogenous seeding occurs via subchondral vascular channels that extend through the vertebral endplates into the discs. These vascular channels have been identified in children up to 8 years of age and, on occasion, have been found in adults up to 30 years of age.[227] Other investigators state that there are vessels that enter the intervertebral disc laterally and have terminal capillaries that ramify in the annulus fibrosus. These vascular channels are arranged in a radial fashion and are independent of the vascular supply of the endplate of the vertebral body. In addition to a direct hematogenous route, intervertebral disc infection in children and young adults also may occur by direct extension through the cartilaginous endplate from the subchondral bone (metaphyseal equivalent) in the form of vertebral osteomyelitis with secondary infection of the disc.

Discitis and vertebral osteomyelitis generally occur as clinically distinct syndromes. Discitis often has a much milder course compared to vertebral osteomyelitis. Partial or complete restoration of the disc height usually occurs with healing, and intervertebral body fusion is not as common as with vertebral osteomyelitis.

There is controversy regarding the proper management of discitis. An infecting organism is occasionally identified by blood culture or disc biopsy in patients with discitis. Some authorities suggest bed rest and intravenous antibiotic therapy after confirmation of the diagnosis and drawing of blood cultures; antibiotics are continued even if the blood cultures are negative. Others hold that open surgical or closed needle biopsy of the abnormal disc space should be performed for culture and sensitivity studies before the institution of antibiotic therapy.

There is usually a rapid response to antibiotic therapy. This usually favorable response supports the proposed bacterial etiology of most cases of discitis. Prolonged immobilization usually is not advocated for the young child who has responded to antibiotics.[228]

Early in the course of discitis, radiographs of the spine are normal. Bone scintigraphy shows increased uptake in the vertebral bodies on each side of the involved disc and may be positive as early as 48 hours after the onset of symptoms.[229] The earliest radiographic finding is a subtle decrease in height of the disc space. The shortest interval between the onset of symptoms and the appearance of radiographic findings is at least 10 days. Within several weeks of the onset of symptoms, radiographs show definite narrowing of the intervertebral disc space and irregular erosions of the adjacent vertebral endplates (Fig. 2-93). Follow-up radiographs after several weeks to months show narrowing of the intervertebral disc space and sclerotic changes in the adjacent vertebral bodies. With healing, a variable degree of the disc height eventually may be restored.[227,230]

MISCELLANEOUS CONDITIONS

Herniated Disc

Intervertebral disc herniation in infants and children is extremely uncommon. It is presumably due to trauma superimposed on early degenerative changes. The onset of symptoms in childhood cases is most often between the ages of 11 and 16 years. There is a slight male predominance. The involved disc is almost always in the lower lumbar region. Many herniated discs in children are related to athletic activities.[231]

Because the index of suspicion for lumbar disc herniation among children is low, there is often a delay in diagnosis. Sciatica, back pain, or both are the initial clinical manifestations. Twenty percent of patients never experience back pain, but virtually all develop sciatica at some time in the course of the disease. Bilateral sciatica occurs in almost half the patients.

The physical findings in disc herniation may include diminished lumbar lordosis, paravertebral muscle spasm, and scoliosis. Some effort is made to hold the lumbar spine rigid in almost every patient. Point tenderness may be elicited over the involved disc space. Straight-leg raising routinely provokes sciatica. Sensation to pin prick may be diminished in the distribution of the L-5 and S-1 dermatomes. The ankle tendon reflexes are diminished or absent in more than half the cases.

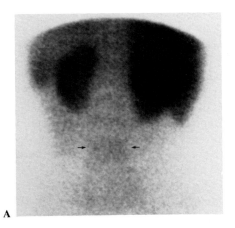

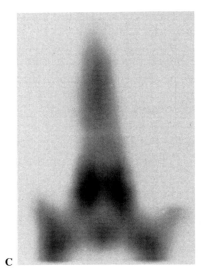

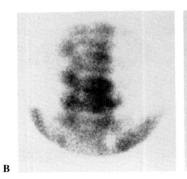 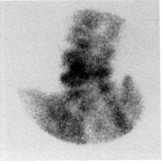

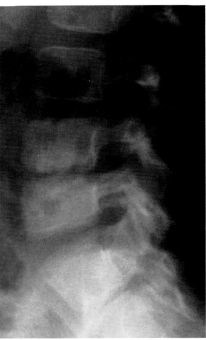

Fig. 2-93 Childhood discitis. (**A**) Posterior blood pool image from bone scintigraphy shows minimally increased activity at the L4–5 level (arrows). (**B**) Oblique delayed pinhole images show markedly increased activity of the L-4 and L-5 vertebral bodies on both sides of the disc space. (**C**) Coronal SPECT image confirms the increased activity at the L4–5 interspace. (**D**) Lateral radiograph of the lumbar spine 2 weeks later shows definite narrowing of the L4–5 interspace. The adjacent vertebral endplates are slightly irregular.

Radiographs in cases of lumbar disc herniation may show loss of the normal lumbar lordosis as a result of muscle spasm and mild to moderate scoliosis. Frequently, radiographs and skeletal scintigraphy are normal. Myelography shows an extradural defect at the level of the involved disc. Disc herniations in children are often quite large and produce a prominent central or lateral extradural mass.

Disc herniation is depicted better on MRI than on any other imaging modality. The normal disc produces low signal intensity on T_1-weighted images and high signal on T_2-weighted images, reflecting the high water content of the nucleus pulposus compared to the adjacent bone marrow. The annulus fibrosus produces lower signal on T_2-weighted images than the central nucleus. Abnormal discs can be classified on MRI as having an annular bulge or as being herniated. The distinction between a bulging annulus fibrosus and a herniated disc is important because a bulging disc is considered less significant clinically and is less often associated with sciatica than a herniated disc. Herniated discs are further characterized as being protruded or extruded or as forming a free fragment.[232–234]

Posterior bulging of the annulus fibrosus is the result of disc degeneration with a grossly intact, albeit lax, annulus fibrosus. Bulging of the annulus is recognized on MRI as a generalized extension of the disc margin beyond the margins of the vertebral endplates, regardless of the signal characteristics of the disc. The margins of the disc are usually smooth and symmetric.

A protruded disc refers to herniation of the nucleus pulposus through a defect in the annulus, producing a focal extension of material at the disc margin. The signal intensity of the parent nucleus pulposus is usually decreased, as is the intensity of the extradural defect, particularly on T_2-weighted images. These protrusions may be located centrally or laterally with respect to the disc space (Fig. 2-94).

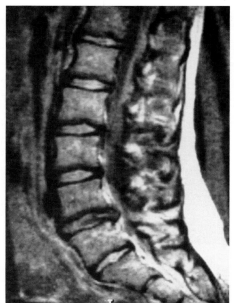

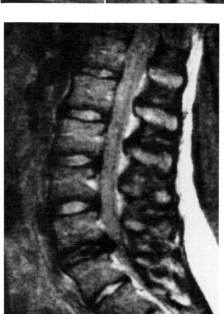

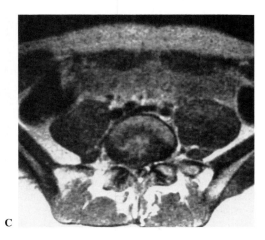

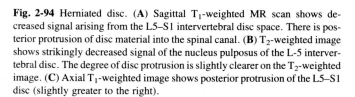

Fig. 2-94 Herniated disc. (**A**) Sagittal T₁-weighted MR scan shows decreased signal arising from the L5–S1 intervertebral disc space. There is posterior protrusion of disc material into the spinal canal. (**B**) T₂-weighted image shows strikingly decreased signal of the nucleus pulposus of the L-5 intervertebral disc. The degree of disc protrusion is slightly clearer on the T₂-weighted image. (**C**) Axial T₁-weighted image shows posterior protrusion of the L5–S1 disc (slightly greater to the right).

An extruded disc refers to more marked herniation of material from the nucleus pulposus, producing an anterior extradural mass that remains attached to the nucleus pulposus, often by way of a high-signal pedicle as seen on T₂-weighted images. The signal intensity of the extruded portion of disc may be increased or decreased on T₂-weighted images. The disc usually remains contained by the posterior longitudinal ligament and the remaining contiguous portions of the annulus fibrosus; these structures are frequently identified as curvilinear areas of decreased signal on T₂-weighted images.

The term *free fragment* refers to disc material that is external to the annulus fibrosus and no longer contiguous with the nucleus pulposus from which it was extruded. Free fragments can lie anterior to the posterior longitudinal ligament, especially if they have migrated behind the vertebral bodies. They also may lie posterior to the posterior longitudinal ligament. Rarely, they may lie intradurally.

Intervertebral Disc Calcification

The precise etiology of intervertebral disc calcification in childhood is unknown, but many cases probably are related to inflammation that causes calcification in the nucleus pulposus. Trauma most often is implicated as the primary causative factor in children. Other conditions that may be associated with disc calcification in children include block vertebrae, vitamin D poisoning, degenerative disease, healing discitis, and alkaptonuria. These conditions are readily distinguished by the clinical history and radiographic appearance. There is an increased frequency of disc calcification in boys, in whom the cervical spine is most often involved. There is a uniform incidence distribution throughout the spine in girls. The average age at diagnosis is approximately 8 years.

Patients with an intervertebral disc space calcification may or may not exhibit symptoms. The clinical findings may include pain, stiffness, limitation of motion, muscle spasm, tenderness, or torticollis. These symptoms are frequent among children with cervical disc calcification but rarely occur in cases of thoracic or lumbar disc calcification. The symptoms usually appear when the calcification, for some unknown reason, begins to resorb or herniate. The clinical symptoms may mimic meningitis, bacterial osteomyelitis, or discitis.

Rupture of the calcific collections into the adjacent vertebral bodies or soft tissues is occasionally identified. The herniation

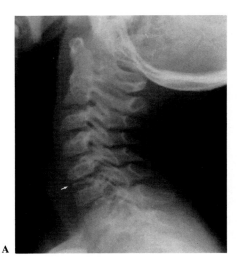 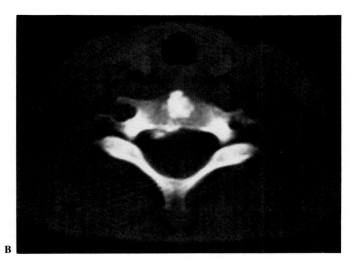

Fig. 2-95 Intervertebral disc calcification in the cervical region. (A) Lateral radiograph of the cervical spine of an 8-year-old boy shows calcification of the C5–6 intervertebral disc (arrow). (B) Unenhanced CT confirms the disc calcification and demonstrates posterior protrusion of a portion of the calcified disc.

may extend anteriorly or posteriorly. This herniation seems to be part of the pathologic process rather than a complication. The herniation undergoes spontaneous resorption with conservative therapy, and the symptoms disappear.

The radiographic appearance of intervertebral disc calcification is usually characteristic. The calcification may be round, oval, flattened, or fragmented. Herniated calcifications may be identified adjacent to the disc space. CT provides superior demonstration of the location and character of the calcifications (Fig. 2-95). MRI is also helpful for detecting protrusion of disc material into the spinal canal.[235,236]

Scheuermann Disease

Scheuermann disease (juvenile or adolescent kyphosis) is a pathologic entity that consists of primary irregularity of the ossification centers of the vertebral endplates. This entity may or may not be associated with symptoms. The changes in the vertebrae include wedging, kyphosis, and Schmorl nodes. The etiology remains unknown, although there is some evidence that the central Schmorl nodes, marginal Schmorl nodes, and irregular ossification of the vertebral endplates are the result of different mechanisms. Many of the changes in Scheuermann disease may be traced to stress changes related to traumatic growth arrest and endplate fractures resulting from the heightened vulnerability of the spine during periods of rapid growth. Marginal Schmorl nodes are due to trauma, and central Schmorl nodes correlate with dynamic stress applied to the spine in the erect position. The irregular ossification, wedging, and kyphosis are probably due to a static load applied to the flexed spine in the sitting position. The irregular endplates are caused by disturbed cell vectoring related to traumatic growth arrest and microfractures.[237,238]

Scheuermann disease occurs in 3% to 5% of otherwise healthy adolescents. Several contiguous vertebrae are usually involved. The disease may occur anywhere from T-4 to L-4, but the greatest frequency is at T-7 to T-10. Lumbar involvement is often accompanied by scoliosis. The disease is slightly more common in boys.

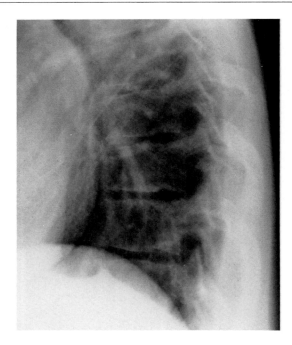

Fig. 2-96 Lateral radiograph of the thoracic spine of an adolescent boy showing irregularity of the superior and inferior endplates of the lower thoracic vertebrae. This has caused mild anterior wedging of these vertebral bodies and has resulted in a mild thoracic kyphosis. This is the usual radiographic appearance of Scheuermann disease.

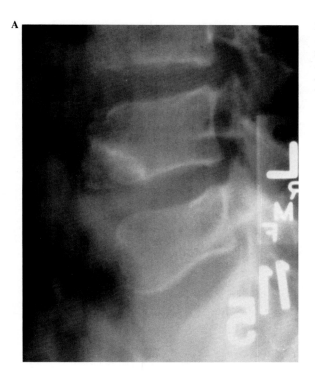

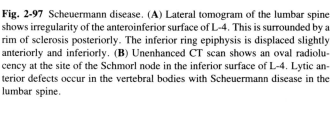

Fig. 2-97 Scheuermann disease. **(A)** Lateral tomogram of the lumbar spine shows irregularity of the anteroinferior surface of L-4. This is surrounded by a rim of sclerosis posteriorly. The inferior ring epiphysis is displaced slightly anteriorly and inferiorly. **(B)** Unenhanced CT scan shows an oval radiolucency at the site of the Schmorl node in the inferior surface of L-4. Lytic anterior defects occur in the vertebral bodies with Scheuermann disease in the lumbar spine.

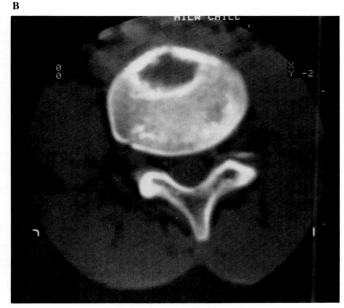

disease, lytic anterior vertebral body defects are identified in the superior or inferior endplates (Fig. 2-97).

Limbus Vertebra

The limbus vertebra is due to protrusion of a portion of the intervertebral disc into the vertebral body between the cartilaginous endplate of the ring epiphysis and the border of the adjacent vertebral rim. Limbus vertebra is asymptomatic and does not cause spinal deformity or growth disturbance. It is important not to mistake this malformation for a destructive lesion or an acute fracture.

Radiographically, the limbus vertebra appears as a triangular osseous density adjacent to the vertebral body endplate. Both the limbus vertebra and the adjacent vertebral body have sclerotic margins; this helps in the differentiation from an acute fracture. This abnormality is most frequently identified along the anterosuperior aspects of the midlumbar vertebral bodies, but it may also occur laterally, posteriorly, or inferiorly.

Spinal Stenosis

Developmental stenosis of the spinal canal results in an overall reduction in the caliber of the spinal canal. This is greatest in the anteroposterior dimension. In the cervical region, stenosis usually becomes symptomatic in adults when a myelopathy occurs as a result of compression of the cervical cord. A prompt diagnosis is necessary to allow for surgical decompression to reduce the risk of neurologic deficits.[239]

Numerical criteria have been determined for the sagittal measurements of the cervical spinal canal.[240] Similar criteria have been developed for measurement of the sagittal diameter of the lumbar spinal canal.[241] In the cervical spine, a myelopathy is more likely to occur if the midsagittal diameter of the cervical spinal canal is 10 mm or less. In the lumbar spine, spinal stenosis is more frequent in the lower lumbar region, particularly at L-4, but may involve the L-3 to L-5 levels. The pedicles are short and enlarged in diameter as well. Patients who have a midsagittal diameter in the lumbar spine of 15 mm or less are prone to develop clinical spinal stenosis (Figs. 2-98 and 2-99).

Radiographically the superior and inferior vertebral margins are irregular, and multiple Schmorl nodes are seen. The intervertebral disc height may be decreased, with kyphosis and wedge-shaped vertebrae developing (Fig. 2-96). The diagnosis of Scheuermann disease is indicated when radiographs show anterior wedging of greater than 5° of three or more contiguous vertebrae and a structural kyphosis of greater than 40°. Endplate erosions and vertebral body wedging are not seen in cases of postural kyphosis. With lumbar Scheuermann

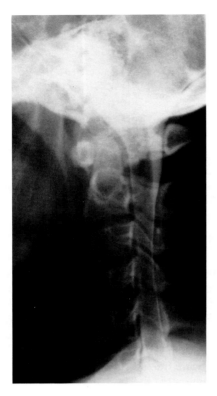

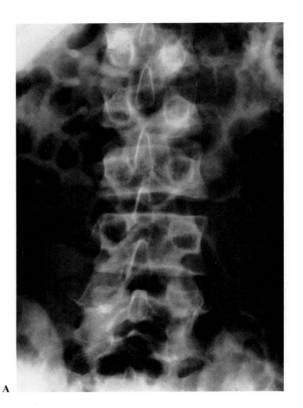

Fig. 2-98 Lateral cervical myelogram showing severe spinal stenosis, which is most marked in the midcervical region. This has narrowed the subarachnoid space and compressed the spinal cord.

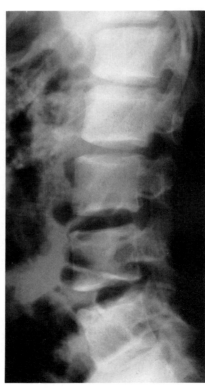

Fig. 2-99 Lumbar spinal stenosis. (**A**) Anteroposterior and (**B**) lateral radiographs of the lumbar spine of an adolescent show foreshortening of the length of the pedicles. The pedicles are also enlarged and rounded in configuration. This has narrowed the spinal canal in the anteroposterior and lateral dimensions.

REFERENCES

1. Moore KL. The articular and skeletal systems. In: *The Developing Human.* 3rd ed. Philadelphia: Saunders; 1982:344–360.

2. Dryden RJ. Duplication of the spinal cord: a discussion of the possible embryogenesis of diplomyelia. *Dev Med Child Neurol.* 1980;22:234–243.

3. Dolan KD. Developmental abnormalities of the cervical spine below the axis. *Radiol Clin North Am.* 1977;15:167–175.

4. Fietti VG, Fielding JW. The Klippel-Feil syndrome: early roentgenographic appearance and progression of the deformity: a report of two cases. *J Bone Joint Surg Am.* 1976;58:891–892.

5. Nasca RJ, Stelling FH, Steel HH. Progression of congenital scoliosis due to hemivertebrae and hemivertebrae with bars. *J Bone Joint Surg Am.* 1975;57:456–466.

6. Lederman HM, Kaufman RA. Congenital absence and hypoplasia of pedicles in the thoracic spine. *Skeletal Radiol.* 1986;15:219–223.

7. Dolan KD. Cervical basilar relationships. *Radiol Clin North Am.* 1977;15:155–166.

8. Hinck VC, Hopkins CE, Savara BS. Diagnostic criteria of basilar impression. *Radiology.* 1961;76:572–585.

9. Calvy TM, Segall HD, Gilles FH, et al. CT anatomy of the craniovertebral junction in infants and children. *AJNR.* 1987;8:489–494.

10. Di Lorenzo N, Fortuna A, Guidetti B. Craniovertebral junction malformations: clinicoradiological findings, long-term results and surgical implications in 63 cases. *J Neurosurg.* 1982;57:603–608.

11. Hinck VC, Hopkins CE. Measurement of the atlanto-dental interval in the adult. *Am J Roentgenol Radium Ther Nucl Med*. 1960;84:945–951.

12. Spillane JD, Pallis C, Jones AM. Developmental abnormalities in the region of the foramen magnum. *Brain*. 1975;80:11–48.

13. McRae DL, Barnum AS. Occipitalization of the atlas. *Am J Roentgenol Radium Ther Nucl Med*. 1953;70:23–46.

14. Doyne HL, Just N, Lander PH. CT recognition of anomalies of the posterior arch of the atlas vertebra: differentiation from fracture. *AJNR*. 1986; 7:176–177.

15. Lombardi G. The occipital vertebra. *Am J Roentgenol Radium Ther Nucl Med*. 1961;86:260–269.

16. Hadley LA. Atlanto-occipital fusion, ossiculum terminale and occipital vertebra as related to basilar impression with neurological symptoms. *Am J Roentgenol Radium Ther Nucl Med*. 1948;59:511–524.

17. Fielding JW, Hensinger RN, Hawkins RJ. Os odontoideum. *J Bone Joint Surg Am*. 1980;62:376–383.

18. Dyck P. Os odontoideum in children: neurological manifestations and surgical management. *Neurosurgery*. 1978;2:93–99.

19. Anderson FM. Occult spinal dysraphism: diagnosis and management. *J Pediatr*. 1968;73:163–177.

20. Roos RAC, Vielvoye GJ, Voormolen JHC, Peters AC. Magnetic resonance imaging in occult spinal dysraphism. *Pediatr Radiol*. 1986; 16:412–416.

21. Scarff TB, Fronczak S. Myelomeningocele: a review and update. *Rehabil Lit*. 1981;42:143–148.

22. Bahnson DH. Myelomeningocele and its problems. *Pediatr Ann*. 1982;11:528–540.

23. Bloch S, Van Rensburg MJ, Danziger J. The Arnold-Chiari malformation. *Clin Radiol*. 1974;25:335–341.

24. Naidich TP, McLone DG, Fulling KH. The Chiari II malformation: part IV: the hindbrain deformity. *Neuroradiology*. 1983;25:179–197.

25. Hall P, Lindseth R, Campbell R. Scoliosis and hydrocephalus in myelocele patients: the effects of ventricular shunting. *J Neurosurg*. 1979;50:174–178.

26. Samuelsson L, Bergstrom K, Thomas K-A, Hemmingsson A, Wallensten R. MR imaging of syringohydromyelia and Chiari malformations in myelomeningocele patients with scoliosis. *AJNR*. 1987;8:539–546.

27. Barnes PD, Lester PD, Yamanashi WS, Prince JR. MRI imaging in infants and children with spinal dysraphism. *AJR*. 1986;147:339–346.

28. Wippold FJ, Citrin C, Barkovich AJ, Sherman JS. Evaluation of MR in spinal dysraphism with lipoma: comparison with metrizamide computed tomography. *Pediatr Radiol*. 1987;17:184–188.

29. Emery JL, Lendon RG. The local cord lesion in neurospinal dysraphism (meningomyelocele). *J Pathol*. 1973;110:83–96.

30. McGuire RA Jr, Metcalf JC, Amundson GM, McGillicudy GT. Anterior sacral meningocele. Case report and review of the literature. *Spine*. 1990;15:612–614.

31. Vade A, Kennard D. Lipomeningomyelocystocele. *AJNR*. 1987;8: 375–377.

32. Wright RL. Congenital dermal sinuses. *Prog Neurol Surg*. 1971; 4:175–191.

33. Harwood-Nash DC, Fitz CR, Resjo M, Chuang S. Congenital spinal and cord lesions in children and computed tomographic metrizamide myelography. *Neuroradiology*. 1978;16:69–70.

34. Bean JR, Walsh JW, Blacker HM. Cervical dermal sinus and intramedullary spinal cord abscess: case report. *Neurosurgery*. 1979;5:60–62.

35. Scotti G, Harwood-Nash DC, Hoffman HJ. Congenital thoracic dermal sinus: diagnosis by computer-assisted metrizamide myelography. *J Comput Assist Tomogr*. 1980;4:675–677.

36. Wright RL. Congenital dermal sinuses. *Prog Neurol Surg*. 1971; 4:175–191.

37. Lemire RJ, Graham CB, Beckwith JB. Skin-covered sacrococcygeal masses in infants and children. *J Pediatr*. 1971;79:948–954.

38. Aoki N. Rapid growth of intraspinal lipoma demonstrated by magnetic resonance imaging. *Surg Neurol*. 1990;34:107–110.

39. Chapman PH. Congenital intraspinal lipoma: anatomic considerations and surgical treatment. *Childs Brain*. 1982;9:37–47.

40. Goyal RN. Epidural lipoma causing compression of the spinal cord. *Surg Neurol*. 1980;14:77–79.

41. Naidich TP, McLone DG, Mutleur S. A new understanding of dorsal dysraphism with lipoma (lipomyeloschisis): radiological evaluation and surgical correction. *AJNR*. 1983;4:103–116.

42. Gold LH, Kieffer SA, Peterson HO. Lipomatous invasion of the spinal cord associated with spinal dysraphism: myelographic evaluation. *Am J Roentgenol Radium Ther Nucl Med*. 1969;107:479–485.

43. Guidetti B, Gagliardo FM. Epidermoid and dermoid cysts: clinical evaluation and late surgical results. *J Neurosurg*. 1977;47:12–18.

44. Tibbs PA, James HE, Rorke LB, Schut L, Bruce DA. Midline hamartomas masquerading as meningomyelocele or teratomas in the newborn infant. *J Pediatr*. 1976;89:928–933.

45. Wilson DA, Prince JR. MR imaging determination of the location of the normal conus medullaris throughout childhood. *AJNR*. 1989;10:259–262.

46. Kaplan JO, Quencer RM. The occult tethered conus syndrome in the adult. *Radiology*. 1980;137:387–391.

47. Balasubramaniam C, Laurent JP, McCluggage C, Oshman D, Cheek WR. Tethered cord syndrome after repair of meningomyelocele. *Childs Nerv Syst*. 1990;6:208–211.

48. Sarwar M, Virapongse C, Bhimani S. Primary tethered cord syndrome: a new hypothesis of its origin. *AJNR*. 1984;5:235–242.

49. Scheible W, James HE, Leopold GR, Hilton SW. Occult spinal dysraphism in infants: screening with high resolution real-time ultrasound. *Radiology*. 1983;146:743–746.

50. Naidich TP, Harwood-Nash DC. Diastematomyelia: hemicords and meningeal sheaths: single and double arachnoid and dural tubes. *AJNR*. 1984; 4:633–636.

51. Han JS, Benson JE, Kaufman B, et al. Demonstration of diastematomyelia and associated abnormalities with MR imaging. *AJNR*. 1985; 6:215–219.

52. Hilal SK, Marton D, Pollak E. Diastematomyelia in children. Radiographic study of 34 cases. *Radiology*. 1974;112:609–621.

53. Levine RS, Geremia GK, McNeill TW. CT demonstration of cervical diastematomyelia. A case report. *J Comput Assist Tomogr*. 1985;9:592–594.

54. Naidich TP, McClone DG, Harwood-Nash DC. Spinal dysraphism. In: Newton TH, Potts DG, eds. *Computed Tomography of the Spine and Spinal Cord*. Sonensalmo, CA: Clavadel; 1983:299–353.

55. Scatliff JH, Kendall BE, Kingsley DP, Britton J, Grant DN, Hayward RD. Closed spinal dysraphism: analysis of clinical, radiological, and surgical findings in 104 consecutive patients. *AJR*. 1989;152:1049–1057.

56. Schlesinger AE, Naidich TP, Quencer RB. Constant hydromyelia and diastematomyelia. *AJNR*. 1986;7:473–477.

57. Thron A, Schroth G. Magnetic resonance imaging (MRI) of diastematomyelia. *Neuroradiology*. 1986;28:371–372.

58. Hans JS, Benson TE, Kaufman B, et al. Demonstration of diastematomyelia and associated abnormalities with MR imaging. *AJNR*. 1985; 6:215–219.

59. Superina RA, Ein SH, Humphreys RP. Cystic duplications of the esophagus and neurenteric cysts. *J Pediatr Surg*. 1984;19:527–530.

60. Guilburd TN, Arieh YB, Peyser E. Spinal intradural enterogenous cyst: report of a case. *Surg Neurol*. 1980;14:359–362.

61. Burrows FG, Sutcliffe J. The split notochord syndrome. *Br J Radiol*. 1968;41:844–847.

62. Gupta DK, Deodhar MC. Split notochord syndrome presenting with meningomyelocele and dorsal enteric fistula. *J Pediatr Surg.* 1987;22:382–383.

63. Alrabeeah A, Gillis DA, Giacomantonio M, Lau H. Neurenteric cysts—a spectrum. *J Pediatr Surg.* 1988;23:752–754.

64. Kallen B, Winberg J. Caudal mesoderm pattern of anomalies: from renal agenesis to sirenomelia. *Teratology.* 1974;9:99–112.

65. Jaramillo D, Lebowitz RL, Hendren WH. The cloacal malformation: radiologic findings and imaging recommendations. *Radiology.* 1990;177:441–448.

66. Pang D, Hoffman HJ. Sacral agenesis with progressive neurological deficit. *Neurosurgery.* 1980;7:118–126.

67. Renshaw TS. Sacral agenesis: a classification and review of twenty-three cases. *J Bone Joint Surg Am.* 1978;60:373–383.

68. Logue V, Edwards MR. Syringomyelia and its surgical treatment—an analysis of 75 patients. *J Neurol Neurosurg Psychiatry.* 1981;44:273–284.

69. Schlesinger EB, Antuenes JL, Michelsen WJ, Louis KM. Hydromyelia: clinical presentation and comparison of modalities of treatment. *J Neurosurg.* 1981;9:356–365.

70. Sherman JL, Barkovich AJ, Citrin CM. The MR appearance of syringomyelia: new observations. *AJNR.* 1986;7:985–995.

71. Wiltse LL, Widell EH, Jackson DW. Fatigue fracture: the basic lesions in isthmic spondylolisthesis. *J Bone Joint Surg Am.* 1975;57:17–22.

72. Grogan JP, Hemminghytt S, Williams AL, Carrera GF, Haughton VM. Spondylolysis studied with computed tomography. *Radiology.* 1982;145:737–742.

73. Wilkinson RH, Hall JE. The sclerotic pedicle: tumor or pseudotumor? *Radiology.* 1974;111:683–688.

74. Rothman SL, Glenn DV Jr. CT multiplanar reconstruction in 253 cases of lumbar spondylolysis. *AJNR.* 1984;5:81–90.

75. Wells RG, Miller JH, Sty JR. Scintigraphic patterns in osteoid osteoma and spondylolysis. *Clin Nucl Med.* 1987;12:39–44.

76. Wiltse LL, Newman PH, Macnab I. Classification of spondylolysis and spondylolisthesis. *Clin Orthop.* 1976;117:23–29.

77. Ravichandran G. A radiologic sign in spondylolisthesis. *AJR.* 1980;134:113–117.

78. Wiltse LL, Winter RB. Terminology and measurement of spondylolisthesis. *J Bone Joint Surg Am.* 1983;65:768–772.

79. Elster AD, Jensen KM. Computed tomography of spondylolisthesis: patterns of associated pathology. *J Comput Assist Tomogr.* 1985;9:867–874.

80. McAlister WH, Shackelford GD. Classification of spinal curvatures. *Radiol Clin North Am.* 1975;13:113–121.

81. Dickson RA, Lawton JO, Archer IA, Butt WP. The pathogenesis of idiopathic scoliosis. Biplanar spinal asymmetry. *J Bone Joint Surg Br.* 1984;66:8–15.

82. McMaster MJ. Infantile idiopathic scoliosis: can it be prevented? *J Bone Joint Surg Br.* 1983;65:612–617.

83. Figueiredo UM, James JIP. Juvenile idiopathic scoliosis. *J Bone Joint Surg Br.* 1981;63:61–66.

84. Rogala EF, Drummond DS, Gurr J. Scoliosis: incidence in natural history. A prospective epidemiologic study. *J Bone Joint Surg Am.* 1978;60:173–176.

85. Smyrnis PN, Valavanis J, Alexopoulos A, Siderakis G, Giannestras NJ. School screening for scoliosis in Athens. *J Bone Joint Surg Br.* 1979;61:215–217.

86. Roth M. Idiopathic scoliosis from the point of view of the neuroradiologist. *J Neuroradiol.* 1981;21:133–138.

87. Lonstein JE, Carlson M. The prediction of curve progression in untreated idiopathic scoliosis during growth. *J Bone Joint Surg Am.* 1984;66:1061–1071.

88. Weinstein SL, Ponseti IV. Curve progression in idiopathic scoliosis. *J Bone Joint Surg Am.* 1983;65:447–455.

89. Bernard TN Jr, Burke SW, Johnston CE III, Roberts JM. Congenital spine deformities. A review of 47 cases. *Orthopedics.* 1985;8:777–783.

90. McMaster MJ. Occult intraspinal anomalies and congenital scoliosis. *J Bone Joint Surg Am.* 1984;66:588–601.

91. Beals RK. Nosologic and genetic aspects of scoliosis. *Clin Orthop.* 1973;93:23–32.

92. Winter RB, Moe JH, Eilers CE. Congenital scoliosis: a study of 234 patients treated and untreated. Part I: natural history. *J Bone Joint Surg Am.* 1968;50:1–15.

93. Lawhon SM, MacEwen GD, Bunnell WP. Orthopaedic aspects of the VATER association. *J Bone Joint Surg Am.* 1986;68:424–429.

94. Roth A, Rosenthal A, Hall JE, et al. Evaluation of kidney anomalies in congenital scoliosis. *Clin Orthop.* 1973;93:95–102.

95. Sirois JL III, Drennan JC. Dystrophic spinal deformity in neurofibromatosis. *J Pediatr Orthop.* 1990;10:522–526.

96. Stillwell DL Jr. Structural deformities of vertebrae: bone adaptation and mottling in experimental scoliosis and kyphosis. *J Bone Joint Surg Am.* 1962;44:611–634.

97. Cobb JR. Outline for the study of scoliosis. *Am Acad Orthop Surg.* 1948;5:261–275.

98. Fergusson AB. *Roentgen Diagnosis of the Extremities and Spine.* New York: Hoeber; 1945.

99. Kittleson AC, Lim LW. Measurement of scoliosis. *Am J Roentgenol Radium Ther Nucl Med.* 1970;108:775–777.

100. George K, Rippstein J. A comparative study of the two popular methods of measuring scoliotic deformity of the spine. *J Bone Joint Surg Am.* 1961;43:809–818.

101. Nash CL, Moe JH. A study of vertebral rotation. *J Bone Joint Surg Am.* 1969;51:223–229.

102. Thomas IT, Frias JL, Williams JL, Friedman WA. Magnetic resonance imaging in the assessment of medullary compression in achondroplasia. *Am J Dis Child.* 1988;142:989–992.

103. Bethem D, Winter RB, Lutter L, et al. Spinal disorders of dwarfism. Review of the literature and report of eighty cases. *J Bone Joint Surg Am.* 1981;63:1412–1425.

104. Rouse GA, Filly RA, Toomey F, Grube GL. Short-limb skeletal dysplasias: evaluation of the fetal spine with sonography and radiography. *Radiology.* 1990;174:177–180.

105. Langer LO Jr, Baumann PA, Gorlin RJ. Achondroplasia. *Am J Roentgenol Radium Ther Nucl Med.* 1967;100:12–26.

106. Wang H, Rosenbaum AE, Reid CS, Zinreich SJ, Pyeritz RE. Pediatric patients with achondroplasia: CT evaluation of the craniocervical junction. *Radiology.* 1987;164:515–519.

107. Kahanovitz N, Rimoin DL, Sillence DO. The clinical spectrum of lumbar spine disease in achondroplasia. *Spine.* 1982;7:137–140.

108. Strauss L. The pathology of gargoylism. Report of a case and review of the literature. *Am J Pathol.* 1948;24:855–887.

109. Mitchell GE, Lourie H, Berne AS. The various causes of scalloped vertebrae with notes on their pathogenesis. *Radiology.* 1967;89:67–74.

110. Langer LO Jr, Carey LS. The roentgenographic features of the KS mucopolysaccharidosis of Morquio (Morquio-Brailsford disease). *Am J Roentgenol Radium Ther Nucl Med.* 1966;97:1–20.

111. Rabinowitz JG, Moseley JE. The lateral lumbar spine in Down syndrome: a new roentgen feature. *Radiology.* 1964;83:74–79.

112. Semine AA, Ertel AN, Goldberg MJ. Cervical-spine instability in children with Down syndrome (trisomy 21). *J Bone Joint Surg Am.* 1978;60:649–652.

113. Shikata J, Mikawa Y, Ikeda T, Yamamuro T. Atlanto-axial subluxation with spondyloschisis in Down syndrome. Case report. *J Bone Joint Surg Am.* 1985;67:1414–1417.

114. Pitt MJ. Rachitic and osteomalacic syndromes. *Radiol Clin North Am.* 1981;19:581–599.

115. Fried JA, Athreya B, Gregg JR. The cervical spine in juvenile rheumatoid arthritis. *Clin Orthop.* 1983;179:102–106.

116. Reynolds J. Roentgenographic and clinical appraisal of sickle cell–hemoglobin C disease. *Am J Roentgenol Radium Ther Nucl Med.* 1962;88:512–522.

117. Moseley JE. Skeletal changes in the anemias. *Semin Roentgenol.* 1974;9:169–184.

118. Swischuk LE. The spine and spinal cord. In: *Emergency Radiology of the Acutely Ill or Injured Child.* 2nd ed. Baltimore: Williams & Wilkins; 1986:556–609.

119. Gaugin LM, Goodman SJ. Cervical spine injuries in infants: problems in management. *J Neurosurg.* 1975;42:179–184.

120. McPhee IB. Spinal fractures and dislocations in children and adolescents. *Spine.* 1981;6:533–537.

121. Penning L. Prevertebral hematoma in cervical spine injury: incidence and etiologic significance. *AJR.* 1981;136:553–561.

122. Clark WM, Gehweiler JA Jr, Laib R. Twelve significant signs of cervical spine trauma. *Skeletal Radiol.* 1979;3:201–205.

123. Locke GR, Gardner JI, Van Epps EF. Atlas-dens interval (ADI) in children: a survey based on 200 normal cervical spines. *Am J Roentgenol Radium Ther Nucl Med.* 1966;97:135–140.

124. Swischuk LE. Anterior displacement of C2 in children: physiologic or pathologic? A helpful differentiation. *Radiology.* 1977;122:759–763.

125. Mirvis SE, Young JW, Lim C, Greenberg J. Hangman's fracture: radiologic assessment in 27 cases. *Radiology.* 1987;163:713–717.

126. Naidich JB, Naidich TP, Garfein C, Liebeshind AL, Hyman RA. The widened interspinous distances: a useful sign of anterior cervical dislocation in the supine frontal projection. *Radiology.* 1977;123:113–116.

127. Dolan KD. Cervical spine injuries below the axis. *Radiol Clin North Am.* 1977;15:247–259.

128. Miller MD, Gehweiler JA, Martinez S, Charlton OP, Daffner RH. Significant new observations on cervical spine trauma. *AJR.* 1978;130:659–663.

129. Allen BL Jr, Ferguson RL, Lehmann TR, O'Brien RP. A mechanistic classification of closed, indirect fractures and dislocations of the lower cervical spine. *Spine.* 1982;7:1–27.

130. Gehweiler JA Jr, Clark WM, Schaff RE, Powers B, Miller MD. Cervical spine trauma: common combined conditions. *Radiology.* 1979;130:77–86.

131. Scher A, Vambeck V. An approach to the radiological examination of the cervico-dorsal junction following injury. *Clin Radiol.* 1977;28:243–246.

132. Lee C, Kim KS, Rogers LF. Triangular cervical vertebral body fractures: diagnostic significance. *AJR.* 1982;138:1123–1132.

133. Schneider RC, Kahn EA. Chronic neurological sequelae of acute trauma to the spine and spinal cord. Part I: the significance of the acute-flexion or "tear drop" fracture dislocation of the cervical spine. *J Bone Joint Surg Am.* 1956;38:985–997.

134. Lynch D, McManus F, Ennis JT. Computed tomography in spinal trauma. *Clin Radiol.* 1986;37:71–76.

135. Kaufman RA, Dunbar JS, Botsford JA, McLaurin RL. Traumatic longitudinal atlanto-occipital distraction injuries in children. *AJNR.* 1982;3:415–419.

136. Bucholz RW, Burkhead WZ. The pathological anatomy of fatal atlanto-occipital dislocations. *J Bone Joint Surg Am.* 1979;61:248–250.

137. Powers B, Miller MD, Kramer RS, Martinez S, Gehweiler JA Jr. Traumatic anterior atlanto-occipital dislocation. *Neurosurgery.* 1979;4:12–17.

138. Schaaf RE, Gehweiler JA Jr, Miller MD, Powers B. Lateral hyperflexion injuries of the cervical spine. *Skeletal Radiol.* 1978;3:73–78.

139. Scher AT. Unilateral locked facet in cervical spine injuries. *AJR.* 1977;129:45–48.

140. Shapiro FR, Youngberg AS, Rothman SLG. The differential diagnosis of traumatic lesions of the occipito-atlantoaxial segment. *Radiol Clin North Am.* 1973;11:505–526.

141. Jefferson G. Fracture of the atlas vertebrae: report of four cases and a review of those previously recorded. *Br J Surg.* 1920;7:407–422.

142. Gehweiler JA Jr, Duff DE, Martinez S, et al. Fractures of the atlas vertebra. *Skeletal Radiol.* 1976;1:97–102.

143. Gehweiler JA, Daffner RH, Roberts L Jr. Malformations of the atlas vertebra simulating the Jefferson fracture. *AJR.* 1983;140:1083–1086.

144. Spence KF Jr, Decker S, Sell KW. Bursting atlantal fracture associated with rupture of the transverse ligament. *J Bone Joint Surg Am.* 1970;52:543–549.

145. Apple JS, Kirks DR, Merten DF, Martinez S. Cervical spine fractures and dislocations in children. *Pediatr Radiol.* 1987;17:45–49.

146. Ehara S, El-Khoury GY, Sato Y. Cervical spine injury in children: radiologic manifestations. *AJR.* 1988;151:1175–1178.

147. Flournoy JG, Cone RO, Saldana JA, Jones MD. Jefferson fracture: presentation of a new diagnostic sign. *Radiology.* 1980;134:88.

148. Kadoya S, Nakamura T, Kobayashi S, Yamamoto I. Magnetic resonance imaging of acute spinal cord injury. Report of three cases. *Neuroradiology.* 1987;29:252–255.

149. Smith GR, Northrop CH, Loop JW. Jumpers fractures: patterns of thoracolumbar spine injuries associated with vertical plunges: a review of 38 cases. *Radiology.* 1977;122:657–663.

150. Ferguson RL, Allen BL Jr. A mechanistic classification of thoracolumbar spine fractures. *Clin Orthop.* 1984;189:77–88.

151. Denis F. Spinal instability as defined by the three column spine concept in acute spinal trauma. *Clin Orthop.* 1984;89:65–76.

152. Holdsworth F. Fractures, dislocations and fracture dislocations of the spine. *J Bone Joint Surg Br.* 1963;45:6–20.

153. Guerra J Jr, Garfin SR, Resnick D. Vertebral burst fractures: CT analysis of the retropulsed fragment. *Radiology.* 1984;153:769–772.

154. Laasonen EM, Riska EB. Preoperative radiological assessment of fractures of the thoracolumbar spine causing traumatic paraplegia. *Skeletal Radiol.* 1977;1:231–234.

155. Denis F. The three column spine and its significance in the classification of acute thoracolumbar spinal injuries. *Spine.* 1983;8:817–831.

156. Escalona-Zapata J. Pathology of spinal cord tumors in children. In: Pascual-Castroviejo I, ed. *Spinal Tumors in Children and Adolescents.* New York: Raven; 1990:11–34.

157. Farwell JR, Dohrman GJ, Flannery JT. Central nervous systems tumors in children. *Cancer.* 1977;40:3123–3132.

158. Di Lorenzo N, Giuffre R, Fortuna A. Primary spinal neoplasms in childhood: analysis of 1234 published cases (including 56 personal cases) by pathology, sex, age, and site. Differences from the situation in adults. *Neurochirurgia (Stuttg).* 1982;25:153–164.

159. Reimer R, Onofrio BM. Astrocytomas of the spinal cord in children and adolescents. *J Neurosurg.* 1985;63:669–675.

160. Purohit AK, Dinakar I, Sundaram C, Ratnakar KS. Anaplastic astrocytoma of the spinal cord presenting with features of raised intracranial pressure. *Childs Nerv Syst.* 1990;6:113–115.

161. DeSousa AL, Kalsbeck JE, Mealey J Jr, Campbell RL, Hockey A. Intraspinal tumors in children. A review of 81 cases. *J Neurosurg.* 1979;51:437–445.

162. Epstein F, Epstein N. Surgical treatment of spinal cord astrocytomas of childhood. A series of 19 patients. *J Neurosurg.* 1982;57:685–689.

163. Citron N, Edgar MA, Sheehy J, Thomas DG. Intramedullary spinal cord tumours presenting as scoliosis. *J Bone Joint Surg Br.* 1984;66:513–517.

164. Handel S, Grossman R, Sarwar M. Computed tomography in the diagnosis of spinal cord astrocytoma. *J Comput Assist Tomogr.* 1978;2: 226–228.

165. Walker HS, Dietrich RB, Flannigan BD, Lufkin RB, Peacock WJ, Kangarloo H. Magnetic resonance imaging of the pediatric spine. *Radio-Graphics.* 1987;7:1129–1152.

166. Duthoy MJ, Lund G. MR imaging of the spine in children. *Eur J Radiol.* 1988;8:188–195.

167. Davis PC, Hoffman JC Jr, Ball TI, et al. Spinal abnormalities in pediatric patients: MR imaging findings compared with clinical, myelographic, and surgical findings. *Radiology.* 1988;166:679–685.

168. Goy AMC, Pinto RS, Raghavendra BN, Epstein FJ, Kricheff II. Intramedullary spinal cord tumors: MR imaging, with emphasis on associated cysts. *Radiology.* 1986;161:381–386.

169. Scotti G, Scialfa G, Colombo N, Landoni L. Magnetic resonance diagnosis of intramedullary tumors of the spinal cord. *Neuroradiology.* 1987; 29:130–135.

170. Okawara S. Ruptured spinal ependymoma simulating bacterial meningitis. *Arch Neurol.* 1983;40:54–55.

171. Dillon WP, Norman D, Newton TH, Bolla K, Mark A. Intradural spinal cord lesions: Gd-DTPA-enhanced MR imaging. *Radiology.* 1989;170: 229–237.

172. Fortuna A, Celli P, Palma L. Oligodendrogliomas of the spinal cord. *Acta Neurochir.* 1980;52:305–329.

173. Garcia JH, Lemmi H. Ultrastructure of oligodendroglioma of spinal cord. *Am J Clin Pathol.* 1970;54:757–765.

174. Fortuna A, Nolletti A, Nardi P, Caruso R. Spinal neuromas and meningomas in children. *Acta Neurochir.* 1981;55:329–341.

175. Burk DL Jr, Brunberg JA, Kanal E, Latchaw RE, Wolf GL. Spinal and paraspinal neurofibromatosis: surface coil MR imaging at 1.5 T. *Radiology.* 1987;162:797–801.

176. Garrison JE, Kasdon DL. Intramedullary spinal teratoma: case report and review of the literature. *Neurosurgery.* 1980;7:509.

177. Herskowitz J, Bielawski MA, Venna N, Sabien TD. Anterior cervical arachnoid cyst simulating syringomyelia. A case with preceding posterior arachnoid cyst. *Arch Neurol.* 1978;35:57–58.

178. Sundaram M, Awward EA. Magnetic resonance imaging of arachnoid cyst destroying the sacrum. *AJR.* 1986;146:359–360.

179. Lundqvist C, Berthelsen B, Sullivan M, Svendsen P, Andersen O. Spinal arteriovenous malformations: neurological aspects and results of embolization. *Acta Neurol Scand.* 1990;82:51–58.

180. Riche MC, Modenesi-Freitas J, Djindjian M, Merland JJ. Arteriovenous malformations (AVM) of the spinal cord in children. A review of 38 cases. *Neuroradiology.* 1982;22:171–180.

181. Dormont D, Gelbert F, Assouline E, et al. MR imaging of spinal cord arteriovenous malformations at 0.5 T: study of 34 cases. *AJNR.* 1988;9: 830–838.

182. Armstrong EA, Harwood-Nash DC, Fitz CR, Chuang SH, Pettersson H, Martin DJ. CT of neuroblastomas and ganglioneuromas in children. *AJR.* 1982;139:571–576.

183. Kumar R, Guinto FC, Madewell JE, David R, Shirkhoda A. Expansile bone lesions of the vertebra. *RadioGraphics.* 1988;8:749–769.

184. Rogalsky RJ, Black B, Reed MH. Orthopaedic manifestations of leukemia in children. *J Bone Joint Surg Am.* 1986;68:494–501.

185. Epstein BS. Vertebral changes in childhood leukemia. *Radiology.* 1957;68:65–69.

186. Schabel SL, Tyminski L, Holland D, Rittenberg GM. The skeletal manifestations of chronic myelogenous leukemia. *Skeletal Radiol.* 1980;5: 145–149.

187. Karasick S, Karasick D, Schilling J. Acute megakaryoblastic leukemia (acute "malignant" myelofibrosis): an unusual cause of osteosclerosis. *Skeletal Radiol.* 1982;9:45–46.

188. Nixon GW, Gwinn JL. The roentgen manifestations of leukemia in infancy. *Radiology.* 1973;107:603–609.

189. McAllister MD, O'Leary DH. CT myelography of subarachnoid leukemic infiltration of the lumbar thecal sac and lumbar nerve roots. *AJNR.* 1987;8:568–569.

190. Jackson RP, Reckling FW, Mautz FA. Osteoid osteoma and osteoblastoma: similar histologic lesions with different natural histories. *Clin Orthop.* 1977;128:303–313.

191. Kirwan W, Hutton PA, Pozo JL, Ransford AO. Osteoid osteoma and benign osteoblastoma of the spine. Clinical presentation and treatment. *J Bone Joint Surg Br.* 1984;66:21–26.

192. Schulman L, Dorfman HD. Nerve fibers in osteoid osteoma. *J Bone Joint Surg Am.* 1970;52:1351–1356.

193. Ransford AO, Pozo JL, Hutton PA, Kirwan EO. The behavior pattern of the scoliosis associated with osteoid osteoma or osteoblastoma of the spine. *J Bone Joint Surg Br.* 1984;66:16–20.

194. Janin Y, Epstein JA, Carras R, Khan A. Osteoid osteomas and osteoblastomas of the spine. *Neurosurgery.* 1981;8:31–38.

195. Freiberger RH, Loitman BS, Halpern M, et al. Osteoid osteoma: a report on 80 cases. *Am J Roentgenol Radium Ther Nucl Med.* 1959;82: 194–205.

196. Wedge JH, Tchang S, MacFadyen DJ. Computed tomography in localization of spinal osteoid osteoma. *Spine.* 1981;6:423–427.

197. Lichtenstein L, Sawyer WR. Benign osteoblastoma. Further observations and report of 20 additional cases. *J Bone Joint Surg Am.* 1964;46: 755–765.

198. Akbarnia BA, Rocholamini SA. Scoliosis caused by benign osteoblastoma of the thoracic or lumbar spine. *J Bone Joint Surg Am.* 1981; 64:1146–1155.

199. Papanicolaou N, Treves S. Bone scintigraphy in the preoperative evaluation of osteoid osteoma and osteoblastoma of the spine. *Ann Radiol.* 1984;27:104–110.

200. Izant RJ Jr, Filston HC. Sacrococcygeal teratomas: analysis of forty-three cases. *Am J Surg.* 1975;130:617–621.

201. Noseworthy J, Lack EE, Kozakewich HP, Vawter GF, Welch KJ. Sacrococcygeal germ cell tumors in childhood: an updated experience with 118 patients. *J Pediatr Surg.* 1981;16:358–364.

202. Whalen TV Jr, Mahour GH, Landing BH, Woolley MM. Sacrococcygeal teratomas in infants and children. *Am J Surg.* 1985;150:373–375.

203. Sheth S, Nussbaum AR, Sanders RC, et al. Prenatal diagnosis of sacrococcygeal teratoma: sonographic pathologic correlation. *Radiology.* 1988;169:131–136.

204. Ein SH, Mancer K, Adeyemi SD. Malignant sacrococcygeal teratoma—endodermal sinus, yolk sac tumor—in infants and children: a 32-year review. *J Pediatr Surg.* 1985;20:473–477.

205. Altman RP, Randolph JG, Lilly JR. Sacrococcygeal teratoma: American Academy of Pediatrics Surgical Section survey, 1973. *J Pediatr Surg.* 1974;9:389–398.

206. Schey WC, Shkolnik A, White H. Clinical and radiographic considerations of sacrococcygeal teratomas: an analysis of 26 new cases and review of the literature. *Radiology.* 1977;125:189–195.

207. Currarino G, Coln D, Votteler T. Triad of anorectal, sacral, and presacral anomalies. *AJR.* 1981;137:395–398.

208. Wells RG, Sty JR. Imaging of sacrococcygeal germ cell tumors. *RadioGraphics.* 1990;10:701–713.

209. Monajati A, Spitzer RM, Wiley JL, Heggeness L. MR imaging of a spinal teratoma. Case report. *J Comput Assist Tomogr.* 1986;10:307–310.

210. Spencer JD. Bone and joint infection in a renal unit. *J Bone Joint Surg Br.* 1986;68:489–493.

211. Donovan RM, Shah KJ. Unusual sites of acute osteomyelitis in childhood. *Clin Radiol.* 1982;33:222–230.

212. Goldman AB, Freiberger RH. Localized infectious and neuropathic diseases. *Semin Roentgenol*. 1979;14:19–32.

213. Kricun ME. Red-yellow marrow conversion: its effects on the location of some solitary bone lesions. *Skeletal Radiol*. 1985;14:10–19.

214. Ratcliffe JF. An evaluation of the intraosseous arterial anastomoses in the human vertebral body at different ages. A microarteriographic study. *J Anat*. 1982;134(pt 2):373–382.

215. Ratcliffe JF. Anatomic basis for the pathogenesis and radiologic features of vertebral osteomyelitis and its differentiation from childhood discitis: a microarteriographic investigation. *Acta Radiol Diagn*. 1985;26:137–143.

216. McCook TA, Felman H, Ayoub E. Streptococcal skeletal infections: observations in infants. *AJR*. 1978;130:465–467.

217. Eismont FJ, Bohlman HH, Soni PL, Goldberg VM, Freehafer AA. Vertebral osteomyelitis in infants. *J Bone Joint Surg Br*. 1982;64:32–35.

218. Digby JM, Kersley JB. Pyogenic nontuberculous spinal infection. An analysis of 30 cases. *J Bone Joint Surg Br*. 1979;61:47–55.

219. Adatepe MH, Powell OM, Isaacs GH, Nichols K, Cefola R. Hematogenous pyogenic vertebral osteomyelitis: diagnostic value of radionuclide bone imaging. *J Nucl Med*. 1986;27:1680–1685.

220. Chan F, Cheng C, Tam PK, Saing H. Sacrococcygeal teratoma: computed tomography evaluation. *J Comput Assist Tomogr*. 1987;11:200–204.

221. Bertino RE, Porter BA, Stimac GK, Tepper SJ. Imaging spinal osteomyelitis and epidural abscess with short T_1 inversion recovery (STIR). *AJNR*. 1988;9:563–564.

222. Post MJ, Quencer RM, Montalvo BM, Katz BH, Eismont FJ, Green BA. Spinal infection: evaluation with MR imaging and intraoperative US. *Radiology*. 1988;169:765–771.

223. Spiegel PG, Kengla KW, Isaacson AS, et al. Intervertebral disc-space inflammation in children. *J Bone Joint Surg Am*. 1972;54:284–296.

224. Smith RF, Taylor TKF. Inflammatory lesions of intervertebral discs in children. *J Bone Joint Surg Am*. 1967;49:1508–1520.

225. Alexander CJ. The aetology of juvenile spondylarthritis (discitis). *Clin Radiol*. 1970;21:178–187.

226. Menelaus MB. Discitis: an inflammation affecting the intervertebral discs in children. *J Bone Joint Surg Br*. 1964;46:16–23.

227. Coventry, MB, Ghormley RK, Kernohan JW. The intervertebral disc: its microscopic anatomy and pathology. Part I: anatomy development and physiology. *J Bone Joint Surg Am*. 1945;27:105–112.

228. Wenger DR, Bobechke WP, Gilday DL. The spectrum of intervertebral disc-space infection in children. *J Bone Joint Surg Am*. 1978;60:100–108.

229. Gates GF. Scintigraphy of discitis. *Clin Nucl Med*. 1977;2:20–25.

230. Kemp HB, Jackson JW, Jeremiah JD, Hall AJ. Pyogenic infection occurring primarily in intervertebral discs. *J Bone Joint Surg Br*. 1973;55:698–714.

231. Hashimoto K, Fujita K, Kojimoto H, Shimomura Y. Lumbar disc herniation in children. *J Pediatr Orthop*. 1990;10:394–396.

232. Modic MT, Masaryk T, Boumphrey F, et al. Lumbar herniated disc disease and canal stenosis: perspective evaluation by surface coil MR, CT, and myelography. *AJR*. 1986;147:757–765.

233. Holtås S, Nordström C-H, Larsson EM, Pettersson H. Case report. MR imaging of intradural disk herniation. *J Comput Assist Tomogr*. 1987;11:353–356.

234. Masaryk TJ, Ross JS, Modic MT, Boumphrey F, Bohlman H, Wilber G. High-resolution MR imaging of sequestered lumbar intervertebral disks. *AJNR*. 1988;9:351–358.

235. Lester JW Jr, Miller WA, Carter MP, Hemphill JM. MR of childhood calcified herniated cervical disk with spontaneous resorption. *AJNR*. 1989;10:S48–S50.

236. McGregor JC, Butler P. Disc calcification in childhood: computed tomographic and magnetic resonance imaging appearances. Case reports. *Br J Radiol*. 1986;59:180–182.

237. Ippolito E, Ponseti IV. Juvenile kyphosis: histological and histochemical studies. *J Bone Joint Surg Am*. 1981;63:175–182.

238. Lowe TG. Scheuermann disease. *J Bone Joint Surg Am*. 1990;72:940–945.

239. Starshak RJ, Kass GA, Samaraweera RN. Developmental stenosis of the cervical spine in children. *Pediatr Radiol*. 1987;17:291–295.

240. Hinck VC, Hopkins CE, Savara BS. Sagittal diameter of the cervical spinal canal in children. *Radiology*. 1962;79:97–108.

241. Hinck VC, Hopkins CE, Savara BS. Sagittal diameter of the lumbar spinal canal in children and adults. *Radiology*. 1965;85:929–937.

Chapter 3

Extracranial Head and Neck

ABNORMALITIES OF THE UPPER AIRWAY

Upper Airway Obstruction

Upper airway obstruction is a common and potentially serious problem in infants and children. It may be caused by a wide spectrum of pathologic disorders. These children usually present with acute respiratory distress associated with stridor, apnea, and, rarely, pulmonary edema. Some may have a more protracted course, however, characterized by recurrent pulmonary infections, obstructive sleep apnea (which may be associated with chronic pulmonary failure), cor pulmonale, and even death. Knowledge of the clinical factors that can help differentiate among the various etiologies of upper airway obstruction is beneficial in selecting and interpreting the imaging studies that are necessary in the evaluation of these children. Abnormalities that are associated with upper airway obstruction may be classified with respect to pathology, patient age, chronicity, or anatomic site. Limiting the differential diagnosis according to the anatomic site of involvement is probably the most useful system (Tables 3-1 to 3-4).

The anatomic divisions of the upper airway are the pharynx, the larynx, and the trachea and major bronchi. Lesions of the pharynx are subdivided into those affecting the nasopharynx, the oropharynx (including the mandible and tongue), and the hypopharynx. Laryngeal abnormalities affect the epiglottis, the aryepiglottic folds, and the glottis. The tracheobronchial tree is anatomically divided into the subglottic trachea, the cervical trachea, the intrathoracic trachea, and the major bronchi. Pathologic conditions will at times overlap the anatomic divisions.

In addition to anatomic considerations, the etiologies of upper airway obstruction in children may be divided into congenital and acquired types. The congenital varieties most often produce chronic symptoms, whereas acquired lesions usually produce acute symptoms. There are exceptions. For example, congenital lesions may be undetected until a superimposed abnormality such as infection or trauma occurs. Although infection and trauma are usually associated with acute symptoms, some acquired lesions may produce slowly progressive symptoms of airway obstruction, such as thyroid enlargement. Slow-growing tumors, like those that occur in the mediastinum, are asymptomatic for a defined period of time until the airway is critically narrowed.[1]

Stridor indicates the presence of partial upper airway obstruction. The term stridor is applied to any form of noisy breathing. It is distinct from the rales and wheezing of lower airway disease and from vocal cord sounds such as grunting. Stridor results from an airway lesion that causes turbulent airflow. Because the airway of infants and young children is relatively flexible, it undergoes changes in cross-sectional area with the normal pressure gradients of the respiratory cycle. The timing and character of stridor differ according to the anatomic site of partial airway obstruction. The normal changes in airway diameter that occur during respiration are accentuated markedly with partial obstruction.

Pressure gradients generated in the airway during the respiratory cycle are opposite above and below the thoracic inlet. During inspiration the intrathoracic pressure decreases, and the intrathoracic trachea increases in diameter. During expiration the intrathoracic pressure increases, and the diameter of the intrathoracic trachea decreases. The pressure in the soft

Table 3-1 Causes of Airway Obstruction in Childhood (Nasal, Oral, and Retropharyngeal)

Etiology	Nasopharyngeal	Oropharyngeal	Retropharyngeal
Congenital	Choanal atresia (bony, membranous) Choanal stenosis Cephalocele Craniofacial anomalies	Glossoptosis (eg, Pierre Robin syndrome) Micrognathia Macroglossia (cretinism, Beckwith-Wiedemann syndrome)	Branchial cleft cyst Cystic hygroma Ectopic thyroid
Inflammatory	Polyps, etc	Abscess, etc	Adenitis Cellulitis Abscess
Neoplastic	Juvenile angiofibroma Rhabdomyosarcoma Teratoma Neuroblastoma Nasopharyngeal carcinoma Lymphoma	Lingual tumor (lymphangioma, hemangioma) Lingular cyst	Neuroblastoma Neurofibromatosis Hemangioma
Traumatic	Foreign body Rhinolith Hematoma	Foreign body Hematoma	Foreign body Hematoma
Idiopathic	Adenoidal enlargement	Tonsillar hypertrophy	Hypothyroidism

Table 3-2 Causes of Airway Obstruction in Childhood (Vallecular and Supraglottic)

Etiology	Vallecular	Supraglottic
Congenital	Congenital cyst Ectopic thyroid Thyroglossal duct cyst	Aryepiglottic fold cyst Laryngomalacia
Inflammatory	Abscess	Epiglottitis Angioneurotic edema
Neoplastic	Teratoma	Cystic hygroma Retention cyst Neurofibroma
Traumatic	Foreign body Hematoma	Hematoma Hemophilia Foreign body Radiation Caustic ingestion Thermal injury

tissues surrounding the cervical airway remains relatively constant during the respiratory cycle. During inspiration the intraluminal pressure in the extrathoracic trachea decreases slightly, causing a slight decrease in airway diameter. During expiration the intraluminal pressure increases, and the extrathoracic airway widens slightly.

When a lesion is located in a portion of the airway that varies in diameter during the respiratory cycle, the degree of luminal obstruction caused by the lesion may vary significantly. Stridor may occur during only one phase of the respiratory cycle. Lesions of the extrathoracic airway most often cause inspiratory stridor because the lumen of this portion of the airway is smaller during inspiration. Lesions of the intrathoracic portion of the airway are most often associated with stridor during the expiratory phase because this portion of the airway is smaller on expiration. Abnormalities that do not change the cross-sectional area of the airway do not cause a

Table 3-3 Causes of Airway Obstruction in Childhood (Glottic, Subglottic, and Tracheal)

Etiology	Glottic	Subglottic	Tracheal
Congenital	Laryngeal web Laryngeal stenosis Vocal cord paralysis	Stenosis	Tracheal stenosis Tracheomalacia
Inflammatory	Laryngitis Diphtheria	Croup	Pseudomembranous tracheitis Diphtheria
Neoplastic	Laryngeal papillomatosis	Hemangioma Papillomatosis Mucocele	Hemangioma Papillomatosis Fibroma Other rare tumors
Traumatic	Hematoma Foreign body	Stricture Granuloma	Foreign body Acquired stenosis Granuloma

Table 3-4 Causes of Airway Compression in Childhood

Etiology	Anterior Compression	Posterior Compression
Congenital	Congenital goiter Thymic cyst	Vascular ring Bronchogenic cyst Pulmonary sling
Inflammatory	Cervical or mediastinal abscess	Adenitis Abscess
Neoplastic	Teratoma (intrathoracic or cervical) Thymoma Thyroid tumors Lymphoma Desmoid tumor	Neurofibroma Bone tumors (eg, Ewing sarcoma)
Traumatic	Hematoma	Esophageal foreign body Esophageal stricture Hematoma

distinction between the inspiratory and expiratory phases. Also, large lesions may produce significant narrowing of the airway in both inspiratory and expiratory phases to result in stridor throughout the respiratory cycle.

The larynx remains relatively rigid during the respiratory cycle and does not change appreciably in caliber. Lesions in the larynx, therefore, typically produce biphasic stridor, although inspiratory stridor usually predominates. The vocal cords are the narrowest point of the larynx and the narrowest segment of the entire airway. This region is a crucial site in infants because even small lesions involving the vocal cords produce significant alterations in the cross-sectional diameter of the airway.

In addition to the presence and character of stridor, there are other clinical findings that may suggest the etiology of upper airway obstruction. Lesions that affect the glottis and vocal cords usually produce vocal abnormalities, such as hoarseness or aphonia. An exception is bilateral vocal cord paralysis because these children have a normal voice. Lesions adjacent to the glottis may produce abnormalities of the voice that are indistinguishable from those due to vocal cord lesions. Nasopharyngeal obstruction may result in nasal speech in older children, although an infant's cry is usually unaffected. Oropharyngeal or supraglottic laryngeal obstructions do not produce vocal abnormalities but may produce muffled phonation. Unilateral vocal cord paralysis results in a weak cry and minimal respiratory distress. Subglottic laryngeal obstruction produces a hoarse-sounding voice. The character of the voice is typically unaffected with tracheal obstruction, such as tracheomalacia.

Cough is frequently present in children with airway obstruction, and the nature of the cough may have diagnostic implications. Nasopharyngeal obstructions are not usually associated with cough except in infants during feeding. Obstructing lesions in the oropharynx or at the base of the tongue may also produce cough related to feeding. A barking cough is highly suggestive of subglottic obstruction, usually due to croup. Epiglottitis may be associated with a cough that has a raspy

character. A harsh, brassy cough frequently accompanies lesions of the intrathoracic trachea.

Feeding difficulties in addition to stridor suggest anatomic disorders such as tracheoesophageal fistula, cleft larynx, vascular ring, or neurologic disease. Feeding difficulties are associated with aspiration of secretions or food. Repeated aspiration often results in pulmonary symptoms.

Signs of respiratory distress occur in some infants and young children with lesions of the airway. These correlate with the severity of the obstruction but not with the location of the abnormality. Inspiratory retraction is an indicator of respiratory distress. Retractions most commonly occur in the presence of upper tracheal obstruction. In infants with nasopharyngeal occlusion, retractions do not occur during open-mouth breathing. Retractions suggest a relatively severe obstruction and are most commonly associated with croup, epiglottitis, laryngomalacia, vocal cord paralysis, and the uncommon laryngeal webs, cysts, and tumors.[1]

The lateral radiograph of the upper airway is the cornerstone of diagnostic imaging techniques for the evaluation of children with suspected upper airway obstruction. An anteroposterior radiograph of the upper airway and anteroposterior and lateral chest radiographs are frequently useful for complete evaluation. Improved visualization of the airway is provided by filtered, high-kilovoltage radiographs. Airway fluoroscopy is sometimes needed to identify a dynamic abnormality, such as tracheomalacia. Barium studies of the pharynx and esophagus are useful for definition of pharyngeal anatomy, demonstration of primary esophageal pathology associated with airway obstruction, and detection of obstructing lesions that are extrinsic to the trachea and esophagus, such as a vascular ring or bronchogenic cyst.

Computed tomography (CT) is valuable in some instances of airway obstruction because of the cross-sectional depiction of the airway and adjacent structures. CT is most useful for evaluation of mass lesions intrinsic or extrinsic to the trachea. Disadvantages of CT include its limited ability to image in the sagittal and coronal planes and to demonstrate dynamic processes.

Magnetic resonance imaging (MRI) provides excellent depiction of pharyngeal and tracheal anatomy in all three orthogonal planes. This technique is well suited for imaging of mass lesions and vascular anomalies. Utilization of this technique is somewhat limited by expense, time of the examination, and the requirement for the child to remain motionless for extended periods of time.[1–4]

Nose and Nasopharynx

The internal nasal cavities extend from the nares anteriorly to the choanae posteriorly. The superior walls of the nasal cavities are derived from the frontal bone and sphenoid bone; the floor is provided by the hard palate. The nasal cavities are surrounded by the paranasal sinuses and communicate with them via ostia located between the turbinates. The frontal sinuses lie superior, the sphenoid sinuses posterior, the ethmoid sinuses lateral, and the maxillary sinuses inferolateral to the nasal cavities. Because of these anatomic relationships, disease processes arising in the nasal cavities frequently secondarily involve the paranasal sinuses, and vice versa.

The nasopharynx is a midline, semirigid, tubular-shaped, inverted muscular sling that forms the most superior portion of the airway. It is continuous with the nasal cavities anteriorly and with the oropharynx inferiorly, through the nasal choanae. A horizontal line drawn along the hard palate and soft palate divides the nasopharynx above from the oropharynx below. Posterosuperiorly, the nasopharynx is bounded by the lower portion of the clivus, the upper cervical spine, and the paravertebral muscles. The medial pterygoid plates provide structural support for the anterolateral nasopharynx; posterolaterally, structural rigidity is provided by the cervical fascia.

Nasal and nasopharyngeal masses that may be associated with upper airway obstruction in children are listed in Table 3-5.[5,6]

Choanal Atresia

Choanal atresia is a congenital obstruction of the posterior nasal passages. The obstruction can be unilateral or bilateral, bony or membranous, complete or incomplete. Choanal atresia results from failure of normal perforation of the oronasal membrane during fetal week 7. In 90% of cases the obstruction is bony, and in approximately 30% the condition is bilateral. Because the neonate is an obligatory nose breather, bilateral choanal atresia is associated with severe respiratory distress in the postpartum period and may, on occasion, cause death. The unilateral type is usually associated with less dramatic symptomatology, and in some cases clinical presentation (unilateral nasal obstruction and rhinorrhea) may not occur until later in infancy.

Table 3-5 Nasal and Nasopharyngeal Masses in Children

Congenital or developmental
  Cephalocele/meningocele
  Glioma
  Dermoid/teratoma
Inflammatory
  Polyp
  Retropharyngeal abscess
Benign neoplasm
  Juvenile angiofibroma
  Teratoma
  Hemangioma
  Fibrous dysplasia/juvenile ossifying fibroma (rare)
  Inverting papilloma (rare)
  Fibrous histiocytoma (rare)
  Chondroma (rare)
  Meningioma (rare)
  Neurofibroma/schwannoma (rare)
Malignant neoplasm
  Rhabdomyosarcoma
  Esthesioneuroblastoma
  Nasopharyngeal carcinoma/lymphoepithelioma
  Osteosarcoma (rare)
  Chondrosarcoma (rare)
  Fibrosarcoma (rare)
  Langerhans cell histiocytosis (rare)
  Hemangiopericytoma (rare)
  Schwannoma (rare)
  Lymphoma (rare)
  Metastatic disease (rare)

Choanal atresia is associated with significant feeding problems because the infant has difficulty sucking and breathing at the same time. Clinically, the diagnosis of choanal atresia can be established by failure to pass a small catheter through the nostrils into the pharynx. This does not, however, differentiate between bony and membranous obstruction; this differentiation is of vital importance for selecting appropriate therapy.[6,7]

The radiographic evaluation of choanal obstruction has changed with the introduction of new imaging techniques. Previously, a choanagram was the imaging procedure of choice. With this technique, contrast medium is placed in the nostril with the infant in the supine position, and a cross-table lateral radiograph is obtained. Normally, the contrast material passes immediately into the nasopharynx and oropharynx. With choanal atresia the contrast material remains in the nasal passages, and the posterior extent defines the level of obstruction (Fig. 3-1).[8,9]

In current practice, CT with bone and soft tissue techniques provides the best diagnostic approach for evaluation of choanal atresia. CT is as accurate as the choanagram in detecting choanal obstruction; in addition, CT can define whether the obstruction is membranous or bony, determine the extent of obstruction, and evaluate coexistent facial anomalies. With CT, the complete anatomic abnormality is easily visualized, and a systematic approach to surgery can be formulated.

In bony choanal atresia, characteristic findings are present on CT. There is medial bowing and thickening of the lateral

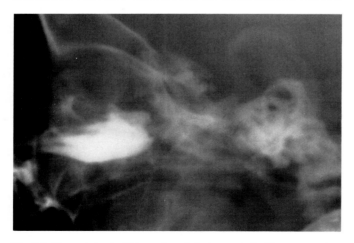

Fig. 3-1 Choanal atresia. This newborn infant presented with severe respiratory distress. Catheters could not be advanced into the nasopharynx. Positive-contrast choanagram demonstrates complete obstruction of the posterior nasal choanae. The choanagram cannot differentiate between membranous and bony choanal atresia.

wall of the nasal cavity, which is composed of the perpendicular plates of the palatine bones and the pterygoid processes. The vomer is enlarged and fused with the lateral walls of the nasal cavity. In membranous atresia bony fusion is not present, although some degree of bony thickening is present. The air passage between the lateral wall of the nasal cavity and the vomer is smaller than normal. Membranous obstruction is located anterior to the pterygoid plates, at the level of the junction of the perpendicular portion of the palatine bone with the pterygoid processes (Fig. 3-2).[10–13]

The evaluation of choanal atresia may be complicated by mucoid impaction proximal to the site of obstruction. The mucous impaction may simulate an intranasal neoplasm on either CT or contrast radiographic studies. Impacted mucus may also lead to an overestimation of the thickness of an obstructing membrane on CT.[10,14] To lessen this pitfall, the nares should be suctioned before imaging and a few drops of phenylephrine nose drops placed in the nares.

Juvenile Angiofibroma

Juvenile angiofibroma is a rare, extremely vascular tumor that occurs in the posterior nasal cavity. It accounts for less than 1% of all head and neck neoplasms in children. Although pathologically benign, these tumors frequently attain a relatively large size and are locally invasive. Juvenile angiofibroma occurs almost exclusively in adolescent boys; only a few cases have been reported in girls.

Signs and symptoms of juvenile angiofibroma are often related to tumor extension into the nasal cavity, orbit, or skull base. A more unusual presentation is due to extension of the tumor into the posterior oral cavity. Most often, the mass is located in the parasagittal plane near the base of the skull and is entirely extracranial.

The clinical signs of juvenile angiofibroma are most often indolent, with many patients in retrospect reporting symptoms of up to 2 years' duration. Nasal obstruction occurs in 80% to 90% of the cases and epistaxis in 70% to 90%. Other potential clinical findings include nasal discharge, facial deformity, exophthalmos, anosmia, and hearing loss. Rhinoscopy shows a deep red, firm, rubbery, lobulated mass that usually occupies one side of the nasal cavity. The surface is often ulcerated or granular. The lesion bleeds briskly if sampled by biopsy. Juvenile angiofibroma is classified histologically as a benign fibromatous or angiofibromatous hamartoma. There is a 25% to 60% recurrence rate after surgical resection.[15,16]

Almost all juvenile angiofibromas arise in the posterior nasopharynx near the pterygopalatine fossa and sphenopalatine foramen. Diagnostic imaging studies may show the tumor to remain localized in the nasopharynx (stage 1) or to extend into the nasal cavity or sphenoid sinus (stage 2). Further tumor extension is common, and may result in involvement of the pterygopalatine fossa (89% of cases), high masseter space, maxillary sinuses, and ethmoid sinuses (stage 3). Typically, even when large, juvenile angiofibroma does not extend far enough posterolaterally to obliterate the fat planes of the

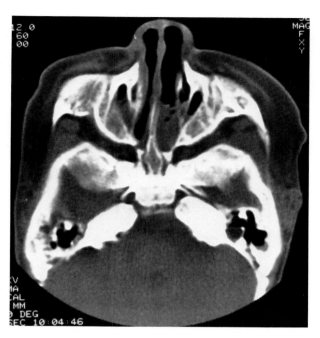

Fig. 3-2 Bilateral choanal atresia in a newborn. CT demonstrates bony atresia on the left and membranous atresia on the right.

carotid sheath. Intracranial involvement (stage 4) usually occurs by extension from the pterygopalatine fossa into the orbit through the inferior orbital fissure and then through the superior orbital fissure into the region of the middle cranial fossa and cavernous sinus.[17]

The diagnostic features of juvenile angiofibroma identified on standard radiography are highly characteristic and include anterior bowing of the posterior wall of the maxillary antrum (antral sign), lateral displacement of the nasal septum, and a large soft tissue mass in the nasal cavity and nasopharynx with or without bony erosion of contiguous structures. The antral sign is the most common abnormality seen on standard radiographs. Bony erosion or destruction with sharp margins is present in about 50% of cases (Fig. 3-3).

CT and MRI provide markedly superior demonstration of tumor morphology and the effects of the tumor on adjacent structures. These techniques are particularly useful for depicting extension of tumor into the sinuses, orbit, and skull base. CT is the superior imaging method for demonstrating bone involvement; MRI offers the capability of direct sagittal imaging and depiction of vascular anatomy without intravenous contrast agents.

CT evaluation of juvenile angiofibroma is usually performed with scanning in both axial and coronal planes. The intense vascularity of the tumor is best appreciated when images are obtained dynamically during, or immediately after, bolus contrast medium administration. Tumor enhancement usually fades rapidly, and delayed scanning may result in poor visualization of the lesion. CT findings include an enhancing pharyngeal mass, anterior bowing of the posterior wall of the

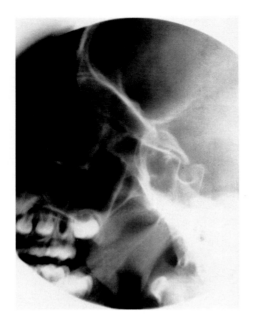

Fig. 3-3 Juvenile angiofibroma. The large retropharyngeal mass has displaced the posterior wall of one maxillary sinus anteriorly. This is the antral sign.

maxillary antrum due to a mass in the pterygopalatine fossa, opacity of one or more of the paranasal sinuses, erosion of the sphenoid bone, erosion of the hard palate, erosion of the medial wall of the maxillary sinus, deviation of the nasal septum, and, rarely, intracranial extension (Fig. 3-4).

Tumor morphology and effects on adjacent structures are also well demonstrated on MRI. The lesion produces a variable degree of increased signal compared to adjacent normal

structures on T_2-weighted images. The vascular nature of the tumor is usually clearly demonstrated on MRI because of signal void from the rapidly flowing blood in the tumor vessels.

As described above, involvement of the paranasal sinuses is a common finding with juvenile angiofibroma. Sinus involvement takes two forms: obstruction of the sinus ostia, and extension of tumor into the sinus cavity. The sphenoid sinus is involved in 60% to 70% of cases, the ethmoid sinus in 35% to 45%, and the maxillary sinus in 25%. Approximately 5% of cases have orbital or intracranial extension.[15,18,19]

Sinus involvement is indicated on standard radiographs by bone destruction or nonspecific sinus opacification. Differentiation of sinus opacification due to obstruction from that due to tumor extension into the sinus is sometimes difficult even with CT and MRI. Fluid may be differentiated from tumor on CT by lack of contrast enhancement; thickened mucosa in an obstructed sinus typically exhibits significant enhancement, however, which may be similar to tumor enhancement. Accurate detection of sinus extension is usually possible with MRI. Mucosal thickening and fluid in the sinus usually produce greater signal intensity than tumor on T_2-weighted images.

Angiography is usually performed in cases of juvenile angiofibroma before surgical treatment to define the extent of the lesion, the degree of vascularity, and the source of the feeding vessels. A reticulated pattern is usually identified in the early arterial phase. A dense homogeneous blush develops that persists into the venous phase. Early draining veins are typically not identified. The major vascular supply usually is from branches arising from the external carotid, maxillary, facial, and ascending pharyngeal arteries. In many cases, embolization of major feeding vessels is performed to facili-

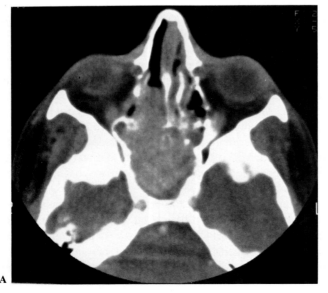

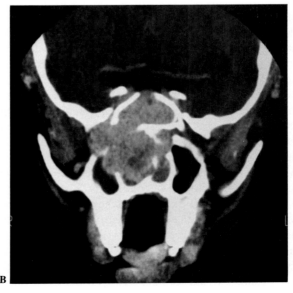

A   B

Fig. 3-4 Juvenile angiofibroma. (**A**) Contrast-enhanced axial and (**B**) coronal CT scans show an enhancing, lobulated mass occupying the nasopharynx and ascending into the sphenoid sinus, right orbit, right maxillary sinus, and floor of the anterior cranial fossa.

tate the surgical approach to this lesion and to decrease blood loss during the procedure (Fig. 3-5).

The most important differential diagnostic consideration in juvenile nasal angiofibroma is the angiomatous polyp. These lesions may be confused even on pathologic examination. In contradistinction to juvenile angiofibroma, however, an angiomatous polyp typically is hypovascular on CT and does not invade the pterygopalatine fossa or sphenoid sinus. It differs from juvenile angiofibroma in both the arterial supply and the ease of surgical removal.[17]

From the radiologic viewpoint, certain conclusions can be made concerning juvenile angiofibroma:[8,20]

1. The lesion originates at the sphenopalatine foramen, enlarges the foramen, and erodes the base of the medial pterygoid plate, the floor of the sphenoid sinus, and the posterior wall of the maxillary antrum. Extension can lead to invasion of the infratemporal fossa, orbit, and middle cranial fossa.
2. The antral sign seen on standard radiographs is not totally reliable because other aggressive or slow-growing benign tumors can produce this finding.
3. When a positive antral sign is identified on plain radiographs, MRI is the modality of choice in the investigation of the lesion.
4. Angiography is not needed for the diagnosis of juvenile angiofibroma but is useful for surgical planning and therapeutic embolization before surgery.

Nasal Polyps

Nasal polyps are uncommon in healthy children but still represent the most common clinically identified nasal masses. Most nasal polyps are of the inflammatory or allergic types. Children with atopy, aspirin-sensitive allergy, cystic fibrosis, Woakes syndrome, and Kartagener syndrome and other forms of dysmotile cilia are prone to nasal polyps; these are often associated with chronic sinusitis. Approximately 10% of children with cystic fibrosis have inflammatory polyps.

The term *nasal polyp* is somewhat of a misnomer; in fact, most nasal polyps are actually herniations of hypertrophic paranasal sinus mucosa that protrude from the sinus ostium. The mucosa of the paranasal sinuses and nasal cavity responds in a similar manner to a variety of long-term insults, such as allergy or chronic infection. The cells undergo metaplasia and an increase in the number of goblet cells. Secretions increase, and edema with polypoid degeneration of the mucosa occurs. The polyps themselves represent protrusions of edematous lamina propria surrounded by hyperplastic secretory mucosa.

Most nasal polyps originate from the middle turbinates and ethmoid sinuses. Those arising from the ethmoid sinuses are often multiple, producing a grapelike appearance. Nasal polyps usually have a glistening gray-white hue and are mobile. Large polyps may protrude through the anterior nares. It is important to remember that embryonal rhabdomyosar-

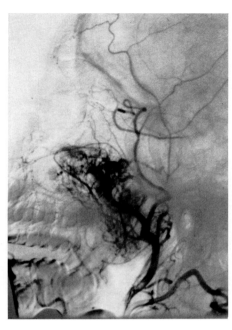

Figure 3-5 Juvenile angiofibroma. External carotid arteriogram shows enlargement of the internal maxillary artery that feeds the hypervascular retropharyngeal tumor.

coma of the botryoid type, when found in the nasal cavity or nasopharynx, may have a similar gross appearance.

Antrochoanal polyp is a relatively unusual abnormality that may produce a nasopharyngeal mass in older children and young adults. In this condition, an antral polyp from within the maxillary sinus enlarges and widens the sinus ostium to prolapse into the nasal cavity. A large antrochoanal polyp may fill the nasopharynx and extend into the oropharynx. The clinical presentation is most often due to obstruction of the nasopharyngeal airway; some cases present as an asymptomatic mass protruding from the nares or extending into the oropharynx. In contradistinction to most nasal polyps, the antrochoanal polyp is usually not associated with allergy; rather, in most instances, chronic maxillary sinusitis is the underlying pathology. Antrochoanal polyps represent between 4% and 6% of all nasal polyps. This type of polyp is usually unilateral, but bilateral maxillary sinus inflammatory disease is found in 30% to 40% of cases.[6,21–23]

Nasal polyps are readily seen on clinical examination. Radiographic studies serve to determine the posterior extension, to detect osseous changes, and to aid in the differential diagnosis. Standard radiographs demonstrate increased density in the nasal cavity. The rounded contour of the polyp is sometimes identified. Cross-sectional imaging with CT or MRI more clearly defines the morphology and composition of the mass. The imaging principles are similar to those of the inflammatory and allergic polyps that occur in the paranasal sinuses.

On unenhanced CT images, a nasal polyp is demonstrated as a homogeneous, rounded mass in the nasal cavity. The

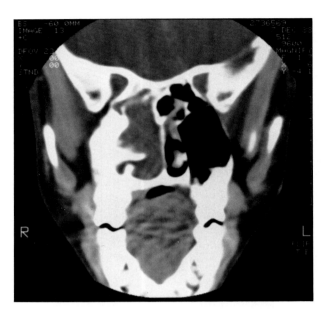

Fig. 3-6 Nasal polyp. Coronal CT shows a soft tissue mass that fills the nasal cavity, displacement of the middle turbinate, and superior and lateral displacement of ethmoid air cells. No true bone destruction is seen. There is sclerosis of the lateral wall of the right maxillary sinus due to chronic sinusitis.

osseous structures are usually normal in appearance. After intravenous contrast medium administration, areas of thickened mucosa may enhance, but the fluid-filled cavity of the polyp does not enhance (Fig. 3-6).[24]

Nasal polyps are easily visualized on MRI. Because the primary cause of polyp formation is the intracellular accumulation of fluid, polyps characteristically demonstrate bright signal intensity on T_2-weighted images. High T_2 signal intensities are present both in cystic fluid collections and in areas of inflammatory mucosal edema. Primary sinonasal neoplasms, however, typically produce intermediate signal on T_2-weighted images and only rarely produce signal approaching the bright signal intensity typical of inflammatory polyps.[25]

The diagnosis of an antrochoanal polyp is usually suggested on frontal and lateral radiographs of the paranasal sinuses. Frontal views show opacification of the maxillary sinus, usually with slight expansion of the walls of the maxillary antrum. A polypoid mass extends from the sinus into the nasal cavity. Lateral radiographs may demonstrate posterior extension of the mass into the nasopharynx.[21,22]

Cross-sectional imaging with CT provides improved characterization of antrochoanal polyps compared to radiographs. The involved maxillary sinus is opacified, and its bony walls are enlarged. The sinus ostium is widened by pressure necrosis, and a soft tissue mass is visible extending through the ostium. With intravenous contrast medium administration, the edematous inflammatory mucosa demonstrates moderate enhancement; the fluid-filled portions of the mass do not enhance. It has been reported that inflammatory hypertrophic mucosa in the maxillary sinus can become sufficiently edematous and redundant to prolapse into the nasal cavity

through the sinus ostium, producing imaging findings that simulate those of antrochoanal polyp.[23]

Nasopharyngeal Teratoma

Benign nasopharyngeal tumors are uncommon in children. Benign neoplasms that may occur in this region include teratoma, osteoma, and hemangioma. The nasopharynx is the most common site of origin of teratomas in the head and neck. There is a female predominance. Nasopharyngeal teratomas most commonly arise in the soft palate or the fossa of Rosenmüller.

A nasopharyngeal teratoma is a congenital neoplasm that can cause significant airway obstruction if the mass interferes with the normal obligate nasal breathing of infants. Occasionally, the tumor stalk is long enough to touch the supraglottic larynx, resulting in coughing or gagging. On examination, a large lobulated mass is usually visible protruding from the nasopharynx into the oral cavity or externally through the anterior nares. Although most of these tumors are pedunculated, the site of attachment in the nasopharynx may be difficult to ascertain.

Nasopharyngeal teratomas are most often covered with skin; if hair is present, they are referred to clinically as hairy polyps (Fig. 3-7). In some instances, the tumor may protrude through a midline facial cleft (epignathus). Communication with the central nervous system through the base of the skull indicates a poor prognosis.

The origin of these tumors is thought to be similar to that of sacrococcygeal teratoma (ie, development from totipotent germ cells) because they occur in an area that remains active in embryologic differentiation until late in fetal life.[26]

The diagnosis of nasopharyngeal teratoma is often suggested on conventional radiographs. Characteristically, a large mass with calcification or ossification is seen in the nasopharynx and oral cavity, causing gross deformity of the maxilla and mandible. The radiographic literature contains little or no information regarding these teratomas. Calcification occurs in at least 60% of sacrococcygeal teratomas, but the frequency in nasopharyngeal teratomas has not been reported. The few scattered case reports in the surgical literature describe calcification or ossification that was seen on plain radiographs (Fig. 3-8).

CT is extremely useful in defining the full extent of the tumor in relationship to other structures. Often, difficulty in maintaining the airway may be so pronounced that immediate surgical attention is needed; CT is deferred until a stable airway is achieved.[27–29]

Malignant Tumors

Primary malignant lesions of the nasopharynx include nasopharyngeal carcinoma, malignant germ cell tumors, rhabdomyosarcoma, lymphoma, and esthesioneuroblastoma. The tumors that are found in this location collectively account for less than 1% of all pediatric malignancies. Rhabdomyosar-

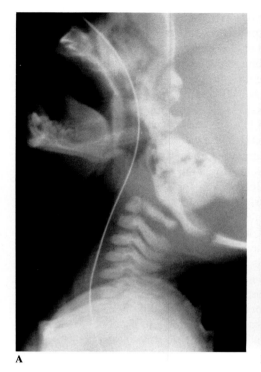
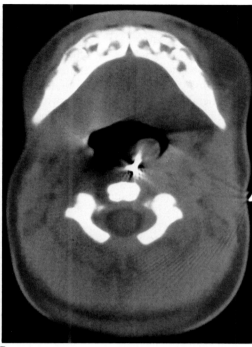

A   B

Fig. 3-7 Nasopharyngeal teratoma (hairy polyp). (**A**) Lateral radiograph and (**B**) axial CT scan demonstrate a round soft tissue mass lying in the posterior left portion of the nasopharynx. A nasogastric tube lies immediately posterior to the mass.

coma is the most common primary nasopharyngeal malignancy in children.[6,30,31]

Epithelial malignancies are uncommon in children. Nasopharyngeal and thyroid carcinomas are the most common epithelial malignancies of the head and neck region in the pediatric age group. Both neoplasms frequently present with cervical lymphadenopathy. The average age of the child with nasopharyngeal carcinoma is 12 years. It is more common in boys. The most common histologic type of nasopharyngeal carcinoma in the pediatric age group is a variant of squamous cell carcinoma with lymphocytic infiltration termed *lymphoepithelial carcinoma* (formerly lymphoepithelioma). It is approximately five times more common in adolescent African-Americans than in whites.[32,33]

Nasal obstruction, cervical adenopathy (often unilateral), epistaxis, cranial nerve palsy, deafness, and pain in the ear are the main clinical manifestations of nasopharyngeal carcinoma. Cervical lymph node metastasis occurs in about 70% of patients. The mass, which is frequently located in the posterior nasopharynx, often involves the fossa of Rosenmüller. Because of its location, the tumor is often difficult to appreciate on the clinical examination.[6,30]

The differential diagnosis of nasopharyngeal carcinoma includes inflammatory disease, sinusitis, and the more common head and neck neoplasms of childhood such as lymphoma with cervical lymph node enlargement and rhabdomyosarcoma. Diagnostic delay results when this tumor is not considered a possible etiology in the presence of early, nonspecific symptoms, yet it is only by early detection, when the tumor is confined to the soft tissues in the nasopharynx, that improved

survival rates can be obtained. The average delay in diagnosis is probably 1 year.[34]

Rhabdomyosarcoma is an aggressive malignant neoplasm that tends to invade adjacent structures. Rhabdomyosarcoma is the most common soft tissue sarcoma of childhood. Forty percent of these tumors occur in the head and neck region. This tumor typically grows rapidly, infiltrates extensively, and metastasizes widely. In order of frequency, the most common

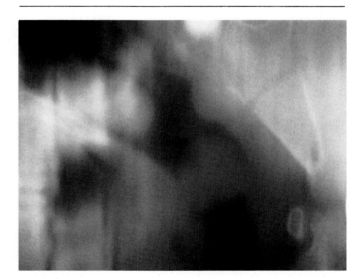

Fig. 3-8 Nasopharyngeal teratoma. Lateral tomogram demonstrates a round, noncalcified, soft tissue mass in the posterior nasopharynx. No specific characterizing features are present.

anatomic locations of rhabdomyosarcoma in the head and neck region are the orbit, the naso-oropharynx, and the aural region. Seventy percent of head and neck rhabdomyosarcomas occur in patients younger than 12 years of age. Histologically, 75% are of the embryonal type, which is associated with an overall better prognosis than the other histologic types (botryoid, alveolar, or pleomorphic). In general, these tumors cannot be totally resected; thus diagnostic biopsy with moderate surgical resection is usually performed.

Rhabdomyosarcoma frequently metastasizes to the cervical lymph nodes. Invasion through the base of the skull with potential meningeal dissemination is common. Nasal obstruction and serous otitis media are common presenting symptoms. Extension into the orbit may cause proptosis with or without a decrease in visual acuity. Some patients present with a bloody nasal discharge. Cranial nerve palsy due to intracranial invasion may be evident at the time of presentation (Fig. 3-9).[6,35]

Malignant lymphoma is one of the more common primary tumors to involve the nasal cavity, paranasal sinuses, tonsils, or nasopharynx in children. The ring of Waldeyer is the most common site of origin of non-Hodgkin lymphoma in the head and neck region. When lymphoma presents in these locations, it is difficult to distinguish clinically from nasopharyngeal carcinoma. The most common variety of lymphoma is the large cell type. Uncommonly, Burkitt (B-cell) lymphoma can occur in the nasopharynx. Hodgkin disease typically involves cervical lymph nodes; extranodal involvement in the head and neck region is rare. The adenoids rarely may be involved with Hodgkin disease.

Esthesioneuroblastoma (olfactory neuroblastoma) is a rare malignant tumor of the nasal fossa in children. It is seen more frequently in adult men. The neoplasm is neural in origin; it arises from the epithelium and nerves of the olfactory mucosa. This specialized epithelium is located on the upper surface of the superior turbinate, the uppermost aspect of the nasal septum, and the inferior surface of the cribriform plate. Therefore, this tumor typically arises high in the nasal cavity. There are two age peaks: 11 to 20 years, and 31 to 40 years. Patients younger than 15 years of age account for approximately 15% of cases. Unilateral nasal obstruction, epistaxis, and epiphora are the most common symptoms. A reddish-gray polypoid mass that bleeds readily is the usual physical finding. These tumors grow slowly, and local recurrences are frequent. Metastasis occurs to cervical lymph nodes, liver, lung, bone, and brain.[36]

Presently, CT and MRI are the imaging modalities that are most useful for evaluating nasopharyngeal malignancies. The imaging findings are usually not tumor specific. Permeative bone destruction in association with a soft tissue mass is virtually diagnostic of a malignant tumor. Imaging studies often show tumor extension into one or more paranasal sinuses or sinus opacification that is due to obstruction. Extension into the infratemporal fossa or pterygopalatine fossa and involvement of the orbit are indicators of aggressive malignant lesions. Tumor extension into these anatomic regions is imaged as a mass with disruption of the soft tissue planes of the infratemporal fossa, pterygopalatine fossa, or parapharyngeal space.

Although the cross-sectional capability of CT has improved the radiographic evaluation of nasopharyngeal pathology, structures having similar soft tissue characteristics remain difficult to differentiate. Because of its greater soft tissue contrast resolution, MRI has improved diagnostic informa-

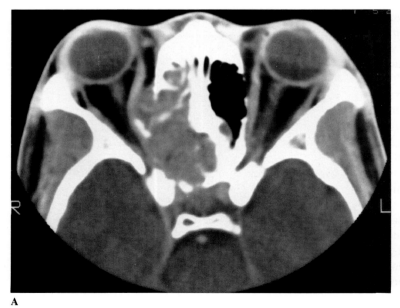
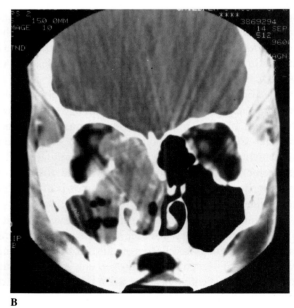

A   **B**

Fig. 3-9 Nasopharyngeal rhabdomyosarcoma. (**A**) Axial and (**B**) coronal contrast-enhanced CT scans demonstrate a large mass arising from the nasopharynx with bony destruction and extension into the paranasal sinuses and right orbit.

tion, especially with the use of paramagnetic agents, such as gadopentetate dimeglumine. The advantages of direct multiplanar imaging with MRI are valuable when tumor extent is evaluated. In the usual case, MRI demonstrates normal and morbid pharyngeal anatomy better than CT. Vascular structures can be differentiated from surrounding tissue without intravenous contrast material, and direct coronal and sagittal images optimally demonstrate the anatomy at the base of the skull. In patients with nasopharyngeal malignancy, MRI is of equal or greater accuracy compared to CT in identifying tumor margins, mass effect, and regional lymph nodes. Both reactive and metastatic nodes are detected with greater sensitivity by MRI, although distinction between the two requires histologic verification. This may be a problem in young children, who frequently have benign cervical adenopathy.[17,37–40]

The mass produced by nasopharyngeal carcinoma can be detected with most imaging techniques. Lymph node enlargement may be demonstrated with CT, MRI, or [67Ga]citrate scintigraphy. Uptake of ^{67}Ga is a nonspecific finding that may occur in benign disease or other head and neck malignancies. Local involvement of bone with destruction at the base of the skull is frequently identified in cases of nasopharyngeal carcinoma and is best seen on CT at bone windows. Radiographs of the skull may show sclerosis of the skull base, but this is a late finding. When bone scintigraphy is performed, hypertrophic osteoarthropathy and local invasive changes are the most common findings.[17,34–36]

CT and especially MRI in the coronal and sagittal planes provide excellent demonstration of the extent of involvement by nasopharyngeal rhabdomyosarcoma and are effective in assessing the response to therapy. Nasopharyngeal rhabdomyosarcoma is typically imaged as a soft tissue mass with malignant permeative bone destruction. CT demonstrates the full extent of bone involvement and delineates the margins of the lesion and associated intracranial and extracranial components. Frequently, the margins of bone destruction are ill defined because of the aggressive growth pattern. Involvement of the base of the skull may be extensive. The tumor shows a variable degree of contrast enhancement on CT. Often the intracranial component will be seen as an extradural-based enhancing soft tissue mass. The mass is usually homogeneous on MR images and produces low to intermediate signal on T_1-weighted images. Moderate signal intensity is produced by these neoplasms on T_2-weighted images, which is in contradistinction to the bright signal of inflammatory changes in adjacent mucosa and sinuses. Meningeal involvement by permeation through adjacent bone or extension through neural foramina is a poor prognostic feature. After therapy, these tumors usually regress and calcify.[25,35,36]

Diagnostic imaging in cases of malignant lymphoma reveals an infiltrating soft tissue mass. The lesion is most often located in the region of the ring of Waldeyer. Most often there is infiltration of more than one site in the ring, but an isolated mass in the nasopharynx or tonsil may occur. This tumor may also arise in the nasal cavity or paranasal sinuses. As with other pharyngeal malignancies, imaging studies usually dem-

onstrate infiltration of adjacent structures and a variable degree of bone destruction.[40]

Esthesioneuroblastoma usually arises high in the nasal fossa, and when the tumor is small the location of the lesion may be the only clue to the diagnosis. A soft tissue mass is identified in the nasal cavity. Unilateral opacification of the ethmoid sinuses, with or without accompanying bone erosion or destruction, is frequent. Extension into the sphenoid and maxillary sinuses, orbit, and anterior cranial fossa is common. When the tumor is large, it is indistinguishable from other nasal malignancies. Distant metastases are uncommon.

The angiographic findings with esthesioneuroblastoma vary from hypervascularity with early draining veins to faint tumor blush. CT shows a contrast-enhancing mass and delineates its extension into adjacent structures. CT may help distinguish the tumor mass from reactive sinusitis. Punctate intratumoral calcifications are occasionally present. An osteoblastic reaction in adjacent structures has been reported but is uncommon.

MRI of esthesioneuroblastoma readily demonstrates the extent of the tumor. The lesion is usually nearly isointense to brain on T_1-weighted images and is moderately hyperintense on T_2-weighted images. Differentiation between tumor invasion of the paranasal sinuses and fluid retention due to obstruction of the ostia is readily identified on MRI.[36,41–43]

Developmental Masses

There is a spectrum of developmental malformations related to abnormalities of closure of the midline facial structures and the central nervous system. These include congenital dermoid cyst and fistula, nasal glioma, heterotopic brain, and intranasal meningoencephalocele. The prevalence of these congenital midline nasal masses is one in every 20,000 to 40,000 live births. A mass presenting in the nasal region in a newborn infant or an intranasal abnormality discovered during the first year of life is the usual clinical presentation of these abnormalities. Any of these lesions that has a significant intranasal component may be associated with signs of obstruction of the nasopharyngeal airway.[5,6]

Nasal dermoid cysts are similar to those found in the orbit and oral cavity. Most arise adjacent to the nasofrontal suture. The mass is usually midline at the bridge of the nose and has a visible superficial component. If the cyst is deep, it may be recognized clinically by the identification of a small indentation at the bridge of the nose. A sinus tract to the skin is frequently present, or there may be a fistulous communication with other adjacent structures. Sixty percent are discovered at birth or shortly thereafter. Secondary infection of a dermoid cyst is an occasional complication.[6,29]

Nasal gliomas occur at the bridge of the nose (as with a dermoid cyst) or near the glabella at the side of the nose (60%), intranasally (30% to 40%), or in both locations (10%). When the lesion arises from the lateral nasal wall, it is sometimes misdiagnosed as a polyp. The term *glioma* is a misnomer because these lesions are not true neoplasms but rather are composed of mature neural tissue. They tend to be firmer in consistency than a dermoid cyst. When a nasal glioma is located entirely in the nasal fossa, it is difficult to differentiate from a nasal cephalocele on the basis of its clinical appearance. A bony defect is usually apparent in cases of cephalocele, however, and by definition there is connection with the subarachnoid space, the ventricular system, or both. Approximately 15% of nasal gliomas are connected by a fibrous stalk to the dura, and an open communication with the cerebrospinal fluid circulation may occur.[5,44]

Meningocele and meningoencephalocele can occur in an anterior location and involve the nasopharynx. These lesions are congenital extracranial herniations of meninges (meningocele) or of meninges and neural tissue (meningoencephalocele). In this location, a pure meningocele without a neural component is rare. Approximately 12% to 13% of all cephaloceles involve the anterior cranial fossa.[45]

The occipitoparietal region is the most frequent site for meningoencephaloceles. Anterior cephaloceles may be categorized as follows: nasofrontal, located between the nasal and frontal bones; nasoethmoid, extending through the embryonic foramen cecum into the nasal cavity; naso-orbital, protruding through the lamina papyracea into the orbit; transethmoidal, protruding through the cribriform plate into the superior meatus; and sphenomaxillary, extending through the supraorbital and infraorbital fissures. A symmetric mass that distorts the external nose or a purely intranasal process is the form of presentation of an anterior meningoencephalocele. Intranasal cephaloceles frequently produce symptomatic nasal airway obstruction; most present at birth.

Heterotopic brain tissue has been reported in the soft palate and pharynx, where, if of sufficient size, it can be responsible for severe respiratory distress in the neonatal period. Because of the rarity of this lesion, if neural tissue is discovered on biopsy of a nasopharyngeal mass then cephalocele is the most likely diagnosis. Differentiation between cephalocele where there is a connection with the central nervous system and heterotopia where this connection is lacking is an important function of diagnostic imaging studies.

The radiographic presentation of nasal glioma is a purely intranasal mass in 30% of cases, a completely extranasal mass in 60% of cases, and a combination of these in the remainder of cases.[44] Radiographs of the paranasal sinuses are usually normal in cases of nasal glioma, or, if a lesion is visualized, it is indistinguishable from a nasal polyp. CT shows a round mass of homogeneous soft tissue attenuation, with no intracranial extension. If the lesion is of sufficient size, it may cause obstruction of the ostium of a paranasal sinus. The radiographic findings and clinical presentation of this lesion often do not allow definitive differentiation from cephaloceles or other local tumors.[46–48]

Radiographic findings in cases of nasal dermoid cyst include broadening or disruption of the nasal bridge of the nose, a sharply demarcated bony defect in the region of the nasofrontal suture or nasal bone, and a soft tissue mass in the nasal cavity. Most frequently, the margins of these lesions are thin and sclerotic. There may be deformity of the crista

galli. CT and MRI aid greatly in the diagnosis. Both imaging modalities show a lobulated mass that is predominantly cystic and may contain fat. On CT, the contents of the cyst do not enhance. The cystic component frequently is hyperintense on both T_1- and T_2-weighted MR images, reflecting its fatty and cystic nature.[43,49]

The radiographic findings with frontonasal meningocele or meningoencephalocele include an osseous defect (described above) and a soft tissue mass in the nasal cavity, nasopharynx, or paranasal sinuses. A variable degree of hypertelorism occurs with nasoethmoidal cephalocele. With nasofrontal cephalocele, lateral displacement or bowing of the superior aspects of the medial orbital walls occurs.[50]

CT, especially in the coronal plane, provides improved definition of the osseous and soft tissue abnormalities of nasofrontal cephaloceles. The mass appears cystic on CT in cases of meningocele, whereas the mass produced by a meningoencephalocele is imaged as a soft tissue lesion that is contiguous with and of similar CT attenuation characteristics as the frontal lobes of the brain. A variable amount of low-attenuation cerebrospinal fluid is usually identified surrounding the herniated brain. Communication with the intracranial subarachnoid spaces may be confirmed by CT cisternography.[6,45]

MRI, especially in the sagittal plane, is well suited for the diagnosis and characterization of anterior meningoencephaloceles (Fig. 3-10). T_1-weighted images usually provide the greatest anatomic detail. MRI findings include a protrusion of brain and a variable amount of surrounding cerebrospinal fluid through an osseous defect in the base of the skull. Other intracranial structures, such as blood vessels, may also protrude through the defect.

MRI and CT may demonstrate associated anomalies in cases of sphenoethmoidal cephalocele, which consist of midline clefts of the upper lip or nose (65%), optic nerve dysplasias (40%), and dysgenesis of the corpus callosum (40%).[51]

Heterotopic brain tissue in the nasopharynx may be demonstrated on a lateral radiograph as a mass related to the soft palate or lateral pharyngeal wall. In general, no osseous defect is identified. CT and MRI more clearly depict the location and composition of the mass. Occasionally, the mass may have low attenuation values on CT, mimicking fluid. CT and MRI usually allow differentiation of nasopharyngeal heterotopic brain from cephalocele and meningocele because no communication of the mass with the brain is observed on imaging studies and because the tissue usually extends laterally rather than being completely midline.[52–58]

Hypertrophied Tonsils and Adenoids

The adenoids are collections of lymphoid tissue that are located in the posterior aspect of the nasopharynx; the tonsils are similar lymphoid aggregates that lie in the oropharynx. Hypertrophy of these tissues is a common cause of upper airway obstruction in children. Mild cases are associated with

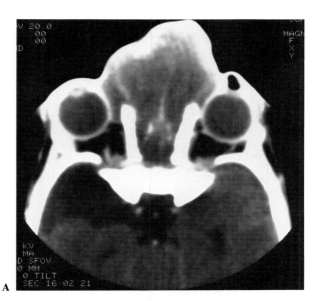

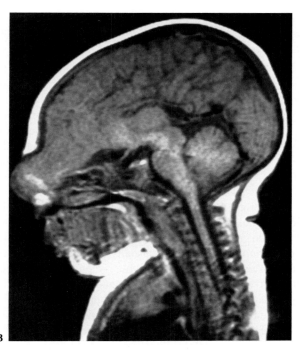

Fig. 3-10 Nasofrontal meningoencephalocele. (**A**) Contrast-enhanced axial CT scan and (**B**) T_1-weighted sagittal MR image demonstrate an osseous defect in the frontal bone. There is extension of brain and meninges through the defect into the nasal cavity. There is marked hypertelorism.

nasal stuffiness. Mouth breathing, noisy respirations while awake, and loud snoring while asleep are all common symptoms. With long-standing significant obstruction, a characteristic adenoid facies may be identified that consists of an open mouth with a flattened nose, small or underdeveloped nostrils, a short upper lip, a thick and everted lower lip, and a bored expression.

A distinct syndrome has been described in young children who develop cor pulmonale due to airway obstruction caused by hypertrophied tonsils and adenoids. These patients have noisy breathing and excessive daytime sleepiness. They have chronic hypoxia, hypercapnia, and acidosis. The signs of airway obstruction can be aggravated by sedation, supine positioning, or acute airway infections. The cause of this syndrome is significant chronic respiratory tract obstruction with hypoxia, hypercapnia, respiratory acidosis, and pulmonary hypertension. Right heart failure is the end result.[6,59]

A lateral radiograph of the nasopharynx obtained with the mouth closed to distend the nasopharynx usually is sufficient for the radiographic evaluation of the tonsils and adenoids. Enlargement of the adenoids and tonsils may be transient as a result of acute infection. In addition, there is marked normal variation in the size of the adenoids and tonsils among children. The radiographic demonstration of prominent adenoids and tonsils is not pathognomonic of disease.

Normally before 3 months of age, adenoidal tissue is sparse and not demonstrable radiographically. After 3 months the adenoids become progressively larger, and it is not unusual to see adenoids greater than 2 cm in thickness in an older child.[60] Large adenoids and tonsils occur in both healthy and ill children. Consequently, radiographs generally do not provide

information that is not clinically suspected. The most common problem radiographically is distinguishing large adenoids from an angiofibroma or other nasopharyngeal tumor. With simple adenoidal hypertrophy, there is normally an air space between the anterior surface of the adenoids and the uvula; with most other pathology this air space is obliterated (Fig. 3-11).[61,62]

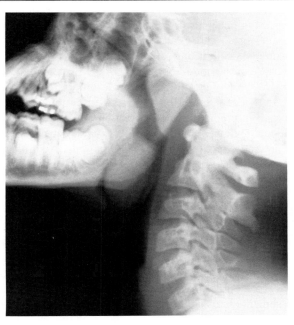

Fig. 3-11 Hypertrophied tonsils and adenoids. Lateral radiograph demonstrates enlargement of the tonsils and slight prominence of the adenoids.

Infectious Mononucleosis

Infectious mononucleosis is a disease caused by infection with Epstein-Barr virus, a type of herpes virus. The epithelial cells of the pharynx are the initial targets of infection of this virus, but shortly thereafter lymphocytes of B lineage soon become infected and become disseminated throughout the lymphatic system to most organs, where they will proliferate until they are checked by activated T cells. In the United States, the disease rarely occurs in children younger than 3 years of age, yet 60% to 80% of young adults are seropositive.

Infectious mononucleosis is often preceded by a 7- to 14-day prodrome of malaise, fatigue, headache, nausea, and abdominal pain. Patients develop fever, sore throat, and tonsillar enlargement (sometimes with exudate). Cervical lymphadenopathy is frequent, usually predominantly involving the posterior cervical chain. Other lymph node groups may also be involved. Epitrochlear lymphadenopathy is particularly consistent with infectious mononucleosis. The liver becomes enlarged in about one-third of patients, but elevations of hepatic enzymes indicating hepatitis are found in approximately 80% of patients. Jaundice is much less common. Splenomegaly is found in about half the patients, although massive enlargement is rare. Conversely, splenic enlargement may be rapid enough to cause left upper quadrant pain and tenderness. These may be the presenting complaints in a minority of cases.

Ancillary clinical findings include edema of the eyelids and skin rashes. The rash is usually maculopapular and is found in 3% to 15% of patients. For some unknown reason, 80% of patients with infectious mononucleosis develop a rash if treated with ampicillin.

The enlargement of the tonsils and adenoids can be massive and may be associated with swelling of the prevertebral soft tissues. Significant airway obstruction can occur in infectious mononucleosis, which can be of sufficient severity to cause hypoxia and death if untreated (Fig. 3-12).[62,63]

Because of the ubiquitous nature of the Epstein-Barr virus, extensive serologic testing has been developed to assess acute infection, recent infection, and past infection. Especially important in predicting acute infection is the presence of an immunoglobulin G (IgG) antibody to viral capsid antigens. This antibody persists for prolonged periods. A similar IgM antibody to viral capsid antigens is identified only with acute infections. Antibodies to Epstein-Barr nuclear antigen are found only in association with remote infections.

The diagnosis of infectious mononucleosis is made on the basis of clinical and laboratory features. Occasionally, the diagnosis may be suggested from lateral radiographs of the neck in an older child or an adolescent. The principal radiographic finding is enlargement of the tonsils and adenoids, which is sometimes massive. Although tonsillar and adenoidal enlargement are usually concomitant and proportional, either may be predominant. The enlargement of the adenoids frequently causes nasal obstruction or can simulate a neoplasm. Prevertebral soft tissue swelling may occur that can simulate a retropharyngeal bacterial infection (cellulitis) or retropharyngeal abscess.

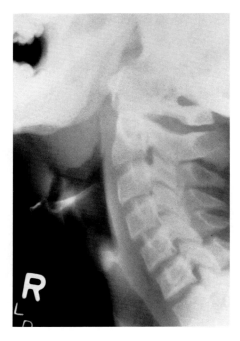

Fig. 3-12 Infectious mononucleosis. Lateral radiograph demonstrates marked enlargement of the tonsils and adenoids, with obliteration of the nasopharyngeal and oropharyngeal portions of the airway.

It is important to recognize that these radiographic findings may be present in cases of infectious mononucleosis for the following reasons: (1) Soft tissue swelling may be of sufficient severity to cause concern about malignancies or suppuration. (2) The diagnosis of infectious mononucleosis may be first suggested by the radiographic findings. (3) Clinically significant, but potentially treatable, upper airway obstruction due to adenoidal or tonsillar swelling may occur with infectious mononucleosis. (4) Surgical treatment such as tonsillectomy or tracheostomy should be avoided unless medical treatment with corticosteroids fails.[63,64]

Oral Cavity and Oropharynx

The oropharynx is continuous with the oral cavity anteriorly, the nasopharynx superiorly, and the hypopharynx inferiorly. The oropharynx is bounded anteriorly by the tongue and laterally by the faucial pillars. It is separated from the nasopharynx by the soft palate and the bar of Passavant. The pharyngoepiglottic folds define the boundary with the hypopharynx. Important structures within the oral cavity and oropharynx include the tongue and the palatine tonsils.

Abnormalities of the Tongue

Macroglossia, or pathologic enlargement of the tongue, can cause airway obstruction. Moderate enlargement of the tongue is seen in Down syndrome, congenital hypothyroidism, and glycogen storage disease. In the neonatal period, asymmetric enlargement of the tongue falls into two large pathologic groups. Lymphangioma is the most common among the solitary mass lesions and is followed in frequency by lingual thyroid, thyroglossal duct cyst, enteric duplication cyst, and hemangioma (Fig. 3-13). Patients with muscular hypertrophy have been reported to have muscle fibers that are four to five times larger in diameter than normal. Later in life, rhabdomyosarcoma may occur as a primary neoplasm in the tongue, but this is extremely rare.

Another extremely rare congenital anomaly of the tongue is complete or almost complete absence of this organ. These infants feed poorly at first, but despite the lack of this primary muscular organ of the oropharyngeal component of swallowing they eventually learn to feed with the aid of gravity. Surprisingly, the sensation of taste in these infants has been found to be normal, and ultimately these children learn to speak, albeit somewhat imperfectly.[65]

Severe macroglossia is manifested by huge and symmetric thickening and overgrowth of the tongue to the point that it protrudes constantly from the open mouth, impeding feeding and making respiration noisy and partially obstructed. In children with Beckwith-Wiedemann syndrome, macroglossia is associated with macrosomia that may be asymmetric,

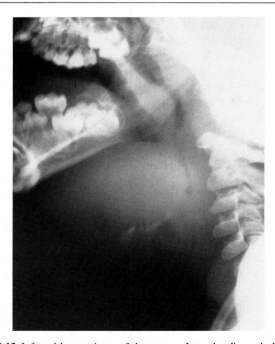

Fig. 3-13 Infected hemangioma of the tongue. Lateral radiograph demonstrates a mass arising from the posterior aspect of the tongue with marked narrowing of the airway.

omphalocele, a variety of other congenital defects, and frequently symptomatic neonatal hypoglycemia. These patients are, later in life, at significant risk for developing malignancies, especially Wilms tumor. Non-neoplastic enlargement of the tongue occurs in Beckwith-Wiedemann syndrome, congenital hypothyroidism, and glycogen storage disease.

Because the tongue is located in a region amenable to clinical inspection, radiographic evaluation is not usually required. A mass located at the base of the tongue is an exception. Such lesions may be first detected on diagnostic imaging. Macroglossia is demonstrated on lateral neck radiographs as diffuse glossal enlargement, usually with some degree of posterior extension into the oropharynx. Focal lesions arising in the tongue most often produce a rounded soft tissue density that projects into the airway. Soft tissue fullness at the base of the tongue should be evaluated with caution because a pseudomass may be produced by the normal lingual tonsils. A lingual thyroid can be demonstrated scintigraphically with ^{123}I or [^{99m}Tc]pertechnetate imaging as a focal ectopic accumulation of the tracer, usually in the base of the tongue.

Noma

Noma (cancrum oris or gangrenous stomatitis) is a rapidly progressive gangrenous process that results in destruction of orofacial tissue. Less common areas of involvement include the eyelids and the perineum. Although the pathogenesis of this disorder has not been clearly established, the pathologic findings and the usual favorable clinical response to antibiotics suggest a bacterial pathogenesis. Despite this, a specific bacterial agent has not been implicated, and it is generally believed that noma results from the effects of normal oral flora on tissues in the presence of markedly compromised host resistance.

Noma is a relatively common disorder in Africa, where it affects malnourished children, frequently after an acute viral illness such as measles. In developed countries, noma is occasionally encountered in children with severe combined immunodeficiency or leukemia and in debilitated elderly patients. A usually fatal form occurs in low–birth weight and ill premature infants (noma neonatorum).

The initial clinical manifestation of noma is usually a small, painful gingival ulceration. This is followed by a rapidly progressive focus of inflammation and tissue necrosis with extension into adjacent structures. Soft tissue and bone alike are destroyed. The process may be halted with appropriate antibiotics and steps to improve the underlying systemic pathology.[66,67]

Radiographic examination is helpful in severe cases of noma to define the severity of osseous and soft tissue destruction. Radiographs of the facial bones show destructive changes of the teeth, maxilla, and mandible. The process may extend superiorly to involve the maxillary sinuses, hard palate, and nose.

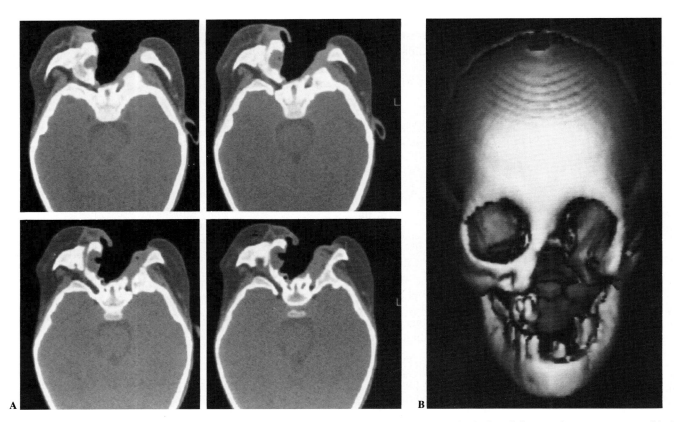

Fig. 3-14 Noma. **(A)** Axial CT and **(B)** a computer-generated three-dimensional reformation show a large defect in the soft tissues and osseous structures of the left midface.

The destructive changes of noma are shown most effectively with CT. Imaging in both axial and coronal planes is usually required. Computer-generated three-dimensional CT may be helpful in planning the complex reconstructive surgery that may be required in these children (Fig. 3-14).[68]

Retropharyngeal Soft Tissues

The retropharynx is a potential space of loose areolar tissue posterior to the pharyngeal mucosal space. The anterior boundary of the retropharyngeal space is defined by the middle layer of the deep cervical fascia. The posterior boundary is the deep layer of the deep cervical fascia. The lateral boundary is formed by the alar fascia. The superior margin is the skull base and the caudal margin is the carina. The carotid space is lateral to the retropharyngeal space and the prevertebral space is posterior.

Retropharyngeal Infections

Retropharyngeal infection is usually a complication of bacterial pharyngitis. Bacterial infections of the retropharynx occur most commonly in early childhood, when the lymph nodes in the prevertebral space communicate with those that drain portions of the nasopharynx and the posterior nasal cavities. Pathologic retropharyngeal enlargement is most often caused by lymphadenopathy and cellulitis. This may progress to abscess formation. Penetrating injury of the pharynx is a less common mechanism for bacterial inoculation.[62] Enlargement of the retropharyngeal soft tissues due to infection produces a variable degree of compression of the oropharynx, hypopharynx, and trachea and may cause airway obstruction.

More than half the cases of retropharyngeal abscess occur between the ages of 6 and 12 months. Most often, an abscess develops from focal suppurative adenitis of a retropharyngeal lymph node. A retropharyngeal abscess also may be due to cervical osteomyelitis or penetrating injury of the pharynx. Congenital piriform sinus fistula is a cause of recurrent retropharyngeal cellulitis and abscess formation. This anomaly may also be associated with recurrent suppurative thyroiditis.[69]

Although retropharyngeal soft tissue thickening in children is most often a result of infection and trauma, rarely neoplasm may be the cause. The most common tumor to involve the retropharyngeal area in children is cystic hygroma, although the retropharyngeal involvement in these cases usually represents extension from a more lateral origin. Other neoplastic lesions that may occur in the retropharyngeal area in children include teratoma, hemangioma, neurofibroma, and adenopathy related to Langerhans cell histiocytosis, metastatic neuroblastoma, lymphoma, or leukemia.[50] Chronic inflammatory adenopathy in this region may occur in tuberculosis, usually as a result of atypical mycobacteria infection (scrofula) and fungal diseases such as histoplasmosis.

Widening of the retropharyngeal space on lateral radiographs of the neck is not a specific finding. As described above, a wide variety of abnormalities may produce this radiographic appearance. The most common cause is pseudothickening due to buckling of the airway when the neck is flexed or when the radiograph is obtained during expiration or swallowing.

The most reliable radiographic sign of true pathologic thickening of the retropharyngeal space is a curved anterior displacement of the posterior pharyngeal airway. In addition, there is obliteration of the usual step-off of the airway at the level of the larynx. Normally, with inspiration, the soft tissues below the level of the larynx are twice as thick as those above. This is due to interposition of the esophagus between the trachea and the prevertebral soft tissues. Radiographically, this produces a step-off in the airway.

The most common pathologic cause of retropharyngeal soft tissue swelling is lymphadenitis (Fig. 3-15). If inflammatory lymph nodes undergo suppuration, this leads to abscess formation. The most reliable radiographic sign of an abscess is gas in the soft tissue fullness (Fig. 3-16); this finding is present in a distinct minority of cases. Inflammation in the retropharyngeal region is associated with muscle spasm, which results in

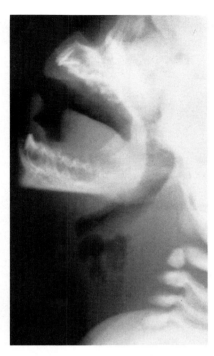

Fig. 3-16 Retropharyngeal abscess. The lateral radiograph of this infant shows marked enlargement of the retropharyngeal soft tissues as well as an irregular gas collection in an abscess cavity.

straightening of the cervical spine and in some cases acute hyperflexion; this is a supplemental radiographic sign of retropharyngeal infection. Flexion of the cervical spine frequently causes pseudosubluxation of C-1 on C-2 and, especially, C-2 on C-3; this should not be mistaken as a sign of injury.

CT is particularly useful in evaluating cases of suspected retropharyngeal abscess. This technique shows a moderately low-attenuation mass, often with an irregular, enhancing margin. Fluid-debris or gas-fluid levels may be present. CT is much more sensitive than standard radiographs in detecting gas in a retropharyngeal abscess (Fig. 3-17).

The differential diagnosis of widening of the retropharyngeal soft tissues includes several uncommon etiologies in addition to typical retropharyngeal infection. The prevertebral space may be widened in trauma to the cervical vertebrae. Less commonly it is thickened in cervical osteomyelitis, primary or metastatic tumors, retropharyngeal goiter, or duplication cyst. An even rarer cause is obstruction of the superior vena cava. CT, MRI, or sonography can be employed if the differential diagnosis is a clinical problem.

Retropharyngeal Tumor

In addition to infectious etiologies, retropharyngeal thickening occurs with various tumors. The most common is cystic hygroma; other tumors include neuroblastoma, ganglioneuroma, neurofibroma, hemangioma, and teratoma. Other causes of noninflammatory retropharyngeal adenopathy include Lan-

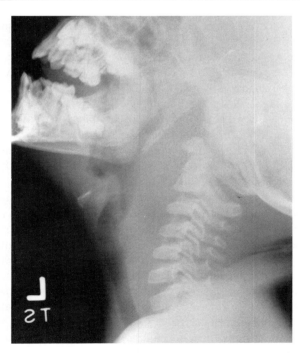

Fig. 3-15 Retropharyngeal lymphadenitis. Lateral radiograph demonstrates thickening of the retropharyngeal soft tissues and anterior displacement of the hypopharynx and upper trachea.

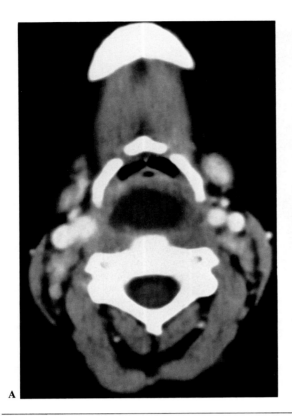

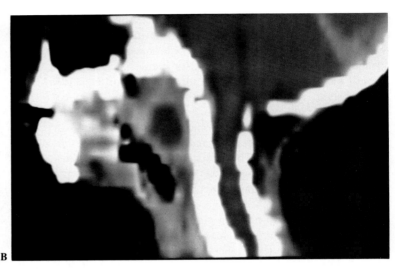

Fig. 3-17 Retropharyngeal abscess. (A) Axial and (B) reformatted sagittal contrast-enhanced CT images demonstrate an oval fluid collection in the retropharyngeal soft tissues.

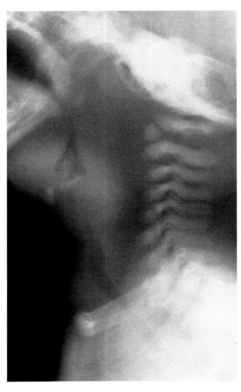

Fig. 3-18 Retropharyngeal cystic hygroma. Lateral radiograph demonstrates marked enlargement of the retropharyngeal soft tissues, causing anterior displacement and narrowing of the upper trachea and pharyngeal airway.

gerhans cell histiocytosis, leukemia, lymphoma, and sinus histiocytosis.

Most lymphangiomas or cystic hygromas occur in the neck. They usually begin in the posterior triangle and sometimes extend into the anterior mediastinum. Rarely, they can present in the mediastinum as an isolated mass. These lesions can be classified into three types: simple, which consist of capillary-size, thin-walled lymphatic channels with considerable connective tissue stroma; cavernous, which are actively growing, dilated lymphatic channels containing a lymphoid stroma; and cystic, which may be single or multiple cystic masses containing serous or milky fluid and little, if any, communication with normal lymphatics.

The usual radiographic findings of retropharyngeal cystic hygroma and lymphangioma include retropharyngeal thickening, airway displacement, and increased soft tissue density (Fig. 3-18). These tumors do not contain calcification, as is found in neuroblastoma and ganglioneuroma; likewise, they lack the ossification and fat seen in teratoma.

The CT appearance of cystic hygroma is a soft tissue mass with low-attenuation cystic regions. Attenuation values of the central areas do not change after bolus injection of contrast material. The mass usually contains septa that enhance after contrast agent administration. Cystic hygroma does not demonstrate invasive characteristics but usually causes displacement of adjacent structures. Uncommonly, a cervical cystic hygroma can be extensive, involving the floor of the mouth, the epiglottis, or the larynx.

Neuroblastoma, ganglioneuroma, and neurofibroma have the same radiographic characteristics in this region as they do in other areas of the body. They appear as masses with fine, stippled calcification (50%). Extension into the neural forami-

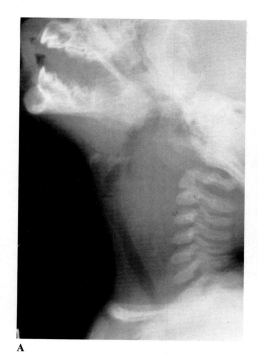
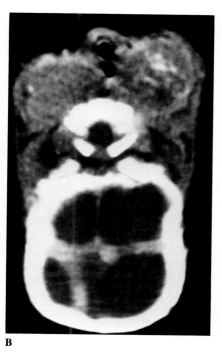

A   B

Fig. 3-19 Metastatic neuroblastoma. **(A)** Lateral radiograph demonstrates thickening of the retropharyngeal soft tissues. Amorphous calcifications are faintly visible in this region. **(B)** Contrast-enhanced CT shows lobulated anterior cervical masses with involvement of the retropharyngeal region. Irregular contrast enhancement and coarse calcifications are present.

na is suggested by enlargement of the foramina and adjacent sclerosis (Fig. 3-19).

Intraspinal involvement with neurogenic tumors in the cervical region can be demonstrated with CT. The punctate calcification that is often present in these neoplasms is easily detected with CT. The intraspinal extension of tumor is more readily demonstrated with MRI, especially in the coronal projection. T_2-Weighted images demonstrate moderate to marked hyperintensity of these neural tumors compared to surrounding muscle and spinal cord. Extension through neural foramina is exquisitely demonstrated with coronal imaging.

Hemangiomas may or may not contain phleboliths. There is frequently an overlying cutaneous hemangioma. Other diseases such as Langerhans cell histiocytosis, lymphoma, and sinus histiocytosis can increase the depth of the retropharyngeal soft tissues. These disease processes share the same radiographic appearance as retropharyngeal cellulitis, inflammatory adenopathy, and abscess.

Larynx and Upper Trachea

Laryngomalacia

Laryngomalacia may be a confusing diagnostic entity, although most pediatricians are aware of its clinical features. Laryngomalacia is the most common congenital abnormality of the larynx. Boys are affected twice as often as girls. In laryngomalacia, there are floppiness of the epiglottis, aryepiglottic folds, and supraglottic aperture caused by a weakness of the cartilage structures supporting the airway

walls. These lead to partial collapse and incomplete obstruction during inspiration. Stridor is usually present from birth but may not appear until 2 months of age. Although the stridor may disappear with crying, it is exacerbated by minor respiratory infections or when the infant is supine. Aside from the inspiratory stridor, the infant is usually healthy. A minority of infants with laryngomalacia have severe dyspnea that can lead to difficulty in nursing, resulting in undernutrition and poor weight gain. The respiratory difficulties in these infants may be of such severity as to cause retractions that may lead to persistent thoracic deformity. In most infants with laryngomalacia, stridor persists for several months to 1 year after birth and then gradually disappears with further growth and development of the airway.[71,72]

Laryngomalacia may be evaluated fluoroscopically, which assesses the changing dynamics of the airway throughout the respiratory cycle. The important findings occur during inspiration. There is distention of the hypopharynx and oropharynx, inferior and posterior bending of the epiglottis, anteroinferior buckling of the aryepiglottic folds, and paradoxic narrowing of the subglottic trachea. In current practice, fiberoptic endoscopy has supplanted fluoroscopic evaluation in cases where clinical diagnostic uncertainty exists.

Epiglottitis

Acute epiglottitis can be a life-threatening disease. Its highest incidence is between 3 and 6 years of age. The disease is characterized by the rapid onset of fever, sore throat, dyspnea, and drooling. The clinical signs of airway obstruction in these patients are severe inspiratory stridor and aphonia. Acute epiglottitis is most often caused by *Hemophilus influenzae* type B. Bacteremia occurs in most patients.

Children with epiglottitis usually show a characteristic position, sitting upright with the chin forward to keep the airway patent. Many pediatric hospitals suggest direct visualization of the epiglottis by an individual who is prepared to perform endotracheal intubation. In addition to acute infectious epiglottitis, enlargement of the epiglottis can also occur with caustic or thermal injuries or unusual entities such as hemophilia, angioneurotic edema, Stevens-Johnson syndrome, and aryepiglottic or epiglottic cysts.

On the lateral neck radiograph, the findings of epiglottitis are characteristic, consisting of enlargement of the epiglottis and aryepiglottic folds. The earliest radiographic sign is rounding of the normally straight anterior surface of the epiglottis. In advanced cases, the swollen epiglottis appears as an upward-pointing thumb, and hence references have been made to the thumb sign. Mild to moderate hypopharyngeal distention may occur but is less marked than that seen in croup. In addition, the laryngeal and subglottic portions of the airway may be indistinct as a result of edema (Fig. 3-20). On frontal radiographs, some cases of epiglottitis demonstrate significant subglottic edema and can be indistinguishable from croup. In these cases, although the primary problem is the supraglottic edema, sufficient edema extends to the subglottic portion of the trachea to produce a funnel-shaped deformity.

Radiographically, infectious epiglottitis cannot be differentiated from enlargement due to thermal or caustic trauma, hemophilia, angioneurotic edema, Stevens-Johnson syn-

drome, and aryepiglottic or epiglottic cysts.[72] Abnormal enlargement of the epiglottis must be differentiated from the so-called omega epiglottis, which is a normal variation. The omega-shaped epiglottis is produced when the lateral portions assume a curved configuration and overlie the body of the epiglottis when viewed on the lateral projection. A simple method to confirm the presence of an omega epiglottis is to determine whether there is abnormal thickening and straightening of the aryepiglottic folds, which occurs in epiglottitis and most other forms of epiglottic pathology. When the hypopharynx is well distended, the normal aryepiglottic folds appear thin and have a stout triangular base. The aryepiglottic folds are normal in cases of omega epiglottis.

Croup

Croup is the most common cause of acute upper airway obstruction in infants and young children. Croup is also referred to as laryngotracheitis; if there is an associated bronchitis, it is termed laryngotracheobronchitis. Although a large segment of the airway is usually involved in croup, the crucial area of narrowing is in the subglottic trachea. The susceptibility to narrowing in this area is thought to be related to the loose attachment of the mucosa in this segment.

Croup is most commonly caused by a viral infection. The major viruses responsible are myxoviruses, parainfluenza type 1, and influenza type A. Croup tends to occur between fall and spring. The age range is from 6 months to 5 years, with most cases occurring between 1 and 3 years.

Although the onset of croup may be abrupt, it usually follows several days of upper respiratory infection. The cough has the character of a seal's bark. Inspiratory stridor predominates. When the disease is severe, the stridor is biphasic. Croup tends to worsen at night and remits during the day. The usual duration is from 4 to 8 days. In most cases, croup is a relatively mild, self-limited disease, but occasionally airway obstruction is sufficiently severe to cause death.

On physical examination, the typical cough of croup is usually apparent. Intercostal, substernal, and supraclavicular retractions are common. The pharynx is usually only slightly inflamed. Other abnormalities that may mimic croup clinically include congenital subglottic stenosis, laryngeal web, subglottic hemangioma, foreign body, and epiglottitis (Figs. 3-21 and 3-22).[70,73]

In a patient with stridor, the role of imaging is to identify the location of the obstruction. In suspected croup, the symptoms clearly indicate that the lesion is in the region of the larynx or lower. The initial radiograph should be a lateral view of the neck. This view is used because the epiglottis and foreign bodies are best seen in this projection and because the most important role of imaging is to rule out these problems.

In croup, lateral neck films frequently confirm the diagnosis. Chest radiographs provide supplementary information. On the lateral neck radiograph, the hypopharynx is frequently distended in children with croup. The distention is a useful sign of upper airway obstruction. Hypopharyngeal distention is a neurogenic response that serves to reduce airway

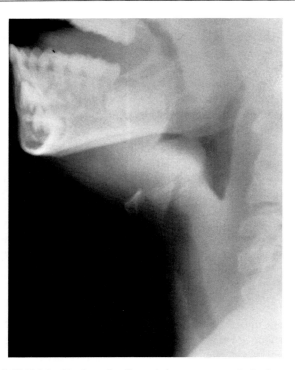

Fig. 3-20 Epiglottitis. Lateral radiograph demonstrates marked enlargement of the epiglottis and aryepiglottic folds.

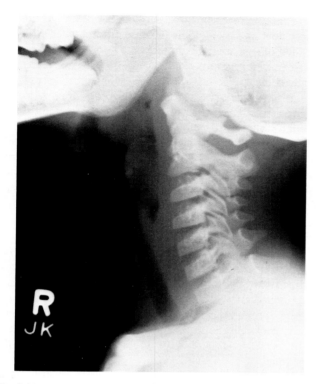

Fig. 3-21 Foreign body. An important abnormality in the differential diagnosis of stridor in children is airway obstruction due to a foreign body. This lateral radiograph demonstrates a pistachio nut lodged in the hypopharynx.

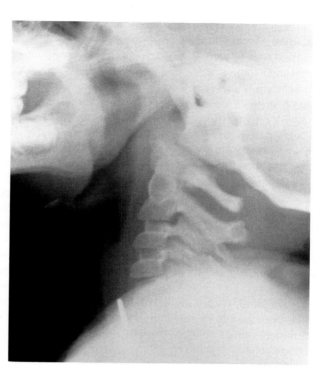

Fig. 3-22 Esophageal foreign body. Secondary tracheal effects may produce stridor in the presence of an esophageal foreign body. This lateral radiograph demonstrates a coin in the proximal esophagus with edema of the posterior wall of the trachea.

resistance; it is not related to pressure differences or to labored respiration. The degree of subglottic narrowing viewed on the lateral film is usually not marked, but a general indistinctness of this portion of the airway is seen (Fig. 3-23). This is due to the looseness of the connective tissue in the lateral walls of the subglottic airway as opposed to the relatively more tightly adherent connective tissue in the anterior and posterior aspects of this portion of the airway. As a result, the narrowing is more readily appreciated on the anteroposterior radiograph because inspiratory collapse occurs primarily from side to side. Instead of the normal parallel walls of the subglottic airway, there is a tapered narrowing that has been likened to the appearance of a steeple. This appearance is considerably less marked on expiration, indicating that the inspiratory collapse is not fixed, as it is in similar-appearing conditions such as subglottic stenosis.[74]

Membranous Croup and Tracheitis

Membranous croup (bacterial tracheitis) is characterized by diffuse inflammation of the larynx, trachea, and bronchi. The name is derived from the adherent or semiadherent mucopurulent membranes (also referred to as pseudomembranes) that are typically present. These membranes are produced by sloughing of the respiratory epithelium and large amounts of mucopurulent secretions and debris. In most cases, bacteria can be cultured from the tracheal secretions or pseudo-

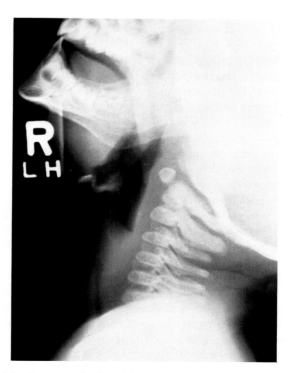

Fig. 3-23 Laryngotracheobronchitis (croup). Lateral radiograph demonstrates edema and narrowing of the subglottic region and upper trachea. The epiglottis is normal.

membranes. *Staphylococcus aureus* is the most commonly isolated organism, although *Hemophilus influenzae* and other organisms may be responsible. It is not clearly known whether membranous croup is due to a primary bacterial infection of the trachea or is a severe form of ordinary croup with superimposed bacterial infection. Membranous tracheitis tends to occur in a slightly older age group than does viral croup.

Children with membranous croup initially have symptoms that are similar to those of uncomplicated viral croup. The more serious nature of this condition is demonstrated by the typical rapid development of more severe inspiratory stridor. The condition of these children generally is more toxic, and they have higher fevers than children with viral croup. Likewise, they are less responsive to racemic epinephrine and supportive therapy.

Laryngeal diphtheria, although rare in the United States, should be considered in the differential diagnosis of membranous croup. This diagnosis is unlikely in children who have been immunized against diphtheria. One fatal case of diphtheria has been seen at our institution within the past 5 years; it occurred in a patient who was not immunized because of religious beliefs.

Involvement of the larynx in cases of diphtheria usually results from extension of the infection from the pharynx, with only rare cases being limited to the larynx or trachea. Laryngeal diphtheria is associated with membrane formation; the membranes are tightly adherent to the deep layers of the airway, in contradistinction to the typical loose attachment of the pseudomembranes found in bacterial tracheitis. In most cases, a gray-white membrane over the tonsils is visible in the posterior pharynx on clinical examination, although there are unusual cases in which the membrane formation is limited to the larynx (Fig. 3-24).[62,70,75]

Radiographically, typical croup is characterized by subglottic edema; the rest of the upper airway is normal. On the lateral radiograph, the subglottic airway has an indistinct increase in density, with blurred margins extending over a variable distance (usually not exceeding 1 to 2 cm). On frontal radiographs the involvement of the lateral walls of the airway is more apparent, causing the subglottic airway to have a steeple or pencil shape.

Subglottic narrowing also occurs in membranous croup, and the findings may be indistinguishable from those in subglottic stenosis or croup. If the diagnosis of membranous tracheitis is to be established radiographically, mucosal swelling and irregularity must be identified inferior to the subglottic region. In addition, when membranes are large and become detached or partially detached, they can be recognized as soft tissue densities of irregular linear configuration in the tracheal lumen. During repeat radiography, the position or configuration of these membranes changes. They may not be seen on follow-up radiographs if they have been expectorated. The mobility of the tracheal membranes can be observed fluoroscopically; in many respects, the appearance may simulate that of a foreign body.

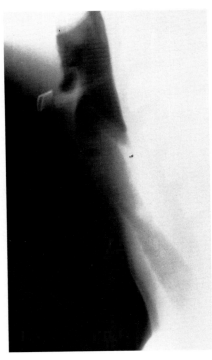

Fig. 3-24 Bacterial tracheitis. Lateral radiograph demonstrates irregular soft tissue densities in the trachea as well as moderate narrowing of the airway.

The radiologic and endoscopic evidence in membranous croup suggests that the involvement is principally in the trachea, although there is an increased incidence of associated pneumonia. Recognizing membranous croup as a distinct entity is important because the presence of pathogens in the tracheal secretions or membranes in most patients indicates the need for specific antibiotic therapy; because there is usually a poor response to racemic epinephrine and supportive therapy that is usually effective in typical croup; and because endoscopic clearing of the pseudomembranes or endotracheal intubation occasionally may be necessary. Membranous croup can be recognized or strongly suggested radiographically, although the radiologic findings can be mistaken for those of a tracheal foreign body.[76]

Subglottic Hemangioma

Hemangioma is the most common subglottic tumor-producing upper respiratory tract obstruction in infants and young children. Inspiratory stridor in these patients starts in infancy as opposed to the later presentation of typical croup. This lesion occurs in the immediate subglottic trachea, usually in a posterior or lateral location. Fifty percent of these children have associated cutaneous hemangiomas.

Initially, stridor associated with subglottic hemangioma is inspiratory, but with increased size of the lesion it becomes biphasic because of the lesion's subglottic location. The stridor is exacerbated by crying or upper respiratory tract inflammation. Most patients present before 6 months of age. These hemangiomas have been demonstrated to regress in size with age. It is impossible to determine the outcome by the initial endoscopic appearance. In general, these lesions enlarge early in life, cease growing spontaneously before 1 year of age, and then slowly involute.[70,77]

Radiographically, the subglottic hemangioma is usually eccentric and deforms the subglottic trachea. It is the asymmetry of the subglottic space that suggests the diagnosis. The lesion most often occurs on the posterior or posterolateral walls of the subglottic trachea. A rounded or lobulated configuration may be visible. An eccentric location of the lesion in the subglottic trachea may be demonstrated on frontal radiographs, but this is most easily demonstrated with CT (Figs. 3-25 and 3-26).

Congenital Laryngeal Stenosis

Congenital laryngeal stenosis results from failure of normal recanalization of the larynx during fetal week 10. Congenital laryngeal stenosis may be membranous (laryngeal web) or cartilaginous. The lesion is further classified according to the level of obstruction as supraglottic, glottic, and subglottic.

A laryngeal web at the level of the glottis is the most common form of congenital laryngeal stenosis. Most often, the web extends across the anterior portion of the vocal cords. A laryngeal web is usually associated with inspiratory and expiratory stridor and a hoarse cry. With severe narrowing, symptoms occur at the time of delivery, and a tracheostomy is mandatory.

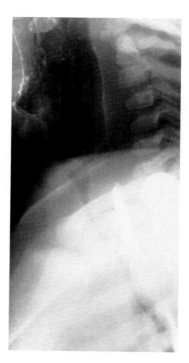

Fig. 3-26 Esophageal foreign body. In addition to subglottic hemangioma, thickening of the posterior soft tissues of the subglottic trachea can be related to the effects of an adjacent foreign body in the upper esophagus, as in this case.

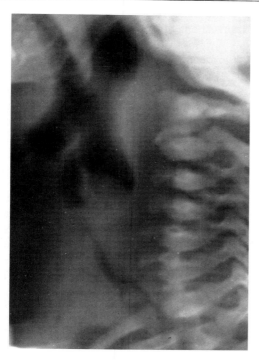

Fig. 3-25 Subglottic hemangioma. Lateral radiograph demonstrates a lobulated soft tissue mass along the posterior aspect of the subglottic trachea.

Nonmembranous congenital laryngeal stenosis usually occurs in the subglottic region. Congenital subglottic stenosis consists of circumferential narrowing of the airway below the vocal cords at the level of the cricoid cartilage. This entity is the most common congenital airway abnormality necessitating early tracheostomy. The presenting symptoms consist of biphasic stridor with a normal cry. Cyanosis may be present if the obstruction is severe. A barking cough similar to that of viral croup may be present. Infection increases the severity of symptoms. Some mild cases of congenital subglottic stenosis may present clinically as prolonged or recurrent croup. The symptoms of congenital subglottic stenosis may not be present at birth, but most often they become apparent by the age of 6 months because the ventilatory requirements of the child increase with greater activity.

Congenital subglottic stenosis may mimic subglottic hemangioma clinically and radiographically. Also, laryngeal stenosis as an acquired lesion can result from physical, thermal, or caustic trauma. Most cases of acquired laryngeal stenosis occur in the subglottic region and are related to tracheal intubation. The subglottic stenosis in these children may be due to thickening of the tracheal wall, membranes, or granuloma formation.[50,71]

Laryngeal webs are not visualized with standard imaging studies and are generally diagnosed by direct visualization or endoscopy. The radiographic appearance of congenital subglottic stenosis is smooth (usually circumferential) narrowing

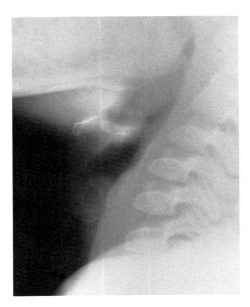

Fig. 3-27 Laryngeal papillomatosis. Lateral radiograph demonstrates multiple irregular masses in the region of the larynx and subglottic trachea.

in the subglottic region. The findings are quite similar to those of croup and subglottic hemangioma. Congenital subglottic stenosis can be differentiated from croup by observing a lack of change in subglottic narrowing on both inspiration and expiration in the former; the degree of subglottic narrowing in croup increases during inspiration and decreases during expiration. Differentiation from subglottic hemangioma is usually possible radiographically because hemangioma typically produces a localized lesion along the posterior and lateral walls of the subglottic larynx, whereas congenital stenosis more often results in circumferential narrowing. CT may be necessary to differentiate the eccentric location of subglottic narrowing that occurs in hemangioma from the circumferential narrowing that occurs in subglottic stenosis.

Laryngeal Papillomatosis

Laryngeal papillomatosis is a histologically benign but clinically aggressive lesion. It is the most common benign tumor of the larynx in childhood. Most children (approximately 65%) who develop laryngeal papillomatosis become symptomatic during the first 7 years of life, and many become symptomatic before the age of 1 year. Hoarseness, aphonia, croupy cough with or without stridor, dyspnea, and progressive cyanosis are the usual order and progression of symptoms and signs. Respiratory difficulty is especially prominent in infants; sudden death can occur.

A viral etiology for laryngeal papillomatosis is suggested by the association of cutaneous verrucae and a later relationship with condyloma acuminatum. Human papillomavirus is specifically implicated as the etiology. A history of maternal condyloma acuminatum of the cervix or vagina has been reported in 50% of the children with laryngeal papillomatosis.

During infancy, the usual pattern of involvement in cases of laryngeal papillomatosis is widespread glottic, ventricular, and supraglottic papillomas. Older children usually have more localized disease, which is often confined to the vocal cords. The overall recurrence rate is approximately 75% (Fig. 3-27).

In addition to papillomatosis, other rare benign tumors of the larynx in children include chondroma, granular cell myoblastoma, plasma cell granuloma, chemodectoma, neurofibroma, and fibroma. Malignant neoplasms of the larynx are extremely rare in children; reported types include lymphosarcoma, fibrosarcoma, rhabdomyosarcoma, and epidermoid carcinoma.[50]

Lateral radiographs of the neck in cases of laryngeal papillomatosis may demonstrate a mulberrylike or cauliflowerlike growth that measures 3 to 6 mm. These are usually clustered and may be multifocal. The anterior third of the true vocal cord is a frequent site, but the lesion may occur anywhere in the hypopharynx, the aryepiglottic folds, the subglottic larynx, the trachea, and even the bronchi. Widespread involvement of the lower respiratory tract has been reported in about 5% of patients. Lesions in the oral cavity may occur. The most diagnostic radiographic finding is the mulberrylike appearance. Improved demonstration of the lesions may be provided with CT. As in other chronic intrinsic diseases of the larynx and airways, however, the diagnosis needs to be confirmed by endoscopy and biopsy.[78-81]

Laryngocele and Saccular Cyst

Laryngocele and saccular cyst are rare congenital abnormalities of the larynx that may cause respiratory tract obstruction in children. Both lesions arise from the saccular appendage of the larynx. A laryngocele freely communicates with the laryngeal lumen and is filled with air; a saccular cyst lacks communication with the laryngeal lumen and is fluid filled. The most common clinical presentation is inspiratory stridor.

The radiographic appearance of laryngocele or saccular cyst is an intrinsic laryngeal mass (Fig. 3-28). The lesion may extend superiorly, producing a large supraglottic component. Because a laryngocele communicates with the laryngeal lumen, the lesion may inflate and deflate intermittently; therefore, radiographs may show marked variation in the size of the mass.

An internal laryngocele is confined to the interior of the larynx and extends posterosuperiorly to the supraglottic larynx. This type represents about 60% of laryngoceles. An external laryngocele extends through the thyrohyoid membrane and presents clinically as a mass in the lateral aspect of the neck. A combined laryngocele has features of both internal and external types.[72,82]

Vocal Cord Paralysis

Vocal cord paralysis is the second most common abnormality of the larynx in infants. With unilateral vocal cord paralysis, symptoms are mild, and the disorder may go unnoticed.

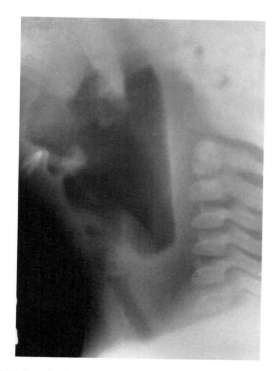

Fig. 3-28 Saccular laryngocele. Lateral radiograph shows a rounded soft tissue density in the upper airway just below the level of the true vocal cords. The lesion is of soft tissue density because the saccular cyst is fluid filled and because communication with the airway is only minimal. Air-filled laryngoceles may also occur. Some lesions contain both air and fluid.

In most cases, however, there is an element of stridor, and the child produces a weak or hoarse cry. Unilateral vocal cord paralysis may result from injury of the recurrent laryngeal nerve at birth. It is more common on the left, reflecting the long course of this nerve under the aortic arch. More uncommonly, it is due to impingement on this nerve by mediastinal tumors, anomalies of the cardiovascular system, or injury from thoracic surgery.

Bilateral vocal cord paralysis is characterized by a normal cry and severe stridor. The paralyzed vocal cords assume a midline or slightly adducted position. This position is relatively fixed, varying little with the respiratory cycle. Because the glottis is the narrowest segment of the airway, significant airway obstruction accompanies bilateral vocal cord paralysis.

Bilateral vocal cord paralysis in infants and young children is most often associated with central nervous system disorders, such as Arnold-Chiari type II malformation. Temporary vocal cord paralysis may occur in Guillain-Barré syndrome. Vocal cord paralysis in the neonate may be related to brain injury, intracranial hemorrhage, or perinatal asphyxia.[83,84]

The radiographic findings in cases of vocal cord paralysis include indistinctness of the cords and laryngeal ventricle. Paradoxic collapse of the subglottic region of the trachea on deep inspiration may be identified fluoroscopically. These findings may mimic croup. In cases of unilateral vocal cord paralysis, fluoroscopic evaluation in the frontal projection shows the paralyzed vocal cord to lie in an abnormal, fixed midline position. With phonation, the normal cord extends toward the midline and then retracts during resting; the paralyzed cord fails to retract normally during the resting phase. When both vocal cords are paralyzed, they lie in a midline position, with only a narrow slitlike air passage extending between them. Endoscopy has limited the necessity for fluoroscopic evaluation in patients with vocal cord paralysis.[83]

PARANASAL SINUSES

Development and Anatomy

The paranasal sinuses are named according to the bones within which they are contained: maxillary, ethmoid, frontal, and sphenoid. The ethmoid sinuses are divided anatomically into anterior, middle, and posterior groups. The paranasal sinuses communicate with the nasal cavity via ostia. The maxillary, anterior ethmoid, and frontal sinuses drain into the middle meatus beneath the middle turbinate; the posterior ethmoid and sphenoid drain into the sphenoethmoid recess (the posterosuperior aspect of the nasal cavity). The nasal mucosa is contiguous with the sinus mucosa through these ostia. The sinus walls are composed of mucosa, periosteum, and bone.

The paranasal sinuses originate as diverticula from the mucosal lining of the lateral nasal walls during gestation months 3 and 4.[85] The maxillary sinuses are the first to develop and are the largest sinuses at birth, measuring approximately $7 \times 4 \times 4$ mm.[86] The ethmoid sinuses are present at birth and continue to develop until approximately the age of 15 years. The rudimentary frontal sinuses remain confined to the nasal cavity and are indistinguishable from the ethmoid air cells until approximately 20 months of age, when pneumatization of the frontal bone begins. The rudimentary sphenoid sinuses also are initially confined to the nasal vault until approximately 3 to 4 years of age, when pneumatization of the sphenoid bone begins. Full development of the maxillary sinuses occurs at 15 to 18 years of age, the frontal sinuses at 15 to 20 years, the ethmoid sinuses at 12 to 15 years, and the sphenoid sinuses at 12 to 15 years. The frontal sinuses are often quite asymmetric and may be absent.[87–89]

The approximate ages at which the paranasal sinuses become radiographically visible are as follows: maxillary, 2 to 3 months; ethmoid, 3 to 6 months; sphenoid, 1 to 2 years; and frontal, 4 to 8 years. The radiographic finding of sinus opacification is of limited usefulness in infants because sinus opacification correlates poorly with clinical disease. Underaeration due to redundant mucosa is a normal and frequent occurrence in infants. Interpretation of sinus radiographs in infants is difficult because of the small sizes of the paranasal sinuses at this age, the frequent occurrence of patient motion, suboptimal positioning or radiographic technique, and overlying soft tissue abnormalities.[89,90]

Congenital Abnormalities

Sinus Hypoplasia

The most common abnormality of sinus development is hypoplasia. Unilateral hypoplasia of a frontal sinus is not uncommon, and bilateral frontal sinus aplasia occurs in approximately 4% of normal individuals.[87] Hypoplasia of the ethmoid and sphenoid sinuses is rare.

The incidence of unilateral maxillary sinus hypoplasia is 1.7%, and that of bilateral hypoplasia is 7.2%.[91] Maxillary sinus hypoplasia is occasionally associated with thalassemia, hemifacial microsomia, and mandibulofacial dysostosis (Treacher Collins syndrome).[87] Unilateral maxillary sinus hypoplasia produces a variable degree of facial asymmetry and enophthalmos.

Radiographs in cases of sinus hypoplasia usually allow an accurate differentiation from acquired sinus pathology. Maxillary sinus hypoplasia results in a sinus cavity that is of decreased dimension in all directions. The orbital floor develops an oblique angle with depression laterally as a result of lack of normal lateral sinus development under the orbit. The lateral wall of the nasal vault is laterally placed, and the inferior turbinate may be enlarged.

Radiographic differentiation between frontal sinus hypoplasia and inflammatory opacification is often difficult because both conditions produce the appearance of sinus clouding on frontal views. The bony margins of the frontal sinuses usually remain visible radiographically despite inflammatory opacification of the sinus air space. The lateral view is often helpful in distinguishing between an opacified normal frontal sinus and a thin hypoplastic sinus.

Inflammatory Disease

Infectious Sinusitis

Viral infections cause most paranasal sinus infections in children. Typical signs and symptoms include fever, nasal congestion, headache, and clear rhinorrhea. Pathologically, there is inflammatory thickening of the nasal and sinus mucosa. Symptoms referable to the paranasal sinuses are usually minimal unless mucosal edema is severe enough to occlude the sinus ostium.

Acute bacterial sinusitis is, in most instances, associated with a predisposing condition. The most common predisposing factor is an antecedent viral upper respiratory infection. Obstruction of the sinus ostia due to mucosal edema and lymphadenopathy is probably the important precipitating factor with viral illnesses. Other obstructive lesions that may lead to acute sinusitis include polyps, foreign bodies, adenoid hyperplasia, tumors, and nasal septal deviation. Diseases that impair the immune system or the mucociliary transport mechanism, such as leukemia, cystic fibrosis, and ciliary dysmotility syndromes, also predispose to acute sinusitis.

Signs and symptoms of acute bacterial rhinosinusitis include fever, cough, mucopurulent discharge, headache, and tenderness over the involved sinuses. The ethmoid and maxillary sinuses are the most frequently involved sinuses in children. The most common infecting organisms include *Streptococcus pneumoniae, Hemophilus influenzae, Staphylococcus aureus, Branhamella catarrhalis*, and various anaerobic organisms such as species of *Peptostreptococcus, Bacteroides*, and *Fusobacterium*.[88,89,92–94] Mixed infections are not uncommon.

Fungal infections of the sinuses are uncommon and most often occur in patients with immunodeficiency states. *Aspergillus* and *Candida* species are the most common fungi recovered from abnormal sinuses. Sinusitis due to *Mucor* species occurs in children with poorly controlled diabetes. Fungal sinus disease may occur as a slow-growing central fungus ball, a slowly progressive invasive disease, or a fulminant infection with vascular invasion.

The spread of sinus infection to adjacent structures produces various complications, some of which are life threatening. The most common pathway for the spread of infection is through the network of small veins that drain the sinus mucosa.[95–98] These mucosal veins communicate with diploic veins in the walls of the sinuses, which in turn join the venous plexi of the periosteum and dura. These veins generally have no valves, and alterations in the direction of flow may occur with sinus infection. The interconnecting venous drainage systems may serve as pathways for spread of infection from the paranasal sinuses to the orbit, intracranial spaces, subperiosteal spaces of the head, skull and facial bones, facial soft tissue structures, and diploic spaces of adjacent and remote osseous structures. Direct spread of infection by inflammatory destruction of the sinus wall is a less common mechanism.

The most frequent complications from acute sinusitis occur in the orbit and periorbital tissues.[92,99] Either reactive inflammatory edema or actual infection of orbital structures may occur. The range of orbital complications that are due to acute sinusitis includes reactive edema, orbital cellulitis, subperiosteal abscess, intraorbital abscess, and optic neuritis. In children, orbital complications most commonly arise from ethmoid sinus disease. Symptoms suggesting spread of sinus disease into the orbit include periorbital edema, proptosis, pain, and chemosis. In some cases, symptoms related to orbital involvement are the initial indication of ethmoid sinusitis.

Septic thrombophlebitis originating in sinus mucosal veins may also provide a pathway for intracranial spread of sinus infection.[95–98] This most often occurs as a complication of frontal sinusitis. By this mechanism, epidural abscess or subdural empyema may occur with or without osteomyelitis of the overlying bone. Subdural empyema is the most common intracranial complication of sinusitis.[93] Subdural empyema due to sinusitis occurs predominantly in adolescent boys.[100] The arachnoid functions as a barrier to bacterial invasion, so that meningitis is an infrequent complication of subdural empyema in children and adults.[95] In infants, however, the immature arachnoid is a less effective barrier, and the incidence of bacterial meningitis accompanying subdural empyema is as high as 75%.[101] In addition to subdural empyema, epidural abscess, and meningitis, other potential intracranial complications of acute sinusitis include brain abscess, cavernous sinus thrombosis, and superior sagittal sinus thrombosis. Intracranial complications of sinusitis are often clinically silent, the symptoms being masked by the dramatic physical findings caused by the overlying sinusitis.[96]

Osteomyelitis may develop in cases of acute sinusitis as a result of either direct invasion or inoculation of the bone via diploic veins.[95] Interconnecting veins are the presumed pathway of organisms in septic emboli that produce calvarial osteomyelitis at sites that are remote from the infected sinus. Frontal bone osteomyelitis due to frontal sinusitis is usually accompanied by pericranial, periorbital, or epidural abscesses.

The extracranial equivalent of an epidural abscess is a subperiosteal abscess.[102] Frontal subperiosteal (pericranial) abscess is usually a complication of frontal sinusitis and, therefore, is a disease of older children and adults. Frontal subperiosteal abscess due to frontal sinusitis was initially described in 1760 by Sir Percivall Pott and is referred to as the Pott puffy tumor.[103] In comparison to the relatively common periorbital and orbital cellulitis, the other extracranial and intracranial complications of acute sinusitis are rare in children.

Chronic sinusitis is uncommon in infants and children. Most often there is an underlying disease process such as cystic fibrosis, ciliary dysmotility, allergy, or immunodeficiency that predisposes to chronic sinus disease, which can produce atrophic, sclerosing, or hypertrophic polypoid changes in the sinus mucosa. Symptoms include chronic

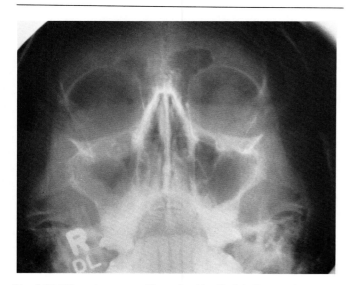

Fig. 3-29 Bilateral acute maxillary sinusitis. Upright Waters view shows marked mucoperiosteal thickening in the maxillary sinuses. There are air-fluid levels in the sinuses.

mucopurulent nasal discharge and congestion. Pain and fever are absent except in an acute exacerbation of otherwise chronic disease. The organisms identified in chronic sinusitis are similar to those seen in acute infections, although there is an increased incidence of *Staphylococcus aureus* infection.

The most important sequela of chronic inflammatory disease of a sinus is mucocele. The cause of a mucocele is long-standing obstruction of the sinus ostium. The ostial obstruction is most often due to chronic infection, but structural abnormalities or tumors are occasionally responsible. Paranasal mucoceles in the pediatric age group most often occur in children with cystic fibrosis or a strong history of atopy.[104,105]

The continued secretion of mucus by the epithelium of an obstructed sinus causes the sinus cavity to eventually become filled with mucoid secretions and thickened mucosa. The increased pressure results in a slow increase in the size of the mucocele, resulting in thinning, remodeling, and expansion of the sinus walls. The mucoperiosteum of the sinus functions as the cyst wall of the mucocele. As the sinus walls expand, the mucocele impinges on adjacent structures such as the orbit, which may cause proptosis. Although thinned, the expanded sinus wall usually remains intact; destruction of a portion of the sinus wall may occur in long-standing disease. If infected, a mucocele is termed a pyocele or pyomucocele.

In children, mucoceles most often occur in the ethmoid sinuses. The clinical presentation is usually related to impingement on the orbit. Potential presenting signs and symptoms include exophthalmos, epiphora, diplopia, headache, and nasal obstruction.

A clinically less significant complication of sinusitis is a mucous retention cyst. This common abnormality results from obstruction of a seromucinous gland. Continued glandular secretion results in a cyst. Retention cysts are asymptomatic unless they become large enough to fill completely the sinus cavity or to obstruct the ostium. A similar, somewhat less common cystic abnormality related to chronic inflammation is a serous cyst. This results from fluid accumulation in the submucosal layers of the mucoperiosteum. A serous cyst cannot be differentiated clinically or radiographically from the more common mucous retention cyst.

The radiographic findings of viral sinusitis include thickening of the nasal turbinates and uniform thickening of the mucoperiosteal lining of the sinus cavity. Air-fluid levels in the sinus may occur but are not common (Fig. 3-29). Mucoperiosteal thickening and air-fluid levels are the radiographic hallmarks of acute bacterial sinusitis.[87,94] Unilateral or asymmetric involvement is more common with bacterial disease compared to viral or allergic sinusitis, which tends to cause fairly symmetric and bilateral involvement of the paranasal sinuses.

CT and MRI are quite sensitive methods for the demonstration of inflammatory sinus disease.[106,107] These studies, however, are not usually required in typical uncomplicated sinusitis. Both these modalities clearly demonstrate sinus fluid and mucoperiosteal thickening. With CT, mucosal thickening

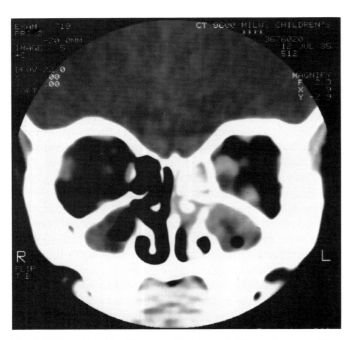

Fig. 3-30 Sinusitis with orbital extension. Coronal CT scan shows opacification of the maxillary sinuses and the left ethmoid air cells. There is a subperiosteal abscess in the medial aspect of the left orbit and inflammatory enlargement of the medial rectus muscle.

is identified as enhancing tissue along the walls of the involved sinus, while entrapped mucus or fluid does not enhance. Air-fluid levels are easily identified when present. Fluid and edematous mucosa produce very bright signal on T_2-weighted MR images.

Abnormalities of the paranasal sinuses have been found in asymptomatic children undergoing CT for unrelated reasons. These studies have demonstrated the frequent occurrence of sinus opacification as an incidental finding. Diament et al[108] found a variable degree of opacification of the maxillary or ethmoid sinuses in about half the asymptomatic children younger than 13 years of age. Glasier et al[109] reported sinus abnormalities in 18% of children older than 1 year without signs or symptoms of sinusitis or recent upper respiratory infection and in 31% of those with evidence of a recent respiratory infection but without clinical manifestations of sinusitis. Seventy-two percent of infants younger than 1 year of age were found to have sinus opacification on CT. Similar findings have been reported in studies that used plain radiographs.[110,111] These studies indicate that close correlation of the imaging findings with the clinical findings is essential. Also, images should be inspected for ancillary signs of sinus infection, such as air-fluid levels or extension into adjacent structures.

Imaging studies are particularly important for the identification and characterization of the various complications of acute sinusitis. Radiographs are of limited usefulness in this regard, aside from documentation of the underlying sinus opacification. CT and MRI are quite sensitive for the detection of

potential complications (Fig. 3-30). The CT and MRI findings of orbital extension from adjacent sinus infection include one or more of the following: thickening of periorbital soft tissues, increased attenuation of orbital fat, enlargement of one or more of the extraocular muscles, increased enhancement of the periosteum, a low-attenuation fluid collection due to subperiosteal or intraorbital abscess formation, and, rarely, optic nerve enlargement. Abnormal fluid collections and inflammatory changes of soft tissue structures produce increased signal on T_2-weighted MR images.

The imaging patterns of the intracranial complications of acute sinusitis are well described.[95] Intracranial empyemas are located adjacent to the calvaria or along the falx and are imaged as crescentic or lentiform, extra-axial, low-attenuation fluid collections on CT or as regions of bright signal on T_2-weighted MR images.[112] With intravenous contrast material, there is sharply defined enhancement of the medial rim of the fluid collection as a result of meningeal inflammation.[113] This enhancing rim helps distinguish an empyema from a subdural hygroma or subacute hematoma.

Four types of subdural empyema can be distinguished. The exudative process may be spread diffusely over the frontoparietal convexity, loculated in focal areas anywhere over the hemisphere (most often over the frontal pole and occipital cortex), collected in the interhemispheric fissure, or collected under the tentorium (Fig. 3-31).[114]

The cerebral cortex adjacent to a subdural empyema is occasionally involved. It may be due to encephalitis or, more

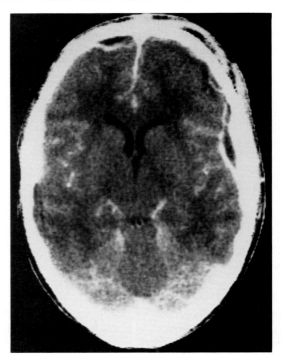

Fig. 3-31 Intracranial empyema due to frontal sinusitis. Contrast-enhanced CT shows bilateral subdural fluid collections—one in the right frontal region and the other in the left temporal region. There is displacement of thickened enhancing meninges.

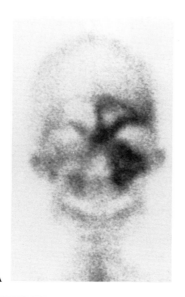

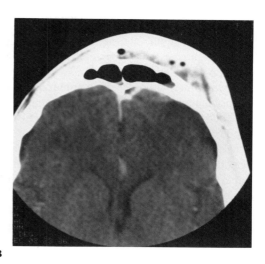

Fig. 3-32 Complicated sinusitis. (**A**) Bone scintigraphy shows markedly increased osseous uptake in the region of the left maxillary sinus and the margins of the left frontal sinus, extending into the adjacent portions of the frontal bone. (**B**) Contrast-enhanced CT shows a small amount of fluid in the frontal sinus. There is a small epidural abscess immediately posterior to the frontal sinus and thickening and enhancement of the meninges. A pericranial abscess is also visible anterior to the frontal sinus.

A

B

commonly, venous infarction resulting from septic thrombophlebitis. These are imaged as superficial areas of low attenuation on unenhanced CT scans. With contrast enhancement, patchy areas of enhancement in the brain parenchyma are usually seen if there is cerebral involvement. Formation of a brain abscess is extremely rare; it is indicated by an enhancing rim that surrounds a central cavity (usually of decreased attenuation) contained in the brain parenchyma, usually in the frontal lobes.[113]

Epidural abscesses most commonly occur adjacent to the frontal sinus. An epidural abscess frequently accompanies calvarial osteomyelitis. As with subdural abscess, an epidural abscess is imaged on CT as a low-attenuation fluid collection adjacent to the calvaria that has an enhancing internal rim. If the epidural abscess crosses the midline, posterior displacement of the falx and superior sagittal sinus serves to confirm that the fluid collection lies in the epidural space (Fig. 3-32).[113] A large epidural abscess displaces and distorts the adjacent brain parenchyma.

A frontal subperiosteal abscess (Pott puffy tumor) is demonstrated on CT as a low-attenuation fluid collection projecting anteriorly adjacent to the frontal bone (Fig. 3-33).[102] There is an enhancing rim along the peripheral aspect of the fluid collection, which represents the thickened, displaced periosteum. Because epidural and subperiosteal abscesses are usually accompanied by osteomyelitis, CT may demonstrate areas of bone destruction. In some cases, air is seen in the epidural or pericranial spaces as a result of a communication with the frontal sinus caused by bone destruction.

Concerning intracranial fluid collections that are complications of acute sinus infection, there are several factors that help differentiate a subdural empyema from an epidural abscess. A subdural abscess typically has a crescentic configuration, whereas an epidural collection is lenticular in shape. The meningeal and superficial cerebral inflammation along the medial aspect of a subdural empyema produces irregular,

inhomogeneous enhancement, whereas the inflamed dura adjacent to an epidural abscess forms a well-defined enhancing medial rim. Anterior epidural abscesses will frequently cross the midline and displace the superior sagittal sinus and falx posteriorly; this does not occur with subdural collections.

MRI offers improved sensitivity over CT for the detection of small subdural and epidural fluid collections. Subdural and epidural abscesses produce increased signal compared to cerebrospinal fluid on T_1-weighted MR images as a result of the shortened T_1-relaxation times of purulent fluid. Therefore, on T_1-weighted images the fluid component of epidural and sub-

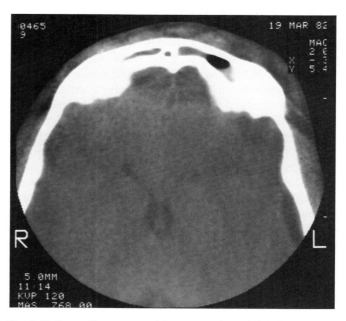

Fig. 3-33 Pott puffy tumor. Axial contrast-enhanced CT shows partial opacification of the frontal sinuses. There is thickening and enhancement of the pericranial soft tissues anterior to the frontal sinus.

dural abscesses is usually approximately isointense to brain and of higher signal intensity than cerebrospinal fluid. On T_2-weighted images, the fluid collections are hyperintense to brain. A well-defined, low-intensity line (the displaced dura) forms the internal border of an epidural abscess. The inflammatory inner membrane of a subdural empyema is usually less well defined and more difficult to demonstrate without intravenous paramagnetic contrast enhancement.

MRI also offers superior sensitivity compared to CT for the detection of intracerebral complications of acute sinusitis. Superficial venous infarcts, cerebral inflammation, and encephalitis, all of which may accompany subdural empyemas, are imaged as areas of decreased signal on T_1-weighted images and high signal on T_2-weighted images.

MRI is quite sensitive for the detection of cerebral abscess. The signal intensity characteristics of the abscess vary somewhat with the degree of maturity. Initially, T_1-weighted images show indistinct decreased intensity, and T_2-weighted images show high intensity. As necrosis develops, the central portion shows a further decrease in intensity on T_1-weighted images and variable isointensity or high intensity on T_2-weighted images. The surrounding edema remains hyperintense. An isointense or hypointense capsule may be visible surrounding a mature abscess.

Imaging of a mucocele demonstrates opacification of the involved sinus with fluid and hypertrophied mucosa. A mucocele may exhibit CT attenuation values ranging from low to high, depending on the contents of the lesion (mucoid material, desquamated epithelium, hemorrhage, or serous fluid). Rim enhancement may be seen, but most of the lesion is composed of fluid and does not enhance. The bony walls are expanded and thinned, but bone destruction does not occur except as a late finding (Fig. 3-34).[105,115,116]

The MR appearance of a mucocele is a well-defined, expansile sinus lesion. The thinned sinus wall produces a low-signal rim surrounding the mass. The MR signal intensities of the contents of the mucocele vary somewhat, depending on the fluid content. Most often, the contents of a mucocele produce low signal intensity on T_1-weighted images, intermediate signal on proton density–weighted images, and high signal on T_2-weighted images. If the proteinaceous secretions in a long-standing mucocele become concentrated, shortening of the T_1-relaxation time may cause an intermediate signal intensity on T_1-weighted images. If the protein concentration becomes very high, first the T_2-weighted signal intensity and then the T_1-weighted signal intensity decrease. The diagnosis of a pyomucocele is suggested by enhancement with intravenous contrast material on CT or enhancement with intravenous gadolinium-DTPA on MRI.

Mucous retention cysts and serous cysts are imaged as well-defined, round, low-attenuation lesions projecting from the sinus wall. The wall of the cyst is too thin to be visualized on CT. There should not be enhancement of the wall or the contents of the cyst with intravenous contrast agents. The MR findings of mucous retention cysts are similar to those of CT. The fluid contents of the cyst produce low signal on T_1-

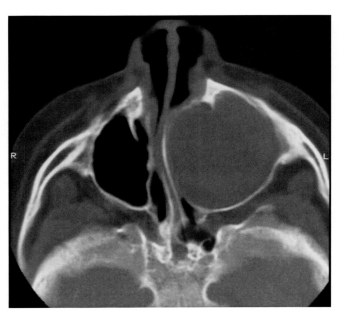

Fig. 3-34 Mucocele. Axial CT shows opacification of the left maxillary sinus. The walls of the sinus cavity are expanded and thinned. The medial wall bulges into the nasal cavity and displaces the nasal septum to the right.

weighted images and high signal on T_2-weighted images. The protein content of a cyst may increase due to infection, thereby resulting in moderate signal intensity on T_1-weighted images.

The radiographic appearance of chronic sinusitis is a variable degree of mucoperiosteal thickening of the involved sinus. Air-fluid levels should not be present. Typically, there is relatively symmetric involvement of the sinuses with chronic sinusitis. With long-standing disease, reactive sclerosing osteitis of the sinus walls may be seen. The mucoperiosteal thickening of chronic sinusitis may also be demonstrated with CT or MRI. The thickened mucosa in chronic sinusitis produces high signal on MRI, but the signal is less than that of the edematous mucosa and free fluid present in acute sinusitis.

Differentiation of chronic sinusitis from a sinus neoplasm may, at times, be difficult. Imaging studies in cases of primary chronic sinusitis usually show a decrease in the size of the involved sinus with thickening of the sinus wall. Tumors tend to cause enlargement of the sinus cavity and thinning of the walls. In cases of secondary chronic sinusitis (eg, due to antrochoanal polyp, polyposis, or other partially obstructing lesion), the size of the involved sinus is variable, but a diffuse increase in wall thickness is frequently present except in cases of mucocele.[117]

Bony erosion may occur in cases of chronic sinusitis. The erosions tend to be relatively small and most often occur in a region of a normal anatomic bony defect, such as the semilunar hiatus, the infraorbital canal, and the ethmoid bulla. Bony erosions seen in malignancies of the paranasal sinuses in children are usually extensive and are not confined to areas of normal anatomic defects.[117]

The radiographic appearance of fungal sinusitis is nodular mucoperiosteal thickening with a variable degree of sinus opacification. The nodular, irregular rim of soft tissue thickening is more readily demonstrated on CT than on standard radiographs. Differentiation from other etiologies of sinus opacification is sometimes possible with CT when focal or diffuse areas of increased attenuation are identified in the sinus on unenhanced scans. These areas are thought to represent calcium deposits in necrotic areas of a mycetoma. These fungal concretions produce an area of significantly decreased signal intensity on T_2-weighted MR images.[118,119]

Osteomyelitis is an uncommon but serious complication of acute or recurrent sinusitis. Radiographs and CT scans may demonstrate areas of bone destruction. Osteomyelitis of the frontal bone is frequently accompanied by epidural and pericranial fluid collections. Calvarial osteomyelitis produces alterations in signal intensity of bone marrow on MRI. Inflammatory marrow changes produce a relative decrease in signal intensity on T_1-weighted images and a relative increase on T_2-weighted images.

Bone scintigraphy is often useful for the evaluation of suspected osteomyelitis.[102] Bone imaging in cases of acute sinusitis with suspected calvarial osteomyelitis must be interpreted with caution because the bony walls of an infected sinus frequently develop a reactive osteitis. Both reactive osteitis and osteomyelitis produce increased tracer uptake on bone scintigraphy. Therefore, bone scintigraphy demonstrates increased tracer uptake in the sinus walls in most cases of acute or chronic sinusitis.. Secondary osteomyelitis is suggested if there is extension of abnormal uptake beyond the sinus wall (eg, superiorly into the frontal bone) or areas of abnormal calvarial tracer accumulation that are remote from the involved paranasal sinuses. Correlation with other imaging modalities is essential for proper interpretation of the scintigraphic abnormalities.

Allergic Sinusitis

Significant allergic rhinitis and sinusitis involve approximately 10% of the population in the United States. This is most often due to a seasonal pollinosis allergy. Approximately 1.5 million school days are lost per year because of allergic rhinosinusitis. Seasonal pollinosis is rare before the age of 4 to 5 years.

Another group of patients have perennial allergic rhinitis and sinusitis. These patients are symptomatic year round. The causative agents, when identifiable, are generally found to be allergens to which the patient is exposed more or less continually. Examples are house dust, feathers, and the dander of household pets.

Uncomplicated allergic sinusitis can produce mucoperiosteal hyperplasia and hypersecretion. Chronic allergic rhinosinusitis is the most common abnormality associated with nasal polyps. Other complications of allergic sinusitis include secondary bacterial infection and mucocele formation.[87,120]

Radiographs in allergic sinusitis demonstrate mild to moderate mucoperiosteal thickening that most commonly involves the maxillary antra. There is also thickening of the nasal turbinates. The distribution of abnormality is typically relatively symmetric, in contradistinction to that in acute bacterial sinusitis. Air-fluid levels occasionally occur, but they are not as common as in acute bacterial sinusitis.

CT and MRI also demonstrate mucoperiosteal thickening and often small fluid collections in the sinuses. These imaging modalities are particularly useful for detection of complications of chronic allergic sinusitis such as polyps and mucoceles. Pansinusitis, polyp formation, and diffuse polyposis are more commonly identified in allergic sinusitis compared to bacterial disease.

Neoplasms

Neoplasms of the paranasal sinuses are infrequent in children. Because the paranasal sinuses are histologically similar to the nasopharynx, similar tumors occur in both locations. Also, tumors that arise in the paranasal sinuses frequently extend into the nasopharynx, and vice versa. Paranasal sinus tumors usually do not produce symptoms until they fill the affected sinus or occlude the ostium. The initial presenting symptoms may also be due to involvement of adjacent structures such as the orbit or nasopharyngeal airway.

Benign paranasal sinus neoplasms that occur in the pediatric age group include inverting papilloma, angiomatous polyp, epidermoid tumor, fibrous dysplasia, and osteoma. The paranasal sinuses are secondarily involved with juvenile angiofibromas that arise in the posterior nasopharynx. The gross morphology of angiomatous polyps in the paranasal sinuses closely resembles that of the juvenile angiofibroma. Chondromas and osteomas occur most commonly in the ethmoid and frontal sinuses. Osteomas of the paranasal sinus are a component of Gardner syndrome. Epidermoid tumors arise as cellular rests in the walls of the frontal sinuses, where they slowly enlarge, causing expansion of the bony margins without destruction.

Malignant epithelial tumors of the paranasal sinuses, such as squamous cell carcinoma, are rare in children. The frontal and ethmoid sinuses may be secondarily involved with esthesioneuroblastoma, which arises in the superior aspect of the nasopharynx. Nonepithelial tumors, which include rhabdomyosarcoma, lymphoma, and malignant fibrous histiocytoma, are the most common primary malignant paranasal sinus tumors in the pediatric age group.[121] Seventy-five percent of paranasal sinus rhabdomyosarcomas occur in the first decade of life, and 7% occur in the second decade. Approximately 10% of head and neck rhabdomyosarcomas occur in the maxillary sinuses. This tumor is characterized by aggressive growth and rapid extension into adjacent structures. Approximately 10% of non-Hodgkin lymphomas occur in the head and neck, with large cell lymphoma being the most common histology. Bone destruction and infiltration along fascial planes into adjacent structures are typical. Malignant fibrous histiocytoma produces a localized bulky mass that may cause symptoms of sinus inflammation as a result of occlusion of the sinus ostium. Metastatic neuroblastoma occasionally involves the paranasal sinuses.

Paranasal sinus osteomas are usually easily visualized on radiographs. These lesions are well demonstrated on CT, which shows a lobulated, nonenhancing mass of high attenuation. A compact osteoma is uniformly ossified, whereas a cancellous osteoma may show tumor components of soft tissue attenuation on bone window CT images. On MRI osteomas produce heterogeneous low to moderate signal intensity on all imaging sequences. Osteomas produce intense focal uptake on blood pool and delayed skeletal scintigraphy.[122]

Small inverting papillomas may be indistinguishable from sinus polyps or cysts. Large tumors result in opacification of the involved sinus on radiographs, sometimes with bone destruction. CT more accurately demonstrates the soft tissue mass, bone destruction, and invasion of adjacent structures.

An angiomatous polyp is imaged on CT as a soft tissue mass. There is minimal contrast enhancement in the periphery of the lesion, and the intense enhancement seen in juvenile angiofibroma is not present. The polyp does not extend into the pterygopalatine fossa and only rarely protrudes into the sphenoid sinus. Vascular flow voids are not present on MRI.[123]

Radiographs of malignant paranasal sinus neoplasms demonstrate partial or complete opacification of one or more sinuses. The hallmark radiographic findings of a malignant lesion are bone destruction and invasion of adjacent structures without sinus cavity expansion. Benign lesions more often remain confined to the sinus cavity or produce bone expansion without permeative destructive bone changes.

Compared to radiographs, CT scans more accurately depict the tumor morphology, bone destruction, and adjacent structure involvement.[124] MRI is not well suited for detecting the osseous changes. Tumor morphology, composition, and extent, however, are well evaluated with this imaging modality.[125] Bone scintigraphy is useful for identifying osseous changes in the region of the sinus neoplasm as well as for detecting distant skeletal metastases.

Imaging of malignant tumors of the paranasal sinuses shows opacification of the involved sinus, destruction of the sinus walls, and invasion of adjacent structures.[35,117] On CT, a variable degree of contrast enhancement of the mass is usually demonstrable. At the time of diagnosis, most malignant tumors of the paranasal sinuses extensively involve the nasal cavity and nasopharynx; therefore, localization of the site of origin to the sinus or the nasal structures is often unclear (Fig. 3-35).

Malignant tumors of the paranasal sinuses usually demonstrate low to intermediate signal intensity on T_1-weighted MR images. Most often, these malignancies produce areas of moderate signal intensity on T_2-weighted images, which may be distinguished from the bright signal areas produced by adjacent inflammatory disease and fluid. These neoplasms

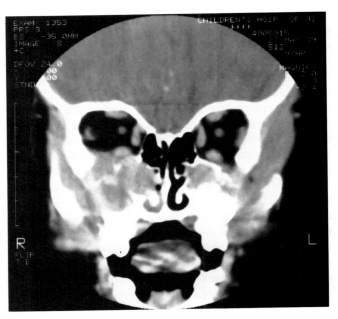

Fig. 3-35 Lymphoma. Coronal contrast-enhanced CT scan shows opacification of the maxillary sinuses with moderately enhancing soft tissue masses. There are areas of bone destruction. The mass arising from the right maxillary sinus extends into the inferior aspect of the orbit.

usually exhibit relatively uniform internal architecture. If hemorrhage occurs in the tumor, an area of increased signal on T_1-weighted images and moderate intensity on T_2-weighted images is produced.[25]

Systemic Disease

Sarcoidosis is an uncommon disease in the pediatric age group. It is a chronic multisystem disease of obscure origin and shows a variable pattern of involvement. Weight loss, cough, fatigue, bone and joint pain, and anemia are the most frequent clinical manifestations. Sarcoidosis can result in granulomatous masses that fill the sinus cavities. The bony walls of the sinuses may be expanded, so that the disease may resemble a malignant neoplasm. The radiographic findings with sarcoidosis include sinus opacification and bone destruction predominantly involving the ethmoid sinuses.

Wegener granulomatosis is characterized by a necrotizing granulomatous vasculitis that involves multiple organ systems. The most severely involved organs are the upper respiratory tract, lungs, and kidneys. The male-to-female ratio is approximately 2:1. Respiratory symptoms are prominent early clinical manifestations. Persistent nasal stuffiness with or without discharge is a frequent early symptom. There are usually crusted or pustular lesions seen in the anterior nares. The lesions are progressively destructive and may result in perforation of the nasal septum, obliteration of the nasal cavity, and ulcerations of the palate and other areas in the upper airway. Involvement of sinus and nasal mucosa may lead to mucosal ulceration and inflammation. Chronic bacterial sinusitis is often superimposed on the granulomatous vasculitis.

The radiographic findings with Wegener granulomatosis include sinus and nasal mucosal thickening, sinus opacification, and areas of bone destruction. The chronic sinusitis may result in thickening of the sinus walls. The osseous and soft tissue abnormalities of the sinus in cases of Wegener granulomatosis are best demonstrated on CT.[122,126]

There are various systemic abnormalities that predispose to sinus inflammatory disease. These include dysmotile cilia syndrome, cystic fibrosis, and primary immunologic disorders. Sinus disease related to compromised immune response is also relatively common in bone marrow transplant patients, those with acquired immunodeficiency syndrome, and those on high-dose chemotherapy. A unique entity develops in a small subset of patients who have received a bone marrow transplant. These patients usually have been treated with monoclonal antibodies to T cells. They develop an Epstein-Barr virus–associated lymphoproliferative disorder of transplanted cells that has a predilection for involvement of the paranasal sinuses and retropharynx. The radiographic findings are those of chronic sinus inflammatory disease.

One or more paranasal sinuses may be involved in children with fibrous dysplasia. In this condition, the normal spongiotic bone of one or more bones is replaced by abnormal fibrous tissue. The bone becomes expanded and may impinge on adjacent structures. The cavity of the paranasal sinus is involved in cases of fibrous dysplasia by extension of a bony lesion into the cavity or by stenosis of the sinus ostium.[124]

CT of facial fibrous dysplasia shows expansion of the diploic spaces. The cortical margins are expanded and thinned but intact. Most often, the tumor matrix demonstrates a ground-glass appearance on CT and radiographs; the matrix consists of a mixture of osseous and fibrous material.[124]

Thalassemia causes severe hypoplasia of the sinuses as a result of enlargement of the marrow spaces. The osseous expansion may also cause ostial obstruction and secondary infection. Radiographs and CT scans demonstrate marked expansion of the marrow-containing bones of the face and calvarium. This results in obliteration of the cavity. The ethmoid sinuses are not involved because they lack marrow spaces.[87,124]

The mucous membranes of the paranasal sinuses are abnormal in patients with cystic fibrosis. The secretory mucous glands produce an excessive amount of abnormal mucus, and the mucosa is thickened. The mucosa of the paranasal sinuses is frequently colonized with *Pseudomonas aeruginosa* and *Staphylococcus aureus*. Acute or chronic sinus infections are common. Obstruction of a sinus ostium by thick, tenacious mucus may lead to the development of a mucocele or pyocele. Polyps of the sinus and nasal mucosa are also common in children with cystic fibrosis (6% to 9%).[89,127]

Radiographs, CT scans, and MR images demonstrate mucosal thickening involving all or most of the paranasal sinuses in virtually all children with cystic fibrosis. Complete opacification of one or more sinuses is common, and correlation with the clinical findings is important in distinguishing acute from chronic disease. Despite the common radiographic evidence of mucosal edema or sinus opacification in children with cystic fibrosis, the incidence of clinical sinusitis is only 11%.[128] Polyps are imaged as round (usually multiple) lesions protruding into a sinus or the nasal cavity.[127]

SOFT TISSUES OF THE NECK

There is a broad spectrum of abnormalities that produce neck masses in children (Table 3-6). The soft tissues of the neck are a common site for the expression of malignancy in childhood. Both primary and metastatic lesions occur in this region. Lymphoma accounts for approximately 55% of pediatric neck malignancies and rhabdomyosarcoma for 10%; the remainder includes fibrosarcoma, thyroid carcinoma, neuroblastoma, squamous cell carcinoma, and primary bone tumors. It must be remembered, however, that 90% of children with abnormal lymph nodes in the head and neck region have a benign process, usually of infectious etiology. Congenital abnormalities also occur in this region; these include thyroglossal duct cysts and sinuses; branchial cleft cysts, sinuses, and fistulae; and fibromatosis of the sternocleidomastoid.[129–131]

Because the differential diagnosis of a cervical mass is lengthy, review of the historical and physical characteristics of the mass is absolutely necessary to indicate the appropriate diagnostic pathway. Lesions present at birth suggest congenital cysts or anomalies. Congenital cysts, however, may remain clinically silent until they become infected and may easily become confused with infectious lymphadenitis or

---

Table 3-6 Etiologies of Neck Masses in Infancy

Inflammatory
  Cervical adenitis
  Abscess
  Tuberculosis
Developmental
  Cysts
  Fistulae
Neoplastic
  Hemangioma
  Lymphangioma (cystic hygroma)
  Lipoma, lipoblastoma
  Lymphoproliferative disease
  Neuroblastoma
  Teratoma
  Thyroid tumor
  Metastatic disease
Idiopathic
  Congenital fibromatosis of the sternocleidomastoid
  Fibrodysplasia ossificans progressiva

abscess formation. Inflammation may be associated with congenital lesions as well as malignant lymphadenopathy; its presence does not always predict benignity. Masses that enlarge slowly over months are generally benign, whereas rapidly enlarging masses, particularly nontender matted nodes, suggest malignancy. Inflamed masses that are painful during eating suggest sialadenitis.

Diffuse, soft, spongy masses may be cystic or vascular malformations such as cystic hygroma or hemangioma. Cystic hygromas transilluminate, whereas a bluish hue suggests a hemangioma. A midline mass that retracts while swallowing describes the more classic thyroglossal duct cyst. The neonate who presents with head tilt and a fibrous tumor in the sternocleidomastoid muscle may have congenital muscular torticollis. Generalized lymphadenopathy is a sign of systemic illness, and signs and symptoms often will lead to the appropriate diagnosis.

Congenital Abnormalities

Thyroglossal Duct Cyst

The thyroid anlage appears as a thickening of the endoderm in the floor of the pharynx during week 4 of fetal development. This structure grows into a bilobed diverticulum that descends in the midline through the region where the tongue muscles and hyoid bone eventually develop. Once the diverticulum reaches the level of thyroid cartilage, it may deviate laterally. Statistically, it most often deviates to the left. As the diverticulum descends it remains attached to the pharynx by a tubular stalk, which is called the thyroglossal duct. Normally, this duct becomes solid and then disintegrates by week 6 of life. The site of origin of this duct in the base of the tongue is called the foramen cecum, and its termination remains as the pyramidal lobe of the thyroid gland.

Remnants of the thyroglossal duct may persist from embryonic life. For unknown reasons, the undifferentiated cells in these remnants may become active and differentiate into columnar, ciliated, or squamous epithelium or into glandular tissue (sebaceous, salivary, or thyroid). When these cell groups are activated, they usually produce a midline mass that is often cystic and contains mucoid material; this represents a thyroglossal duct cyst. Occasionally, the cyst or another part of the duct will create a sinus tract to the skin surface, nearly always in the midline.

Overall, clinically apparent thyroglossal duct cysts and sinuses are relatively uncommon, but thyroglossal duct cyst is the most common midline neck mass in children. Accumulated secretions can produce a cyst at any level from the foramen cecum to the thyroid, although most occur just above or below the hyoid bone. In most cases there is no spontaneous communication with the skin, but communication with the skin occasionally occurs with infection. Most external communications are the result of incomplete surgical excision. Under these circumstances, formation of a draining sinus is related to the residual secretions of the thyroglossal mucosa.

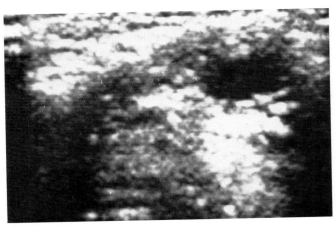

Fig. 3-36 Thyroglossal duct cyst. Transverse sonogram of the anterior neck shows a small cyst in the midline with good through-transmission.

Carcinoma (most often papillary thyroid carcinoma) can occur in these cysts.[50,132–135]

Radiographically, thyroglossal duct cyst is best visualized on lateral views of the neck and appears as a sharply demarcated, round to oval soft tissue structure. Thyroglossal duct cysts located above the larynx may produce an airway obstruction. Demonstration of fistulous tracts can be accomplished by the injection of contrast material.[50]

The sonographic appearance of a thyroglossal duct cyst is relatively specific. An anechoic, well-marginated, cystic mass with good through-transmission is found near the midline. These lesions may occur at any level from the base of the tongue to the thyroid (Fig. 3-36).

An infected thyroglossal duct cyst usually exhibits scattered internal echoes on sonography. The wall may become thick and irregular. In some cases, a heterogeneous, complex mass is imaged. An infected thyroglossal duct cyst cannot usually be differentiated from an abscess or other complex neck mass, although the midline location indicates that this lesion should be included in the differential diagnosis.[136]

The CT appearance of a thyroglossal duct cyst is a well-circumscribed, low-attenuation lesion with peripheral rim enhancement. The mass is usually in a midline location. Inflammation can alter the density of the cyst so that it approaches or equals that of soft tissue. At times, septations may be noted. Alterations in the adjacent soft tissues can be produced by inflammatory changes. A thyroglossal duct cyst produces high signal intensity on T_2-weighted MR images.

Most thyroglossal cysts (about 65%) are located below the hyoid bone in the region of the thyrohyoid membrane; 20% are suprahyoid, and 15% are at the level of the hyoid bone. Those cysts located below the level of the hyoid bone are usually imbedded in the strap muscles.[137,138]

Branchial Cleft Cysts

Early in embryogenesis, there are five transverse mesodermal bars in the developing neck that are separated by clefts.

Each of these clefts is in contact with related outpouchings from the pharynx; the two are separated only by a thin membrane. Later in embryogenesis, the second, third, and fourth clefts coalesce to form a common chamber called the cervical sinus. This is due to caudal growth of the second branchial arch, which overlaps the third and fourth clefts. The lateral branchial anomalies that arise from the second cleft in the cervical sinus are therefore seen throughout the neck. Most arise from the second cleft and pouch. Because the second branchial pouch forms the palatine fossae and the tonsils, fistulae to the pharynx are likely to occur at this point, but they drain into the pharynx anywhere from the piriform sinus to the tonsillar fossa.[139]

Some authorities believe that branchial cleft cysts, sinuses, and fistulae arise from branchial cleft remnants and that all are lined with stratified squamous epithelium. Branchial cleft cysts constitute approximately 20% of neck masses in children. Most of these arise from the second branchial cleft; other anomalies related to the second branchial cleft include cutaneous sinuses that drain externally along the anterior border of the sternocleidomastoid muscle near the angle of the mandible fistulae between the pharynx and neck, and pharyngeal diverticula arising from the tonsillar fossa, piriform sinus, or vallecula. Most branchial cleft cysts are located in the upper third of the neck, and fistula formation is present in less than 15%.

Defects of the first branchial cleft are of two types: a duplication of the membranous external auditory canal (cystic mass anterior and inferior to the ear lobe), and an anomalous external auditory canal with deformity of the ear cartilage (a large cystic mass over the parotid and upper neck). Malformations of the third branchial cleft are rare and consist of cysts, sinuses, or fistulae. They occur along the lower third of the neck and are located near the midline.[50]

Clinically, a branchial cleft sinus or fistula presents as a 2- to 3-mm slit in the skin anterior to the lower third of the sternocleidomastoid muscle. These lesions may be identified in the newborn infant. The sinus is a portal of entry for pathogens.

Branchial cleft cysts can present at any age and usually are located adjacent to the middle third of the sternocleidomastoid muscle. The most common time for presentation is the early school years. Palpation of a rounded mass that is nontender and only slightly movable in the appropriate location makes a branchial cleft cyst a likely diagnosis. If the patient is seen during an acute respiratory infection, the mass may be mistaken for lymphadenopathy. Also, because of the adjacent lymph node chain, the cyst may enlarge concomitantly with the lymph nodes. Clinical observation of lymph nodes decreasing in size after infection while the mass persists is a useful clue.[132,140,141]

Radiographically, the findings of a branchial cleft cyst are nonspecific. Radiographs show a soft tissue mass. On CT, a branchial cleft cyst is imaged as a well-circumscribed, low-attenuation structure. The course and extent of branchial cleft sinuses and fistulae can be demonstrated by cannulating the orifice of the sinus tract at the skin surface and injecting it with water-soluble contrast material (Fig. 3-37). Most branchial cleft cysts and sinuses are easily treated with surgical resection; if there is delay in treatment, however, the therapeutic approach is frequently complicated by infection.[50]

Branchial cleft cysts demonstrate cystic sonographic characteristics but may also contain low-level echoes due to superimposed infection. The usual location, anterior to the carotid sheath and sternocleidomastoid muscle and separate from the thyroid gland, can be explained by the embryologic derivation. It is difficult in certain circumstances to differentiate branchial cleft cyst from an abscess or other hypoechoic mass such as lymphadenopathy.[141–143]

CT demonstrates a noninflamed branchial cleft cyst as a well-defined low-attenuation mass surrounded by a thin wall of slightly higher attenuation. The wall shows only minimal enhancement with intravenous contrast media. An infected cyst usually exhibits higher attenuation values than clear fluid. The wall is ill defined, and there is prominent irregular rim enhancement.

A branchial cleft cyst produces bright signal on T_2-weighted MR images. The lesion may be hypointense or slightly hyperintense to muscle on T_1-weighted images. Noninflamed cysts typically have thin, well-defined walls. Current or previous infection usually is associated with a thick, irregular wall. Inflammatory changes in the adjacent soft tissues cause increased signal intensity on T_2-weighted images.

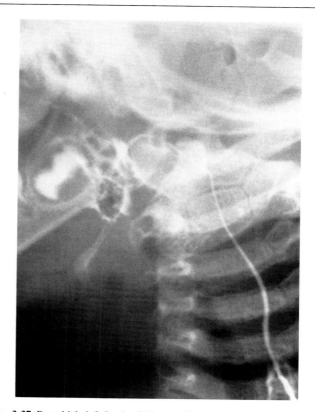

Fig. 3-37 Branchial cleft fistula. Oblique radiograph of the upper neck after contrast agent injection through the external opening of a fistula shows communication of the tract with the nasopharynx at the level of the adenoids.

Congenital Fibromatosis of the Sternocleidomastoid

Congenital fibromatosis of the sternocleidomastoid refers to a unilateral contracture of the sternocleidomastoid muscle that is usually associated with torticollis. Other terms for this condition include congenital muscular torticollis and congenital wry neck. Two theories of the etiology of this condition have been proposed: birth trauma with hemorrhage and eventual fibrosis of the sternocleidomastoid, and intrauterine malposition with vascular occlusive events in the muscle resulting in edema, muscle fiber degeneration, and fibrosis. At least 40% of infants with this condition have a history of difficult delivery. This entity has been reported in infants who have been delivered by cesarean section, suggesting a prenatal cause in some cases. About 75% of cases occur on the right side, and 20% are accompanied by congenital hip dislocation.

The classic clinical presentation of congenital muscular torticollis includes a tight sternocleidomastoid muscle, restricted range of neck motion, facial asymmetry, and plagiocephaly. The head is tilted toward the side of the muscular contracture, but the chin is turned toward the opposite side. A mass may be palpated, representing contracture and fibrosis of the sternocleidomastoid. The mass is usually nontender, firm, mobile beneath the skin, and located in the body of the sternocleidomastoid muscle. The clinical features may be absent or minimal at birth but are usually discovered during the first 2 months of life.

In those cases in which the typical clinical findings are absent, the condition may be confused with other causes of neck masses or torticollis. In approximately half the infants with congenital fibromatosis of the sternocleidomastoid, a discrete mass is not recognized on physical examination despite the presence of torticollis. Likewise, in some cases a mass is palpable, but the other clinical features are absent or go unrecognized. The differential diagnosis of congenital muscular torticollis and neck masses in infancy is presented in Tables 3-6 and 3-7. The timely diagnosis of this condition is important for the prompt initiation of appropriate therapy and to prevent unnecessary biopsy or more aggressive surgical therapy.[144]

Radiographs should be obtained in all infants with torticollis to detect structural defects of the cervical spine. There are several abnormalities of the cervical spine that can result in clinical torticollis in infants (Table 3-7). In true congenital muscular torticollis, the cervical spine is structurally normal.

The diagnosis of congenital fibromatosis of the sternocleidomastoid can be confirmed with sonography. The sternocleidomastoid muscles are well visualized with high-frequency ultrasound transducers. In those cases of congenital muscular torticollis with a palpable mass, sonography confirms that the mass is contained in the sternocleidomastoid muscle. The mass usually exhibits echogenicity similar to that of normal muscle, or it may be slightly hypoechoic. In most cases, the superior and inferior margins of the mass have a tapered appearance, where the mass blends with the normal portions of the muscle.[136]

As discussed above, there are several abnormalities of the soft tissue structures in the neck that may result in clinical torticollis or a palpable mass. Because of the ability of CT to distinguish among the various tissues and bony structures of the neck, this modality is uniquely suited for evaluation of clinically equivocal cases. In congenital muscular torticollis, CT demonstrates abnormal enlargement of the sternocleidomastoid as the cause of the palpable mass. The area of enlargement is usually in the inferior half of the muscle. The attenuation values of the mass are similar to those of normal muscle. Calcification in the mass or the remainder of the muscle does not occur (Fig. 3-38).

Fibrodysplasia ossificans progressiva may also result in enlargement of the sternocleidomastoid or other neck muscles. The CT appearance of fibrodysplasia ossificans progressiva is usually distinctive. In the acute phase, enlarged, hypodense muscles are imaged. If intravenous contrast medium is used, marked nonuniform enhancement is typically identified; this is not present in congenital muscular torticollis. CT performed during the quiescent phase demonstrates areas of soft tissue ossification.

CT is also helpful in differentiating this condition from infantile neck masses that arise from structures other than muscle. Lymphadenopathy results from an inflammatory mass or metastatic disease (neuroblastoma). A matted mass of nodes in either of these conditions is usually poorly marginated. Although adjacent muscle may be secondarily involved, the extramuscular origin of the abnormality is usually apparent on CT. In addition, areas of calcification may be detected in either inflammatory or neoplastic lymphadenopathy.

CT is also useful in evaluating primary cervical neoplasms that may occur in infancy. Hemangioma, for example, demonstrates marked contrast enhancement on dynamic CT. Cystic hygroma is imaged as a mass composed of multiple, irregular, fluid-containing cavities. These lesions usually are located in the posterior cervical triangle of the neck behind the sternocleidomastoid muscle. Lipoblastoma shows a fatty, sep-

---

Table 3-7 Etiologies of Congenital Torticollis

Skeletal
  Klippel-Feil anomaly
  Unilateral atlanto-occipital synostosis
  Unilateral basilar impression
  Unilateral occipital condyle hypoplasia
  Odontoid anomaly
Muscular
  Congenital fibromatosis of the sternocleidomastoid
  Fibrodysplasia ossificans progressiva
Skin
  Pterygium coli (skin web)
Central nervous system
  Posterior fossa tumor
  Spinal cord tumor
  Syringomyelia

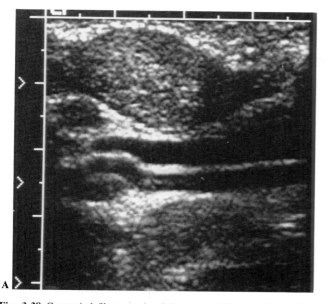
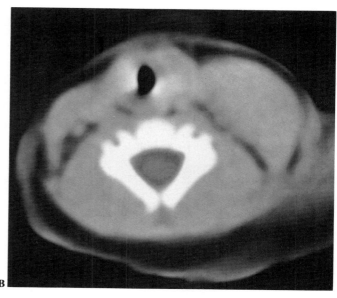

Fig. 3-38 Congenital fibromatosis of the sternocleidomastoid muscle. (**A**) Longitudinal sonogram shows an oval mass in the midportion of the left sternocleidomastoid muscle. The superior and inferior margins of the lesion have a tapered appearance. (**B**) Axial CT confirms that the mass lies in the sternocleidomastoid muscle. The lesion has CT attenuation characteristics similar to those of normal muscle.

tated, lobulated mass on CT. Teratoma may also contain areas of fat, but most of the mass is usually of soft tissue density, and regions of ossification or calcification are demonstrated. With most neoplasms, CT may show displacement or invasion of muscles, but the extramuscular origin of the mass is usually clear.[145]

Fibrodysplasia Ossificans Progressiva

Fibrodysplasia ossificans progressiva is a rare disorder in which there is intermittent progressive ossification of the soft tissues. It was formerly known as myositis ossificans progressiva. The great majority of affected patients present during childhood, but there is often a delay in diagnosis because of lack of familiarity with this condition.

An autosomal dominant pattern of inheritance has been determined in fibrodysplasia ossificans progressiva; most cases are sporadic, however. Advanced paternal age has been associated in some cases. One case of possible maternal germ cell mutation associated with phenytoin therapy has been reported.[146] Most patients present before the age of 5 years.[147]

The initial presentation of fibrodysplasia ossificans progressiva is usually multiple, firm, soft tissue masses, most commonly involving the back and neck. Other relatively common areas of involvement include the shoulders, chest, hips, elbows, knees, and jaw. The lumps are often warm, red, and painful; they may develop over a period of several hours. Fever and elevated erythrocyte sedimentation rate are frequently present. The small lumps may coalesce into a large mass. Firmness and lack of mobility of the affected structure usually develop. There is often a history of predisposing soft tissue trauma, intramuscular injection, or other forms of

injury. Biopsy of the lesion or attempts at surgical excision result in exacerbation of the condition.

There are several important associated physical findings that aid in establishing the diagnosis of this disorder. Microdactyly of the great toes, often with hallux valgus, is present at birth in most patients. Approximately 50% of the affected children also have hypoplastic first metacarpals and clinodactyly of the fifth finger. Broad-necked femurs and ankylosis of the cervical vertebrae may also occur. Deafness, baldness, and, rarely, retardation have been reported.

Radiographs in cases of fibrodysplasia ossificans progressiva demonstrate nonspecific soft tissue swelling during the acute phase. As acute lesions subside, a cloudlike area of calcification may be visualized in the center of the lesion. Eventually, definite ossification is visible with recognizable cortex and bone trabeculae. An ossified lesion adjacent to bone may blend with the cortex and have the radiographic appearance of an exostosis (Fig. 3-39).

CT is more sensitive and specific than standard radiography in the evaluation of the masses that occur in fibrodysplasia ossificans progressiva. In the acute phase, CT demonstrates enlarged hypodense muscles. Other soft tissue structures may also be involved. CT with intravenous contrast medium usually shows marked nonuniform enhancement in the involved areas. CT performed during the quiescent phase clearly demonstrates the area of soft tissue ossification. Ossification may occur in muscles, tendons, ligaments, joint capsules, and fasciae. Muscle groups that are enlarged and hypodense during the acute phase usually are found to be only slightly enlarged during the quiescent phase. The CT attenuation values of involved muscles usually return to nearly normal during the quiescent phase, except in the areas of ossification.[146,148]

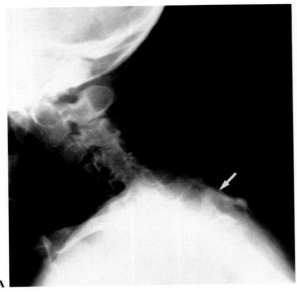

A

Fig. 3-39 Fibrodysplasia ossificans progressiva. Lateral radiographs of the **(A)** neck and **(B)** chest show areas of ossification (arrow in **A**) in the soft tissues.

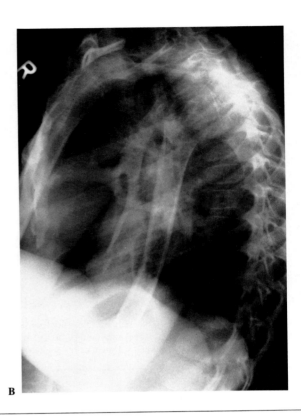

B

Benign Tumors

Cystic Hygroma

Cystic hygromas are anomalies of the lymphatic system that are characterized by single or multiple cysts in the soft tissues, most commonly in the neck. Therefore, cystic hygroma is a type of lymphangioma. The most common sites of involvement are the posterior triangle of the neck and the supraclavicular fossa.

A cystic hygroma is frequently found in association with chromosomal abnormalities (chiefly Turner syndrome). This is especially true in aborti: The reported incidence of cystic hygroma is 1 in 200 spontaneously aborted fetuses.[149] The exact cause of this lesion is unknown. Two theories have been put forward. One suggests that buds develop from lymphatic endothelium and eventually canalize to form cysts. The other suggests that the lesion results from sequestration of the primitive jugular lymphatic sac.

Most cases of cystic hygroma present clinically as an otherwise asymptomatic neck mass. Although cystic hygroma is a benign lesion, extensive infiltration into adjacent tissues is common, and symptoms are related to the effects on the involved structures. The child may exhibit severe respiratory distress, dysphagia, or vascular compression. Large cystic hygromas arising from the neck can extend into the mediastinum or dissect posteriorly into the retropharyngeal space. Cystic hygroma is the most common tumor of the retropharyngeal space in children.

In approximately 30% to 50% of patients with cystic hygroma, the soft tissue mass is identified at birth. Most of the remainder of the patients present clinically early in infancy.

Occasionally, a lesion may spontaneously regress. Usually the tumor grows in proportion to the infant's growth. A sudden increase in size of the lesion is generally the result of infection or hemorrhage.[50,132]

Sonography is well suited for imaging of cystic hygroma of the neck, and the sonographic findings are relatively specific. These lesions appear as multilocular, predominantly cystic masses containing septa of variable thickness (Fig. 3-40). Solid echogenic components of variable sizes arise from the cyst walls and septa. The cysts are most often uniformly anechoic, but internal echoes may be produced by hemorrhage. Large cystic hygromas may have ill-defined borders and may dissect between normal tissue planes. Cystic hygroma of the neck has been diagnosed with prenatal ultrasound.[136,150–152]

The CT appearance of a cystic hygroma is a multiloculated, low-attenuation mass that is usually located in the posterior triangle of the neck. The cystic components are usually approximately of water density, although slightly increased attenuation may be produced by hemorrhage. Large lesions tend to be poorly circumscribed and may infiltrate adjacent fascial planes.

MRI is well suited for imaging of cystic hygroma because of the excellent depiction of soft-tissue structures and the capability for imaging in various planes. The cystic components of the lesion produce bright signal on T_2-weighted images. The T_1 characteristics are determined by the composition of the cysts. If there is relatively clear fluid, the cysts produce low signal on T_1-weighted images; hemorrhage or infection may cause higher signal intensities.[153]

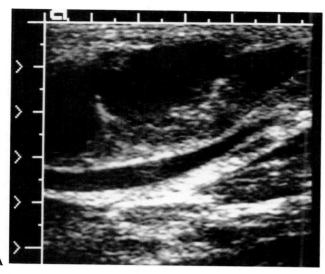

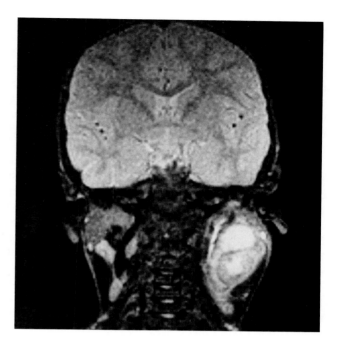

Fig. 3-40 Cystic hygroma. **(A)** Longitudinal sonogram of the anterolateral aspect of the neck shows a multiloculated, predominantly cystic mass. Layering of debris is visible in the dependent portion of the lesion. The neck vessels are draped around the posterior aspect of the mass. **(B)** Coronal T$_2$-weighted MR image shows the cystic hygroma as a septated area of high signal in the left upper neck. The fibrous septa produce low signal.

Cervical Teratoma

Cervical teratoma typically presents in the newborn as a large neck mass either anterior or lateral in location. There is a tendency for involvement of the right side of the neck. Respiratory distress in the neonatal period may result from partial airway obstruction. Also, maternal polyhydramnios may result from mechanical interference with the fetal swallowing mechanism. Polyhydramnios is more likely to occur if the teratoma is larger than 10 cm.[29,154,155]

Imaging studies in cases of cervical teratoma serve to differentiate this lesion from other childhood neck masses and also to determine the effects of the mass on adjacent structures. The diagnosis of teratoma may be suggested on standard radiographs by areas of calcification or ossification (Fig. 3-41). Cross-sectional imaging studies are usually most efficacious for establishing the correct diagnosis, however.

Sonography in cases of teratoma demonstrates a complex mass. Anechoic cystic components are frequently demonstrated. Areas of calcification or ossification result in acoustic shadowing. Similar sonographic features have been reported in utero.[156]

The typical CT appearance of a cervical teratoma is a large, heterogeneous mass. Areas of calcification are usually visible; these range from faint amorphous calcifications to areas of dense ossification. Cystic components and areas of fat attenuation are also common.

Malignant Tumors

Lymphoid tumors account for at least 50% of malignancies involving the neck and extracranial portions of the head in

children. The presenting site in Hodgkin disease is almost invariably nodal, and the cervical and supraclavicular regions are the most common locations of Hodgkin disease in pediatric patients. Conversely, the most common primary site of disease in non-Hodgkin lymphoma of the head and neck in children is extranodal structures. Initial presentation with cervical lymphadenopathy is roughly twice as common in Hodgkin disease compared to non-Hodgkin lymphoma. With both types, cervical lymphadenopathy is frequently unilateral,

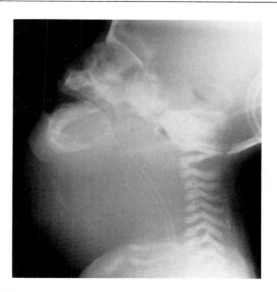

Fig. 3-41 Teratoma. Lateral radiograph of a newborn demonstrates a large anterior neck mass that contains irregular areas of calcification.

and upper cervical lymph nodes are more frequently involved than lower cervical nodes. The head and neck region accounts for approximately 5% to 10% of the primary sites of involvement in children with non-Hodgkin lymphoma. The Waldeyer ring areas and other nasopharyngeal structures represent relatively frequent primary sites of non-Hodgkin lymphoma in the head and neck. Other sites of potential involvement include the paranasal sinuses, orbit, maxilla, mandible, and, rarely, the thyroid gland.

American Burkitt lymphoma is a rare type of non-Hodgkin lymphoma that may involve head and neck structures in children. Only 20% of children with American Burkitt lymphoma present with primary head and neck disease; 12% present with an enlarged cervical lymph node, and 8% have extranodal head and neck disease. American Burkitt lymphoma is distinct from the African variety, which classically occurs as an extranodal mass involving the jaw.[157]

Rhabdomyosarcoma is the second most common pediatric neoplasm occurring in the neck and extracranial head. The most frequent sites include the orbit, nasopharynx, paranasal sinuses, oral cavity, middle ear, mastoid, and infratemporal fossa. The head and neck region is the most common site of occurrence of rhabdomyosarcoma in children. These tumors frequently attain a large size and present as a lateral neck mass. Rhabdomyosarcoma frequently is associated with bone destruction, and those lesions that are located adjacent to the skull base may extend intracranially. Metastases to regional lymph nodes are frequently present at the time of diagnosis.

Fibrosarcoma, neurofibrosarcoma, thyroid malignancies, and primary neuroblastoma each account for approximately 5% of extracranial head and neck malignancies in children. Squamous cell carcinoma accounts for approximately 4%. Other rare head and neck malignancies in children include primary bone tumors, melanoma, malignant fibrous histiocytoma (Fig. 3-42), malignant hemangiopericytoma, malignant hemangioendothelioma, parotid tumors, Schwann cell tumors, and malignant germ cell tumors.[158,159]

The cervical lymph nodes are a relatively common site for metastatic disease in head and neck malignancies. Approximately 30% of children who have rhabdomyosarcoma of the head and neck have cervical lymph node involvement. Conversely, about one of six children with malignant cervical lymphadenopathy have rhabdomyosarcoma of the nasopharynx as the primary lesion. Neuroblastoma and thyroid carcinoma are frequently metastatic to the cervical lymph nodes. It is important to remember, however, that at least 90% of children with abnormal lymph nodes in the head and neck region have a benign lesion, most often of infectious etiology.[31,160,161]

Imaging studies in Hodgkin disease usually demonstrate nonspecific lymphadenopathy. The enlarged cervical lymph nodes are frequently unilateral. In most cases, a group of nodes coalesce to form an isolated matted mass. Standard radiographs show only soft tissue fullness without calcification and are of little value. Sonography demonstrates enlargement of one or more cervical lymph nodes. The involved nodes are relatively hypoechoic.

Cervical lymph node involvement with Hodgkin disease is especially well demonstrated on CT and MRI. The involved nodes are enlarged, are usually of homogeneous attenuation, and may demonstrate slight contrast enhancement on CT (Fig. 3-43). Rarely, the nodes involved in Hodgkin disease are hypodense with respect to muscle. These nodes may show enhancing peripheral margins. This hypodensity correlates with tissue necrosis. Gallium-67 scintigraphy demonstrates abnormal increased uptake in involved nodes. Studies have indicated an overall accuracy of 96% of ^{67}Ga imaging in defining or excluding sites of active lymphoma.[162]

A significant problem with lymphoma, especially Hodgkin disease, is the tendency for masses to persist after therapy. CT

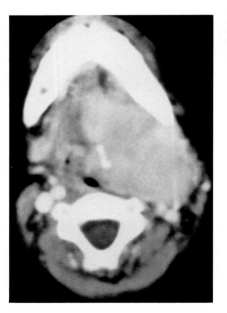

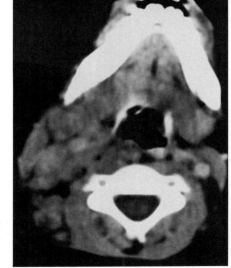

Fig. 3-42 Malignant fibrous histiocytoma. Contrast-enhanced CT of the upper neck demonstrates a homogeneous, enhancing mass in the left side of the neck.

Fig. 3-43 Lymphoma. Contrast-enhanced CT demonstrates lymphadenopathy involving the anterior and posterior cervical triangles on the right.

in these patients usually reveals a persistent mass either in the neck or mediastinum that may represent active tumor or necrotic and fibrotic tissue. Data are accumulating that indicate the disappearance of ^{67}Ga uptake in the mediastinum or neck corresponds to tumor regression, usually with fibrosis of the involved lymph nodes, whereas persistent ^{67}Ga uptake indicates active disease.[163]

In contradistinction to Hodgkin disease, non-Hodgkin lymphoma most often demonstrates a solitary mass of extranodal origin on imaging studies. Lymphadenopathy is a secondary finding. Cross-sectional imaging with CT or MRI usually provides the most satisfactory depiction of non-Hodgkin lymphoma in the head and neck region. These studies demonstrate a soft tissue mass that frequently invades adjacent structures. Bone destruction is common. The lesion usually demonstrates moderate contrast enhancement on CT and is imaged on MRI as a relatively hyperintense mass on T_2-weighted images.

Standard radiographs in cases of rhabdomyosarcoma of the head and neck structures demonstrate a noncalcified soft tissue mass. Those lesions located in the face or adjacent to the skull base frequently are associated with bone destruction, permeative bone changes, or enlargement of neural foramina. These osseous abnormalities are best evaluated with CT. The soft tissue mass demonstrates variable contrast enhancement on CT. The CT study should include evaluation of the neck for evidence of metastatic lymphadenopathy.[164]

Infection: Cervical Adenitis

Cervical adenitis in children is most often associated with a viral upper respiratory infection or a bacterial infection of the tonsils, teeth, pharynx, middle ear, or skin. Microorganisms enter the lymphatic fluid in the infected tissues and spread to regional lymph nodes. The involved nodes develop inflammatory changes that result in enlargement, tenderness, warmth, and redness. Groups of involved nodes sometimes become matted together. In severe cases there is abundant infiltration of leukocytes, and an abscess develops.

Cervical adenitis can be classified into three general categories: acute unilateral adenitis, acute bilateral adenitis, and subacute or chronic adenitis. Most cases of acute unilateral adenitis are due to *Staphylococcus aureus* or group A β-hemolytic streptococci. Infections with these organisms tend to progress rapidly; abscess formation is not uncommon.

Acute bilateral adenitis is most often due to a viral upper respiratory infection or streptococcal pharyngitis; abscess formation is uncommon. Acute bilateral adenitis, which predominantly affects nodes in the posterior triangle, is classically associated with rubella and infectious mononucleosis.

Subacute or chronic adenitis in children is most often caused by cat-scratch disease, nontuberculous (atypical) mycobacterial infection, or toxoplasmosis. About 80% of nontuberculous mycobacterial cervical adenitis occurs in children between the ages of 1 and 5 years. The adenitis is unilateral and is often localized to a single tonsillar or submandibular node. If untreated, the involved nodes eventually become

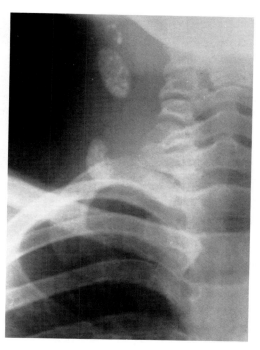

Fig. 3-44 Tuberculosis with scrofula. Enlarged calcified cervical lymph nodes are visible in this patient with tuberculosis.

fluctuant (over the course of a few months). Radiographic evidence of pulmonary involvement is rare in cases of atypical mycobacterial adenitis.

Cervical tuberculous adenitis (scrofula) most often produces clinical findings similar to those of nontuberculous mycobacterial adenitis. Compared to nontuberculous mycobacterial infections, tuberculous adenitis more commonly involves the posterior triangle or supraclavicular nodes, is occasionally bilateral (about 10% of cases), and is often associated with radiographic evidence of pulmonary disease (Fig. 3-44).[165,166]

Cervical abscesses are most often caused by suppuration of inflammatory adenopathy, as described above. Abscesses may also be related to primary infection of other neck structures, such as the thyroid gland, neck muscles, or salivary glands. Another important etiology of a neck abscess is secondary infection of a pre-existing congenital malformation, such as a dermoid cyst, thyroglossal duct cyst, or branchial cleft cyst.

Acute suppurative thyroiditis is an uncommon condition. It is usually preceded by respiratory tract infection and may progress to thyroid abscess. Anaerobic organisms, especially *Eikenella corrodens*, are the causative organisms. This would suggest that the infection arises from a patent thyroglossal duct remnant with spread of oral flora to the thyroid. The thyroid gland is exquisitely tender, swollen, and erythematous. The patient has dysphagia and limitation of head motion. Surprisingly, systemic manifestations are extremely rare.[167]

Both CT and sonography represent valuable methods for evaluating cervical infections, particularly complex or widespread infections that are difficult to assess clinically. The

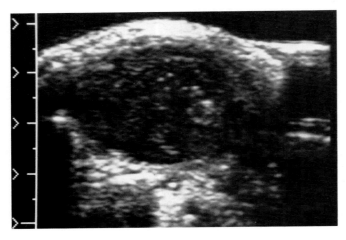

Fig. 3-45 Lymphadenopathy in cervical adenitis. Transverse sonogram shows a group of enlarged lymph nodes in the left side of the neck anterior to the neck vessels.

major role of cross-sectional imaging studies is to distinguish cellulitis or adenitis from abscess. This represents important information for directing medical or surgical management.

The sonographic appearance of uncomplicated cervical adenitis is one or more discrete, enlarged, oval lymph nodes. The nodes frequently have a homogeneous hypoechoic appearance but lack back wall acoustic enhancement (Fig. 3-45). A group of inflamed nodes may form a poorly defined inflammatory mass that usually exhibits mixed echogenicity. Sonography does not allow differentiation of inflammatory from malignant adenopathy.

An abscessed node or an abscess in an adherent group of nodes has a variable sonographic appearance. The presence of fluid is reliably shown as an anechoic lesion with prominent distal acoustic enhancement. Scattered internal echoes are frequently present in an abscess, however, as a result of debris (Fig. 3-46). In addition, nonabscessed inflammatory nodes are often relatively hypoechoic and may exhibit some degree of acoustic enhancement. Unlike uncomplicated adenopathy, an abscess usually demonstrates an irregular, thickened wall. Visualization of a fluid-debris level, when present, is definitive of a fluid-containing structure that is most likely to represent an abscess. Equivocal cases require additional imaging studies or needle aspiration.[136]

Enlarged cervical lymph nodes in adenitis are well demonstrated on CT. In most cases, one node or a group of nodes shows nonspecific enlargement. CT does not allow accurate differentiation of inflammatory from neoplastic adenopathy. The involved nodes most often retain an oval shape and produce CT attenuation values similar to those of normal lymph nodes on both unenhanced and enhanced scans. Inflammatory changes in adjacent soft tissue structures may result in ill-defined borders of the involved nodes. In some cases, a group of inflamed nodes coalesces to form an inflammatory mass that usually demonstrates heterogeneous contrast enhancement.

An abscess may form in a single inflammatory node, in an inflammatory mass of nodes, or in other neck structures such as the thyroid gland, neck muscles, or developmental cysts. The CT appearance of an abscess is a nonenhancing, low-attenuation area surrounded by an enhancing, irregular wall of variable thickness (Figs. 3-47 and 3-48). The lesion may have a single cystic or a multiloculated appearance. An air-fluid level or a fluid-debris level may be present.[168,169]

An element of cellulitis frequently accompanies cervical adenitis or cervical abscess. The CT indications of cellulitis include soft tissue swelling, obliteration of fat planes, and heterogeneous enhancement of soft tissue structures. Cellulitis may also occur as an isolated abnormality, most often being due to trauma or a skin infection.

An advantage of CT over sonography in the evaluation of cervical infections is its greater utility in demonstrating complications such as airway encroachment, osteomyelitis, vascular compression, venous thrombosis, and extension into the face, paranasal sinuses, or orbit. One or more of these complications occurs in up to 25% of children with severe neck infections. In addition, CT is best suited for the detection of mediastinal or intracranial extension of infection.

An important role of CT in cases of cervical infection is the demarcation of secondary effects on major neck vessels. Dynamic contrast enhancement is required for optimal visualization of vascular structures. Large abscesses or inflammatory masses frequently cause some degree of vascular displacement. Extrinsic compression of the jugular vein may cause narrowing or occlusion. Rarely, thrombosis of the jugular vein may result from an adjacent infection; this is imaged on CT as a nonenhancing segment of the vein or a filling defect in the vein.[137,169]

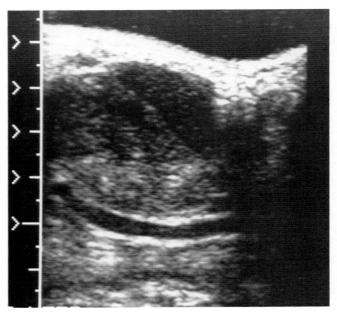

Fig. 3-46 Cervical abscess. Longitudinal sonogram shows a fluid-debris level in the dependent portion of this cervical abscess.

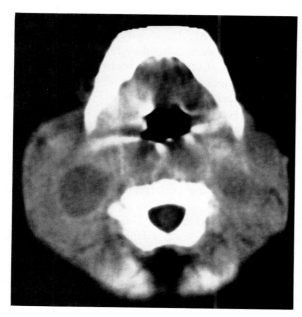

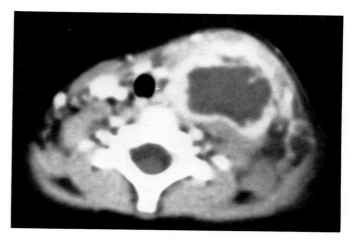

Fig. 3-48 Mature abscess. Contrast-enhanced CT shows a thick, irregular, enhancing pseudocapsule surrounding a low-attenuation fluid collection in this left cervical abscess.

Fig. 3-47 Cervical adenopathy with abscess formation. Contrast-enhanced CT shows multiple, enlarged, conglomerate lymph nodes in both sides of the neck and involvement of the retropharyngeal region. Areas of abscess formation are indicated by regions of relatively decreased attenuation and a surrounding, slightly enhancing pseudocapsule.

The presence of a large cervical abscess or inflammatory mass frequently causes displacement of the carotid artery. Mild narrowing may occur, but severe narrowing or occlusion of the carotid is rare because of the inherent strength of the arterial wall. CT demonstration of vascular involvement in cases of neck infection is important for proper surgical planning.

A rare complication of cervical infection is a secondary mycotic aneurysm. This results from destruction of a portion of the arterial wall by an adjacent infectious process. Unenhanced CT shows a low-attenuation mass that is indistinguishable from a simple cervical abscess. Dynamic contrast-enhanced CT, however, indicates the aneurysmal component of the mass as an area of intense enhancement (Fig. 3-49).

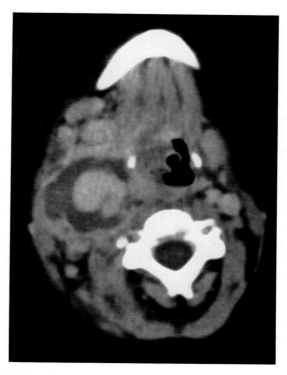

Fig. 3-49 Mycotic aneurysm. Contrast-enhanced CT shows an irregular mass in the right side of the neck with a central area of enhancement. There is a thick rind of nonenhancing material, which probably represents thrombus; external to this an enhancing pseudocapsule is visible.

THYROID

Thyroid pathology in children encompasses the same spectrum of conditions that affect adults. In addition, there are abnormalities that are unique to the pediatric age group. Diagnostic imaging serves an important role in the evaluation of most pediatric thyroid abnormalities; close correlation with clinical findings and laboratory studies, however, is required for specific diagnoses. Scintigraphic techniques that are available for evaluation of the thyroid provide both anatomic and functional information while imparting a relatively small radiation dose. Sonography, CT, and MRI provide anatomic information and allow some degree of tissue characterization. Radiographs are sometimes useful for demonstrating calcifications and the effects of large thyroid masses on the airway.

Imaging

The thyroid gland is made up of right and left lobes and an inferior connecting isthmus. The normal thyroid weighs approximately 1 g in the neonate and 20 g in the adult. The normal adult gland measures approximately $2 \times 2 \times 4$ cm. The thyroid wraps around the anterior and lateral aspects of the cervical trachea, with the upper margin of the isthmus lying just inferior to the cricoid cartilage and the lateral lobes lying adjacent to the thyroid cartilage. The sternocleidomastoid muscles and carotid sheaths are situated lateral and posterior to the lateral thyroid lobes. The four parathyroid glands lie adjacent to the posterior surfaces of the lateral lobes.

Thyroid scintigraphy can be performed with either ^{123}I or [99mTc]pertechnetate. In special circumstances, ^{131}I and ^{201}Tl are utilized. Radioactive iodine is trapped, organified, and utilized for hormone synthesis in the same manner as dietary iodine. Technetium-99m in the form of sodium pertechnetate is trapped by the thyroid in a manner analagous to iodine but is not organified. Both these radiopharmaceuticals are well suited for gamma-camera imaging. The radiation dose to the thyroid is somewhat less with ^{99m}Tc compared to [123]I.[170,171]

Iodine-123 scintigraphy is performed with tracer administered orally in capsule form. Images are obtained 2 to 4 hours after administration. The study usually includes a determination of ^{123}I thyroid uptake values. In North America, the range of normal 24-hour ^{123}I thyroid uptake values is approximately 10% to 40%, and the normal 4-hour uptake is in the range of 5% to 15% of the ingested dose.[172,173]

Functional assessment of thyroid uptake may also be performed with [99mTc]pertechnetate. Thyroid counts are obtained at 2, 10, and 15 minutes after intravenous injection of the radiopharmaceutical, and counts over the thigh are obtained at 16 minutes. Uptake ratios are calculated as follows: 10-minute thyroid count:2-minute thyroid count, and 15-minute thyroid count:16-minute thigh count. Criteria for interpretation of these uptake ratios are listed in Table 3-8.[174]

Pinhole images of the thyroid are obtained 2 to 4 hours after oral administration of ^{123}I or 10 to 30 minutes after intravenous administration of [99mTc]pertechnetate. Anterior and oblique projections are obtained routinely and may be supplemented with lateral views. If the gland is not visualized, additional images of the upper chest, upper neck, and mouth should be obtained to search for ectopic tissue. The scintigraphic appearance of the normal thyroid gland is a bilobed structure that shows homogenous tracer uptake.

On CT, the normal thyroid gland is visible as a bilobed structure of higher attenuation than adjacent muscles (as a result of the normal physiologic iodine content). After intravenous contrast agent administration, the thyroid demonstrates greater enhancement than neck muscles because of its rich blood supply. Contrast enhancement allows improved visualization of neck vessels that lie adjacent to the thyroid. On both unenhanced and enhanced CT scans, the thyroid should appear homogeneous and have sharp borders.

Excellent visualization of the thyroid is usually obtained with high-frequency ultrasound transducers. The normal gland is homogenous and moderately echogenic. The thyroid is normally more echogenic than adjacent muscles. The adjacent carotid and jugular vessels are well demonstrated sonographically.

The normal thyroid is imaged on MRI as a homogeneous structure with smooth, sharply delineated margins. The gland is bordered medially by tracheal cartilage, anterolaterally by the sternocleidomastoid and sternothyroid muscles, and posteriorly by fat and vascular structures. On T_1-weighted images, the signal intensity of the thyroid is similar to or slightly greater than that of adjacent neck muscles. On T_2-weighted images, signal intensity is much greater than that of adjacent muscles and equal to or slightly less than that of adjacent fat. The normal gland may appear slightly inhomogeneous on T_2-weighted images.

Neonatal Hypothyroidism

Neonatal hypothyroidism (congenital hypothyroidism) occurs with an incidence of approximately 1 in 4000 births.[175–179] The various etiologies of this disorder include defective thyroid development (dysgenesis), defective thyroid hormone synthesis, hypothalamic or pituitary abnormalities, intrauterine exposure to goitrogens, and maternal dietary iodine deficiency. Most affected infants do not have clinically detectable symptoms at birth; the majority of cases are discovered by routine screening of neonates for levels of blood thyroid hormone or thyroid-stimulating hormone.[175] Signs and symptoms that may be present in cases of hypothyroidism include abnormal facies, macroglossia, umbilical hernia, feeding problems, lethargy, respiratory abnormalities, dry skin, jaundice, subnormal temperature, constipation, and an enlarged posterior fontanelle.[176,180] This last finding reflects the retarded skeletal maturation that is common in congenital hypothyroidism. There is an increased incidence of neonatal hypothyroidism in infants with Down syndrome.[181]

Thyroid dysgenesis is the most common etiology of neonatal hypothyroidism (congenital hypothyroidism), accounting for approximately 80% of cases.[172] Thyroid dysgenesis consists of a developmental defect of the gland. There are three main types: aplasia (athyreosis), which accounts for approximately 25%; thyroid ectopia, which accounts for about 75%; and hypoplasia, which is rare.[171,182] There is an increased incidence of thyroid dysgenesis in girls.[183]

The next most common etiology of neonatal hypothyroidism is dyshormonogenesis, which accounts for 10% to 15% of

Table 3-8 Criteria for Interpretation of [99mTc]Pertechnetate Uptake Values in Children

Condition	10-min thyroid: 2-min thyroid		15-min thyroid: 16-min thigh
Hyperthyroid	>1.2	or	>4.7
Euthyroid	1.0–1.2		3.0–4.7
Hypothyroid	<1.0	and	<3.0

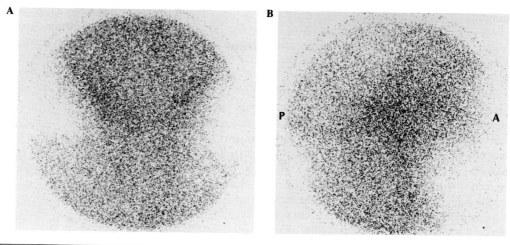

Fig. 3-50 Athyreosis. (**A**) Anterior and (**B**) lateral views of the neck after intravenous administration of [^{99m}Tc]pertechnetate show no identifiable thyroid activity. Faint salivary gland activity is visible superimposed on diffuse soft tissue activity. P, posterior; A, anterior.

cases.[174] In this condition, defective thyroid hormone synthesis results from an enzyme defect or deficiency that may occur anywhere along the pathway of biochemical steps that produce T_3 and T_4 from tyrosine in the thyroid gland. The most common abnormality is an organification defect, in which a deficient thyroid peroxidase fails to oxidize (organify) iodide to iodine. Dyshormonogenesis demonstrates an autosomal recessive pattern of inheritance.

Secondary and tertiary hypothyroidism result from deficiency of thyroid-stimulating hormone or thyroid-releasing hormone. Idiopathic pituitary aplasia or congenital midline brain defects, such as septo-optic dysplasia, are associated with this etiology of hypothyroidism. Secondary and tertiary hypothyroidism account for less than 5% of cases of neonatal hypothyroidism.

Neonatal hypothyroidism due to maternal dietary iodine deficiency was relatively common in the past but now accounts for less than 1% of cases in the United States. Hypothyroidism may also be related to exposure to excess iodine as a result of the Wolff-Chaikoff effect. This increased iodine exposure may be related to use of iodine-containing skin antiseptics, radiologic contrast agents, or iodine-containing medications. Some cases of neonatal hypothyroidism have been linked to maternal antibodies to thyroid.[184] Also, maternal usage of antithyroid medications may produce abnormal thyroid function in the newborn.

Laboratory studies provide relatively specific diagnoses in some cases of neonatal hypothyroidism. Both thyroid hormone (T_3 and T_4) and thyroid-stimulating hormone levels are decreased in secondary and tertiary hypothyroidism. The evaluation of thyroid-stimulating hormone response to exogenously administered thyroid-releasing hormone helps separate hypothalamic from pituitary etiologies. All cases of primary hypothyroidism demonstrate decreased thyroid hormone levels and increased thyroid-stimulating hormone levels. Laboratory evaluation, however, usually does not allow differentiation among the various etiologies of primary hypothyroidism. An occasional exception is athyreosis, in which absence of measurable plasma thyroglobulin may be diagnostic.[185,186]

Thyroid anatomy in cases of neonatal hypothyroidism may be characterized into four types on the basis of the scintigraphic findings: normal size and location, normal location with increased size or uptake, ectopic location, and no detectable thyroid tissue.[171,187,188]

Lack of detectable thyroid activity in the presence of elevated blood thyroid-stimulating hormone levels indicates thyroid aplasia (athyreosis). Nonvisualization of the thyroid combined with severely decreased thyroid-stimulating hormone levels indicates secondary or tertiary hypothyroidism (Fig. 3-50).

A normally located thyroid gland may be small (hypoplastic), normal, or large. Hyperstimulated, enlarged thyroid glands usually demonstrate intense uptake of tracer compared to background activity, and the margins of the lateral lobes develop a rounded appearance. The most common cause of an enlarged, normally positioned thyroid in the neonate is dyshormonogenesis (Fig. 3-51). Iodine deficiency, iodine

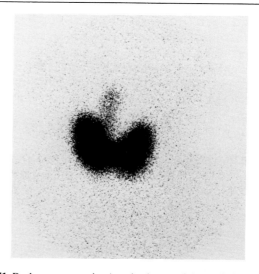

Fig. 3-51 Dyshormonogenesis. Anterior image of the neck from [^{99m}Tc]pertechnetate thyroid scintigraphy in a neonate demonstrates enlargement of the thyroid gland with rounding of the contours. There is also uptake in the pyramidal lobe.

excess, and exposure to antithyroid medication in utero may also result in an enlarged thyroid gland. In less severe presentations of these conditions, the appearance of the thyroid gland is often within normal limits.

In some cases of dyshormonogenesis, the scintigraphic findings help isolate the specific enzymatic defect. Trapping defects and a thyroid that is unresponsive to thyroid-stimulating hormone (rare) produce markedly decreased uptake or nonvisualization of the thyroid. Documentation of an organification defect can be obtained by performing the perchlorate washout test.[189] In this condition, iodide is trapped in the thyroid but is not organified. Administration of perchlorate ion, which is also trapped by the thyroid, results in displacement of unorganified iodide from the gland. This is detected scintigraphically by sequential determinations of ^{123}I thyroid uptake values before and after oral administration of potassium perchlorate. A decrease in thyroid ^{123}I content of more than 10% to 15% after perchlorate administration is considered positive.

Ectopic thyroid is usually demonstrated scintigraphically as a round or oval area of uptake in the midline of the upper neck. The ectopic gland may be located in the lingual, sublingual, or prelaryngeal areas (Fig. 3-52).[190] Mediastinal or lateral cervical locations are rare. Thyroid activity may be identified in two or more locations, most commonly being found in the lingual and sublingual regions. Demonstration of an ectopic gland mandates lifelong thyroid supplementation to prevent complications from enlargement of lingual or sublingual thyroid masses, even if laboratory studies indicate borderline or compensated hypothyroidism.[191]

Sonography may be utilized to determine the presence or absence of the thyroid gland in neonates with hypothyroidism. The normal thyroid gland should be identifiable in neonates and infants if high-frequency transducers are utilized. Failure to demonstrate the gland in a normal position should prompt a search of the neck and upper mediastinum for ectopic tissue. Lingual thyroid tissue has been identified sonographically as a solid mass of homogeneous low-level echogenicity at the base of the tongue.[192] Sonography is particularly helpful in children with equivocal scintigraphic studies.[193]

Thyroiditis

Thyroiditis is a nonspecific term that refers to inflammation or infection of the thyroid gland. The etiologies of thyroiditis are varied and include autoimmune disease, radiation injury, infectious disease, and idiopathic disorders. Imaging studies usually do not allow definitive diagnosis of most cases of thyroiditis but rather provide confirmatory or supplemental information, which must be correlated with the clinical findings.

Chronic Lymphocytic Thyroiditis

Chronic lymphocytic thyroiditis (Hashimoto thyroiditis or autoimmune thyroiditis) is the most common form of thyroid disease in children and adolescents, having an estimated incidence of between 1% and 5% of all children.[194,195] This disorder is the most common cause of hypothyroidism in children.[196]

Chronic lymphocytic thyroiditis is an autoimmune disorder, but the basic immunologic defect remains unsettled. Circulating antibodies to thyroid are present, and there is an abnormal population of suppressor T lymphocytes.[197] Interference with normal thyroid hormone biosynthesis occurs to a variable degree and may result in subclinical or overt hypothyroidism. Chronic lymphocytic thyroiditis and Graves disease are the two important forms of autoimmune thyroid disease; considerable overlap of the clinical, immunologic, and pathologic features of these two disorders has been documented.[198,199]

The histologic findings in chronic lymphocytic thyroiditis include diffuse lymphocytic infiltration, obliteration of follicles, and a variable degree of fibrosis. This disorder is more

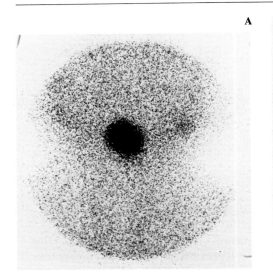
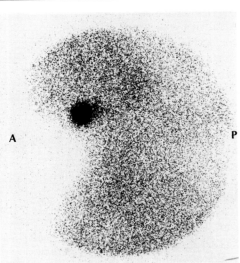

Fig. 3-52 Ectopic thyroid. (**A**) Anterior and (**B**) lateral images with [99mTc]pertechnetate thyroid scintigraphy show no identifiable thyroid uptake in the normal location of the gland. There is a single round focus of uptake at the base of the tongue, indicating lingual ectopic thyroid. A, anterior; P, posterior.

common in girls (female-to-male ratio, 4:1 to 5:1). The peak incidence occurs in adolescence; disease in children younger than 5 to 6 years of age is unusual.[195,200] A family history of thyroid disease is often present.[201] There is an increased incidence in children with congenital rubella. Chronic lymphocytic thyroiditis is sometimes associated with other endocrine and autoimmune disorders. The association of Addison disease with insulin-dependent diabetes mellitus or autoimmune thyroid disease (or both) is known as Schmidt syndrome or type II polyglandular autoimmune disease. Autoimmune thyroid disease is also associated with pernicious anemia, vitiligo, and alopecia. Chronic lymphocytic thyroiditis is associated with some chromosomal abnormalities, especially Turner and Down syndromes.

The clinical presentation of chronic lymphocytic thyroiditis is variable.[195,202] Nonspecific thyromegaly is the most common presenting complaint. This disorder accounts for one-third to two-thirds of nontoxic goiters in children. In most patients, the thyroid is diffusely enlarged, firm, and nontender. An irregular or lobulated surface is sometimes palpated. Most affected children are clinically euthyroid; signs of hypothyroidism are sometimes present. Thyroid hormone levels are most often decreased, particularly if the disorder has been present for months or years. Serum thyroid-stimulating hormone concentrations are usually slightly to moderately elevated. Transient hyperthyroidism occurs in 3% to 5% of pediatric cases of chronic lymphocytic thyroiditis. Serum levels of antibodies to thyroid and microsomes are elevated in most patients. This is not true in children as often as in adults; therefore, the presence of low titers of antibody to thyroid in children does not exclude the diagnosis of chronic lymphocytic thyroiditis.[203]

The findings on thyroid scintigraphy in children with chronic lymphocytic thyroiditis vary, depending on the severity and stage of disease. In most cases, the gland is mildly enlarged. An irregular or mottled uptake pattern is identified in about 50% of cases (Fig. 3-53). Fifteen percent to 20% of scans demonstrate normal homogeneous uptake; this is most common in early or mild cases. A discrete area of decreased uptake occurs in 15% to 20% of cases. Nodules that do not accumulate radiopharmaceutical should be regarded with the same level of suspicion as those in patients without the diagnosis of thyroiditis for three reasons: (1) A malignant thyroid nodule may occur in a gland affected by chronic lymphocytic thyroiditis (although the question of an increased incidence of malignancy with this disorder is not yet resolved); (2) thyroid malignancy is sometimes associated with elevated serum titers of antibodies to thyroid, which may lead to a mistaken clinical diagnosis of thyroiditis; and (3) lymphocytic infiltration of thyroid tissue can accompany thyroid malignancy and result in misleading histologic evidence of thyroiditis on biopsy.

Uptake values of ^{123}I and ^{99m}Tc are usually decreased in chronic lymphocytic thyroiditis, particularly in those patients with significant hypothyroidism. Uptake values are elevated in a minority of patients; this most often occurs early in the course of the disease process, when the thyroid is still capable

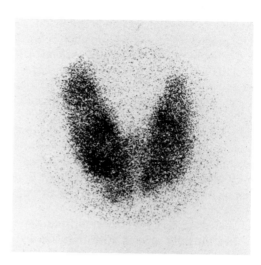

Fig. 3-53 Thyroiditis. Thyroid [99mTc]pertechnetate scintigraphy shows enlargement and heterogeneity of the thyroid gland.

of responding to stimulation by thyroid-stimulating hormone. The perchlorate washout test is positive in about half the patients with chronic lymphocytic thyroiditis, indicating that defective organification is a component of the disease process.

Sonography in cases of suspected chronic lymphocytic thyroiditis may be useful to substantiate the diffuse nature of the abnormality. Although the thyroid is usually enlarged, the echogenicity of the gland is decreased. The adjacent neck muscles can be used as an internal standard because the normal thyroid is of greater echogenicity than surrounding muscle. In many cases, the echo pattern is patchy or irregular. In general, sonography cannot differentiate chronic lymphocytic thyroiditis from other diffuse thyroid disorders.[193,204,205]

MRI in cases of chronic lymphocytic thyroiditis usually demonstrates diffuse high signal intensity on T_2-weighted images (indicated by signal greater than that of surrounding fat). Signal intensity on T_1-weighted images is variable. Linear bands of fibrosis may be visible as areas of very low signal on all pulse sequences.

Bacterial Thyroiditis

Bacterial thyroiditis (acute suppurative thyroiditis) is rare. There frequently is a pre-existing thyroid abnormality. It is usually preceded by an upper respiratory infection or otitis media. Recurrent episodes or the detection of mixed bacterial flora suggest that the infection arises from a thyroglossal duct remnant. Some pediatric cases have been related to fistulae originating from the piriform sinus.[206]

The classic clinical findings of bacterial thyroiditis are pain, swelling, hoarseness, and dysphagia. The thyroid is usually exquisitely tender. There may be marked limitation of head movement. Despite the severity of the local infection, systemic manifestations are often lacking. The most common organisms include anaerobes, staphylococci, streptococci, and *Eikenella corrodens*.[207,208]

Thyroid abscess is extremely rare in childhood. Thyroiditis infrequently progresses to abscess formation before the age of 10 years. There are usually associated systemic signs of illness (eg, chills and fever). Frequently, the firmness of the thyroid on physical examination suggests the possibility of an abscess or neoplasm. Fluctuation may be difficult to detect clinically.[206]

Thyroid scintigraphy in cases of bacterial thyroiditis demonstrates inhomogeneous uptake in the involved lobe. Scintigraphic cold areas may be produced by focal areas of infection or abscess formation. Scintigraphy is useful for differentiating thyroid infection from infectious abnormalities of other neck structures.

Barium studies are useful to detect piriform sinus fistulae. These fistulae virtually always arise from the left piriform sinus, and the associated thyroiditis involves the left lobe. The fistulous tract extends from the apex of the piriform sinus to the thyroid or perithyroid space. These fistulae are frequently associated with recurrent episodes of acute bacterial thyroiditis.[206,209]

Sonography early in the course of acute bacterial thyroiditis demonstrates irregular enlargement of one or both lobes and diffuse decreased echogenicity of the involved thyroid lobe. There are frequently scattered focal areas of increased or decreased echogenicity, and the gland has an irregular sonographic appearance. Abscess formation is indicated by a hypoechoic area, usually with irregular margins and internal debris. Fluid-debris levels may be imaged in the abscess cavity.[210]

The CT findings of bacterial thyroiditis correlate with those described for sonography. Initially, the involved portion of the gland appears inhomogeneous and decreased in attenuation compared to normal thyroid tissue on contrast-enhanced images. There may be enlargement of the affected portion of the thyroid. There is frequently poor definition of the surrounding tissue planes. Abscess formation is indicated by an area of low attenuation that does not enhance with intravenous contrast medium administration and sometimes exhibits a multilocular appearance (Fig. 3-54).[211]

Subacute Thyroiditis

Subacute thyroiditis (de Quervain thyroiditis or granulomatous thyroiditis) refers to inflammation of the thyroid gland in association with a viral infection. In many cases, there is a history of a preceding upper respiratory viral illness. There is usually some degree of pain in the region of the thyroid gland that may be accompanied by fever, hoarseness, or

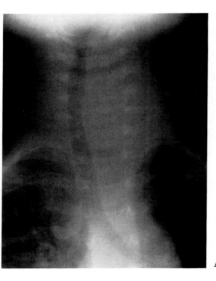

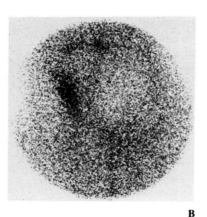

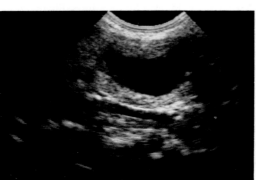

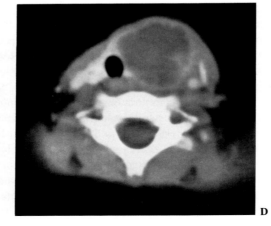

Fig. 3-54 Thyroid abscess. **(A)** Anteroposterior radiograph demonstrates a mass of soft tissue density along the left side of the neck, causing rightward deviation of the trachea. **(B)** Thyroid scintigraphy shows no appreciable uptake in the left lobe of the thyroid; the right lobe is displaced to the right. There is a photopenic region corresponding to the expected location of the left lobe of the thyroid. **(C)** Longitudinal sonogram shows a cystic mass in the region of the left lobe of the thyroid with irregular walls and projections of soft tissue in the lesion. **(D)** Contrast-enhanced CT scan shows a thin enhancing rim surrounding a nonenhancing, low-attenuation fluid collection in the left lobe of the thyroid gland. The normal intense enhancement in the right lobe is visible. The trachea is shifted toward the right.

A

B

C

D

dysphagia. This disorder is rare in young children and most often occurs in women between the ages of 15 and 50.[212]

Subacute thyroiditis typically progresses through distinct pathophysiologic phases that determine the clinical, laboratory, and imaging findings. An initial destructive phase is associated with disruption of thyroid follicles, release of preformed thyroid hormone, and elevation of blood T_3 and T_4 levels. The thyroid-stimulating hormone levels are suppressed, and radionuclide thyroid uptake determinations performed at this time are depressed. Depletion of preformed thyroid hormone stores, low levels of thyroid-stimulating hormone, and follicular cell destruction combine to result in eventual decrease in thyroid hormone levels to normal or subnormal values; this phase usually lasts for a few weeks. As T_3 and T_4 levels fall, levels of thyroid-stimulating hormone increase. As healing occurs, radionuclide uptake values may climb into the hyperthyroid range, particularly if levels of thyroid-stimulating hormone are significantly elevated. Clinical recovery and normalization of laboratory values usually occur within 3 to 6 months following the onset of symptoms. Residual thyromegaly or mild hypothyroidism persists in about 10% of patients.[213]

Scintigraphy in cases of subacute thyroiditis demonstrates patchy, inhomogeneous uptake in the involved portions of the gland. A relatively localized area of abnormality may be identified early in the course of the disease, with subsequent scans showing progression to other areas. Rarely, subacute thyroiditis may present as a painless cold nodule.[214] Frequently, one lobe is more severely involved than the other. Enlargement of the thyroid is usually relatively mild.[215]

During the initial phase of subacute thyroiditis, sonography demonstrates inhomogeneous, hypoechoic changes. These abnormalities may involve irregularly shaped focal regions, an entire lobe, or the entire gland. Sonography after clinical resolution of the disease demonstrates a return to a normal appearance in most patients, but residual diffuse thyroid hypoechogenicity or focal hypoechoic lesions are sometimes identified.[216,217]

Silent Thyroiditis

Silent thyroiditis (subacute lymphocytic thyroiditis or painless thyroiditis) probably represents an autoimmune process, although the specific etiology is unknown. Serum levels of antibodies to thyroid are almost always present. This condition is differentiated from chronic lymphocytic thyroiditis and subacute thyroiditis by differences in the clinical and laboratory findings during the course of the disorder.[215]

The laboratory findings in silent thyroiditis are similar to those in subacute thyroiditis. An initial hyperthyroid phase results from release of preformed thyroid hormone. This is followed by a temporary hypothyroid phase and eventual recovery. The absence of pain and giant cell infiltration differentiates this condition from subacute thyroiditis.

Imaging studies are most often normal in cases of silent thyroiditis. Occasionally, slight thyromegaly is demonstrated.

Also, nonspecific diffuse or focal areas of inhomogenicity may be noted.

Irradiation Thyroiditis

Irradiation thyroiditis represents an occasional complication of ^{131}I therapy. There may be some degree of local neck discomfort. If the gland is already enlarged, acute edematous changes may result in compression of adjacent structures, such as the trachea. Release of preformed thyroid hormone may produce thyrotoxicosis. The greatest risk period for this condition occurs 10 to 14 days after ^{131}I administration.[218]

Imaging studies are usually not required in patients with irradiation thyroiditis. When performed, they show diffuse enlargement of the gland. Thyroid parenchymal edema may produce diffuse inhomogeneity on scintigraphy, decreased enhancement on CT, diffuse hypoechogenicity on sonography, and increased signal on T_2-weighted MR images.

Graves Disease

Graves disease is an autoimmune disorder that is the most common cause of hyperthyroidism in children. Graves disease results from circulating immunoglobulins of the IgG class that bind to the thyroid follicular cell plasma membrane and cause stimulation of the gland in a manner similar to thyroid-stimulating hormone.[219] Normal thyroid regulatory mechanisms are overriden by the stimulatory immunoglobulins.

Clinical findings in Graves disease include diffuse thyroid gland enlargement, thyrotoxicosis, infiltrative ophthalmopathy, and, rarely, infiltrative dermopathy. Enlargement of the thymus, splenomegaly, lymphadenopathy, and peripheral lymphocytosis are also common findings in Graves disease. In most cases, diffuse enlargement of the thyroid gland is identifiable on physical examination. Symptoms include irritability, restlessness, tremor, voracious appetite, and weight loss or lack of weight gain. The earliest signs in children may be emotional disturbances, which are frequently accompanied by hyperactivity.

A rare clinical presentation of hyperthyroidism is thyroid storm. This is manifested by an abrupt onset with hyperthermia, severe tachycardia, and restlessness. There can be rapid progression to delerium, coma, and death.

Ophthalmopathy in cases of Graves disease is suggested by exophthalmos that is rarely severe. Clinical signs of thyroid ophthalmopathy include Graefe sign (lagging of the upper eyelid with downward gaze), Möbius sign (impairment of convergence), and Stellwag sign (retraction of the upper eyelid and infrequent blinking). The ophthalmopathy may parallel the clinical course of thyrotoxicosis and goiter or may run an independent course that is unaffected by antithyroid medication.

Graves disease is much more common in girls than in boys. A positive family history is present in somewhat less than half the patients. Adolescence is the most common age group;

presentation before the age of 3 years is rare. A self-limiting form of Graves disease may occur in neonates as a result of transplacental passage of thyroid-stimulating immunoglobulins from a mother with hyperthyroidism.

Both T_4 and T_3 are secreted at increased rates in Graves disease; there is often a disproportionate increase in T_3 secretion. Values of thyroid-stimulating hormone are decreased. Thyroid uptake values for ^{123}I and ^{99m}Tc are elevated. If iodide turnover is extremely rapid, the 24-hour ^{123}I uptake values may be normal while the 4- to 6-hour uptake values are markedly increased.

Thyroid scintigraphy in Graves disease demonstrates diffuse, homogeneous enlargement of the gland. Uptake may be noted in the pyramidal lobe. One value of scintigraphy in Graves disease is to exclude other causes of thyrotoxicosis, such as toxic adenoma (Plummer disease), toxic multinodular goiter, hyperfunctioning thyroid carcinoma, and acute suppurative thyroiditis. There are also unusual cases of chronic lymphocytic thyroiditis or subacute thyroiditis that are accompanied by some degree of hyperthyroidism. Scintigraphy in these various conditions demonstrates focal abnormalities or an inhomogeneous appearance of the gland, and uptake values are usually subnormal.

Sonography in Graves disease shows diffuse, relatively symmetric enlargement of the thyroid gland. The uniform echo pattern of normal thyroid tissue is usually maintained. Sonography is a simple method for accurate determination of thyroid gland size and morphology in children with Graves disease (Fig. 3-55).[193]

MRI in Graves disease also demonstrates diffuse enlargement of the thyroid gland. The borders may be somewhat lobulated. Signal intensity compared to normal thyroid gland is increased on both T_1- and T_2-weighted images. The appearance of the gland varies from homogeneous to minimally heterogeneous.[220] The degree of abnormally increased signal of the thyroid gland on MR scans appears to correlate with Graves disease activity (ie, T_4 levels), and uptake values with radionuclides show a linear correlation with MR thyroid signal intensity.

Determination of uptake values with ^{99m}Tc may be utilized as a predictor of long-term remission in children with Graves disease who are treated with antithyroid drugs such as propylthiouracil or methimazole.[221] These agents inhibit organification of iodide but do not interfere with the stimulation of the iodine-trapping mechanism that is caused by circulating thyroid-stimulating antibodies. Therefore, despite normalization of thyroid hormone levels with medical therapy for Graves disease, [^{99m}Tc]pertechnetate uptake values remain elevated because of the continued effect of thyroid-stimulating antibodies on the trapping mechanism. The [^{99m}Tc]pertechnetate uptake determination may, therefore, be utilized as an assay of thyroid immunoglobulin stimulation in vivo. Normalization of [^{99m}Tc]pertechnetate uptake ratios during medical therapy indicates an excellent prognosis for normal thyroid function after withdrawal of medication. Failure of uptake values to normalize indicates a high likelihood of early relapse of hyperthyroidism with cessation of medical therapy.

Goiter

Goiter is a nonspecific term that refers to enlargement of the thyroid gland. The enlargement may be due to an increase in the number or size of normal thyroid cells (usually resulting from hyperstimulation) or an infiltrative process (Table 3-9). The causes of goiter that have already been discussed include dyshormonogenesis, chronic lymphocytic thyroiditis, and

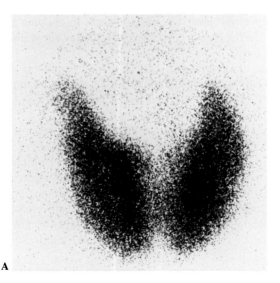
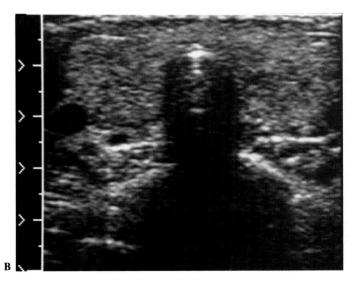

Fig. 3-55 Graves disease. (**A**) Thyroid scintigraphy shows diffuse enlargement of the thyroid gland without focal abnormalities. (**B**) Transverse sonogram shows enlargement of the thyroid with rounding of the borders of the gland. The thyroid parenchyma exhibits normal echogenicity.

Table 3-9 Differential Diagnoses of Goiter

Chronic lymphocytic thyroiditis
Graves disease
Simple goiter
Multinodular goiter
Iodine deficiency
Dyshormonogenesis
Neoplasm
Acute suppurative thyroiditis
Subacute thyroiditis
Iodine excess

Graves disease. Goiter and alterations in thyroid gland function are sometimes related to abnormal dietary iodine uptake, either deficient (endemic goiter) or excessive (iodide goiter). Goiter in neonates may be produced by dyshormonogenesis, neonatal Graves disease, maternal ingestion of antithyroid medications or iodides, or transplacental passage of thyroid-stimulating antibody with maternal Graves disease.

Simple goiter (diffuse nontoxic goiter or colloid goiter) is a condition in which excessive replication of epithelial cells and generation of new follicles occur in euthyroid patients with no evidence of inflammation or neoplasm. The pathogenesis of increased follicular replication may be related to stimulation by thyroid-stimulating hormone (as in iodine shortage), immunologic extrathyroidal growth factors, or local thyroidal tissue growth–regulating factors.[222] The gland is diffusely enlarged and exhibits a normal response to thyroid-stimulating hormone. This condition is more common in girls and has a peak incidence in adolescence. Physical examination demonstrates mild to moderate enlargement of a smooth, firm, and nontender thyroid gland.[203]

Long-standing, diffuse, nontoxic goiter frequently progresses to a multinodular form in which there is anatomic and functional heterogeneity; this is termed nontoxic multinodular goiter. Cystic areas, hemorrhage, and fibrosis may be present. The gradual transition of a simple diffuse goiter into a multinodular type occurs by several mechanisms. Scarring and accumulation of interstitial tissue form an inelastic network that isolates populations of growing follicles. Also, epithelial cell clones may replicate at different rates; those with higher than average rates may form nodules that consist of follicles that are histologically identical to those in non-nodular thyroid tissue. Formation of true adenomas is the least common cause of nodules in this type of goiter.[222] Portions of the gland frequently attain some degree of functional autonomy from control by thyroid-stimulating hormone. Autonomous hyperfunction may eventually become sufficient to result in thyrotoxicosis; this is referred to as toxic multinodular goiter.

Diagnostic imaging in cases of diffuse nontoxic goiter demonstrates nonspecific enlargement of the thyroid gland. Some degree of heterogeneity of ^{99m}Tc or ^{123}I uptake may be identified as a result of regional variability of structure and function among the follicles of the goitrous thyroid. Imaging techniques do not usually allow differentiation of this condition from other causes of diffuse thyroid enlargement. Imaging studies are more often useful in the evaluation of multinodular goiter, particularly in the differentation of this condition from a thyroid neoplasm.

Scintigraphy of multinodular goiter demonstrates a patchy distribution of tracer and thyroid enlargement. The heterogeneous appearance is due, at least in part, to marked variation in iodine metabolism in the follicles in different nodules. Areas of cyst formation or hemorrhage produce cold lesions. Areas of autonomous function may result in one or more discrete areas of increased tracer accumulation. If sufficient nodular hyperfunction occurs, the remainder of the gland will be suppressed and not visualized scintigraphically. In these unusual cases, scintigraphy after stimulation with thyroid-stimulating hormone allows visualization of the remainder of the thyroid in addition to the hot lesions.

Sonography of multinodular goiter demonstrates an inhomogeneous echo pattern in an enlarged thyroid gland. Cystic areas are well demonstrated sonographically. In most cases, many more nodules are identified sonographically than are clinically palpable; high-frequency sonography may detect nodules as small as 2 to 3 mm.

Multinodular goiter produces an inhomogeneous appearance on both CT and MRI. Areas of adenomatous hyperplasia typically are hypointense or isointense to normal thyroid on T_1-weighted images and hyperintense on T_2-weighted images. There is usually marked heterogeneity on T_2-weighted images. Areas of hemorrhage or cyst formation produce high signal on both T_1- and T_2-weighted MR scans.[223] These are identified on CT as nonenhancing areas of decreased attenuation.

The major importance of identifying multinodular goiter with imaging techniques relates to the lower incidence of malignancy in these patients (1% to 6%) compared to the higher incidence of malignancy in patients with a solitary cold nodule (15% to 25%).[224] CT and MRI also provide excellent depiction of the effects of the enlarged gland on adjacent structures and can detect substernal extension of the enlarged thyroid.[225]

Thyroid Neoplasms

Solitary nodules of the thyroid gland are rare in the pediatric age group; solitary nodules are detected in about 1% of asymptomatic children. Most solitary thyroid nodules in children are produced by benign lesions, with follicular adenoma being by far the most frequent diagnosis. Other benign adenomas that may occur in the thyroid include embryonal, fetal, microfollicular, macrofollicular, papillary, and Hürthle cell types. Mixed histology may be present. Non-neoplastic abnormalities that may produce a solitary palpable thyroid nodule include thyroglossal duct cyst, colloid cyst, and chronic lymphocytic thyroiditis.

Thyroid malignancies account for about 5% of head and neck malignancies in children[226]; these lesions are twice as common in girls.[227] Between 20% and 40% of solitary thyroid nodules in the pediatric age group are malignant.[190,228] These malignancies may arise from follicular epithelium or from parafollicular cells. Carcinomas of follicular origin are classified histologically as papillary, follicular, and anaplastic. The papillary type (about 80%) represents the most common thyroid malignancy in pediatrics.[229] Anaplastic carcinomas of the thyroid are extremely rare in children. Carcinoma arising from parafollicular cells is termed medullary carcinoma; this type accounts for less than 5% of thyroid malignancies in pediatrics.[227–231]

By far the most common clinical presentation of pediatric thyroid neoplasms, whether benign or malignant, is a palpable painless nodule. Pain and sudden enlargement may sometimes result from spontaneous hemorrhage into a nodule; most thyroid cysts are probably produced by this mechanism. Palpation of benign lesions usually demonstrates a soft, compressible, well-circumscribed nodule. Tenderness to palpation suggests an inflammatory component or recent hemorrhage.

Thyroid adenomas are capable of some degree of function and usually remain responsive to thyroid-stimulating hormone. Occasionally, one or more adenomas may lose their responsiveness to thyroid-stimulating hormone control and produce excessive thyroid hormone. This abnormality is termed toxic adenoma (toxic uninodular goiter or Plummer disease). Toxic adenoma is rare in pediatrics.

The differential diagnosis of a hyperfunctioning thyroid nodule in the pediatric age group includes adenoma, adenomatous goiter, thyroid hyperplasia, colloid goiter, and papillary adenocarcinoma (rare). These conditions are differentiated by clinical findings, thyroid function tests, thyroid scintigraphy, suppressibility with exogenous thyroid hormone administration, and, in some cases, histologic examination. There is a marked female predominance in cases of hyperfunctioning thyroid nodules. The initial presenting complaint is usually a mass or fullness in the neck. Many of these patients are clinically euthyroid. Signs and symptoms of hyperthyroidism, when present, are typically mild (ie, tachycardia and wide pulse pressure). In contrast to Graves disease, eye signs, neuromuscular abnormalities, and gastrointestinal symptoms are usually absent. Mild to moderate elevation of thyroid hormone levels is usually present. In many cases, 24-hour iodine uptake values are not suppressible by administration of exogenous thyroid hormone; also, the response of thyroid-stimulating hormone to stimulation with thyroid-releasing hormone is often blunted.[232–234]

Thyroid malignancies also most often present as a solitary, painless nodule; cervical lymphadenopathy is the initial presenting complaint in a significant number of cases, however. There are several factors ascertainable from history and physical examination that increase the chances that a palpable thyroid nodule is malignant. These include a history of prior significant radiation exposure, large size of the nodule, a nodule of hard consistency, rapid increase in size, fixation to surrounding structures, cervical lymphadenopathy, and vocal cord paralysis.[235] Radiation is known to be an important inducer of thyroid cancer. The interval between the irradiation and the discovery of the thyroid tumor can be long, in some cases as long as 40 years.

Serum calcitonin levels are frequently elevated in cases of medullary thyroid carcinoma.[227] Medullary carcinoma is often associated with other endocrine abnormalities, such as multiple endocrine adenomatosis or multiple endocrine neoplasia types 2a and 2b (MEN-2a and MEN-2b).[236] In multiple endocrine neoplasia type 2a (Sipple syndrome) there is an association of medullary carcinoma of the thyroid with pheochromocytoma and hyperplasia of the parathyroid glands. Multiple endocrine neoplasia type 2b (mucosal neuroma syndrome) is a syndrome of multiple neuromas with medullary carcinoma of the thyroid and pheochromocytoma. The neuromas most often occur on the tongue, buccal mucosa, lips, and conjunctivae.[237,238]

Scintigraphy plays an important role in the evaluation of the solitary palpable thyroid nodule.[239] Nodules are classified scintigraphically according to the degree of radionuclide accumulation as cold, warm, or hot. Cold lesions produce a photopenic area on scintigraphy, warm nodules demonstrate uptake that is approximately equal to or slightly greater than that in the remainder of the gland, and hot lesions demonstrate definitely increased tracer accumulation, sometimes with suppression of other thyroid activity.

Demonstration of a hot nodule scintigraphically almost always indicates a benign functional adenoma.[231] There are, however, rare well-differentiated thyroid carcinomas that present as a hot nodule.[240] Also, in some thyroid neoplasms, the trapping mechanism is maintained despite failure of organification. These lesions may be visualized as hot nodules on [^{99m}Tc]pertechnetate scintigraphy and as cold nodules on ^{123}I scintigraphy; this represents the so-called discordant nodule.[227] Therefore, a follow-up examination with ^{123}I scintigraphy should be performed in cases in which a solitary thyroid nodule demonstrates increased uptake of [^{99m}Tc]pertechnetate (Fig. 3-56).

Many warm or hot thyroid nodules actually represent pseudonodules in a diseased gland. In this situation, the areas of apparent increased uptake represent accumulation in relatively normal thyroid tissue surrounded by areas of diseased thyroid tissue. This finding has been identified in 3% to 4% of patients with chronic lymphocytic thyroiditis. Also, lymphoid follicles and follicular cysts result in cold nodules in 10% to 15% of patients with chronic lymphocytic thyroiditis.[241]

Hot (hyperfunctioning) thyroid nodules may be classified as autonomous or thyroid-stimulating hormone dependent. The presence of an autonomous nodule is suggested scintigraphically by suppression (poor uptake) of the extranodular thyroid tissue. The autonomous nature of a thyroid nodule may be documented by thyroid scintigraphy and uptake determinations after exogenous administration of thyroid hormone. Uptake in normal thyroid tissue will be suppressed, whereas the autonomous nodule will remain hot. Usually, the uptake values are unaltered or are only mildly suppressed.[232,233]

An autonomously functioning adenoma (toxic adenoma) is imaged scintigraphically as a warm or hot nodule. In some

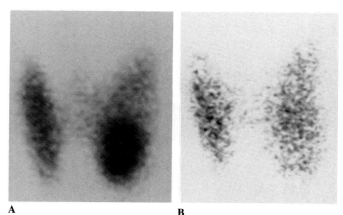

Fig. 3-56 Discordant nodule. **(A)** [⁹⁹ᵐTc]Pertechnetate scintigraphy shows a hot nodule in the inferior aspect of the left lobe of the thyroid. **(B)** Iodine-123 scintigraphy shows failure of accumulation of iodine in the lesion in the left lobe of the thyroid; therefore, a malignant lesion cannot be ruled out. Biopsy demonstrated a benign adenoma.

cases, it may cause sufficient suppression of the remainder of the gland to result in lack of visible tracer uptake other than in the nodule itself.[232] In this instance, repeat scintigraphy after stimulation with exogenous thyroid-stimulating hormone usually allows visualization of the remainder of the gland. This is important before surgery to rule out the presence of hemiagenesis (unilateral absence of the thyroid).[242] Hemiagenesis may also be studied with sonography because the normal thyroid tissue is easily identifiable as a well-defined organ with uniform echotexture that is more echogenic than surrounding muscle. In hemiagenesis, no such tissue can be identified on the side of scintigraphic nonvisualization.[243]

Cold nodules must be considered malignant until proven otherwise. Most cold nodules are benign, however. Most surgical series indicate that only 20% to 30% of cold nodules are malignant.[230] The differential diagnosis of a solitary cold thyroid nodule in the pediatric age group (in approximate decreasing order of incidence) includes follicular adenoma, thyroid carcinoma, chronic lymphocytic thyroiditis, thyroglossal duct cyst, colloid cyst, and abscess. Demonstration of tracer uptake in cervical lymph nodes is a reliable scintigraphic indicator of thyroid carcinoma. This may precede clinical detection of lymphadenopathy.[244] Warm nodules are usually approached clinically with the same level of suspicion as cold nodules.[231,245]

Sonography also plays an important role in the evaluation of thyroid nodules. Sonography allows accurate localization of a palpable nodule and provides some degree of tissue characterization. Also, it is not uncommon for sonography to demonstrate the presence of multiple nodules where only a single nodule is clinically palpable, thus indicating a lesser likelihood of malignancy.

Sonographic demonstration of a cystic thyroid lesion almost always indicates a benign process. Most thyroid cysts result from colloid or hemorrhagic necrosis in multinodular goiters or benign adenomas. The cyst walls are typically irregular, but the cyst is free of material in the cavity. Projections of solid tissue from the walls are sometimes identified sonographically. The presence of malignancy in a thyroid cyst is rare. True primary thyroid cysts are rare and typically demonstrate purely anechoic contents and smooth walls. The presence of a nonlayering projection from the wall of a cystic thyroid nodule indicates that malignancy cannot absolutely be excluded, and in most such cases percutaneous needle aspiration biopsy is performed.[193]

Solid thyroid nodules that are hyperechoic with respect to normal thyroid most commonly represent benign adenomas, although thyroid carcinoma may rarely be hyperechoic. Adenomas usually are relatively well defined. A hypoechoic halo surrounding the nodule may also be identified and is generally considered a sign of benignity, particularly if the halo is not irregular or incomplete. The incidence of malignancy in thyroid nodules with a mixed echoic pattern is relatively low, with the most likely diagnosis being nodular goiter or benign adenoma.

Most malignant thyroid nodules are hypoechoic compared to normal thyroid tissue, although adenomas may also have this appearance. Approximately one-quarter of thyroid nodules that demonstrate an isoechoic consistency in comparison to surrounding thyroid tissue are malignant. This pattern appears to be particularly common in follicular adenomas and follicular thyroid carcinoma. Malignant thyroid nodules usually have irregular or infiltrative margins. Extension of the mass beyond the thyroid may be present. The sonographic evaluation of any thyroid nodule in a child should include a search for cervical lymphadenopathy.[246]

As with sonography, CT provides excellent spatial resolution for evaluation of the thyroid. The high iodine content of the thyroid gland provides inherent contrast for separation from adjacent structures. CT is particularly useful in the evaluation of large thyroid masses or goiters for depiction of retrotracheal or superior mediastinal extension. CT is the most sensitive imaging modality for the detection of calcification in a thyroid mass.

Most thyroid nodules are imaged on unenhanced CT as low-attenuation lesions, sometimes with a surrounding rim. There are no reliable CT criteria to differentiate benign from malignant thyroid masses unless there is evidence of invasion of adjacent structures or lymphadenopathy. Simple cysts demonstrate attenuation values approximately equal to those of water. Because most cystic thyroid masses represent degenerated adenomas, the attenuation value of the cyst contents is usually somewhat higher than that of water. With intravenous contrast agent administration, the contents of a cyst do not enhance, although the surrounding rim often enhances (Fig. 3-57). Metastatic thyroid disease likewise can be detected with ¹³¹I scintigraphy after ablative thyroid surgery (Fig. 3-58).

MRI provides information similar to that from CT in the evaluation of thyroid nodules. Both techniques are most useful for defining the extent of large tumors and for demonstrating infiltration and displacement of adjacent structures. Advan-

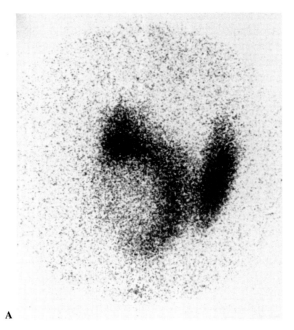

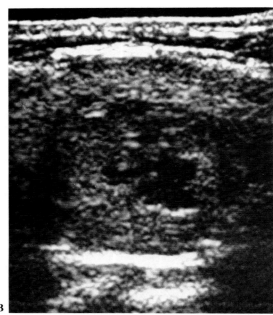

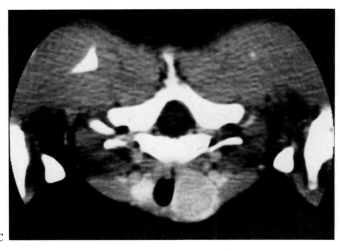

Fig. 3-57 Thyroid adenoma. (**A**) Thyroid scintigraphy shows a cold lesion in the right lobe of the thyroid with displacement of normal tissue. (**B**) Longitudinal sonogram shows a right thyroid mass that is of slightly decreased echogenicity compared to the normal thyroid tissue visible anterior to the lesion. The central portion of the mass contains an irregular cavity due to hemorrhage. (**C**) Contrast-enhanced CT shows a mass in the right lobe of the thyroid with rounded contours and displacement of normal structures. The mass enhances slightly less than the normal thyroid tissue visible on the left.

tages of MRI include its ability to image in the direct sagittal and coronal planes and the excellent inherent contrast between tumor and adjacent muscles and vascular structures.[247,248]

Both thyroid adenomas and carcinomas are imaged on MRI as approximately isointense lesions on T_1-weighted images and as markedly hyperintense lesions on T_2-weighted images. Carcinomas tend to be somewhat heterogeneous on T_2-weighted images, and invasion of adjacent structures may be effectively imaged with MRI. Lymphadenopathy is also well demonstrated, but MRI does not differentiate benign from malignant adenopathy. Lymph nodes produce lower signal than surrounding fat on T_1-weighted images and greater signal than fat on T_2-weighted images. In general, nodes greater than 1.5 cm in diameter should be considered abnormal.[248]

The MR appearance of cystic thyroid nodules is variable. High signal intensity on both T_1- and T_2-weighted images suggests hemorrhage into a cyst or adenoma. Colloid degeneration in an adenoma may also produce this appearance as a result of the short T_1 of proteinaceous fluids. Simple cysts are hypointense on T_1-weighted images and hyperintense on T_2-weighted images.

PARATHYROID

Parathyroid imaging is most often performed for the localization of a parathyroid adenoma in cases of hyperparathyroidism. Primary hyperparathyroidism is rare in children; only 1% to 2% of these patients are younger than 20 years at diagnosis. This condition results from excessive secretion of parathyroid hormone by hyperplastic glands or by one or more autonomous parathyroid adenomas. Approximately 80% of adult cases are due to a single autonomous parathyroid adenoma, and 15% result from idiopathic parathyroid chief cell hyperplasia. Hyperplasia may be proportionately more frequent than adenoma in children. Although most cases of primary hyperparathyroidism occur as an isolated endocrinopathy, this condition is sometimes associated with multiple endocrine neoplasia types 1 and 2.

Primary hyperparathyroidism in the adult age group is most frequently detected as asymptomatic hypercalcemia that is

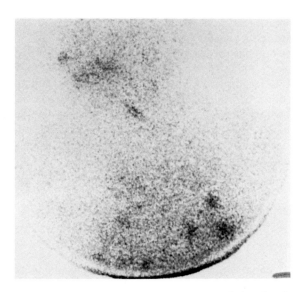

Fig. 3-58 Metastatic thyroid carcinoma. Iodine-131 scintigraphy after thyroidectomy for carcinoma shows multiple foci of tracer uptake due to metastatic disease in the lungs and neck. A chest radiograph was normal.

---

incidentally discovered on routine blood chemistry screening. In the pediatric population, routine blood screening is not usually performed, and most cases are not detected in the asymptomatic phase. The most common (about 37%) initial presentation of primary hyperparathyroidism in children is nephrolithiasis (approximately 6% of children with nephrolithiasis have primary hyperparathyroidism). Other presenting signs and symptoms include gastrointestinal complaints (anorexia, nausea, vomiting, and constipation), bone or joint pain, weakness, pathologic fracture, and hypertension. Pediatric cases that are detected with asymptomatic hypercalcemia usually have a family history of primary hyperparathyroidism that has prompted laboratory investigation.[249,250]

The parathyroid glands originate from the third and fourth pharyngeal pouches. Tissue arising from the third pharyngeal pouch migrates caudally in association with the thymus and gives rise to the inferior parathyroid glands. The fourth pharyngeal pouch gives rise to the superior parathyroid glands. There is considerable normal variation in the location of the parathyroid glands, particularly the inferior glands. The most common ectopic location is adjacent to the superior pole of the thymus. There is less variation in position of the superior parathyroid glands, with 99% being located posterior to the upper pole of the thyroid gland or adjacent to the cricoid cartilage.

The main functions of parathyroid imaging are to locate parathyroid adenomas and to detect ectopic glands for presurgical planning. Dual-isotope subtraction scintigraphy provides a relatively sensitive method for parathyroid imaging. This technique utilizes images obtained with a radiopharmaceutical that is taken up by both thyroid and parathyroid tissue (^{201}Tl) and additional images produced with a radiopharmaceutical that is taken up only by thyroid tissue ([^{99m}Tc]-pertechnetate or ^{123}I). Digital subtraction of the two images by computer results in removal of thyroid tissue from the resulting image and allows visualization of parathyroid tissue.[224,251]

Absolute immobilization of the neck is essential during the examination to allow for precise image subtraction. Sensitivities of approximately 85% to 95% for the detection of parathyroid adenomas have been reported with this technique. (Fig. 3-59).[251,252] False-positive results may be produced by ^{201}Tl accumulation in thyroid lesions such as adenomas or carcinomas. In general, at least 300 mg or 1 mL of parathyroid tissue is required for reliable visualization on dual-isotope subtraction scintigraphy. The normal adult parathyroid gland weighs approximately 40 mg and measures 5 × 3 × 1 mm, so that normal-size parathyroid glands are not reliably visualized on scintigraphy.

A parathyroid adenoma is usually imaged as an area of excess ^{201}Tl uptake adjacent to the thyroid gland. Multiple sites of activity suggest the presence of parathyroid hyperplasia or multiple adenomas. An ectopic parathyroid gland presents as a focal accumulation of ^{201}Tl that is remote from the thyroid gland.

Sonography with high-resolution equipment is sometimes useful for visualization of parathyroid adenomas or enlarged hyperplastic glands.[253,254] Sonography is most sensitive for the detection of normally positioned parathyroid glands but has poor sensitivity for detecting ectopic lesions. Sonography probably provides increased sensitivity compared to scintigraphy for visualization of normally located hyperplastic parathyroid glands.[255]

A hyperplastic or adenomatous parathyroid gland is most often imaged sonographically as an oval, homogeneous mass

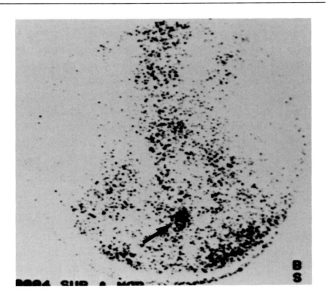

Fig. 3-59 Parathyroid adenoma. [^{99m}Tc]Pertechnetate-[^{201}Tl]thallium subtracted image shows a focus of abnormal tracer accumulation (arrow) at the base of the neck in this child with hypercalcemia.

with moderate or low echogenicity. Most often, the gland is visualized anterior to the longus colli muscle, posterior to the thyroid gland, and medial to the carotid artery. Normal parathyroid glands should measure approximately 5 mm in diameter in adults and are proportionately smaller in children.

Hyperplastic parathyroid glands and adenomas may also be imaged with CT. Parathyroid adenomas are sometimes best demonstrated on unenhanced scans, where they appear as lesions of lower attenuation than thyroid tissue. The degree of enhancement with intravenous contrast material is variable; in some cases enhancement produces attenuation similar to that of the surrounding thyroid gland and may obscure the lesion. The most common locations for an ectopic parathyroid gland are along the tracheoesophageal groove and adjacent to the thymus. CT is particularly useful for visualization of parathyroid adenomas that occur in the mediastinum.[252,256]

The parathyroid glands usually lie in the retrothyroidal fat between the thyroid gland and the longus colli muscle; this fat plane serves as an important anatomic landmark for MRI of the parathyroid glands. Normal parathyroid glands are usually not visualized on MRI. Enlarged parathyroids are usually most satisfactorily identified on T_1-weighted images, which allow good contrast with surrounding fat. Hyperplastic parathyroid glands and adenomas are usually approximately isointense to thyroid tissue and neck muscles on T_1-weighted images. Most parathyroid adenomas demonstrate high signal on T_2-weighted images, but the surrounding fat may obscure parathyroid tissue. Hemorrhage in an adenoma results in high signal intensity on both T_1- and T_2-weighted images. Adenomas produce low signal intensity on both T_1- and T_2-weighted images.[257,258]

EYE AND ORBIT

The eye and orbit in childhood may be involved in a wide variety of pathologic processes. Infection, usually due to an adjacent sinusitis, is the most common clinical orbital abnormality in pediatrics. Various orbital neoplasms occur in children, including dermoid cyst, hemangioma, lymphangioma, rhabdomyosarcoma, optic nerve glioma, neurofibroma, and metastatic disease most often from neuroblastoma. Various developmental abnormalities of the optic nerve, globe, and surrounding osseous structures are encountered. Orbital trauma and orbital pathology related to systemic diseases exhibit clinical and radiologic patterns similar to those in adults.

The most important imaging modalities for the evaluation of the pediatric orbit are CT and MRI. The orbital fat provides excellent inherent contrast for depiction of the orbital soft tissue structures with CT. Also, the cross-sectional imaging provided by CT is well suited for demonstrating the complex anatomy of orbital structures. This advantage is shared by MRI, which has the additional capability of direct sagittal imaging. MRI is particularly well suited for imaging of the intracanalicular and intracranial portions of the optic nerves

and optic tracts, areas where artifact from dense bone obscures the soft tissues on CT.

Radiographs are of limited usefulness with most orbital pathology, although plain films provide important information in orbital trauma and osseous dysplasias. Bone scintigraphy is sometimes helpful for detection of orbital osseous involvement with infection, metastatic disease, or bone infarction in sickle cell disease. Angiography or radionuclide flow studies are occasionally utilized for the evaluation of suspected orbital vascular abnormalities or vascular neoplasms.

Developmental Abnormalities

Coloboma

Congenital ocular coloboma is a developmental abnormality that results from defective closure of the embryonic choroidal fissure during gestation week 5 or 6. This defective closure results in defects that can involve any ocular structure from the optic nerve to the iris. If only the most proximal portion of the fissure fails to close, an isolated optic nerve coloboma is produced. Failure of closure of other segments of the choroidal fissure produces iridic, lenticular, ciliary body, or retinochoroidal colobomas. Colobomas typically occur in the inferomedial quadrant of the globe, corresponding to the line of closure of the fetal choroidal fissure.[259,260]

In retinochoroidal coloboma, there are thinning and outward bulging of the sclera. Colobomas range in size from small defects to large lesions involving the entire length of the choroidal fissure. In some cases, there are extreme ectasia of the sclera and expansion into the orbit, resulting in formation of an intraorbital cyst that communicates with the vitreous of a small globe; this is termed microphthalmos with cyst.[261] Developmental abnormalities in the contralateral eye are common in children with microphthalmos with cyst. Another specific type of coloboma is the morning glory syndrome; this consists of a coloboma of the optic nerve head associated with retinovascular and pigmentary changes and peripapillary gliosis.[262] The optic disc is enlarged, excavated, and funnel shaped and has an elevated rim, thereby resembling the flower for which it is named. Most cases of morning glory anomaly are unilateral.

Ocular coloboma may affect one or both eyes. Most cases arise sporadically, although rare familial cases have been reported. Ocular coloboma occurs with increased frequency in children with midline craniocerebral defects (eg, cleft palate, sphenoethmoidal cephalocele, and agenesis of the corpus callosum). Colobomas have also been associated with a wide variety of syndromes and chromosomal disorders. Visual acuity in affected individuals ranges from nearly normal to total blindness.[259,263]

Simple retinochoroidal coloboma is imaged on CT or MRI as a bulge of the sclera along the inferomedial aspect of the globe. There are thinning and eversion of the sclera at the margins of the defect.[259] In microphthalmos with cyst the globe is

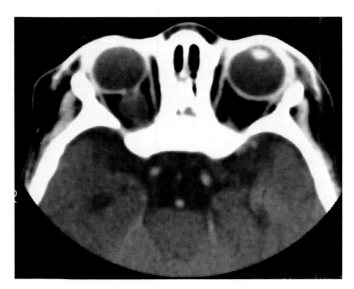

Fig. 3-60 Coloboma. Axial CT shows a cystic intraconal right orbital mass associated with a defect in the posterior aspect of the sclera. The globe is somewhat small.

small, and a large cystic intraorbital mass lies adjacent to the globe.[261] The cystic mass is lined by a capsule that represents the thinned sclera. The cyst contents are homogeneous and produce CT attenuation values and MR signal approximately equal to those of normal vitreous. Contrast enhancement does not occur (Fig. 3-60). With continuous thin sections, communication of the cyst with the vitreous cavity of the globe should be demonstrable at some level. This continuity with the globe, along with the presence of microphthalmos and imaging characteristics of cyst contents similar to those of vitreous, serves to differentiate this condition from other cystic orbital masses such as cephalocele, dermoid cyst, and arachnoid cyst.

In morning glory anomaly, CT and MRI demonstrate a funnel-shaped coloboma in the region of the optic nerve head.[263] The retrobulbar portions of the optic nerves are generally normal. Retinal detachment and subretinal exudate occur in approximately 38% of cases.[262] Subretinal exudate of sufficient size may be visualized on CT or MRI as thickening of the subretinal space.

Coats Disease

Coats disease is a primary vascular abnormality of the retina in which telangiectatic vessels leak serum and lipid that accumulate in the subretinal space. The resulting retinal detachment may produce clinical findings that are similar or identical to those of retinoblastoma.[264,265] Coats disease is generally unilateral; 10% to 15% of cases are bilateral. It affects predominantly boys. Although the anomaly is present at birth, clinical presentation typically does not occur until 6 to 8 years of age. The most frequent presenting clinical signs are blurring of vision, leukocoria, and strabismus.[266,267]

CT in Coats disease demonstrates a variable degree of obliteration of the vitreous cavity by subretinal exudate that is

of increased attenuation compared to vitreous.[264,266] Although the retina itself is too thin to be imaged, interposition of the retina between the vitreous and the exudate often produces a distinct boundary. The subretinal exudate is homogeneous and does not show contrast enhancement. The globe is of normal size, and calcification does not occur. The lack of calcification and lack of contrast enhancement aid in differentiating Coats disease from retinoblastoma. Differentiation from unilateral noncalcifying retinoblastoma is not absolute with CT, however.

MRI may provide additional information that is helpful in the diagnosis of Coats disease. The subretinal exudate has been reported to produce increased signal on both T_1- and T_2-weighted MR images. This appearance may be related to the presence of lipid in the effusion.[268,269]

Persistent Hyperplastic Primary Vitreous

Persistent hyperplastic primary vitreous (PHPV) is a developmental ocular abnormality in which portions of the embryonic hyaloid vascular system (primary vitreous) fail to regress normally.[270] There is also associated hyperplasia of embryonic connective tissue in the globe. The dysplastic vessels are friable, and intravitreal hemorrhage may occur.[265] Persistent hyperplastic primary vitreous is usually (90%) unilateral and is manifested clinically by leukocoria in a microphthalmic eye. The natural course of untreated persistent hyperplastic primary vitreous includes development of glaucoma and eventual buphthalmos or phthisis.[271]

CT in persistent hyperplastic primary vitreous demonstrates increased attenuation of all or portions of the vitreous cavity of the affected globe (Fig. 3-61). The globe is usually microphthalmic. The vascular nature of the abnormality usually results in significant enhancement with intravenous contrast agents.

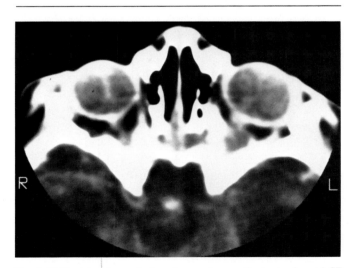

Fig. 3-61 Persistent hyperplastic primary vitreous. Contrast-enhanced CT shows an enhancing linear structure extending through the midportion of the vitreous cavity of the right globe. A similar structure is faintly visible on the left as well. The ocular abnormalities in this child occurred in association with type 2 lissencephaly.

In some cases, a tubular density extending between the optic nerve head and the lens is visualized on CT. This structure corresponds to persistent fetal fibrovascular tissue along the hyaloid artery. Hemorrhage may produce a fluid-fluid level in the subhyaloid or subretinal spaces. Calcification does not occur.[268,272]

The embryonic hyaloid connective tissue in the vitreous can be detected with sonography. It presents as a triangular structure with the apex at the optic disc and the base at the posterior surface of the lens. Flow in the hyaloid vessels can be detected with color-flow Doppler imaging.[270]

MRI in cases of persistent hyperplastic primary vitreous has been reported to demonstrate abnormally increased signal in the vitreous of the affected globe on both T_1- and T_2-weighted images. This is due to the proteinaceous nature of the vascular primary vitreous. Layering of fluid may also be identified, as with CT.[271]

Calvarial Abnormalities

There are several dysostoses of the skull that may produce orbital abnormalities. Dysostoses with significant orbital manifestations include craniosynostosis, the acrocephalosyndactyly syndromes, craniofacial dysplasia, and mandibulofacial dysplasia. Coronal craniosynostosis produces a shallow orbit with an oval configuration (harlequin eye). Bilateral coronal craniosynostosis may produce hypertelorism. Metopic craniosynostosis produces hypotelorism and an oval configuration of the orbital margins in which the orbits are angled upward and medially. This produces a unique appearance on anteroposterior skull radiographs referred to as quizzical eyes. Total craniosynostosis (cloverleaf skull) produces shallow, deformed orbits (Fig. 3-62).

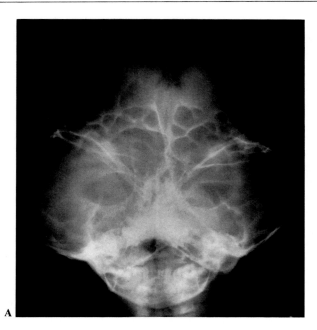

A

Fig. 3-62 Craniosynostosis. (**A**) Anteroposterior radiograph of the skull demonstrates severe cloverleaf skull deformity. (**B**) Computer-generated three-dimensional CT reformation shows the calvarial abnormality. The orbits are shallow, and there is bulging of the anterior and middle cranial fossae into the orbital cavities. (**C**) Sagittal CT reconstruction shows the osseous encroachment into the orbit, which causes marked proptosis.

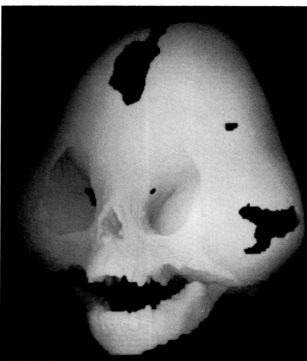

B

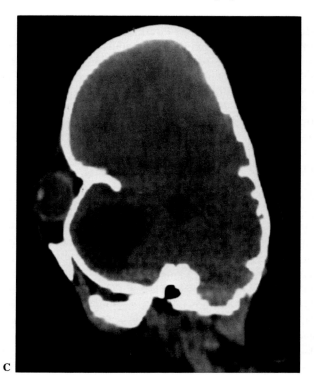

C

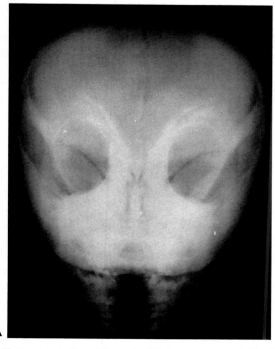
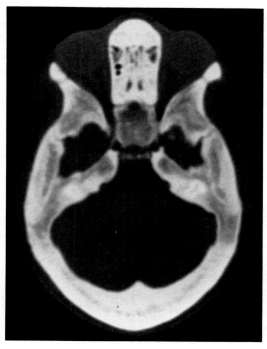

A   B

Fig. 3-63 Craniometaphyseal dysplasia. **(A)** Anteroposterior skull radiograph shows marked calvarial thickening and narrowing of the orbital fissures. **(B)** Axial CT demonstrates the severity of calvarial thickening. The bony overgrowth causes encroachment on the orbits, resulting in proptosis, and narrowing of the optic canals.

Conditions that produce thickening of the base of the skull or facial bones may cause orbital pathology. Most important, thickening of the lesser wing of the sphenoid bone may narrow the optic canal and cause impingement on the optic nerve. Osseous thickening may result in impingement on other nerves and vascular structures as well. With marked osseous thickening the orbits become shallow, and exophthalmos occurs. Conditions that may result in thickening of the bony walls of the orbits include osteopetrosis congenita, idiopathic hypercalcemia, craniometaphyseal dysplasia (Fig. 3-63), and fibrous dysplasia.

Standard radiographs play an important role in the evaluation and classification of the various developmental osseous abnormalities that affect the orbit. Special radiographic positions are required for visualization of the optic canals. Superior imaging of the optic canal is provided by thin-section high-resolution CT. MRI is the best imaging modality for visualization of the optic nerve itself as it travels through the optic canal.

Orbital osseous dysplasia may occur in patients with neurofibromatosis type 1, although orbital involvement is infrequent compared to the osseous abnormalities that occur in the axial and appendicular skeleton in these patients. Osseous dysplasia frequently occurs concomitantly with orbital-facial plexiform neurofibroma. Orbital osseous dysplasia in neurofibromatosis consists of one or more of the following: hypoplasia of the greater wing of the sphenoid, hypoplasia and elevation of the lesser wing of the sphenoid, enlargement of the middle cranial fossa with extension into the posterior orbit,

deformity and decreased size of the ipsilateral ethmoid and maxillary sinuses, and enlargement of the orbit and the superior and inferior orbital fissures.[273,274] Imaging techniques for the evaluation of these abnormalities include radiography, CT, and three-dimensional CT reformation (Fig. 3-64).

Orbital abnormalities frequently accompany congenital oblique facial clefts (Fig. 3-65). Microphthalmia or anophthalmia frequently are present on the side of the facial cleft. CT is useful for depiction of the complex osseous defects and also

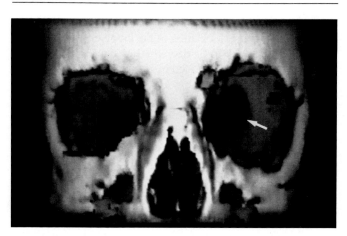

Fig. 3-64 Neurofibromatosis type 1. Computer-generated three-dimensional CT reformation of the orbits demonstrates an osseous defect in the posterior wall of the left orbit (arrow) as well as slight enlargement in the overall dimensions of the left orbit.

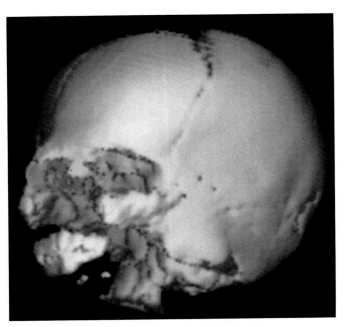

Fig. 3-65 Oblique facial cleft. Computer-generated three-dimensional CT reformation of the left side of the skull demonstrates an oblique facial cleft with absence of a portion of the maxilla and the floor of the left orbit.

demonstrates the degree of microphthalmia and the position of the globe. Three-dimensional CT reformations provide useful information for planning of corrective surgical procedures.

Fibrous Dysplasia

In fibrous dysplasia, there is replacement of normal bony spongiosa by an abnormal proliferation of fibrous tissue. This results in diffuse thickening of the affected bone. Fibrous dysplasia occurs in both monostotic and polyostotic forms. Involvement of one or more of the bones surrounding the orbit may result in proptosis, impaired vision due to optic nerve impingement, or extraocular muscle palsy.

Radiographs of the orbit in fibrous dysplasia demonstrate diffuse sclerosis and thickening of the involved osseous structures. The orbital cavity is decreased in size. Adjacent paranasal sinuses may be decreased in size as well. CT also shows the pattern of bone thickening and demonstrates an irregular internal structure of the involved bones, showing mixed areas of ossified and unossified fibrous tissue. Cystic changes may be seen.[275] Bone scintigraphy is often helpful to document areas of involvement with fibrous dysplasia in the facial bones and base of the skull. The involved bones demonstrate markedly increased tracer uptake.

Cephalocele

A cephalocele represents a congenital malformation that may have orbital effects. Fronto-ethmoidal and sphenoidal cephaloceles frequently protrude between the orbits, producing hypertelorism. Defects in the osseous walls of one or both orbits may occur. A rare type of cephalocele occurs directly through a defect in the roof of the orbit. Sphenoidal cephaloceles may be accompanied by midline clefts of the upper lip or nose, optic nerve dysplasias, and dysgenesis of the corpus callosum.[275,276]

Standard radiographs in children with an anterior cephalocele often demonstrate hypertelorism. The osseous defect may or may not be identifiable on plain radiographs. CT demonstrates protrusion of cerebrospinal fluid and brain tissue through a cranial osseous defect. Both coronal and axial images are often required to demonstrate accurately the orbital abnormalities. MRI is ideally suited for demonstration of a cephalocele, with sagittal images being particularly helpful. The cephalocele is imaged as a thin-walled sac containing cerebrospinal fluid. A variable amount of brain protrudes through the osseous defect into the sac. Islands of disorganized neuroglial tissue may be visualized along the walls of the sac (Fig. 3-66).[276] Angiography is occasionally performed for definition of vascular anatomy in the region of the cephalocele for preoperative planning.

Optic Nerve Hypoplasia

Optic nerve hypoplasia is an uncommon, but important, cause of defective vision in children. Optic nerve hypoplasia may be associated with various central nervous system anomalies, including septo-optic dysplasia, hydrocephalus, cephalocele, porencephaly, and schizencephaly as well as bone dysplasias (Fig. 3-67).[277–279] In most cases, both optic nerves are affected. Ocular abnormalities associated with optic nerve hypoplasia include microphthalmia, coloboma, blepharophimosis, ocular motor nerve palsies, aniridia, and retinal vascular malformations.[280]

Septo-optic dysplasia is a developmental abnormality involving the optic nerves and midline intracranial structures. The septum pellucidum is absent, the optic nerves are hypoplastic, and the pituitary is frequently hypoplastic. Other midline defects such as cleft palate may also be present. Clinical findings include poor vision and hypopituitarism, frequently with isolated growth hormone deficiency. Ophthalmoscopic examination demonstrates hypoplasia of the optic disc.

Evaluation of the orbits in children with optic nerve hypoplasia with CT or plain films demonstrates small optic canals. CT and MRI demonstrate small optic nerves. Coronal images with either imaging modality are essential for accurate evaluation of optic nerve size. The coexistent intracranial abnormalities also can be demonstrated with either CT or MRI.[281,282] In cases of septo-optic dysplasia, CT and MRI show absence of the septum pellucidum and hypoplasia of the pituitary gland.

Orbital Infection

Orbital infection in children and adults is most commonly due to extension of infection from an adjacent paranasal

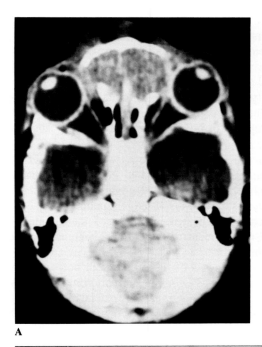

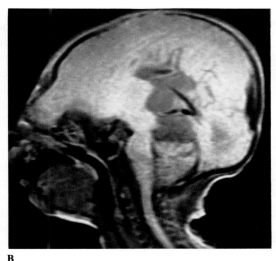

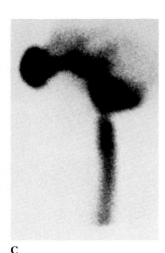

B   C

Fig. 3-66 Nasofrontal cephalocele. (**A**) CT shows defects in the medial walls of both orbits with lateral displacement of the globes. (**B**) T_1-weighted sagittal MR image confirms the presence of a nasofrontal cephalocele. (**C**) Radionuclide cisternography shows extension of labeled cerebrospinal fluid into the meningoencephalocele.

A

sinus.[283] The ethmoid sinuses are the most common primary focus in young children. Concomitant maxillary sinusitis is frequently present. As the frontal sinuses develop in older children and adolescents, they also become a relatively common source of orbital infection. Orbital extension of an infectious abnormality from the sphenoid sinus occurs uncommonly. Orbital infection may also result from spread from an adjacent soft tissue infection of the face, sometimes after minor trauma or an insect bite.[284] Hematogenous inoculation from a remote site is uncommon; this mechanism most often occurs in infants and young children.[285] The most common organisms responsible for orbital infection in the pediatric population include staphylococci, streptococci, and pneumococci. Orbital infection with *Hemophilus influenzae* type 6 may occur in infants and toddlers.[285,286]

Clinical findings in orbital infection include lid edema, ocular pain, proptosis, and limitation of ocular movements. Some degree of visual loss may occur. Fever and elevation of the white blood cell count are usually present. Intracranial complications may produce various neurologic findings.[283,286,287]

The most common manifestations of orbital involvement in an adjacent infection are reactive inflammatory edema (orbital cellulitis in situ) and true orbital cellulitis. The former refers to secondary inflammatory changes in the orbit as a response to infection of the skin, paranasal sinuses, oral cavity, or lacrimal apparatus. With true orbital cellulitis, there is actual infection of orbital structures.[283] Although these two abnormalities cannot be absolutely differentiated radiographically, the clinical and imaging findings are usually more marked with orbital cellulitis. In most children with paranasal sinusitis and periorbital swelling, the pathophysiologic mechanism of orbital involvement is probably as follows: sinusitis causes increased pressure in the sinuses, which results in venous obstruction and, ultimately, inflammatory edema of the periorbital structures without actual spread of infection outside the confines of the sinuses.[283,285]

Reactive inflammatory edema and simple orbital cellulitis are most commonly confined to the preseptal structures (eyelids and face).[286] Radiographs may be helpful in determining whether an underlying sinusitis is present. Both CT and MRI, however, provide superior demonstration of sinus disease and orbital involvement.[288,289] In most cases, CT or MRI demon-

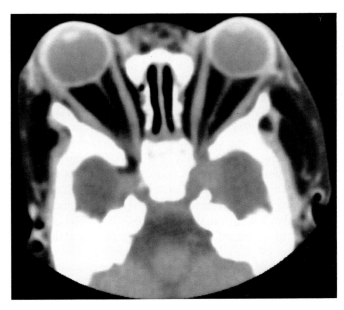

Fig. 3-67 Bilateral optic nerve hypoplasia. CT shows small optic nerves in a patient with bone dysplasia.

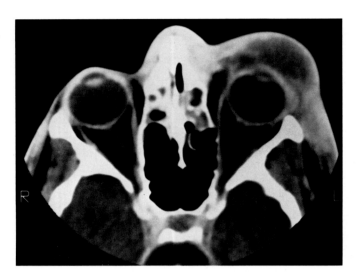

Fig. 3-68 Preseptal cellulitis. Contrast-enhanced CT shows marked thickening of the left periorbital soft tissues. The abnormality is confined to structures anterior to the orbital septum.

strates thickening of the preseptal soft tissue structures without involvement of the orbit proper (Fig. 3-68).

Involvement of postseptal structures occurs in the form of edema of the orbital fat and extraocular muscles. The most common area of involvement is the extraconal fat adjacent to the ethmoid sinuses.[290] Inflammatory edema or cellulitis of orbital fat produces increased attenuation on CT and increased signal on T_2-weighted MR images. Involvement of extraocular muscles is indicated by enlargement and contrast enhancement on CT (Fig. 3-69) or by enlargement and increased signal on T_2-weighted MR images.

Orbital cellulitis is sometimes complicated by abscess formation. In most cases, the abscess is localized in the subperiosteal space and occurs secondary to extension from an adjacent sinusitis. Subperiosteal abscesses are most commonly located along the medial orbital wall in children and may be located medially, superiorly, and inferiorly in adolescents and adults. It is uncommon for an abscess to arise in the intraconal space.

CT in cases of subperiosteal abscess shows displacement of the thickened periosteal membrane away from the orbital wall.[288,290,291] The underlying fluid collection is usually of relatively low attenuation (Fig. 3-70). With intravenous contrast medium, the displaced periosteum enhances while the fluid collection is unchanged in attenuation. This is an important finding in the differentiation of subperiosteal abscess from simple edema of soft tissue structures.[288,290] The orbital fat adjacent to a subperiosteal abscess usually is of increased attenuation on CT, indicating inflammation. There is also some degree of displacement of the adjacent extraocular muscle with or without enlargement and increased contrast enhancement.

The same anatomic changes that are identified on CT in subperiosteal abscess may be demonstrated on MRI

(Fig. 3-71). As with CT, demonstration of the thickened, displaced periosteal membrane and the underlying fluid collection is essential in differentiating subperiosteal abscess from simple orbital cellulitis or inflammatory edema. Axial CT images and axial or sagittal MR images best demonstrate the superficial (periorbital) changes in orbital cellulitis. Coronal images are most sensitive for the detection of involvement of the orbit proper with inflammation, infection, or abscess formation.

Abscesses in the intraconal space are uncommon. CT in these cases demonstrates an intraconal inflammatory mass, usually with enhancing margins. The globe, optic nerve, and extraocular muscles may be displaced by the mass. Adjacent soft tissue edema is indicated by increased attenuation of orbital fat and enlargement of the extraocular muscles and optic nerve complex.[289,292]

Osteitis or osteomyelitis of the orbital wall bordering an infected sinus can occur as a complication of orbital and sinus infection. Sinus infection, however, may extend into the orbit without infection or destruction of the orbital wall via normal small openings through which bridging veins pass. When bone necrosis occurs in cases of sinusitis, it results from osteomyelitis or bone infarction caused by interruption of the blood supply from increased pressure in the sinus.

Radiographs in cases of osteomyelitis of the orbital wall demonstrate opacification of the involved sinus, but osseous abnormalities are usually not visible unless the process is advanced. CT may demonstrate areas of bone destruction. These images, however, must be examined with caution because the medial wall of the orbit is normally quite thin, and apparent bony defects may be seen with improper window and level settings.

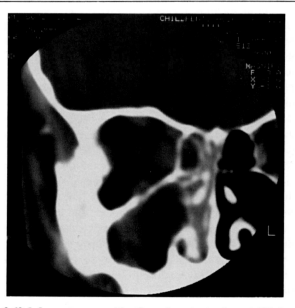

Fig. 3-69 Inflammatory myositis. Coronal contrast-enhanced CT demonstrates opacification of the right nasal cavity, ethmoid air cells, and maxillary sinus due to sinusitis. The medial rectus muscle is enlarged as a result of secondary inflammatory myositis.

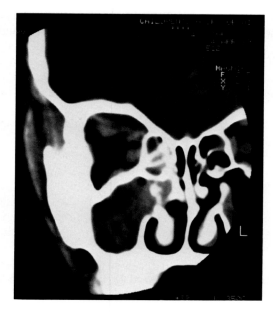

Fig. 3-70 Subperiosteal abscess. Coronal contrast-enhanced CT shows changes of sinusitis in the right maxillary and ethmoid sinuses. There is a superior right orbital subperiosteal abscess. Faint enhancement of the periosteal membrane is visible.

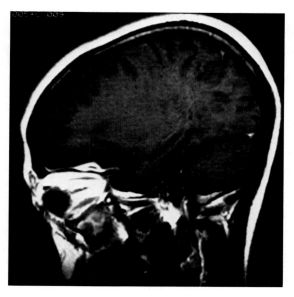

Fig. 3-71 Orbital cellulitis with intracranial extension. Sagittal T_1-weighted MR image with intravenous gadopentetate dimeglumine shows thickening of the extraconal soft tissues in the superior aspect of the orbit. There is also increased signal arising from the meninges at the base of the frontal lobe and a small intracranial epidural abscess.

The most sensitive imaging modality for detection of osteitis or osteomyelitis of the orbital wall is bone scintigraphy. The involved bony structures produce increased tracer accumulation (Fig. 3-72). Other foci of bone involvement in the face and skull may also be identified. In those cases in which infection has resulted in interruption of the osseous blood supply, the appearance on scintigraphy is decreased tracer uptake (cold or infarctive osteomyelitis).

Mucocele is a relatively uncommon sequela of chronic sinus disease that often produces proptosis or other orbital abnormalities. There is an increased incidence of mucoceles in patients with cystic fibrosis. In children, mucoceles most commonly arise from the anterior ethmoid air cells or frontal sinus, but they may occur in any of the paranasal sinuses. As a mucocele slowly enlarges, it may protrude into the orbit through a bony defect in the orbital wall, or the orbital wall may be thinned and gradually displaced into the orbit. Proptosis may be the presenting symptom of a mucocele.

Plain radiographs with small mucoceles may simply demonstrate nonspecific opacification of the involved sinus. As the mucocele increases in size, expansion and thinning of the sinus walls may be identified. CT clearly demonstrates the expanded, thinned sinus walls and homogeneous soft tissue attenuation within. An enhancing capsule may be identified, but the contents of the mucocele in the capsule should not enhance with intravenous contrast agents. Although MRI is not well suited for demonstrating the bony abnormalities of mucocele, this imaging technique is particularly useful in differentiating a mucocele from a paranasal sinus neoplasm. Mucoceles typically demonstrate high signal intensity on both

T_1- and T_2-weighted images. If the contents of the mucocele become inspissated and desiccated, areas of signal void may be demonstrated on MRI on all pulsing sequences despite CT evidence of high-attenuation material filling the sinus cavity.[293]

One of the important roles for imaging studies in patients with orbital infection is the detection of intracranial extension. Direct intracranial extension by destruction of the superior

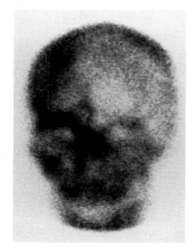

Fig. 3-72 Osteomyelitis. Anterior image of the face and skull with bone scintigraphy shows abnormal tracer accumulation in the walls of the right maxillary, ethmoid, and frontal sinuses as well as extension of abnormality into the more superior aspects of the right frontal bone.

wall of the orbit is unusual. More commonly, intracranial extension occurs via the small bridging veins that extend through the walls of the sinuses, orbits, and calvaria. Intracranial complications include epidural abscess, subdural abscess, meningitis, cerebritis, brain abscess, and cavernous sinus thrombosis. In general, these complications may be detected and characterized with either contrast-enhanced CT or MRI.

Endophthalmitis (infection of the globe) may occur by direct extension of infection from adjacent structures or by hematogeneous inoculation. Most cases result as a complication of eye surgery or trauma.[294] CT demonstrates sclerouveal thickening and enhancement. There is frequently increased attenuation of the vitreous (Fig. 3-73). CT is also useful for identification of intraocular foreign bodies that may be associated with infection.

Toxocara canis endophthalmitis (visceral larva migrans) is associated with ingestion of eggs of the nematode *T canis*. There is usually a history of close contact with dogs, particularly puppies. Similar disease can be produced by *T cati*, a cat nematode. A granulomatous uveitis results in a subretinal exudate, retinal detachment, and a variable degree of organized vitreous. The average patient age at presentation is 6 years. *Toxocara* endophthalmitis may produce leukocoria that is clinically indistinguishable from retinoblastoma.[295]

CT imaging in *Toxocara* endophthalmitis demonstrates a variable degree of obliteration of the vitreous cavity by homogeneous material of increased attenuation.[265,296] Calcification does not occur, and the subretinal collection does not enhance. There are often thickening and contrast enhancement of the sclera. Occasionally, enhancement of the contracted retina may be visible.[268] The proteinaceous subretinal exudate of *T canis* endophthalmitis produces high signal intensity on both T_1- and T_2-weighted MR images.

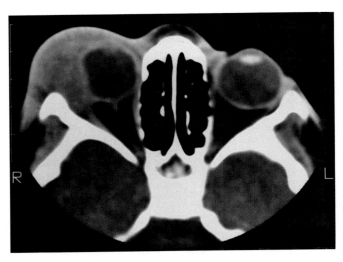

Fig. 3-74 Dacryoadenitis. Axial CT demonstrates marked enlargement of the right lacrimal gland with compression of the globe. Surgical drainage demonstrated bacterial infection of the lacrimal gland.

Dacryoadenitis refers to inflammation of the lacrimal gland. Dacryoadenitis may occur as an isolated process, as part of a diffuse inflammatory process of the orbit, or as a manifestation of a systemic disease. Lacrimal gland inflammation in children most often occurs as part of a postviral syndrome. Infectious etiologies of acute dacryoadenitis include mumps, infectious mononucleosis, Gram-positive bacterial infection, and fungal infection.

CT and MRI in cases of acute dacryoadenitis frequently show nonspecific enlargement of the lacrimal gland (Fig. 3-74). With abscess formation, CT shows a central nonenhancing area surrounded by the irregularly enhancing, enlarged lacrimal gland.[297]

Ocular Masses

Retinoblastoma

Retinoblastoma is a malignant neoplasm of childhood that arises from neuroectodermal cells in the retina that normally differentiate into photoreceptor cells.[298] The incidence of retinoblastoma is 1 in 18,000 live births. There are two genetic forms of retinoblastoma. Approximately 40% of cases represent a hereditary form, with about 10% of these representing inheritance from parents and 30% arising from a sporadic germ cell line mutation. Approximately 60% of cases of retinoblastoma are the result of a somatic cell mutation and are not heritable.[299] The heritable type of retinoblastoma is frequently multicentric, there being bilateral tumors or multiple tumor foci in one globe. These patients are also at increased risk of developing pinealoma (trilateral retinoblastoma), which is histologically indistinguishable from retinoblastoma.[300] All bilateral cases and approximately 10%

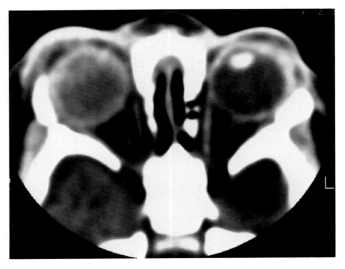

Fig. 3-73 Endophthalmitis. Contrast-enhanced CT shows abnormally increased attenuation of the vitreous cavity of the right globe and slight thickening of the periorbital soft tissues. The lens has been destroyed by infection.

Table 3-10 Flow Diagram of Retinoblastoma

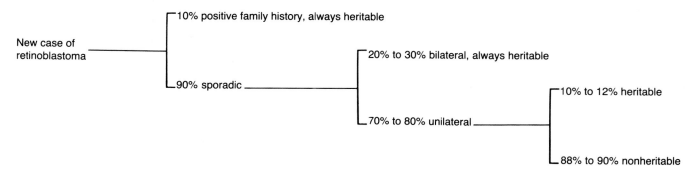

Source: Reprinted from SS Donaldson and PR Egbert, "Retinoblastoma" in *Principles and Practice of Pediatric Oncology* (p 557) by PA Pizzo and DG Poplack (eds) with permission of J.B. Lippincott Company, © 1989.

of unilateral cases are of the hereditary genetic form (Table 3-10). Bilateral hereditary cases have an average age of onset of 12 months, and unilateral cases of either genetic form have an average age of onset of 25 months.[301]

Patients with the hereditary form of retinoblastoma demonstrate a propensity for the development of nonocular tumors, most commonly a sarcoma (usually osteosarcoma).[302,303] Of these second malignant tumors, however, 25% to 35% occur outside the radiation field or develop in nonirradiated patients.[304,305] The incidence of second malignant tumors increases with time. In irradiated patients, the incidence approaches 20% at 10 years, 50% at 20 years, and 90% at 30 years. In nonirradiated patients, the incidence of second malignancies is 10% at 10 years, 30% at 20 years, and 68% at 30 years.[306] An increased incidence of retinoblastoma has been documented in patients with partial deletion of the long arm of chromosome 13.[307]

Retinoblastomas may be classified into one of three types on the basis of tumor morphology[299]: endophytic retinoblastoma, where the mass breaks through the internal limiting membrane of the retina and extends into the vitreous cavity (most common); exophytic retinoblastoma, where the tumor grows in the subretinal space (uncommon; this produces retinal elevation, subretinal exudate, and, rarely, subretinal hemorrhage)[268]; and diffuse infiltrating retinoblastoma, where the tumor cells spread throughout the retina, infiltrate adjacent structures, and may simulate an inflammatory or hemorrhagic condition (rare).

Small tumors limited to the retina have the best prognosis.[298] Retinoblastoma may invade the optic nerve or extend through the sclera into the orbit.[308] Metastasis to the central nervous system may occur by cerebrospinal fluid dissemination. Hematogeneous metastases probably result from invasion of the highly vascular choroid. The most common sites for distant metastasis include bone, bone marrow, liver, and lymph nodes.[307] Osseous metastases produce permeative destructive changes that appear radiographically similar to metastatic neuroblastoma.[309]

The most common clinical sign associated with retinoblastoma is leukocoria, which is identified in approximately 60% of patients.[310] Other potential clinical findings include strabismus, decreased vision, glaucoma, and nystagmus.[298] Ophthalmoscopic examination demonstrates a pinkish-white or gray-white retinal-based mass. In endophytic retinoblastoma, the lobulated mass extends into the vitreous cavity. With exophytic retinoblastoma, ophthalmoscopy demonstrates retinal detachment, but the tumor mass may not be visible. The diffuse type of retinoblastoma may be confused with inflammatory or hemorrhagic conditions ophthalmoscopically and radiographically.

Imaging procedures are generally performed in cases of retinoblastoma for confirmation of the diagnosis, characterization of tumor morphology, and detection of local extension or distant metastases.[265,307,311,312] Evaluation with CT should include unenhanced and enhanced images; the axial projection is usually most advantageous. The mass is typically identified along the posterior aspect of the globe, and in most cases the lobulated tumor is visible extending into the vitreous cavity. Tumor calcification is detectable on CT in at least 80% to 90% of cases (Fig. 3-75). The calcification is thought to result from formation of DNA-calcium complexes as DNA is released from necrotic tumor cells. The calcifications are irregular and range from punctate to conglomerate. Detectable calcification is frequently lacking in small tumors (less than 4 mm) and in the infiltrating type of retinoblastoma. The tumor usually demonstrates some degree of contrast enhancement. Associated areas of subretinal effusion or hemorrhage do not enhance.[268] Infiltration of the sclera produces thickening and increased contrast enhancement. Extension of the tumor into the optic nerve is indicated by enlargement of the nerve.[313] Intracranial extension may be direct or, more commonly, via cerebrospinal fluid dissemination from the subarachnoid space surrounding the optic nerve. Meningeal implants typically demonstrate significant contrast enhancement on CT. The contralateral globe should be closely inspected for evidence of additional primary lesions.

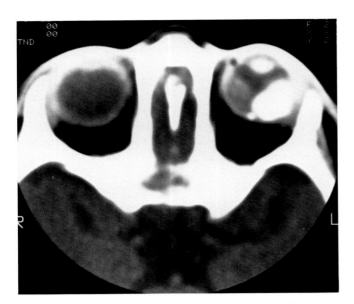

Fig. 3-75 Retinoblastoma. Unenhanced CT shows a densely calcified mass in the posterolateral aspect of the left globe. A second component, without significant calcification, is visible in the medial aspect of the globe.

Retinoblastoma has been reported to appear on T_1-weighted MR images as isointense to slightly hyperintense areas with respect to vitreous. The lesion is hypointense to vitreous on T_2-weighted images. Although small calcifications are poorly demonstrated on MRI, large calcifications may be recognized as areas of signal void. Differentiation of subretinal effusion or hemorrhage from the primary tumor appears to be somewhat easier with MRI compared to CT because the subretinal fluid collection produces high signal on both T_1- and T_2-weighted images. Enlargement of the optic nerve indicates posterior extension of the neoplasm.[313] Intracranial metastases may also be identified on MRI.

There are several abnormalities that must be considered clinically and radiographically in the differential diagnosis of an ocular mass thought to represent retinoblastoma.[265,272] These include persistent hyperplastic primary vitreous, Coats disease, retinochoroidal coloboma, optic nerve head drusen, *Toxocara canis* endophthalmitis, retinal glial tumors, and medulloepithelioma. CT demonstration of tumor calcification is particularly helpful in the differential diagnosis because most lesions, other than retinoblastoma, do not calcify or do not calcify until later in childhood. Optic disc drusen may calcify; these lesions, however, are quite small and occur in the region of the optic disc.[314] Retinoblastoma may invade but does not arise in the optic disc. The globe is typically of normal size in retinoblastoma, whereas some degree of microphthalmos is typically present in persistent hyperplastic primary vitreous and retinochoroidal coloboma.

Medulloepithelioma

Medulloepithelioma is a rare congenital tumor that arises from the ciliary epithelium. Both benign and malignant forms

occur, with approximately two-thirds of cases showing malignant histologic features. Benign and malignant teratoid forms of medulloepithelioma also occur. The average age at presentation in cases of medulloepithelioma is approximately 4 years.[299,315] Medulloepithelioma affects only one eye. Boys and girls are equally affected, and no racial predilection has been observed.

Because the tumor arises from the ciliary body, medulloepithelioma is usually located in the anterior aspect of the globe adjacent to the posterolateral aspect of the lens. Evaluation with CT demonstrates an anteriorly placed, enhancing intraocular mass.[316] The mass produces moderate signal intensity on T_1-weighted MR images and high signal on T_2-weighted images. The lack of calcification and the anterior location help distinguish this neoplasm from retinoblastoma. Also, medulloepithelioma is a unilateral tumor, and the family history is negative for similar ocular tumors.

Glial Tumors

Glial tumors of the retina (most often astrocytic hamartoma of the optic nerve head) occur in more than 50% of cases of tuberous sclerosis.[317] These tumors are also rarely associated with neurofibromatosis and retinitis pigmentosa. Retinal glial tumors are usually flat lesions that are identified ophthalmoscopically. In rare cases a nodule may form, which can, on occasion, contain calcification.

Most retinal glial tumors are too small to be imaged with CT or MRI. If the tumor is of sufficient size, it may be identified as a small retinal-based nodule. Radiographic differentiation from retinoblastoma is generally not possible. The presence of clinical or radiographic manifestations of tuberous sclerosis is helpful.[318]

Orbital Masses

Dermoid Tumor

Dermoid tumor is the most common orbital neoplasm in children, accounting for approximately 45% of pediatric orbital and periorbital masses.[299,319] A dermoid tumor is composed of two germ layers: ectoderm and mesoderm. This tumor contains skin and adnexal appendages such as hair follicles, sebaceous glands, and sweat glands. Solid dermoid tumors contain a thick matrix of fibroadipose tissue. A dermoid cyst consists of an epithelial-lined cavity that contains a cheesy, keratinous material. The cystic variety accounts for most orbital dermoid tumors.

These tumors usually arise along fetal cleavage planes, such as the cranial sutures.[320] Dermoid tumors are most commonly located in the anterior aspect of the extraconal orbital space. Approximately 60% lie in the upper temporal quadrant and 25% in the upper nasal quadrant.[318,321] Deep orbital locations are uncommon.

The clinical presentation of dermoid tumor is usually a painless, slow-growing mass. The globe may be displaced by

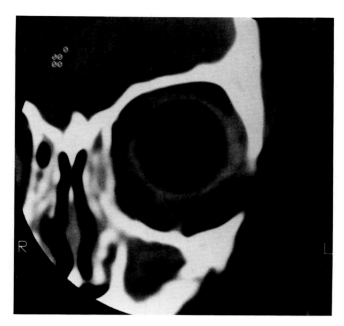

Fig. 3-76 Dermoid cyst. Coronal contrast-enhanced CT shows a dermoid cyst inferior to the left globe. The demonstration of a capsule surrounding a lesion of relatively low attenuation is suggestive of the correct diagnosis.

large lesions. Deep orbital dermoid tumors frequently cause proptosis. In some cases, minor trauma results in rupture of the cyst, and a secondary inflammatory response develops in adjacent tissues that can mimic orbital cellulitis clinically.[322] Epibulbar dermoid tumors are frequently present in children with Goldenhar syndrome. In this syndrome, congenital defects of the eyes, ears, face, mandible, and vertebral column are found. In addition to epibulbar dermoid cysts, colobomas of the upper lid, iris, and choroid occur. There is a frequent association with microphthalmos.[323]

The typical CT appearance of a dermoid tumor is a well-defined extraconal or periorbital mass (Fig. 3-76). There is often erosion of the adjacent orbital wall, but the bone maintains a well-corticated margin.[324] If enough lipid material is contained in the lesion, negative attenuation values are produced, and the CT appearance is virtually pathognomonic.[322,325] It is not unusual, however, for a dermoid tumor to be approximately of the same CT attenuation value as muscle. Areas of calcification are occasionally present. The contents of a dermoid cyst should not enhance with intravenous contrast agents, but some degree of enhancement of the capsule may be identified.

The MR appearance of dermoid tumors is somewhat variable, depending on the fat content. In those lesions with significant fat content, high signal is produced on T_1-weighted MR images. This appearance is in contrast to most neoplasms, particularly malignancies, which typically produce low or moderate signal intensity on T_1-weighted images.[326] Demonstration of a fat-fluid level in a dermoid tumor has been reported.[327] Dermoids with low fat content may have MR signal characteristics similar to those of muscle.

Orbital Teratoma

Orbital teratoma is a congenital tumor that is usually benign.[328] Teratomas contain tissue from all three germ layers. Orbital teratoma is a rare lesion, having an incidence of 1% of all pediatric orbital masses. This lesion is more common in girls. Many cases are clinically evident at birth, sometimes presenting as a large intraorbital mass.[329] A tendency for rapid enlargement of these tumors after birth has been reported (Fig. 3-77).[330] The mass most often arises in the posterior aspect of the intraconal space adjacent to the orbital apex.

Imaging with CT or MRI helps determine the degree of orbital involvement and extension into adjacent structures.[329] The mass usually arises in the muscle cone adjacent to the optic nerve. The teratoid nature of the mass is suggested if areas of fat, cartilage, or bone are identified. The tumor may be cystic or partially cystic in composition. The lesion may have only soft tissue characteristics, however (Fig. 3-78). Teratomas may produce bone erosion or expansion with well-defined margins, but they usually do not cause frank bone destruction.[331] These tumors sometimes extend through the orbital fissures and produce an hourglass- or dumbbell-shaped appearance. The optic canal is enlarged in some cases.

Capillary Hemangioma

Capillary hemangioma is a relatively common orbital neoplasm in children, accounting for approximately 5% to 15% of all pediatric orbital masses. Approximately 95% of orbital hemangiomas are diagnosed by 6 months of age.[332] They are more common in girls. Most pediatric orbital capillary hemangiomas regress spontaneously during the first few years

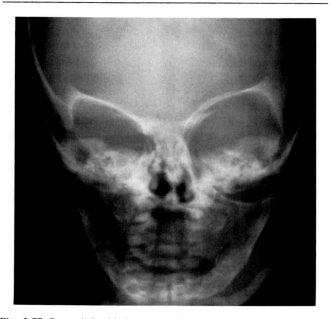

Fig. 3-77 Congenital orbital teratoma. Anteroposterior radiograph of the skull in a neonate shows marked enlargement of the bony margins of the left orbit due to a large, clinically obvious mass.

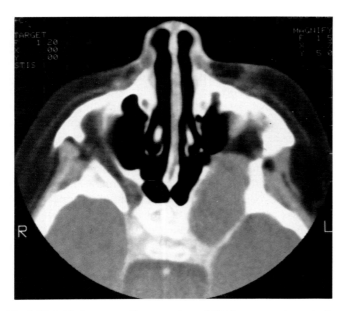

Fig. 3-78 Orbital teratoma. Contrast-enhanced CT shows an oval mass in the posterior aspect of the left orbit. There are remodeling and displacement of the adjacent osseous structures.

of life; large lesions, however, may cause significant visual compromise if not treated.[299] The most common location is the superior nasal quadrant.[333] Occasionally, capillary hemangiomas may extend intracranially through the superior orbital fissure, optic canal, or orbital roof.[323]

Approximately 90% of orbital capillary hemangiomas have an anterior or periorbital component. Conversely, a significant number (about 75%) of clinically obvious superficial capillary hemangiomas extend into the orbit proper. Clinical findings include tumor enlargement during crying, a dark vascular colorization of the subcutaneous orbital and periorbital tissue, and superficial strawberry hemangiomas elsewhere on the body (about 25% of cases).[332]

CT imaging of capillary hemangiomas typically demonstrates a soft tissue prominence corresponding to the superficial component of the tumor. Extension into the orbit is indicated by visualization of an enhancing mass. The mass is usually confined to the extraconal space. Contrast enhancement may be approximately equal to or much greater than that of normal muscle. The margination of the tumor is also variable. Most of these lesions are poorly encapsulated, and infiltration of orbital structures may occur (Fig. 3-79). In some cases, the tumor is well marginated. Phleboliths are occasionally present.[323,334]

A capillary hemangioma is demonstrated on MRI as a soft-tissue mass that is isointense to muscle on T_1-weighted images and markedly hyperintense on T_2-weighted images. Internal septations of lower signal intensity may be present. The lesion typically exhibits intense enhancement with paramagnetic contrast material.

Radionuclide-labeled red blood cell scintigraphy may be utilized to confirm the diagnosis of capillary hemangioma. The vascular nature of the mass is indicated by rapid and intense accumulation of tracer in the lesion.

Cavernous Hemangioma

Cavernous hemangioma most often presents in older children and adults, in contradistinction to the capillary type. This lesion accounts for less than 2% of pediatric orbital masses. Unlike capillary hemangiomas, these tumors demonstrate slowly progressive enlargement and do not spontaneously involute. Cavernous hemangiomas may be located anywhere in the orbit but most commonly occur in the intraconal space.[333] These tumors are surrounded by a fibrous pseudocapsule; therefore, adjacent structures are displaced but not invaded.[323,335]

The CT appearance of cavernous hemangioma is a well-defined, round, high-attenuation mass. The pattern of contrast enhancement is somewhat variable because of the typically slow intratumoral circulation. Dynamic CT imaging may be utilized to document this slow circulation and to differentiate this lesion from capillary hemangiomas, which show rapid circulation.[323] Cavernous hemangiomas are usually isointense to muscle on T_1-weighted MR images and hyperintense on T_2-weighted MR images.

A   B

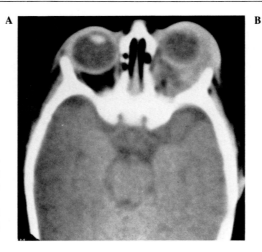

Fig. 3-79 Capillary hemangioma. **(A)** Contrast-enhanced CT shows an enhancing infiltrative lesion involving the periorbital and deep orbital structures on the left. There is moderate proptosis. **(B)** Labeled red blood cell scan (anterior image) shows increased blood pool activity, confirming the vascular nature of the mass.

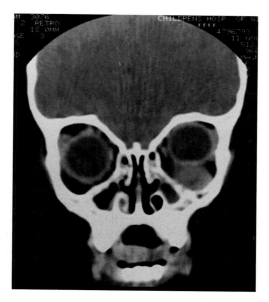

Fig. 3-80 Lymphangioma. Coronal unenhanced CT shows a slightly heterogeneous mass inferior to the left globe. There are no specific identifying characteristics in the appearance of this lesion.

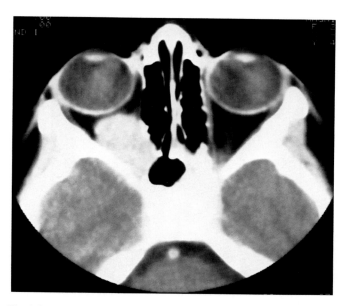

Fig. 3-81 Lymphangioma. Contrast-enhanced CT shows a right orbital mass. The relatively marked contrast enhancement is typical of orbital lymphangioma because of the rich vascular supply.

Lymphangioma

Lymphangioma is a vascular tumor of the orbit that usually presents during the first few years of life. Lymphangioma accounts for less than 2% of pediatric orbital masses. This tumor usually enlarges gradually, but progression slows as general body growth decreases in late adolescence and early adulthood. Spontaneous bleeding occurs more commonly with lymphangioma compared to hemangioma.[335] Orbital lymphangiomas may noticeably increase in size during upper respiratory infections.[336] A superficial component of the tumor is frequently clinically identifiable; proptosis is the clinical hallmark of extension into the orbit.[337]

Lymphangioma is imaged on CT as a heterogeneous mass of relatively high attenuation that is most often confined to the extraconal space (Fig. 3-80).[323] These lesions are usually somewhat infiltrative and, therefore, often demonstrate ill-defined margins.[338] Contrast enhancement is variable, with at least 50% of lymphangiomas exhibiting significant enhancement on CT (Fig. 3-81). Lymphangiomas are typically imaged on MRI as lesions of increased signal on both T_1- and T_2-weighted images.[339] Fluid-fluid levels may be seen if hemorrhage has occurred in the lesion.

Primary Orbital Varix

Primary orbital varices are congenital venous malformations in which there is proliferation of venous elements and massive dilatation of one or more orbital veins. The superior or inferior ophthalmic veins are most commonly involved. The usual clinical presentation is unilateral proptosis.

An orbital varix is imaged on CT and MRI as a well-defined, markedly enhancing mass. The lesion usually lies predominantly or totally in the intraconal space. Phleboliths may be present. In some cases, the lesion is not visible on routine imaging. In this situation, when there is a clinical suspicion of orbital varix, imaging should be repeated with a provocative maneuver such as jugular vein compression or the Valsalva maneuver.[323]

Arteriovenous Malformation

An arteriovenous malformation is the least common orbital vascular abnormality. These lesions may be congenital, spontaneous, or secondary to penetrating trauma. CT imaging shows an irregular, enhancing mass with large vascular structures. The diagnosis is confirmed with angiography.

Rhabdomyosarcoma

Rhabdomyosarcoma is the most common primary malignant orbital tumor in childhood. Because most space-occupying orbital lesions are benign, rhabdomyosarcoma accounts for only 3% to 4% of all pediatric orbital masses. There is an increased incidence in whites. Ninety percent of patients are younger than 16 years of age.[299,340] A rare association with neurofibromatosis has been reported.[341] There are three major histologic types of rhabdomyosarcoma. The most common is embryonal (75%), the alveolar type is less common (15%), and undifferentiated or pleomorphic rhabdomyosarcoma is the least frequent type (10%).[340]

Most rhabdomyosarcomas of the eye arise in the orbit proper (71%); the lids (22%) and conjunctivae (7%) are less common sites.[342] Rapidly progressive unilateral proptosis is the most common clinical finding. Other clinical findings include ptosis, periorbital edema, ophthalmoplegia, pain, and decreased visual acuity.

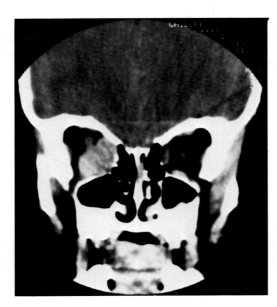

Fig. 3-82 Rhabdomyosarcoma. Coronal CT shows a large soft tissue mass in the inferomedial aspect of the right orbit.

Rhabdomyosarcomas arise from undifferentiated mesenchyma. Although these tumors may contain elements of skeletal muscle, they do not characteristically arise from mature striated muscle. The alveolar type may be an exception because there is evidence that this type arises from mature muscle.[343] Diagnostic imaging, therefore, typically demonstrates the mass to lie in the intraconal or extraconal spaces (or both), but primary involvement of the extraocular muscles is uncommon (Fig. 3-82).

On CT, orbital rhabdomyosarcoma may demonstrate significant enhancement with intravenous contrast material. Some degree of bone destruction is frequently present. Tumor extension into an adjacent sinus, the nasal cavity, or the anterior cranial fossa may occur. Preseptal extension is relatively common; this serves as a differential point from neuroblastoma, which rarely extends into the preseptal space.[338] Metastases may occur to the lungs, bone marrow, or, rarely, cervical lymph nodes. The radiologic differential diagnosis includes other aggressive orbital neoplasms such as neuroblastoma, lymphoma, and Langerhans cell histiocytosis.[344]

On T_1-weighted MR images, orbital rhabdomyosarcoma is hypointense to fat and approximately isointense to muscle. The lesion is hyperintense to fat and muscle on T_2-weighted images. Prominent heterogeneous enhancement occurs with intravenous paramagnetic contrast material. As with CT, MRI often shows bone destruction and invasion of the paranasal sinuses or pharynx.

Neurofibroma and Schwannoma

Neurofibroma and schwannoma are peripheral nerve sheath tumors that may arise in the lid or orbit. These may occur as isolated lesions or in association with neurofibromatosis type 1. Schwannoma is an encapsulated tumor and is typically imaged on CT as a sharply marginated, oval or fusiform mass. Schwannomas are most frequently located in the intraconal space.[345] There is usually moderate to marked enhancement with intravenous contrast agents; enhancement may vary from homogeneous to inhomogeneous.[323] The appearance of a solitary neurofibroma is similar or identical to that of schwannoma on imaging studies.[334] Capsular calcification occasionally occurs.

Plexiform neurofibroma is the most common orbital mass in children with neurofibromatosis type 1.[274] In addition to plexiform neurofibroma, other orbital manifestations of neurofibromatosis include orbital osseous dysplasia, optic neoplasms (optic glioma, perioptic meningioma, neurofibroma, and schwannoma), and buphthalmos (congenital glaucoma).[273] These orbital abnormalities are relatively rare, being found in only 9 of 149 patients with neurofibromatosis in one series.[346]

Plexiform neurofibroma is a congenital lesion with clinical presentation in early childhood. This benign tumor is composed of all the elements of a peripheral nerve. The lesions are relatively vascular and diffusely infiltrate normal soft tissue structures. Involvement of deep orbital structures with plexiform neurofibroma is typically accompanied by clinically identifiable abnormalities of the lids and periorbital soft tissues.[274,347]

Plexiform neurofibroma is imaged on CT as an irregular mass of soft tissue attenuation with infiltrative margins. Inhomogeneous contrast enhancement is typically identified (Fig. 3-83). Thickening and enlargement of the eyelids, periorbital soft tissues, or extraocular muscles indicate infiltration of these structures with tumor.[273,347] CT may also demonstrate increased attenuation of the intraconal fat and enhancement, irregularity, and nodular thickening of the optic nerve sheath complex.[274] In children with buphthalmos associated with neurofibromatosis type 1, the globe is enlarged, and there is uveal and scleral thickening and enhancement with contrast material.[273,274]

On MRI, plexiform neurofibromas are isointense to muscle on T_1-weighted images and hyperintense on T_2-weighted images. There usually is marked enhancement with intravenous paramagnetic contrast material. The margins of the mass are irregular, and there may be infiltration of adjacent soft-tissue structures.

Optic Nerve Glioma

Optic nerve glioma of childhood is a low-grade astrocytic neoplasm that is distinct from the malignant optic glioma that occurs in adults. Retrochiasmatic gliomas usually exhibit a more aggressive growth pattern than prechiasmatic gliomas.[348] The peak age of presentation is approximately 5 years.[349,350] The incidence is slightly increased in girls. Optic nerve glioma accounts for approximately 2% of pediatric orbital masses. Approximately 25% of children with optic nerve gliomas have, or later develop, other stigmata of neurofibromatosis type 1.[351,352] Conversely, the reported inci-

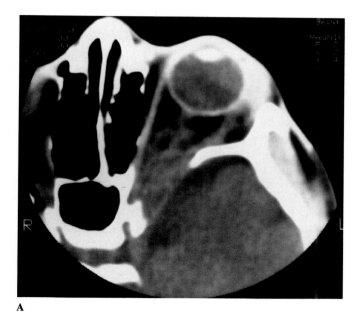

A

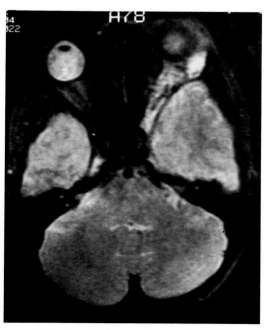

B

Fig. 3-83 Plexiform neurofibroma. **(A)** Axial CT shows an infiltrative left orbital tumor as well as a bony defect in the posterior wall of the orbit. **(B)** T$_2$-weighted MR image shows the infiltrative lesion, which produces moderate hyperintensity.

dence of optic nerve glioma in patients with known neurofibromatosis ranges from 1% to 15%.[353,354] The identification of bilateral optic nerve gliomas is virtually pathognomonic of neurofibromatosis type 1.[355,356]

Optic gliomas may arise anywhere along the anterior visual pathway. Approximately 30% to 40% of the tumors are confined to the intraorbital portion of the optic nerve at the time of diagnosis. Involvement of the intracranial portion of the optic nerve or optic chiasm has important implications for surgical

and radiation therapy. Disease may also spread into the optic tracts, lateral geniculate nuclei, and optic radiations, leading to the term *visual pathway glioma*.[357] Optic nerve glioma is manifested clinically by nonpulsatile proptosis and severe visual loss. Young children rarely complain of the slow and progressive visual loss that is characteristic of these tumors. More commonly, these children are brought to medical attention because of strabismus, nystagmus, or developmental difficulties. Many children with neurofibromatosis type 1 are often visually asymptomatic when the diagnosis is made, with the tumor being identified during the course of screening studies. Mild or moderate proptosis occurs with primary intraorbital tumors, but less than 20% of patients with intracranial tumors have proptosis. Visual acuity is frequently reduced to less than 20/200. The visual field deficit is typically of the central scotoma type. Visual loss begins earlier with chiasmatic disease compared to gliomas that are confined to the optic nerve. Invasion of the third ventricle and hypothalamus from a chiasmatic lesion may be associated with increased intracranial pressure, hypopituitarism, obesity, dwarfism, diabetes insipidus, or precocious puberty.[358]

Optic nerve tumors, such as glioma and meningioma, tend to produce significant visual impairment early in the disease process, while proptosis is still minimal. Most other orbital masses do not cause visual impairment until proptosis is marked.

Optic nerve glioma is most often imaged on CT as symmetric fusiform enlargement of the involved optic nerve.[346,350,359] Moderate contrast enhancement of the lesion is usually identified.[338] In some cases, rim enhancement may occur. Contrast enhancement is usually less intense than that which occurs in meningiomas. When confined to the intraorbital portion of the optic nerve, the tumor typically has a fusiform shape, tapering at both ends. The dura surrounding the optic nerve is stretched but generally is not penetrated by the tumor, so that the mass is usually well circumscribed. The tumor may cause elongation of the optic nerve, producing a kinked appearance. Low-attenuation cystic areas may occur in the tumor, either in the form of multiple small cysts or as a single large cyst with thick, irregular walls. In most cases, the optic nerve itself cannot be differentiated from the surrounding glioma on CT. Some investigators have suggested that, in the optic glioma that occurs in patients with neurofibromatosis type 1, the tumor can be differentiated from the nerve itself on CT more often than in those patients without neurofibromatosis (Fig. 3-84). This may be related to circumferential perineural extension of the tumor, which occurs in patients with neurofibromatosis, as opposed to intraneural tumor growth, which is typical of optic gliomas that occurs in non-neurofibromatosis patients.[360]

An essential role of diagnostic imaging in cases of optic glioma is the detection of intracranial extension of tumor. Thin-section CT provides superior demonstration of the size of the optic canals compared to plain radiographs. Improved visualization of the intracranial portion of the optic nerve, the optic chiasm, and the anterior optic tracts can be achieved with

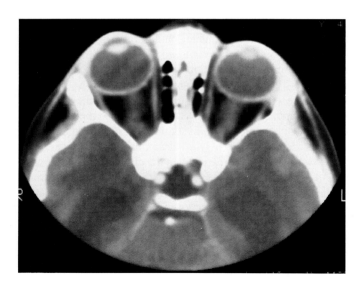

Fig. 3-84 Bilateral optic nerve gliomas in a patient with neurofibromatosis type 1. Contrast-enhanced CT shows enlargement and slight tortuosity of the optic nerve complexes bilaterally. The circumferential character of the neoplasm is apparent.

CT performed after intrathecal administration of water-soluble contrast material. In patients with neurofibromatosis type 1, dysplastic enlargement of the optic canal may occur with an underlying normal optic nerve.[360]

As mentioned previously, optic gliomas may extend posterior to the chiasm to involve the optic tracts, lateral geniculate bodies, and optic radiations. Involvement of these structures is indicated by enlargement and abnormal CT attenuation characteristics. Increased contrast enhancement (sometimes marked) is frequently present.[357,361] Glioma may also arise in the optic chiasm; there is an increased incidence of chiasmal glioma in patients with neurofibromatosis type 1.[346] In the presence of a mass in the region of the chiasm, demonstration of extension into the optic nerves or postchiasmal visual pathways helps differentiate an optic chiasmal glioma from other suprasellar tumors or hypothalamic gliomas.[357,362]

MRI is ideally suited for evaluation of optic gliomas.[363] MRI provides multiplanar imaging capability and allows excellent visualization of the intracanalicular and intracranial portions of the optic nerve without the need for intrathecal contrast agent administration (Fig. 3-85). T_1-weighted or intermediate images are best suited for depiction of optic nerve and chiasm anatomy. T_2-weighted images are superior for demonstration of disease in the optic radiations. Optic nerve glioma is typically isointense to gray matter on both T_1- and T_2-weighted imaging sequences. Large optic nerve gliomas may be hyperintense to gray matter on T_2-weighted images. Involvement of retrochiasmal optic pathways is demonstrated as areas of increased signal on T_2-weighted images.[358] MRI offers greater sensitivity in comparison to CT for the detection of retrochiasmal involvement.

Optic Nerve Sheath Meningioma

Optic nerve sheath meningioma is a rare tumor that tends to be somewhat more aggressive in children than in adults. Rapid growth and sarcomatous degeneration are common.[364] This tumor probably arises from the meningeal covering of the optic nerve sheath.[365] Approximately 80% of cases are unilateral; bilateral lesions are more common in patients with neurofibromatosis type 1.[366]

The CT findings in cases of optic nerve sheath meningioma usually allow distinction from optic nerve glioma.[359] The tumor often arises eccentrically from the side of the optic nerve. The lesion is usually of slightly higher attenuation than the nerve itself on unenhanced scans and demonstrates intense enhancement after intravenous contrast medium administration. In contradistinction to optic nerve glioma, dural penetration usually occurs, producing irregular margins on CT. Calcification is occasionally present. In some cases, meningioma grows to surround the optic nerve. CT then demonstrates a thick cuff of tumor surrounding the lower-attenuation optic nerve, often with an area of more marked tumor mass anteriorly or at the orbital apex.[367] Optic nerve sheath meningioma may involve the optic chiasm and, rarely, the posterior optic pathways.[368]

Orbital meningioma typically demonstrates high signal intensity on T_2-weighted MR images. Cystic components may be identified. The same principles relating to tumor morphology as described with CT apply to MRI. MRI is relatively insensitive for the detection of calcification, which is an important CT finding in the differentiation of meningioma

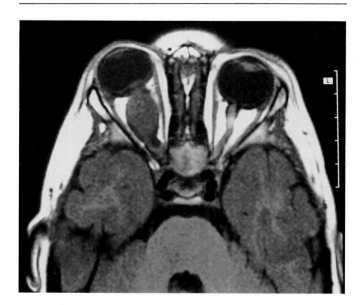

Fig. 3-85 Optic nerve glioma in a patient with neurofibromatosis type 1. Axial T_1-weighted MR image shows fusiform enlargement of the intraorbital and intracanalicular portions of the right optic nerve. The left optic nerve is normal.

from optic nerve glioma. Densely calcified lesions generally produce low signal intensity on both T_1- and T_2-weighted MR images. Posterior extension into the optic tracts, lateral geniculate bodies, and optic radiations produces increased signal in these structures on T_2-weighted images.[326,368]

Metastatic Disease

The most common tumors associated with orbital metastases in children are neuroblastoma and Ewing tumor.[369] In both these diseases, the metastases primarily involve the bony structures that make up the orbital walls. Metastatic lesions are usually present concomitantly elsewhere in the skull and skeleton. There are unusual cases in which metastatic neuroblastoma infiltrates orbital soft tissue structures. Orbital neuroblastoma is bilateral in more than 50% of cases. There are instances in which exophthalmos due to metastatic disease is the initial clinical presentation of neuroblastoma with a primary lesion located in the abdomen.

Bone scintigraphy is routinely utilized in the evaluation of patients with Ewing tumor and neuroblastoma for the detection of osseous metastases. As elsewhere in the skeleton, orbital involvement is usually indicated by areas of increased tracer accumulation. Plain radiographs may be normal or demonstrate permeative osseous destruction. The bony metastases frequently result in expansile lesions that protrude into the orbit and cause proptosis. These masses typically remain confined by the periosteum and, therefore, protrude into the extraconal space but do not invade soft tissue structures of the orbit.

On CT, the extraconal mass of metastatic neuroblastoma is usually of relatively high attenuation and may have ill-defined borders (Fig. 3-86).[338] Extension into the preseptal space does not usually occur except in advanced disease, a feature that aids in differentiating this entity from rhabdomyosarcoma. Bone-window images show permeative destruction. Ocular metastases are imaged as areas of abnormally high attenuation, usually projecting into the vitreous cavity.[370]

MRI in cases of orbital metastatic neuroblastoma demonstrates obliteration of the marrow spaces in the orbital walls by low-signal material on T_1-weighted images. The extraconal orbital metastatic deposits typically produce low signal on T_1-weighted images and high signal on T_2-weighted images. The T_2-weighted sequences are best suited for differentiation of the tumor deposits from normal structures and for the detection of invasion of normal orbital components.

Orbital abnormality in leukemia and metastatic lymphoma may occur secondary to neoplastic infiltration of orbital soft tissue structures, orbital hemorrhage, or opportunistic infection.[338] Myeloid leukemia and Burkitt lymphoma appear to have a particular predilection for orbital involvement.[371] In most cases, diffuse infiltration of orbital structures occurs, and CT or MRI demonstrates extraocular muscle enlargement,

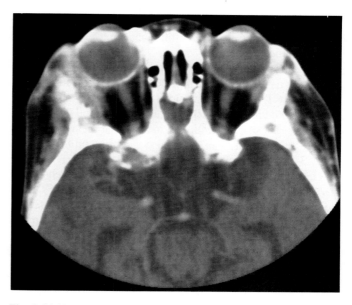

Fig. 3-86 Metastatic neuroblastoma. Contrast-enhanced CT demonstrates marked destruction of the orbital walls, with soft tissue components extending into the extraconal lateral orbital spaces as well as intracranially and into the infratemporal fossae.

scleral thickening, or abnormal fat attenuation or signal (Fig. 3-87). In some cases of leukemia, a relatively localized orbital mass of leukemic cells may occur, usually in the anterior orbit.[372]

Ocular metastases are quite rare. Involvement of the eye usually occurs by hematogenous seeding of the highly vas-

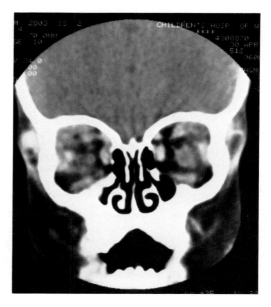

Fig. 3-87 Histiocytic lymphoma. Contrast-enhanced coronal CT shows diffuse infiltration of orbital structures in this patient with histiocytic lymphoma.

cular uveal tract (the layer between the retina and sclera). The posterior temporal portion of the uveal tract is probably the most common site.

Ocular metastases are imaged on CT and MRI as one or more soft tissue masses that project into the vitreous. Detection with CT is frequently aided by contrast enhancement. There may be retinal detachment and a subretinal fluid collection. The lack of calcification in most ocular metastases helps in the differentiation of these lesions from retinoblastoma (Fig. 3-88).

The orbit may be secondarily involved by extension of paranasal sinus tumors or primary bone tumors.[373,374] Bone neoplasms that may arise in the orbital walls include Ewing tumor and osteoma. Paranasal sinus and nasal cavity tumors that tend to expand into the orbit in children include juvenile angiofibroma, rhabdomyosarcoma, and lymphoma. CT and MRI usually are the most useful imaging modalities for evaluation of these lesions and assessing the degree of orbital involvement. Radionuclide flow studies and angiography are helpful in the diagnosis of juvenile angiofibroma.

The orbit is frequently involved in cases of Langerhans cell histiocytosis when lesions in the bony orbital walls protrude into the orbit to cause proptosis.[375] Although orbital wall lesions may be difficult to detect on plain radiographs, lesions with the typical radiographic features of Langerhans cell histiocytosis may be identified elsewhere in the skull on plain radiographs. Bone scintigraphy, if performed, may be normal or show faint areas of increased tracer accumulation. CT is probaby best suited for evaluation of these lesions. Bone-window images demonstrate a lucent area in the diploic space

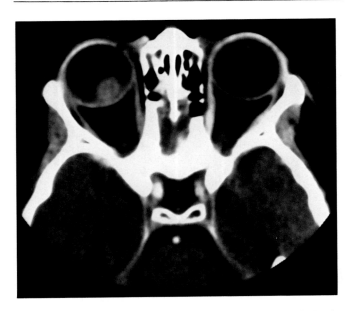

Fig. 3-88 Ocular recurrence in a patient with acute lymphoblastic leukemia. CT demonstrates an intraocular mass in the right globe as well as slight thickening of the uveal-scleral soft tissues posteriorly.

of the involved bone that has thin sclerotic margins. A soft tissue mass extending from this area usually remains confined to the extraconal space.[338] Although the osseous changes are not well demonstrated on MRI, there is usually excellent depiction of the soft tissue component, which has increased signal on T_2-weighted images. Diffuse infiltration of orbital soft tissue structures may occur with fulminant Langerhans cell histiocytosis.

Lacrimal Gland Masses

Approximately 50% of space-occupying lesions arising in the lacrimal gland are of the lymphoid-inflammatory type.[376] This includes a spectrum of abnormalities: dacryoadenitis, nonspecific lymphocytic infiltration, lymphocytic hyperplasia, idiopathic pseudotumor, leukemic infiltration, and primary malignant lymphoma.[349] Although the lacrimal gland is the most common site of primary orbital lymphoma, this is a rare neoplasm in the pediatric age group. Lymphocytic infiltration of the lacrimal gland may occur in patients with connective tissue disease. The lacrimal gland is a relatively common site of leukemic infiltration; this typically produces bilateral abnormality (Fig. 3-89). The lacrimal gland is a common site of involvement in idiopathic inflammatory pseudotumor.

Current imaging modalities, in general, do not allow accurate distinction between benign and malignant lacrimal gland masses, but some findings are helpful in narrowing the differential diagnosis.[349,376,377] Acute dacryoadenitis and lymphoid hyperplasia typically are relatively homogeneous and have well-defined margins on CT and MRI. Gland enlargement may be marked, resulting in displacement and deformation but not invasion of the globe. The margins of the enlarged lacrimal gland are usually ill defined in cases of inflammatory pseudotumor. There may be irregular contrast enhancement. Leukemic infiltration produces nonspecific lacrimal gland enlargement that is usually bilateral.

Primary malignant lymphoma that involves the lacrimal gland is unilateral, and the margins of the enlarged gland are usually somewhat ill defined. Although some aggressive malignant lymphomas produce frank destruction of bone, most of these tumors tend to mold themselves around existing orbital structures and may cause displacement but generally not extensive infiltration or bony erosion. The globe is displaced medially and anteriorly. Contrast enhancement is identified on CT scans.

Lacrimal gland lymphoma is imaged as a mass of low intensity on T_1-weighted MR images and increased intensity on T_2-weighted images. The MR signal characteristics in general do not allow distinction between a benign and a malignant lesion. On T_2-weighted images, however, pseudotumor is generally isointense or only minimally hyperintense to fat, in contrast to the usual hyperintense appearance of most neoplasms.

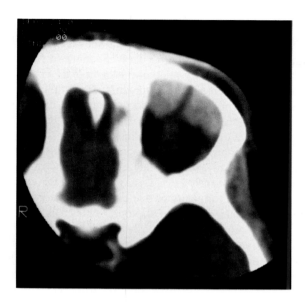

Fig. 3-89 Leukemic infiltration of the lacrimal gland. Axial CT shows lobular enlargement of the left lacrimal gland.

The most common epithelial cell neoplasm of the lacrimal gland in children is the benign mixed cell tumor (pleomorphic adenoma). This tumor is similar to those neoplasms of the same histology that occur in the salivary glands. As opposed to lymphoma, the mixed cell tumor is encapsulated, and imaging with CT or MRI typically demonstrates a sharply marginated lacrimal gland mass. On CT, these lesions are generally of relatively high attenuation and demonstrate some degree of contrast enhancement. Low-attenuation cystic components may be identified.[376] The globe is displaced inferiorly and medially. Five percent to 10% of mixed cell tumors are malignant, in which case imaging usually demonstrates poorly defined margins and evidence of invasion of adjacent structures. Lacrimal gland carcinoma is rare in pediatrics.

Inflammatory Disease and Orbital Manifestations of Systemic Disease

Orbital Pseudotumor

Orbital pseudotumor is a nongranulomatous inflammatory disorder of unknown etiology. Although this condition is usually encountered in adults, more than 16% of cases occur in children and adolescents.[378] The clinical presentation is proptosis, painful ophthalmoparesis, and, occasionally, a palpable mass.[379] Orbital involvement may be unilateral or bilateral. Histologic examination demonstrates nonspecific round cell infiltration of orbital fat, muscles, sclera, or lacrimal gland. Orbital infiltration that is radiographically identi-

cal to pseudotumor has been identified in children with Wegener granulomatosis and sarcoidosis.[380,381]

The CT findings in orbital pseudotumor are varied (Fig. 3-90). Most cases demonstrate relatively localized involvement of the immediate retrobulbar area. There are increased attenuation of the orbital fat, irregular thickening and increased attenuation of the uveal-scleral margins and the optic nerve. These structures show moderate contrast enhancement. The extraocular muscles may be enlarged and demonstrate irregular, thickened margins and abnormal contrast enhancement. In some cases, there is diffuse involvement of virtually all orbital structures, which results in marked proptosis. Sometimes relatively localized involvement of the lacrimal gland may occur. An unusual presentation is a relatively well-defined, focal mass in either the intraconal or the extraconal space.[379]

Some cases of orbital pseudotumor consist of isolated involvement of one or more extraocular muscles (myositic pseudotumor). CT demonstrates diffuse enlargement of the involved muscle. The margins are somewhat irregular and usually show abnormal contrast enhancement. The thickening and irregularity also involve the muscle tendons, which helps in differentiating orbital pseudotumor from thyroid ophthalmopathy.[382] In the latter condition, the enlargement of the muscle spares the tendons.

MRI in orbital pseudotumor, as with CT, demonstrates uveal-scleral thickening, extraocular muscle enlargement, and irregular muscle insertions. These areas of involvement characteristically are approximately isointense to extraocular muscles and hypointense to orbital fat on T_1-weighted images and are approximately isointense to orbital fat on T_2-weighted

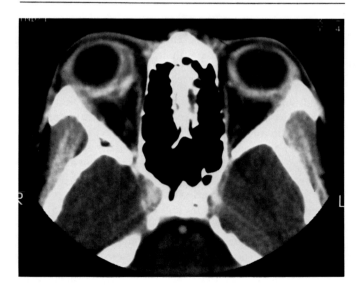

Fig. 3-90 Orbital pseudotumor. Contrast-enhanced CT shows marked thickening and irregular enhancement of the scleral structures, extraocular muscles, and optic nerve complexes bilaterally. There is also evidence of fluid in the space of Tenon.

images. Fat in the involved orbit usually has a decrease in signal intensity on T_1-weighted images in comparison to normal fat on the contralateral side. The signal characteristics of orbital pseudotumor on MRI are similar to those of other benign inflammatory abnormalities, such as orbital cellulitis and infectious myositis. The relatively modest increase in signal on T_2-weighted images allows differentiation from most malignant neoplasms, which generally produce markedly increased signal on T_2-weighted images.[383]

Thyroid Ophthalmopathy

Approximately 5% of patients with Graves disease are younger than 15 years of age. Of these children, only a small number develop orbital involvement. In thyroid ophthalmopathy, one or more of the extraocular muscles become enlarged and edematous. Histologic examination demonstrates mononuclear inflammatory cell infiltration and some degree of muscle fiber necrosis. An autoimmune process due to circulating antithyroglobulin complexes has been implicated; elevated thyroid hormone levels alone do not produce ophthalmopathy. The severity of orbital involvement has little or no relation to the degree of thyroid dysfunction. The condition may be unilateral or bilateral and may involve one or more of the extraocular muscles in any combination. There is an unexplained propensity for involvement of the inferior and medial rectus muscles.[384]

Orbital imaging in cases of suspected thyroid ophthalmopathy should be performed with either CT or MRI.[384] Both coronal and axial imaging planes are essential for accurate depiction of muscle morphology. These imaging procedures confirm muscle enlargement as the etiology of clinically apparent proptosis. Enlargement is most prominent in the midsection of the affected extraocular muscle, with relative sparing of the tendinous origins and insertions; this has been termed the Coke-bottle sign. This appearance contrasts with that of orbital myositic pseudotumor, in which the tendinous portions of the muscles are also enlarged.

On unenhanced CT scans, the involved muscles in thyroid ophthalmopathy may show slightly decreased attenuation compared to normal muscles. Prominent contrast enhancement of the involved muscles may be identified in some cases (Fig. 3-91). Iodinated contrast material usually adds no significant diagnostic information in cases of thyroid ophthalmopathy, however, and the iodine load may interfere with subsequent biochemical thyroid studies. The lacrimal gland is enlarged in some cases of thyroid ophthalmopathy.

In most children with thyroid ophthalmopathy, orbital involvement is bilateral and symmetric. In 10% to 30% of affected patients, however, unilateral or asymmetric involvement occurs. In both symmetric and asymmetric presentations, the inferior and medial rectus muscles are the most frequently involved and are typically the most markedly enlarged. Unilateral, isolated enlargement of a single rectus muscle (usually the inferior rectus) has been reported in some cases of thyroid ophthalmopathy.

Optic Neuritis

Optic neuritis is a general term that indicates optic nerve inflammation, degeneration, or demyelination. In childhood, this condition is usually related to a neurologic or systemic disease such as meningitis, encephalitis, or multiple sclerosis. In some cases, a viral illness accompanies or precedes the clinical symptoms. Exogenous toxins, such as lead or chloramphenicol, are sometimes implicated.

The most important role for diagnostic imaging in cases of optic neuritis is to exclude other conditions that may have similar clinical findings. CT may demonstrate cylindric enlargement and tortuosity of one or both optic nerves.[385] In some cases, enlargement of the optic chiasm is also present.[386,387] Coronal scans are essential for accurate depiction of optic nerve size.[388] Abnormal enhancement is sometimes identified in the involved nerve. When optic nerve enlargement is marked and unilateral, correlation with the clinical findings is required for differentiation from an optic nerve neoplasm. The differential diagnosis of an enlarged optic nerve in childhood includes optic nerve glioma, optic sheath meningioma, nerve infiltration by lymphoma or leukemia, sarcoidosis, and optic neuritis.

As with CT, MRI in cases of optic neuritis is normal or demonstrates a variable degree of enlargement of the optic nerve.[387] In some cases, a subtle abnormal increase in signal on T_2-weighted images is identified; this finding is difficult to appreciate in most cases because the central fat surrounding the optic nerve produces relatively intense signal on T_2-weighted images and tends to obscure the nerve abnormality (Fig. 3-92).[388]

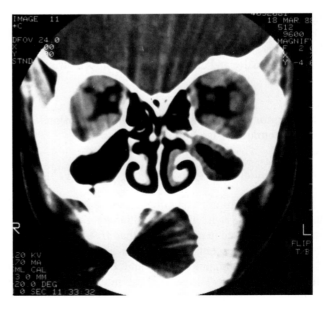

Fig. 3-91 Thyroid ophthalmopathy. Contrast-enhanced coronal CT shows enlargement of the extraocular muscles and edema in the extraconal fat bilaterally.

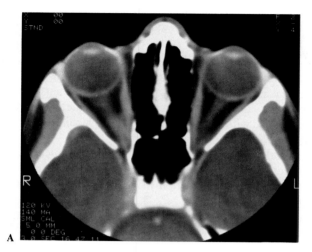

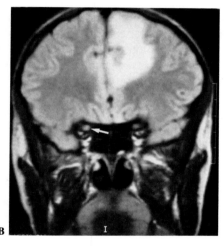

Fig. 3-92 Optic neuritis. **(A)** Contrast-enhanced axial CT shows enlargement and slight irregularity of the right optic nerve complex in this patient with acute disseminated encephalomyelitis. **(B)** Coronal T$_2$-weighted MR image shows slight enlargement and increased signal arising from the right optic nerve complex. A large area of edema in the frontal lobe is also visible.

Enlargement of the optic nerve complex may occur in cases of increased intracranial pressure. This is due to distention of the subarachnoid spaces surrounding the nerves rather than to enlargement of the nerves themselves. The prominent rim of cerebrospinal fluid surrounding the nerves can be imaged on MRI or CT cisternography. The nerve sheaths are usually tortuous on axial images. Elevation of the optic discs may also be visible.[389]

Optic Atrophy and Hypoplasia

Optic atrophy may develop after traumatic, degenerative, neoplastic, or vascular insult to the optic nerve. Optic atrophy is relatively common in children with cerebral palsy. Demonstration of optic atrophy on imaging studies is usually an incidental finding. Absolute measurements of optic nerve diameter are of limited usefulness because reliable data do not exist for the range of normal optic nerve size in children. In cases with unilateral involvement, the uninvolved optic nerve provides an internal standard. Acquired optic atrophy is differentiated from developmental optic nerve hypoplasia by the clinical history and the presence or absence of intracranial anomalies.

Sickle Cell Disease

Several abnormalities may cause orbital symptoms in children with sickle cell disease. In these patients, pain, proptosis, and lid edema may indicate the presence of orbital cellulitis, osteomyelitis, orbital apex syndrome, or bone infarction of the orbital wall. Differentiation of infections from vaso-occlusive orbital abnormalities is important in these cases because the approach to treatment is quite different.

If performed promptly after the development of symptoms, bone scintigraphy may be utilized to establish the diagnosis of an orbital wall infarct.[390,391] As elsewhere in the skeleton, bone infarction is manifested by areas of decreased tracer accumulation. Within 48 to 72 hours, revascularization results in nonspecific increased tracer accumulation. Osteomyelitis involving the orbital walls may be detected on bone scintigraphy as areas of increased tracer accumulation; unless scanning is performed promptly, however, the findings do not allow differentiation from a revascularizing bone infarct. CT scanning in cases of orbital wall infarction in sickle cell disease frequently demonstrates soft tissue abnormalities similar or identical to those of orbital cellulitis, such as edema of the peripheral orbital fat, extraocular muscle displacement, and proptosis (Fig. 3-93).[391]

Orbital apex syndrome is held to result from red cell sludging in small vessels supplying the optic nerve; this produces orbital pain and clinical findings of optic neuritis. An additional factor is vaso-occlusion in other small orbital vessels, resulting in edema of orbital fat and muscles and compression of the optic nerve.[392] CT in cases of orbital apex syndrome may be normal or demonstrate increased attenuation of orbital fat. Bone scintigraphy in these cases is normal unless there is concomitant bone infarction.

Trauma

It is estimated that 160,000 school-age children per year experience eye trauma in the United States.[393] Approximately 1 in every 119 children sustains an eye injury severe enough to require hospital treatment each year.[394] Hyphema and globe lacerations are the most common clinically encountered sequelae of eye trauma in children.[395] Injuries for which diagnostic imaging procedures are helpful include fracture, foreign body, and penetrating injury.

Fractures are the most common indication for imaging of the orbit after trauma. The orbital walls may be involved by

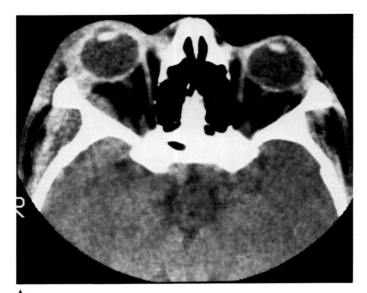

A

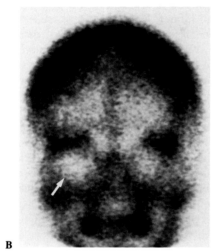

B

Fig. 3-93 Orbital infarction in sickle cell disease. (A) Contrast-enhanced axial CT scan shows thickening of the extraconal soft tissues in the right lateral orbit. The CT findings do not allow accurate distinction between an infectious and infarctive etiology. (B) Bone scintigraphy (anterior image) shows a relative photopenic appearance of the right orbit (arrow), confirming the presence of bone infarction. Abnormal increased uptake throughout the remainder of the skull is due to the chronic anemia.

extension of a fracture line from facial or skull trauma remote to the orbit, such as inferior extension of a frontal bone fracture or orbital wall involvement in a Le Fort facial fracture. A direct blow to the orbital margin may also produce a fracture. The term *blowout fracture* refers to fracture of an orbital wall with intact orbital rims resulting from a blow to the eye by an object that is too large to enter the orbit. The mechanism of this injury is thought to be a sudden increase in intraorbital pressure due to a blow to the globe, resulting in rupture of orbital contents through the orbital wall. It has also been suggested that a blow to the inferior orbital rim may produce a similar fracture of the orbital floor as a result of buckling.

Clinical findings with blowout fractures include periorbital ecchymoses, infraorbital hypesthesia, enophthalmos, impaired extraocular muscle movement, and vertical diplopia. Diplopia is the most common symptom. The orbital floor is the most common site of a blowout fracture; the medial wall is a somewhat less common site, and the roof accounts for the fewest cases. Blowout fractures that involve the orbital floor are associated with a blowout fracture of the medial wall of the orbit in 20% to 50% of the cases.

Most orbital fractures are detectable with technically adequate radiographs. CT is often indicated for better definition of the fracture and for detection of soft tissue abnormalities. Direct coronal CT imaging generally provides the most useful information. Additional direct oblique sagittal CT scans may be helpful in some patients with fractures of the orbital roof or floor.

Bone-window images with CT generally allow excellent visualization of the fracture line. Fracture fragments may be displaced into the adjacent maxillary or ethmoid sinuses. Areas of edema and hemorrhage are identified in the orbit. Intracranial abnormalities frequently accompany orbital roof fractures. A particularly important role for CT evaluation of patients with blowout fractures is demonstration of the status of the adjacent inferior rectus muscle. Restriction of rectus muscle movement may result from incarceration of the muscle by fracture fragments or herniation of the adjacent orbital fat pad through the fracture site. Also, a fracture fragment may be displaced into the orbital cavity and impinge on a rectus muscle, resulting in limitation of eye movement.[396]

CT is an excellent modality for the evaluation of penetrating injuries of the eye and orbit. Soft tissue injuries, hematoma formation, and osseous injuries are well demonstrated. CT is quite sensitive for the detection and localization of intraocular and intraorbital foreign bodies (Fig. 3-94).

CT is sometimes useful for detection of hemorrhagic choroidal detachment, which may occur with blunt trauma or penetrating injury of the eye. Acute hemorrhagic choroidal detachment is imaged on CT as an irregular, crescentic collection of high attenuation compared to vitreous. As the blood is resorbed, the attenuation values decrease.[397]

PAROTID GLAND

The parotid gland is composed of two lobes: one deep and the other superficial. Anteriorly, the gland opposes the masseter muscle and the posterior surface of the ramus of the mandible. Medially, the deep lobe abuts the parapharyngeal space just lateral to the wall of the nasopharynx and oropharynx. The posterior margins of the parotid gland abut the carotid sheath and a portion of the sternocleidomastoid and digastric muscles.

The parotid gland is drained by the duct of Stensen, which courses anterior and lateral to the masseter muscle. The duct then passes through the buccinator space and enters the oral cavity adjacent to the upper third molar. The facial nerve and

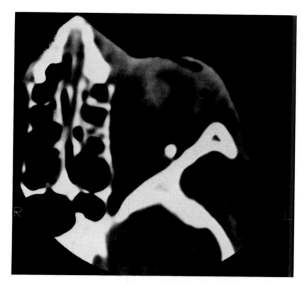

Fig. 3-94 Orbital trauma. Axial CT shows a metallic foreign body posterior to the globe. There are areas of hemorrhage and air visible in the deformed globe. Air and hemorrhage are also visible in the orbit proper.

its branches are deeply embedded in the gland; these relationships are important considerations in any surgical procedure.

There are various pathologic conditions that enlarge the parotid. These include localized inflammatory disease, systemic autoimmune illness, and neoplastic disease. These entities are differentiated by clinical history and physical examination. The inflammatory masses are often transient, recurrent, and painful and may be associated with other autoimmune symptoms.

Neoplastic masses, on the other hand, are discrete, palpable masses that may be associated with cranial nerve VII palsy and cervical adenopathy. In general, CT and MRI are the imaging modalities of choice to evaluate a possible neoplasm or a large parotid mass.[398,399] These studies will determine whether a mass lesion is intrinsic or extrinsic to the gland and whether cranial nerve VII is encased. They also will determine the extent of involvement of the deep lobe.

Differentiation between benign and malignant tumors is often difficult on CT. A benign lesion, however, will often demonstrate high density and have sharply demarcated borders, whereas the malignant masses are more infiltrative in nature. Most parotid neoplasms are located in the superficial portion of the gland. Clinically, they present as a painless mass anterior to the lower portion of the ear lobe. Approximately 10% of the tumors will be located in the deep lobe behind the mandible. Because of the proximity of this portion of the gland to the parapharyngeal space, masses that arise in the deep lobe often project into the oropharynx.

In the pediatric population, half of all parotid tumors are benign hemangiomas (Fig. 3-95). These masses appear by 1 month of age and involute by 5 years of age. On CT, they appear as well-demarcated masses that show dense contrast enhancement. Lymphangiomas or cystic hygromas are also commonly found in pediatric patients with a parotid mass. Half of these are present at birth; and 90% are present by 2 years of age. They most often involve the surrounding structures and are rarely confined to the parotid gland. On CT, they have attenuation values less than those of the gland and show slight enhancement. Malignant tumors of the parotid gland are uncommon in the pediatric age group; the most common are mucoepidermoid carcinoma and acinous cell carcinoma.

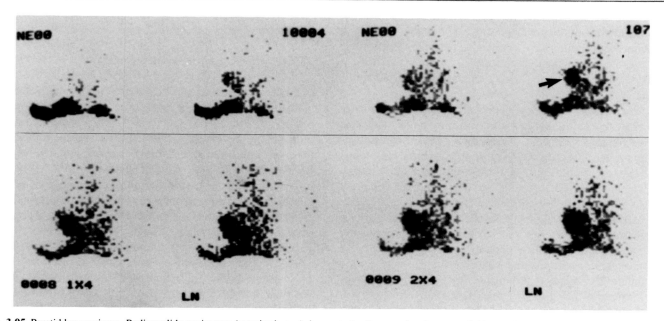

Fig. 3-95 Parotid hemangioma. Radionuclide angiogram (anterior image) demonstrates the vascular character of this parotid hemangioma in a newborn.

Inflammatory masses of the parotid gland may be due to infection, recurrent sialadenitis, sialosis, and noninflammatory abnormalities. Of the infectious group, the most common form is chronic recurrent sialadenitis. Acute sialadenitis usually is due to infection with mumps virus. Noninfectious etiologies include autoimmune disease, which may be isolated to the gland (eg, Mikulicz disease), or, if there are systemic complications, diseases such as Sjögren syndrome. Sialosis and sarcoidosis are two of the noninfectious etiologies of parotid gland enlargement. CT evaluation of these masses will not differentiate one from the other, but sialography will help make these distinctions.

Acute suppurative sialadenitis is most often a disease of debilitated adults. About 35% to 40% of cases, however, occur in neonates. Premature infants are most often affected. Dehydration is thought to play an important role in the pathogenesis. The organisms responsible for the infection may include staphylococci, *P. aeruginosa*, streptococci, pneumococci, and *E. coli*. The infection is usually localized to one or both parotid glands. The other salivary glands are less frequently involved.

Sialography is contraindicated during the acute phase of suppurative sialadenitis. CT shows enlargement and increased attenuation values of the involved salivary gland. There is usually diffuse increased contrast enhancement. With MRI, the edema produced by acute sialadenitis usually causes diffusely increased signal intensity of the gland on T_2-weighted images; lower signal intensity occurs if there is marked cellular infiltration, however.

Chronic recurrent sialadenitis presents clinically as repeated unilateral, painful enlargement of the parotid gland with a milky discharge. Sialography demonstrates pooling of contrast material in ectatic parotid ducts. In some cases, sialectasis, that is, narrowing and irregularity of the ductal system, is seen (Fig. 3-96). CT will show an enlarged but dense gland. Calculi are occasionally identified, and large cysts or mucoceles may occasionally develop.

Patients with sialosis have a nontender but enlarged gland as well as some underlying illness, such as chronic liver disease, diabetes, or malnutrition. Another etiology is postirradiation change.

In sarcoidosis, the parotid glands are enlarged and multinodular in appearance but painless. In autoimmune disorders such as Sjögren syndrome or Mikulicz disease, the glands have a similar appearance. In primary Sjögren (sicca) complex, patients demonstrate keratoconjunctivitis and xerostomia with parotid enlargement. Secondary Sjögren complex consists of the sicca complex with connective tissue disease such as rheumatoid arthritis, systemic lupus erythematosus, scleroderma, or periarteritis nodosa. Thirty percent of patients with Sjögren syndrome have parotid involvement.

Both Sjögren syndrome and Mikulicz disease cause recurrent unilateral or bilateral parotid swelling. Boys are involved more commonly than girls, whereas in the adult form there is a female predominance. On sialography, there is destruction of

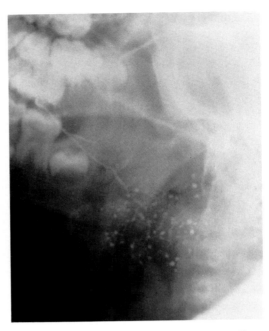

Fig. 3-96 Sialectasis. Parotid sialogram shows multiple, small saccular collections due to ectatic ducts scattered throughout the gland.

the duct with saccule formation and, occasionally, extravasation of contrast medium.

Viral infections frequently cause glandular swelling. These include infections with mumps virus (most common), cytomegalovirus, influenza virus, and coxsackievirus. These different types of infection must correlate with systemic patterns in their differentiation.

NASOLACRIMAL APPARATUS

Epiphora

The lacrimal gland is located in the upper outer quadrant of the orbit. Tears flow from the gland to the lateral aspect of the globe and then enter the superior and inferior canaliculi of the lacrimal sac. The sac drains inferiorly through the nasolacrimal duct into the nasal cavity. There are several indentations in this ductal system. The most prominent of these lies inferior to and in front of the opening into the nasal cavity and is called the valve of Krause.

Tears are secreted by the lacrimal glands, which are situated lateral and superior to the globes. Under normal circumstances, the tears either evaporate from the surface of the globe or drain into the lacrimal passages, where they pass into the inferior meatus of the nose. Epiphora refers to an abnormal overflow of tears. It has two causes: excessive lacrimation and obstruction of the drainage apparatus. Obstruction of the nasolacrimal system may be due to congenital stenosis, inflammatory processes, trauma (including ocular foreign bodies), and tumors. The obstruction caused by these disease processes can be complete or incomplete. Approximately 90% of nasolacrimal obstructions are complete. The most common site of obstruction is at the junction of the lacrimal sac with the nasolacrimal duct. The second most common site of obstruction is in the common canaliculus. Less frequent sites of obstruction occur within the nasolacrimal sac or duct.

Epiphora is a difficult clinical problem to evaluate in a noninvasive manner. Radionuclide dacryocystography is a relatively simple technique to evaluate this clinical problem. With this technique, the site of anatomic obstruction usually can be clearly delineated. If the radionuclide technique is inconclusive, positive contrast dacryocystography can be performed. This is, however, a difficult procedure to perform in most children.

Nasolacrimal Mucocele

A lacrimal sac mucocele is an uncommon mass that occurs in the medial canthal region of the orbits of children. It may connect with an intranasal cyst through an enlarged mucus-filled nasolacrimal duct, thereby forming a nasolacrimal mucocele. This lesion also has been termed a congenital dacryocystocele.

Clinically, patients with a lacrimal sac mucocele present with a nontender mass in the medial canthus of the eye that does not have induration or discoloration. Protrusion of a nasolacrimal mucocele into the nasal cavity may be identified clinically as a smooth cystic-appearing mass in the inferior aspect of the nasal cavity. If this obtains sufficient size, it may obstruct the nasal passage and may even bow the nasal septum to the contralateral side, partially obstructing the contralateral nasal passage as well.

Imaging of these infants is best achieved with CT. The triad of a cystic-appearing mass in the medial canthus of the eye, dilatation of the nasolacrimal duct, and a contiguous submucosal mass in the ipsilateral nasal cavity is diagnostic of a nasolacrimal mucocele. This constellation of imaging findings aids in differentiating this lesion from other causes of swelling at the medial canthus of the eye.[400,401]

TEMPORAL BONE

The temporal bone is a complex structure that can be involved in malformations, infections, trauma, and neoplasms. A discussion of the embryology and anatomy of the temporal bone is beyond the scope of this text. There are several eloquent discussions of this subject in the literature.[402,403]

Congenital Malformations

A prompt diagnosis of bilateral congenital hearing loss is crucial because speech and language development will be markedly retarded if this condition goes unrecognized or untreated. Such auditory sensory deprivation results in stunting of intellectual growth, impairment of intellectual maturity, limitation of development of creative and occupational skills, and diminution in quality of life. Unilateral hearing loss may be difficult to detect in the neonatal period.

Although the external ear is readily available for clinical examination, there is a poor correlation between the visible deformity of the auricle and malformations that might exist in the middle or inner ear. Similarly, if there is stenosis or atresia of the external auditory canal, the status of the middle and inner ears cannot be adequately assessed.

CT has had a significant effect on management of congenital ear malformations. It is only with this modality that the true extent of malformations of the temporal bone can be assessed.

Infants with anomalies of the calvaria, face, spine, and skeleton may also have an associated hearing deficit. For example, patients with anomalies of the inner ear usually have no identifiable abnormality of the external ear, but in more than 95% of cases there are anomalies in other parts of the body.

External Auditory Canal

Dysplasia of the external auditory canal is probably the result of failure of development or failure of canalization of the meatal plate, which is a solid core of epithelial cells that develops between the primary external meatus and the endodermal outpouching from the pharynx that ultimately gives rise to the middle ear cavity. Because most of the first and second branchial arches as well as the first pharyngeal pouch are developing concurrently with the meatal plate, anomalies of the middle ear and mastoid process are the rule rather than the exception. Anomalies of the inner ear are less commonly associated.[404]

Atresia of the external auditory canal is slightly more common in boys and is bilateral in approximately 30% of cases. A family history can be elicited in approximately 15% of cases. The auricle is almost invariably deformed. Concurrent deformity of the jaw usually implies a complicated type of atresia.[405] The atresia of the external canal may be either membranous or bony; some osseous atresias are incomplete (Fig. 3-97). Rarely, congenital stenosis of the canal may occur in a patient with a normal-appearing auricle. Although atresia of the external canal is usually an isolated phenomenon, a number of malformation syndromes have atresia of the external canal as one of their manifestations.

In most cases of atresia of the external auditory canal, the cartilaginous and osseous portions of the canal are absent. In the usual situation, a malformed auricle terminates on a bony overgrowth arising from the squamous portion of the temporal bone. This is referred to as the atresia plate (Fig. 3-98). In many cases, there is associated deformity of the ossicular chain, most commonly fusion of the malleus and incus in the epitympanic recess with absence of the malleoincudal joint.

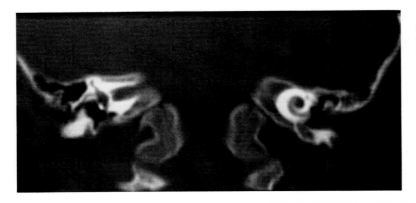

Fig. 3-97 Atresia of the external auditory canal. Coronal CT scan demonstrates soft tissue material filling the right external auditory canal to the level of the tympanic membrane. The external ear was markedly deformed. The middle ear cavity is small and the malleus is slightly hypoplastic.

Frequently, the manubrium of the malleus is absent, and the short process of the malleus is fused to the atresia plate.

Of significant concern to the surgeon is the course of the facial nerve canal. The labyrinthine segment of the canal is usually normal in cases of atresia of the external auditory canal, but the tympanic and mastoid segments are usually anomalous. In particular, the mastoid segment of the canal is more anterior in location than is normal.[406]

Dysplasia of the Middle Ear

Dysplasia with deformity of the ossicular chain is commonly associated with dysplasia of the external auditory canal. Isolated anomalies of the ossicular chain without accompanying malformations of the external ear are not uncommon, however.[407] The clinical presentation is that of a conductive hearing loss. There is no sex predominance, and the right and left ears are involved equally. The mandibular condyle and ramus may be hypoplastic.

Among the isolated congenital malformations of the ossicular chain, disconnection of the incudostapedial articulation is the most common.[408] Less common are fixations of the malleus or incus (or both), and most rare are congenital fixations of the stapes.

Syndrome-Related Hearing Impairment

A number of well-defined syndromes have a definite association with various malformations of the skull, spine, and skeleton (Table 3-11).

Fig. 3-98 Unilateral atresia of the external auditory canal. Coronal CT shows the bony margins of the external auditory canal to be absent. The malformed auricle ends in a dense bony plate. The ossicles are malformed and sit more posteriorly in the epitympanic recess than normal.

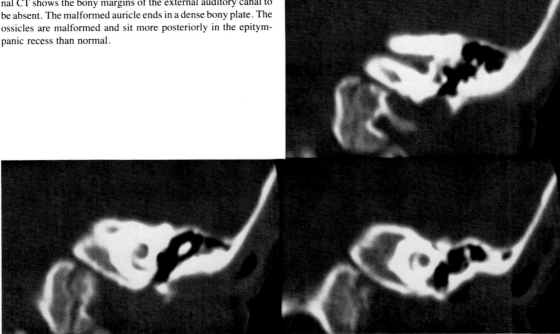

Otofacial Cranial Syndromes

Mandibulofacial Dysplasia (Treacher Collins Syndrome). Patients with mandibulofacial dysplasia have defective eyes, ears, and mandible. The ocular fissures are slanted downward, and there is a notch at the junction of the outer and middle thirds of the lower eyelid. The eyelashes are sparse or absent in the lower eyelids. The mandible is small and the chin receding, and there is a considerable degree of overbite.

The ears are always malformed, and there is frequent atresia of the external auditory canal. A conductive hearing loss is present in the great majority of cases. This disorder is inherited as an autosomal dominant condition, but approximately 60% of cases are sporadic fresh mutations.

The external auditory canal is anomalous in most cases. The anomalies range from mild stenosis to complete bony atresia (Fig. 3-99). The mastoid is usually underdeveloped and sclerotic. The ossicles are fused into a conglomerate mass that itself may be fused to the atresia plate of the external canal, to the epitympanic recess, or to both. The course of the facial nerve canal is abnormal, being more anteriorly placed than usual. The oval window is usually occluded as a result of dysplasia of the stapes.

Hemifacial Microsomia. This disorder may be a variant of mandibulofacial dysplasia with unilateral involvement. Clinically, there is fairly severe unilateral mandibular and maxillary hypoplasia. Macrostomia and microtia are associated with either atresia or severe stenosis of the external auditory canal. Another related disorder is acrofacial dysplasia, in which man-

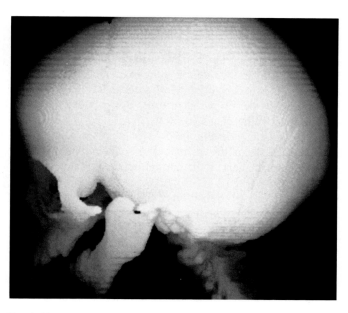

Fig. 3-99 Mandibulofacial dysplasia with bilateral atresia of the external auditory canal. Three-dimensional CT image shows severe micrognathia with relative overgrowth of the coronary process and hypoplasia of the mandibular condyle. The midportion of the zygomatic arch is absent. The external auditory canals are thick. In the middle ear cavities, the ossicles are fused to the atresia plate.

dibulofacial dysplasia occurs with preaxial reduction of the upper limbs. This disorder is inherited as an autosomal recessive condition.

Radiographically, the mandible and maxilla are markedly hypoplastic on the involved side. The external auditory canal is severely stenotic or atretic. More rarely it may be vertically oriented, with the external auditory meatus appearing in the neck. The tegmen of the temporal bone is markedly displaced inferiorly. The ossicles are also markedly deformed.

Craniofacial Syndromes

Crouzon Disease. Crouzon disease (craniofacial dysplasia) is frequently inherited as an autosomal dominant characteristic, although cases have been reported that lack a positive family history. The cranium is deformed as a result of bilateral coronal craniosynostosis, but other sutures may also be affected. Facial abnormalities include a parrot-beak deformity of the nose, hypoplasia of the maxillae, protrusion of the mandible, and exophthalmos.

The auricular manifestations of Crouzon disease include stenosis of the external auditory canal or bony atresia of the canal, a small tympanic cavity, and fixation of the ossicular chain (as a result of ankylosis of the malleus) to the walls of the epitympanic recess or fixation of the stapes to the promontory.

Apert Disease. Apert disease (acrocephaly-syndactyly) is rarely associated with anomalies of the ear, aside from an occasional case of fixation of the stapes to the promontory.

Table 3-11 Syndromes with Related Hearing Loss

Syndrome	External Ear	Middle Ear	Ossicles	Inner Ear
Otocranial-facial (ear-face-skull) syndromes				
Apert disease	0	0	+	0
Crouzon disease	+ + +	+ + +	+ +	0
Hemifacial microsomia	+ + +	+ + +	+ +	0
Mandibulofacial dysplasia	+ +	+ + +	+ +	0
Otocervical (ear-neck-shoulder) syndromes				
Cleidocranial dysplasia	+ +	+ +	0	0
Goldenhar syndrome	+ + +	+ + +	+ +	+ +
Klippel-Feil syndrome	+ +	+ +	+ +	+ + +
Sprengel deformity	0	0	+ +	0
Turner syndrome	0	0	+ +	0
Wildervanck syndrome	0	0	0	+ + +
Otoskeletal (ear-face-limb) syndromes				
Craniometaphyseal dysplasia	+	+ +	0	+ +
Frontometaphyseal dysplasia	0	0	+	+ +
Osteogenesis imperfecta	0	0	+	0
Osteopetrosis	+ +	+ +	+	+ + +

```
    0  =  not involved
    +  =  mild involvement
  + +  =  moderate involvement
+ + +  =  severe involvement
```

Otocervical Syndromes

Klippel-Feil Syndrome. Klippel-Feil syndrome is an association of short neck, low hairline, and limitation of neck mobility. Its estimated incidence is approximately 1 in 42,000 live births. Approximately 30% of patients have hearing loss that is usually sensorineural in type. Some patients present with conductive hearing loss.

Most of the ear anomalies involve the inner ear. These range from hypoplasia of the cochlea and semicircular canals to complete replacement of the normal inner ear structures by a simple otocyst (Fig. 3-100). Middle ear anomalies are also variable, ranging from fixation of the stapes to microtia with atresia of the external auditory canal.[409]

Wildervanck Syndrome. Wildervanck syndrome (cervical-oculoacoustic syndrome) is a rare association of Klippel-Feil–like fusions of the cervical or thoracic spine, congenital deafness, and retraction of the globe of one or both eyes. Paralysis of cranial nerve VI is also a frequent finding. This disorder occurs almost exclusively in girls. The radiographic findings show severe malformation of the inner ear structures, frequently with replacement by a large simple otocyst. The stapes is usually thickened and fixed.[410,411]

Goldenhar Syndrome. Goldenhar syndrome (oculo-auricular-vertebral syndrome) is an association of ocular anomalies, including epibulbar dermoid and coloboma, with auricular and vertebral anomalies. The spinal anomalies most commonly are hemivertebrae or block vertebrae. Occipitalization of the atlas also occurs. There is usually unilateral hypoplasia of the maxilla and mandible.

The auricular anomalies include microtia, atresia of the external auditory canal, severe dysplasia of the middle ear cavity with a narrow tympanic cavity, and absence of the ossicles. The inner ear anomalies include hypoplasia of the cochlea. The internal auditory canal is short and sharply angulated superiorly.

Otoskeletal Syndromes

Craniometaphyseal Dysplasia. Craniometaphyseal dysplasia is an autosomal recessive condition that is manifested by progressive enlargement of the metaphyses of the long bones and marked overgrowth of the craniofacial skeleton. There is progressive hearing loss in this disorder that may be sensorineural, conductive, or mixed in type. It is believed to be due to hyperostotic involvement of the otic capsule and bony proliferation in the tympanic cavity.

There is marked sclerosis of the base of the skull and calvaria with narrowing and constriction of the internal auditory canals, the external auditory canals, and the tympanic cavities (Fig. 3-101). Constriction of the facial nerve canals causes a high incidence of facial nerve paralysis, which is frequently bilateral.

Frontometaphyseal Dysplasia. Frontometaphyseal dysplasia is in many regards similar to craniometaphyseal dysplasia. There are excessive enlargement of the supraorbital ridges, absence of the frontal sinus, and micrognathia. These features distinguish these two entities.

The hyperostosis of the calvaria and skull base infiltrates the temporal bone and surrounds the cochlea. The internal

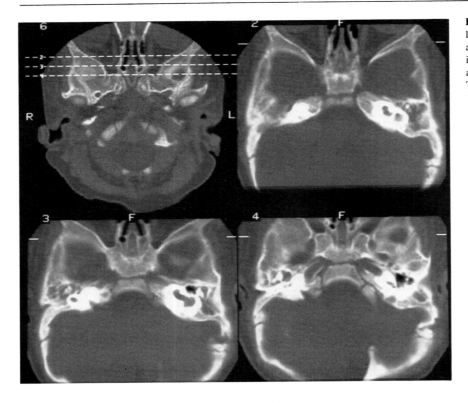

Fig. 3-100 Klippel-Feil syndrome. Axial CT shows the left inner ear to be a large simple otocyst. The internal auditory canal is absent. The right internal auditory canal is hypoplastic and is directed posteriorly. The cochlea is absent. The middle ear cavity on the right is opacified. The ossicles appear to be relatively normally formed.

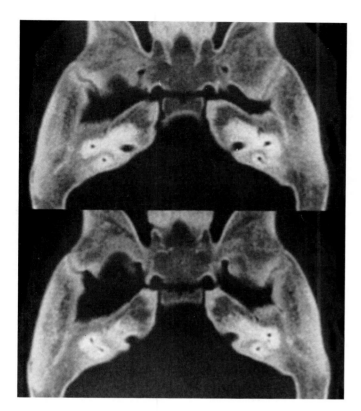

Fig. 3-101 Craniometaphyseal dysplasia. This 3-year-old girl had the classic cranial and long bone findings of craniometaphyseal dysplasia. She had bilateral neurosensory hearing loss. Axial CT demonstrates marked thickening of the calvaria and skull base with narrowing of the internal auditory canals. The semicircular canals stand out as radiolucent ovals in the dense bone.

auditory canal and facial nerve canals are not involved. The ossicles, however, are deformed.

Osteopetrosis. Osteopetrosis congenita is an autosomal recessive skeletal disorder that causes a marked increase in bone density. Numerous neural foramina are compressed by the expansion of the bone. The hyperostosis impinges on the neural foramina, including the internal auditory canal and the facial nerve canal. These canals are progressively narrowed by sclerotic bone, which also covers the oval and round windows.

A similar encroachment occurs in other conditions that cause hypostosis. These include endosteal hyperostosis (van Buchem syndrome), sclerosteosis, and hyperphosphatasia. A conductive hearing loss occurs in autosomal dominant osteogenesis imperfecta as a result of fixation of the stapes foot plate.

Temporal Bone Trauma

Fractures of the petrous portion of the temporal bone are classified on the basis of whether they do or do not involve the labyrinth. Labyrinthine fractures are further subdivided into tympanolabyrinthine fractures and pure labyrinthine fractures. The extralabyrinthine fractures are further subdivided depending on involvement or lack of involvement of the middle ear cavity (Table 3-12).

Clinically, a patient with a tympanolabyrinthine fracture has otorrhagia with laceration of the tympanic membrane, sensorineural hearing loss, and facial nerve palsy. These fractures may be axial, posterior oblique, or combined (Fig. 3-102).

Pure labyrinthine fractures do not involve the middle ear cavity, so that there will be no otorrhagia or laceration of the tympanic membrane. Nevertheless, sensorineural hearing loss and possible facial nerve palsy may occur. These fractures may be radiating transverse fractures or isolated fractures.

With extralabyrinthine fractures, the inner ear is spared. If the middle ear is involved, the patient will have a conductive hearing loss and otorrhagia with laceration of the tympanic membrane but no facial nerve palsy. These fractures are fur-

Table 3-12 Fractures of the Petrous Bone

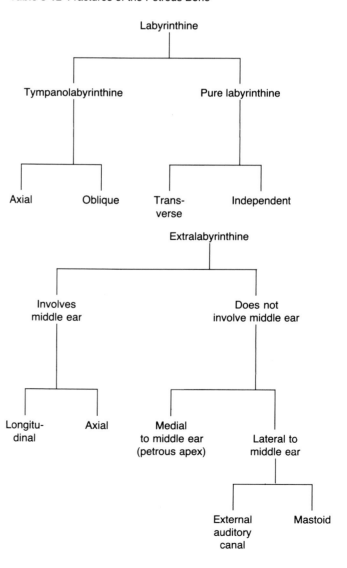

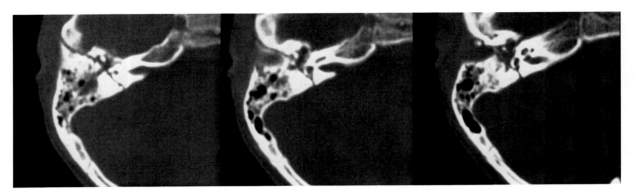

Fig. 3-102 Tympanolabyrinthine fracture. Axial CT demonstrates a posterior oblique tympanolabyrinthine fracture extending from the lateral margin of the temporal bone posteriorly and medially through the middle ear cavity and the labyrinth. There is disruption of the malleoincudal articulation.

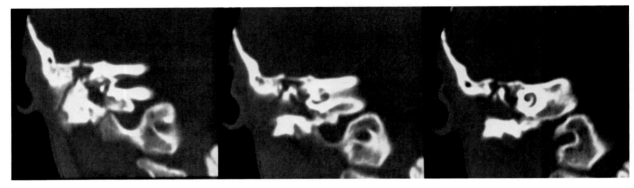

Fig. 3-103 Extralabyrinthine fracture. Coronal CT demonstrates a fracture line extending through the tegmen of the temporal bone with extension inferiorly and laterally through the middle ear cavity. There is disruption of the malleoincudal articulation. The middle ear cavity and external auditory canal are filled with blood.

ther subdivided into anterior and posterior axial fractures (Fig. 3-103).

Extralabyrinthine fractures that do not involve the middle ear cavity may be divided into three types. Fractures of the apex of the petrous bone frequently have lesions of adjacent cranial nerves, especially V and VI. Fractures of the mastoid bone may be accompanied by isolated facial nerve palsy. Isolated fractures of the external auditory canal show clinical evidence of a bloody discharge from the ear (Fig. 3-104).

Lesions of the ossicular chain can be isolated or associated with a fracture of the temporal bone. The suspensory mechanism of the incus is fragile, and therefore the incus is the segment that is most vulnerable to disruption. The most common ossicular lesion is disruption of the incudostapedial joint. Disruption of the malleoincudal articulation occurs less commonly.[412,413]

Infections

Otitis media is common in children. Its clinical features and appearance on physical examination are well known to pedi-

atricians. It is the complications of otitis media that require imaging procedures.

Mastoiditis is the most common complication of acute otitis media. Mastoiditis occurs when inflammation extends from the middle ear cavity through the aditus ad antrum into the mastoid air cells. Mastoid effusions frequently accompany acute otitis media. With severe acute otitis media accompanied by mastoiditis, there are pain, tenderness, and erythema of the postauricular area. The inflammatory exudate may extend under the periosteum of the mastoid, causing the pinna of the ear to be displaced inferiorly and anteriorly. Frequently, the posterosuperior wall of the external auditory canal may be swollen or sagging. Mastoiditis may also break through the tip of the mastoid process to extend into the neck, a so-called Bezold abscess (Fig. 3-105).

Rarely, mastoiditis may extend through the tegmen to produce subperiosteal abscesses in either the floor of the middle cranial fossa or the anterior portion of the posterior cranial fossa (Fig. 3-106). Even more rarely in children, inflammation of the petrous apex (ie, petrositis) may occur. The clinical manifestations are otitis media associated with an ipsilateral cranial nerve VI palsy and pain in the ipsilateral orbit.

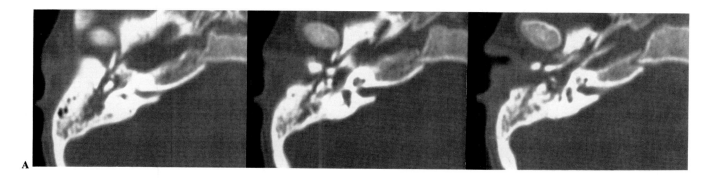

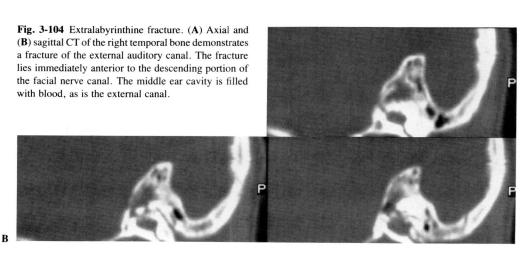

Fig. 3-104 Extralabyrinthine fracture. (**A**) Axial and (**B**) sagittal CT of the right temporal bone demonstrates a fracture of the external auditory canal. The fracture lies immediately anterior to the descending portion of the facial nerve canal. The middle ear cavity is filled with blood, as is the external canal.

Plain radiographs of cases of mastoiditis demonstrate clouding of the mastoid air cells. In chronic mastoiditis, there is coalescence of the mastoid air cells with persistent opacification. Subperiosteal abscesses that extend extracranially or intracranially are seen on CT as localized soft tissue densities with enhancing margins. A subperiosteal abscess complicating petrositis presents as an extradural fluid collection with an enhancing membrane at the apex of the petrous bone in the anteromedial portion of the middle cranial fossa. There may be partial destruction of the petrous apex (Fig. 3-107).

Tumors

The temporal bone may be involved with both benign and malignant tumors. Most common among the benign tumors are congenital cholesteatomas. These lesions represent congenital nests of epithelial tissue in the middle ear cavity. Clinically, they present as white, cystlike structures beneath an intact tympanic membrane. On CT, these lesions present as localized soft tissue densities in the middle ear cavity. They may present in the epitympanum, the tympanic cavity (Fig. 3-108), the hypotympanum (Fig. 3-109), or a combination of these locations. The ossicles may be displaced but are rarely destroyed. Ossicular destruction may occur in acquired

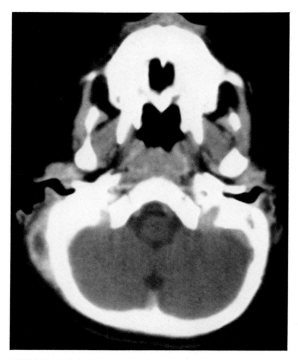

Fig. 3-105 Mastoiditis. Contrast-enhanced axial CT shows an enhancing oval abscess adjacent to the periosteum of the right mastoid. This extends caudally into the neck and represents a Bezold abscess.

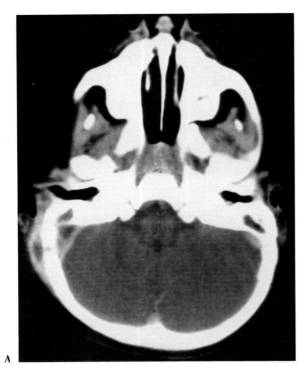
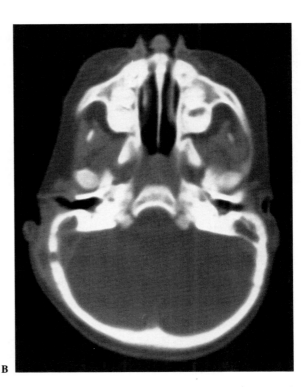

Fig. 3-106 Mastoiditis with extracranial and intracranial subperiosteal abscess. **(A)** Contrast-enhanced axial CT demonstrates enhancing margins of a subperiosteal abscess extending from the right mastoid both extracranially and intracranially. **(B)** Bone-window image shows a focal area of destruction of the posterior aspect of the temporal bone.

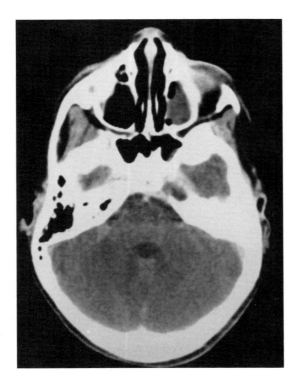
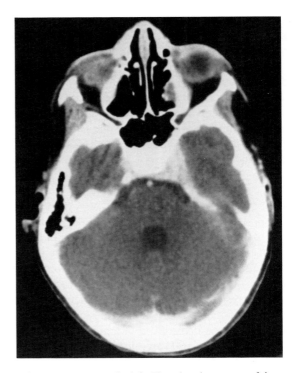

Fig. 3-107 Petrositis. Contrast-enhanced axial CT scans demonstrate a destructive lesion at the petrous apex on the left. There is enhancement of the margins surrounding the petrous apex extending into the left cavernous sinus. The left mastoid is opaque.

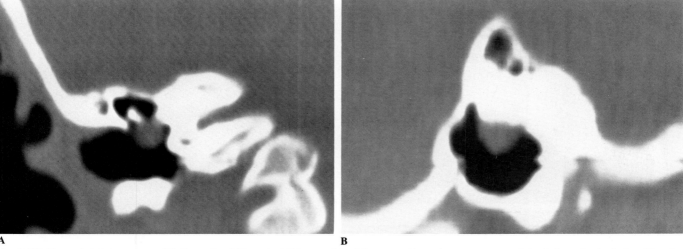

A   **B**

Fig. 3-108 Congenital cholesteatoma. (**A**) Coronal and (**B**) sagittal CT scans of the right temporal bone demonstrate a rounded soft tissue density in the midportion of the tympanic cavity. The ossicles are not destroyed.

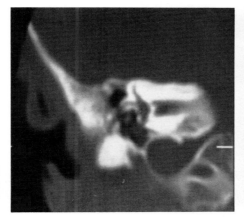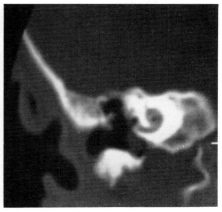

Fig. 3-109 Congenital cholesteatoma. This small cholesteatoma is located in the inferoanterior aspect of the hypotympanum, with a small portion extending into the tympanic cavity.

cholesteatoma; this is a complication of chronic otitis media (Fig. 3-110).

Langerhan cell histiocytosis has a predilection for involvement of the mastoid. Although the mastoid may be an isolated site of disease, lesions elsewhere in the calvaria are frequen.. Extraskeletal disease is found in more advanced states. The disease may be found in skin, liver, spleen, or lungs.

Radiographically, there is an erosion in the mastoid process with a nonenhancing soft tissue mass adjacent to the erosion. The lesion most commonly involves the mastoid and external canal. Involvement of the middle ear cavity is extremely rare. It is not unusual for the destructive process to heal completely after appropriate chemotherapy.

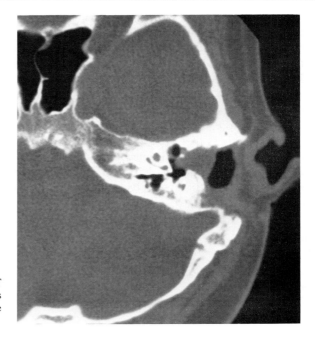

Fig. 3-110 Chronic middle ear infection with acquired cholesteatoma. Axial CT demonstrates a large soft tissue mass that fills most of the middle ear cavity and extends through the perforated tympanic membrane into the external canal. The majority of the ossicular chain has been destroyed. The mastoid is small and sclerotic.

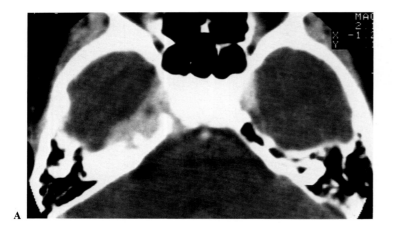

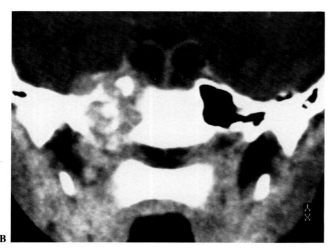

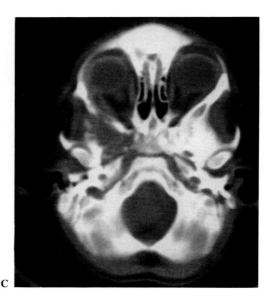

Fig. 3-111 Middle ear rhabdomyosarcoma. **(A)** Axial and **(B)** coronal CT images demonstrate an intensely enhancing mass at the apex of the right temporal bone. The lesion extends both intracranially and extracranially. There is extensive destruction of the base of the skull. **(C)** The bone destruction is more clearly seen on the axial image of the skull base, which demonstrates destruction not only of the floor of the middle cranial fossa but also of the posterior aspect of the right orbit.

Rhabdomyosarcoma is the most common malignant tumor of the temporal bone in childhood. The temporal bone is the third most common site of this tumor in the head and neck. Most cases occur before the age of 12 years, with the peak incidence being at 3 to 6 years. Clinical symptoms are discharge from the ear, pain in the ear, and cranial nerve palsies. Cranial nerves VII and VIII are the most commonly involved. With further medial extension, cranial nerve VI may be involved.

Imaging findings are a soft tissue mass in the middle ear cavity with marked destruction of the contiguous bone (Fig. 3-111). This is best seen with CT. The lesion shows fairly intense contrast enhancement. Dissemination in the cerebrospinal fluid pathways has been reported with this tumor. Widespread metastases to lymph nodes and lung may also develop.

REFERENCES

1. Edwards DK. The child with stridor. In: Hilton S, Edwards DK, Hilton JW, eds. *Practical Pediatric Radiology.* Philadelphia: Saunders; 1984:3–47.

2. Grunebaum M. Respiratory stridor—a challenge for the pediatric radiologist. *Clin Radiol.* 1973;24:485–490.

3. Swischuk LE. The chest. In: *Emergency Radiology of the Acutely Ill or Injured Child.* Baltimore: Williams & Wilkins; 1979:1–115.

4. Holinger LD. Etiology of stridor in the neonate, infant, and child. *Ann Otol Rhinol Laryngol.* 1980;89(5 pt 1):397–400.

5. Dupin CL, LeJeune FE Jr. Nasal masses in infants and children. *South Med J.* 1978;71:124–128.

6. Myer CM, Cotton RT. Nasal obstruction in the pediatric patient. *Pediatrics.* 1983;72:766–777.

7. Stahl RS, Jurkiewicz MJ. Congenital posterior choanal atresia. *Pediatrics.* 1985;76:429–436.

8. Shaffer K, Haughton V, Farley G, Friedman J. Pitfalls in the radiographic diagnosis of angiofibroma. *Radiology.* 1978;127:425–428.

9. Williams HJ. Posterior choanal atresia. *Am J Roentgenol Radium Ther Nucl Med.* 1971;112:1–11.

10. Slovis TL, Renfro B, Watts FB, Kuhns LR, Belenky W, Spoylar J. Choanal atresia: precise CT evaluation. *Radiology.* 1985;155:345–348.

11. Chinwuba C, Wallman J, Strand R. Nasal airway obstruction: CT assessment. *Radiology.* 1986;159:503–506.

12. Crockett DM, Healy GB, McGill TJ, Friedman EM. Computed tomography in the evaluation of choanal atresia in infants and children. *Laryngoscope.* 1987;97:174–183.

13. Tadmor R, Ravid M, Millet D, Leventon G. Computed tomographic demonstration of choanal atresia. *AJNR.* 1984;5:743–745.

14. Kleinman P, Winchester P. Case reports. Pseudotumor of the nasal fossa secondary to mucoid impaction in choanal atresia. *Pediatr Radiol.* 1975;4:47–48.

15. Davis KR. Embolization of epistaxis and juvenile nasopharyngeal angiofibromas. *AJNR.* 1986;7:953–962.

16. Lasjaunias P, Picard L, Manelfe C, Moret J, Doyon D. Angiofibroma of the nasopharynx. A review of 53 cases treated by embolisation. The role of

pretherapeutic angiography. Pathophysical hypothesis. *J Neuroradiol.* 1980;7:73–95.

17. Smoker WRK, Gentry LR. Computed tomography of the nasopharynx and related spaces. *Semin Ultrasound Comput Tomogr Magn Resonance.* 1986;7:107–130.

18. Sessions RB, Bryan RN, Naclerio RM, Alford BR. Radiographic staging of juvenile angiofibroma. *Head Neck Surg.* 1981;3:279–283.

19. Roberson GH, Price AC, Davis JM, Gulati A. Therapeutic embolization of juvenile angiofibroma. *AJR.* 1979;133:657–663.

20. Lloyd GA, Phelps PD. Juvenile angiofibroma: imaging by magnetic resonance, CT and conventional techniques. *Clin Otolaryngol.* 1986; 11:247–259.

21. Towbin R, Dunbar JS, Bove K. Antrochoanal polyps. *AJR.* 1979; 132:27–31.

22. Johnson JT, Effron MZ, Schramm VL Jr. Nasal masses in children. *Postgrad Med.* 1982;72:87–91.

23. Nino-Murcia M, Rao VM, Mikaelian DO, Som P. Acute sinusitis mimicking antrochoanal polyp. *AJNR.* 1986;7:513–516.

24. Som PM, Sacher M, Lawson W, Biller HF. CT appearance distinguishing benign nasal polyps from malignancies. *J Comput Assist Tomogr.* 1987;11:129–133.

25. Som PM, Shapiro MD, Biller HF, Sasaki C, Lawson W. Sinonasal tumors and inflammatory tissues: differentiation with MR imaging. *Radiology.* 1988;167:803–808.

26. Alter AD, Cove JK. Congenital nasopharyngeal teratoma: report of a case and review of the literature. *J Pediatr Surg.* 1987;22:179–181.

27. Howell CG, Van Tassel P, El Gammal T. High resolution computed tomography in neonatal nasopharyngeal teratoma. *J Comput Assist Tomogr.* 1984;8:1179–1181.

28. Senac MO, Segall HD. CT diagnosis of an atypical nasopharyngeal teratoma in a newborn. *AJNR.* 1987;8:710–712.

29. Holt GR, Holt JE, Weaver RG. Dermoids and teratomas of the head and neck. *Ear Nose Throat J.* 1979;58:520–531.

30. Neel HB. Nasopharyngeal carcinoma. Clinical presentation, diagnosis, treatment and prognosis. *Otolaryngol Clin North Am.* 1985;18: 479–490.

31. Cunningham MJ, Myers EN, Bluestone CD. Malignant tumors of the head and neck in children: a twenty-year review. *Int J Pediatr Otorhinolaryngol.* 1987;13:279–292.

32. Heffer DK. Problems in pediatric otorhinolaryngic pathology. IV. Epithelial and lymphoid tumors of the sinonasal tract and nasopharynx. *Int J Pediatr Otorhinolaryngol.* 1983;6:219–237.

33. Morales P, Bosch A, Salaverry S, Correa JN, Martinez I. Cancer of nasopharynx in young patients. *J Surg Oncol.* 1984;27:181–185.

34. Bass IS, Haller JO, Berdon WE, Barlow B, Carsen G, Khakoo Y. Nasopharyngeal carcinoma: clinical and radiographic findings in children. *Radiology.* 1985;156:651–654.

35. Latack JT, Hutchinson RJ, Heyn RM. Imaging of rhabdomyosarcomas of the head and neck. *AJNR.* 1987;8:353–359.

36. Newbill ET, Jones ME, Cantrell RW. Esthesioneuroblastoma. Diagnosis and management. *South Med J.* 1985;78:275–282.

37. Dillon WP, Mills CM, Kjos B, DeGroot J, Brant-Zawadzki M. Magnetic resonance imaging of the nasopharynx. *Radiology.* 1984; 152:731–738.

38. Dillon WP. Magnetic resonance imaging of head and neck tumors. *Cardiovasc Intervent Radiol.* 1986;8:275–282.

39. Dietrich RB, Lufkin RB, Kangarloo H, Hanafee WN, Wilson GH. Head and neck MR imaging in the pediatric patient. *Radiology.* 1986; 159:769–776.

40. Lee YY, Van Tassel P, Nauert C, North LB, Jung BS. Lymphomas of the head and neck: CT findings at initial presentation. *AJNR.* 1987;8:665–671.

41. Schroth G, Gawehn J, Marquardt B, Schabet M. MR imaging of esthesioneuroblastoma. *J Comput Assist Tomogr.* 1986;10:316–319.

42. Regenbogen VS, Zinreich SJ, Kim KS, et al. Hyperostotic esthesioneuroblastoma: CT and MR findings. *J Comput Assist Tomogr.* 1988;12:52–56.

43. Som PM. Sinonasal cavity. In: Som PM, Bergeron RT, eds. *Head and Neck Imaging.* 2nd ed. St Louis: Mosby; 1991;51–276.

44. Kudo A, Lewis JS. Nasal gliomas. *Arch Otolaryngol.* 1971; 94:351–355.

45. Whelan MA, Reede DL, Lin JP, Edwards JH. The base of the brain. In: Bergeron RT, Osborn AG, Som PM, eds. *Head and Neck Imaging: Excluding the Brain.* St Louis: Mosby; 1984:531–574.

46. Bradley PJ, Singh SD. Nasal glioma. *J Laryngol Otol.* 1985; 99:247–252.

47. Patterson K, Kapur S, Chandra RS. ''Nasal gliomas'' and related brain heterotopias: a pathologist's perspective. *Pediatr Pathol.* 1986; 5:353-362.

48. Younus M, Coode PE. Nasal glioma and encephalocele: two separate entities: report of two cases. *J Neurosurg.* 1986;64:516–519.

49. Okuda Y, Oi S. Nasal dermal sinus and dermoid cyst with intrafalcial extension: case report and review of literature. *Childs Nerv Syst.* 1987; 3:40–43.

50. Hayden KC Jr, Swischuck LE. Head and neck lesions in children. In: Bergeron RT, Osborn AG, Som PM, eds. *Head and Neck Imaging: Excluding the Brain.* St Louis: Mosby; 1984:681–727.

51. Naidich TP, Zimmerman RA. Common congenital malformations of the brain. In: Brant-Zawadzki M, Norma D, eds. *Magnetic Resonance Imaging of the Central Nervous System.* New York: Raven Press; 1987:131–150.

52. Seibert RW, Seibert JJ, Jimenez JF, Angtuaco EJ. Nasopharyngeal brain heterotopia—a cause of upper airway obstruction in infancy. *Laryngoscope.* 1984;94:818–819.

53. Lusk RP, Lee PC. Magnetic resonance imaging of congenital midline nasal masses. *Otolaryngol Head Neck Surg.* 1986;95(3 pt 1):303–306.

54. Barkovich AJ, Vandermarck P, Edwards MS, Cogen PH. Congenital nasal masses: CT and MR imaging features in 16 cases. *AJR.* 1991;156: 587–598.

55. Love GL, Riehl PA. Intranasal encephalocele masking as a nasal polyp in an adult patient. *Arch Otolaryngol.* 1983;109:420–421.

56. Lusk RP, Dunn VD. Magnetic resonance imaging in encephaloceles. *Ann Otol Rhinol Laryngol.* 1986;95(4 pt 1):432–433.

57. David DJ, Sheffield L, Simpson D, White J. Frontoethmoidal meningoencephaloceles: morphology and treatment. *Br J Plast Surg.* 1984; 37:271–284.

58. Lloyd GA, Lund VJ, Phelps PD, Howard DJ. Magnetic resonance imaging in the evaluation of nose and paranasal sinus disease. *Br J Radiol.* 1987;60:957–968.

59. Cayler GG, Johnson EE, Lewis BE, Kortzeborn JD, Jordan J, Fricker GA. Heart failure due to enlarged tonsils and adenoids. The cardiorespiratory syndrome of increased airway resistance. *Am J Dis Child.* 1969;118:708–717.

60. Capitanio MA, Kirkpatrick JA. Nasopharyngeal lymphoid tissues. Roentgen observations in 257 children two years of age or less. *Radiology.* 1970;96:389–391.

61. Swischuk LE. The chest. In: *Emergency Radiology of the Acutely Ill or Injured Child.* Baltimore: Williams & Wilkins; 1979:116–131.

62. Strife JL. Upper airway and tracheal obstruction in infants and children. *Radiol Clin North Am.* 1988;26:309–322.

63. Kaplan JM, Keller MS, Troy S. Nasopharyngeal obstruction in infectious mononucleosis. *Am Fam Physician.* 1987;35:205–209.

64. Sato Y, Dunbar JS. Abnormalities of the pharynx and prevertebral soft tissues in infectious mononucleosis. *AJR.* 1980;134:149–152.

65. Ardran GM, Kemp FH. Aglossia congenita. *Arch Dis Child.* 1956;31:400–407.

66. Enwonwu CO. Infectious oral necrosis (cancrum oris) in Nigerian children: a review. *Community Dent Oral Epidemiol.* 1985;13:190–194.

67. Rotbart HA, Levin MJ, Jones JF, et al. Noma in children with severe combined immunodeficiency. *J Pediatr.* 1986;109:596–600.

68. Wells RG, Sty JR, Starshak RJ. CT findings in noma. *J Comput Assist Tomogr.* 1988;12:711–712.

69. DeLozier HL, Sofferman RA. Pyriform sinus fistula: an unusual cause of recurrent retropharyngeal abscess and cellulitis. *Ann Otol Rhinol Laryngol.* 1986;95(4 pt 1):377–382.

70. Hen J Jr. Current management of upper airway obstruction. *Pediatr Ann.* 1986;15:274–294.

71. Cotton RT, Richardson MA. Congenital laryngeal anomalies. *Otolaryngol Clin North Am.* 1981;14:203–218.

72. McCook TA, Kirks DR. Epiglottic enlargement in infants and young children: another radiologic look. *Pediatr Radiol.* 1982;12:227–234.

73. Dunbar JS. Upper respiratory tract obstruction in infants and children. *Am J Roentgenol Radium Ther Nucl Med.* 1970;109:225–246.

74. Edwards DK. The child with stridor. In: Hilton S, Edwards DK, Hilton JW, eds. *Practical Pediatric Radiology.* Philadelphia: Saunders; 1984:3–47.

75. Liston SL, Gehrz RC, Siegel LG, Tilelli J. Bacterial tracheitis. *Am J Dis Child.* 1983;137:764–767.

76. Han BK, Dunbar JS, Striker TW. Membranous laryngotracheobronchitis (membranous croup). *AJR.* 1979;133:53–58.

77. Leikensohn JR, Benton C, Cotton R. Subglottic hemangioma. *J Otolaryngol.* 1976;5:487–492.

78. Holinger PH, Schild JA. Laryngeal papilloma: review of etiology and therapy. *Laryngoscope.* 1968;78:1462–1474.

79. Kramer SS, Wehunt WD, Stocker JT, Kashima H. Pulmonary manifestations of juvenile laryngotracheal papillomatosis. *AJR.* 1985;144:687–694.

80. Cohen SR, Geller KA, Seltzer S, Thompson JW. Papilloma of the larynx and tracheobronchial tree in children: a retrospective study. *Ann Otol Rhinol Laryngol.* 1980;89(6 pt 1):497–503.

81. Borkowsky W, Martin D, Lawrence HS. Juvenile laryngeal papillomatosis with pulmonary spread. Regression following transfer factor therapy. *Am J Dis Child.* 1984;138:667–669.

82. Donegan JO, Strife JL, Seid AB, Cotton RT, Dunbar JS. Internal laryngocele and saccular cysts in children. *Ann Otol Rhinol Laryngol.* 1980;89(5 pt 1):409–413.

83. Williams JL, Capitanio MA, Turtz MG. Vocal cord paralysis; radiologic observations in 21 infants and young children. *AJR.* 1977;128:649–651.

84. Holinger PC, Holinger LD, Reichert TJ, Holinger PH. Respiratory obstruction and apnea in infants with bilateral abductor vocal cord paralysis, meningomyelocele, hydrocephalus, and Arnold-Chiari malformation. *J Pediatr.* 1978;92:368–373.

85. Schaeffer JP. *The Embryology, Development and Anatomy of the Nose, Paranasal Sinuses, Naso-Lacrimal Passageways and Olfactory Organ in Man.* Philadelphia: Blakiston's Son; 1920.

86. Ritter FN. *The Paranasal Sinuses: Anatomy and Surgical Technique.* St Louis: Mosby; 1973.

87. Som PM. The paranasal sinuses. In: Bergerson RT, Osborn AG, Som PM, eds. *Head and Neck Imaging: Excluding the Brain.* St Louis: Mosby; 1984:1–142.

88. Wald ER. Acute sinusitis in children. *Pediatr Infect Dis.* 1983;2:61–68.

89. Hawkins DB. Advances in sinus disease in pediatrics. *Otolaryngol Clin North Am.* 1989;22:553–568.

90. Silverman FN. The face and individual cranial structures. In: Silverman FN, ed. *Caffey's Pediatric X-Ray Diagnosis. An Integrated Imaging Approach.* 8th ed. Chicago: Year Book Medical; 1985:97–103.

91. Karmody CS, Carter B, Vincent ME. Developmental anomalies of the maxillary sinus. *Trans Am Acad Ophthalmol Otolaryngol.* 1977;84(4 pt 1):723–728.

92. Wald ER. Acute sinusitis and orbital complications in children. *Am J Otolaryngol.* 1983;4:424–427.

93. Sable NS, Hengerer A, Powell KR. Acute frontal sinusitis with intracranial complications. *Pediatr Infect Dis.* 1984;3:58–61.

94. Wald ER, Milmoe GJ, Bowen AD, Ledesma-Medina T, Salamon N, Givestone CD. Acute maxillary sinusitis in children. *N Engl J Med.* 1981;304:749–754.

95. Wenig BL, Goldstein MN, Abramson AL. Frontal sinusitis and its intracranial complications. *Int J Pediatr Otorhinolaryngol.* 1983;5:285–302.

96. Harrington PC. Complications of sinusitis. *Ear Nose Throat J.* 1984;63:163–171.

97. Remmler D, Boles R. Intracranial complications of frontal sinusitis. *Laryngoscope.* 1980;90(11 pt 1):1814–1824.

98. Courville CB. Subdural empyema secondary to purulent frontal sinusitis. A clinicopathologic study of forty-two cases verified at autopsy. *Arch Otolaryngol.* 1944;39:211–230.

99. Morgan PR, Morrison WV. Complications of frontal and ethmoid sinusitis. *Laryngoscope.* 1980;90:661–666.

100. Kaufman DM, Litman N, Miller MH. Sinusitis: induced subdural empyema. *Neurology.* 1983;33:123–132.

101. Farmer TW, Wise GR. Subdural empyema in infants, children and adults. *Neurology.* 1973;23:254–261.

102. Wells RG, Sty JR, Landers AD. Radiological evaluation of Pott puffy tumor. *JAMA.* 1986;255:1331–1333.

103. Pott P. *The Chirurgical Works of Percivall Pott.* London: Hayes W. Clarke & B. Collins; 1965.

104. Guttenplan MD, Wetmore RF. Paranasal sinus mucocele in cystic fibrosis. *Clin Pediatr.* 1989;28:429–430.

105. Timon CI, O'Dwyer TP. Ethmoidal mucoceles in children. *J Laryngol Otol.* 1989;103:284–286.

106. Carter BL, Bankoff MS, Fisk JD. Computed tomographic detection of sinusitis responsible for intracranial and extracranial infections. *Radiology.* 1983;147:739–742.

107. Conner BL, Roach ES, Laster W, Georgitis JW. Magnetic resonance imaging of the paranasal sinuses: frequency and type of abnormalities. *Ann Allergy.* 1989;62:457–460.

108. Diament MJ, Senac MO Jr, Gilsanz V, Baker S, Gillespie T, Larsson S. Prevalence of incidental paranasal sinuses opacification in pediatric patients: a CT study. *J Comput Assist Tomogr.* 1987;11:426–431.

109. Glasier CM, Ascher DP, Williams KD. Incidental paranasal sinus abnormalities on CT of children: clinical correlation. *AJNR.* 1986;7:861–864.

110. Odita JC, Akamaguna AI, Ogisi FO, Amu OD, Ugbodaga CI. Pneumatisation of the maxillary sinus in normal and symptomatic children. *Pediatr Radiol.* 1986;16:365–367.

111. Shopfner CE, Rossi JO. Roentgen evaluation of the paranasal sinuses in children. *Am J Roentgenol Radium Ther Nucl Med.* 1973;118:176–186.

112. Sadhu VK, Handel SF, Pinto RS, Glass TF. Neuroradiologic diagnosis of subdural empyema and CT limitations. *AJNR.* 1980;1:39–44.

113. Zimmerman RD, Leeds NE, Danziger A. Subdural empyema: CT findings. *Radiology.* 1984;150:417–422.

114. Wald ER, Pang D, Milmoe GJ, Schramm VI. Sinusitis and its complications in the pediatric patient. *Pediatr Clin North Am.* 1981;28:777–796.

115. Hesselink JR, Weber AL, New PFJ, Davis KR, Roberson GH, Taveras JM. Evaluation of mucoceles of the paranasal sinuses with computed tomography. *Radiology.* 1979;133:397–400.

116. Som PM, Shugar JM. The CT classification of ethmoid mucoceles. *J Comput Assist Tomogr.* 1980;4:199–203.

117. Silver AJ, Baredes S, Bello JA, Blitzer A, Hilal SK. The opacified maxillary sinus: CT findings in chronic sinusitis and malignant tumors. *Radiology.* 1987;163:205–210.

118. Kopp W, Fotter R, Steiner H, Beaufort I, Stammberger H. Aspergillosis of the paranasal sinuses. *Radiology.* 1985;156:715–716.

119. Zinreich ST, Kennedy DW, Malat J, et al. Fungal sinusitis: diagnosis with CT and MR imaging. *Radiology.* 1988;169:439–444.

120. Stahl RH. Allergic disorders of the nose and paranasal sinuses. *Otolaryngol Clin North Am.* 1974;7:703–718.

121. Feldman BA. Rhabdomyosarcoma of the head and neck. *Laryngoscope.* 1982;92:424–440.

122. Hasso AN, Vignaud J. Pathology of the paranasal sinuses, nasal cavity and facial bones. In: Newton TH, Hasso AN, Dillon WP, eds. *Computed Tomography of the Head and Neck.* New York: Raven; 1988:7.1–7.32.

123. Som PM, Cohen BA, Sacher M, Choi I, Bryan NR. The angiomatous polyp and the angiofibroma: two different lesions. *Radiology.* 1982;144:329–334.

124. Weber AL, Stanton AC. Malignant tumors of the paranasal sinuses: radiologic, clinical, and histopathologic evaluation of 200 cases. *Head Neck Surg.* 1984;6:761–776.

125. Lund VJ, Howard DJ, Lloyd GAS, Cheesman AD. Magnetic resonance imaging of paranasal sinus tumors for craniofacial resection. *Head Neck.* 1989;11:279–283.

126. Paling MR, Roberts RL, Fauci AS. Paranasal sinus obliteration in Wegener granulomatosis. *Radiology.* 1982;144:539–543.

127. Amodio JB, Berdon WE, Abramason S, Baker D. Cystic fibrosis in childhood: pulmonary, paranasal sinus, and skeletal manifestations. *Semin Roentgenol.* 1987;22:125–135.

128. Cepero R, Smith RJ, Catlin FI, Bressler KL, Furuta GT, Shandera KC. Cystic fibrosis—an otolaryngologic perspective. *Otolaryngol Head Neck Surg.* 1987;97:356–360.

129. Jaffe BF, Jaff N. Diagnosis and treatment of head and neck tumors in children. *Pediatrics.* 1973;51:731–740.

130. Damion J, Hybels RL. The neck mass: 1. General concepts and congenital causes. *Postgrad Med.* 1987;81:75–93.

131. Damion J, Hybels RL. The neck mass: 2. Inflammatory and neoplastic causes. *Postgrad Med.* 1987;81:97–103, 106–107.

132. Pounds LA. Neck masses of congenital origin. *Pediatr Clin North Am.* 1981;28:841–844.

133. Solomon JR, Rangecroft L. Thyroglossal-duct lesions in childhood. *J Pediatr Surg.* 1984;19:555–561.

134. Noyek AM, Friedberg J. Thyroglossal duct and ectopic thyroid disorders. *Otolaryngol Clin North Am.* 1981;14:187–201.

135. Rohn RD, Rubio T. Neck pain due to acute suppurative thyroiditis and thyroglossal duct abscess. *J Adolesc Health Care.* 1980;1:155–158.

136. Kraus R, Han BK, Babcock DS, Oestreich AE. Sonography of neck masses in children. *AJR.* 1986;146:609–613.

137. Reede DL, Bergeron RT, Som PM. CT of thyroglossal duct cysts. *Radiology.* 1985;157:121–125.

138. Reede DL, Bergeron RT, Osborn AG. CT of the soft tissues of the neck. In: Bergeron RT, Osborn AG, Som PM, eds. *Head and Neck Imaging: Excluding the Brain.* St Louis: Mosby; 1984:491–530.

139. Himalstein MR. Branchial cysts and fistulas. *Ear Nose Throat J.* 1980;59:47–54.

140. Chandler JR, Mitchell B. Branchial cleft cysts, sinuses and fistulas. *Otolaryngol Clin North Am.* 1981;14:175–186.

141. Telander RL, Deane SA. Thyroglossal and branchial cleft cysts and sinuses. *Surg Clin North Am.* 1977;57:779–791.

142. Badami JP, Athey PA. Sonography in the diagnosis of branchial cysts. *AJR.* 1981;137:1245–1248.

143. Simpson RA. Lateral cervical cysts and fistulas. *Laryngoscope.* 1969;79:30–59.

144. Morrison DL, MacEwen GD. Congenital muscular torticollis: observations regarding clinical findings, associated conditions, and results of treatment. *J Pediatr Orthop.* 1982;2:500–505.

145. Sty JR, Wells RG, Schroeder BA. Congenital muscular torticollis: computed tomographic observations. *Am J Dis Child.* 1987;141:243–244. Letter.

146. Lindhout D, Golding RP, Taets van Amerongen AH. Fibrodysplasia ossificans progressiva: current concepts and the role of CT in acute changes. *Pediatr Radiol.* 1985;15:211–213.

147. Connor JM, Evans DAP. Fibrodysplasia ossificans progressiva: the clinical features and natural history of 34 patients. *J Bone Joint Surg.* 1982;64:76–83.

148. Wells RG, Sty JR. Fibrodysplasia ossificans progressiva: an infant neck mass. *Wis Med J.* 1986;85:9–11.

149. Byrne J, Blanc WA, Warburton D, Wigger J. The significance of cystic hygroma in fetuses. *Hum Pathol.* 1984;15:61–67.

150. Sheth S, Nussbaum AR, Hutchins GM, Sanders RC. Cystic hygromas in children: sonographic-pathologic correlation. *Radiology.* 1987;162:821–824.

151. Chervenak FA, Isaacson G, Tortora M. A sonographic study of fetal cystic hygromas. *J Clin Ultrasound.* 1985;13:311–315.

152. Garden AS, Benzie RJ, Miskin M, Gardner HA. Fetal cystic hygroma colli: antenatal diagnosis, significance, and management. *Am J Obstet Gynecol.* 1986;154:221–225.

153. Siegel MJ, Glazer HS, St Amour TE, Rosenthal DD. Lymphangiomas in children. MR imaging. *Radiology.* 1989;170:467–470.

154. Lack EE. Extragonadal germ cell tumors of the head and neck region: review of 16 cases. *Hum Pathol.* 1985;16:56–64.

155. Hajdu SI, Faruque AA, Hajdu EO, Morgan WS. Teratoma of the neck in infants. *Am J Dis Child.* 1966;111:412–416.

156. Trecet JC, Claramunt V, Larraz J, Ruiz E, Zuzuarregui M, Ugalde FJ. Prenatal ultrasound diagnosis of fetal teratoma of the neck. *J Clin Ultrasound.* 1984;12:509–511.

157. Levine PH, Kamaraju LS, Connelly RR, et al. The American Burkitt's Lymphoma Registry: eight years experience. *Cancer.* 1982;49:1016–1022.

158. Jaffe BJ. Pediatric head and neck tumors: a study of 178 cases. *Laryngoscope.* 1973;83:1644–1651.

159. Miller JH, DeClerck YA. Orbit, paranasal sinuses, pharynx, thyroid, and soft tissues of the neck. In: Miller JH, ed. *Imaging in Pediatric Oncology.* Baltimore: Williams & Wilkins; 1985:116–136.

160. May M. Neck masses in children: diagnosis and treatment. *Pediatr Ann.* 1976;5:518–535.

161. Donaldson SS, Castro JR, Wilbur JR, Jesse RH Jr. Rhabdomyosarcoma of the head and neck in children. Combination treatment by surgery, irradiation and chemotherapy. *Cancer.* 1973;31:26–35.

162. Anderson KC, Leonard RC, Canellos GP, Skarin AT, Kaplan WD. High-dose gallium imaging in lymphoma. *Am J Med.* 1983;75:327–331.

163. Drossman SR, Schiff RG, Kronfeld GD, McNamara J, Leonidas JC. Lymphoma of the mediastinum and neck: evaluation with Ga-67 imaging and CT correlation. *Radiology.* 1990;174:171–175.

164. Danziger J, Handel SF, Jing BS, Wallace S. Computerized tomography in rhabdomyosarcoma of the head and neck. *Cancer.* 1979;44:463–467.

165. Marcy SM. Infections of lymph nodes of the head and neck. *Pediatr Infect Dis.* 1983;2:397–405.

166. Saitz EW. Cervical lymphadenitis caused by atypical mycobacterium. *Pediatr Clin North Am.* 1981;28:823–839.

167. Wojtowycz M, Duck SD, Lipton M, Sty JR, Young LW. Radiological case of the month. Acute suppurative thyroiditis. *Am J Dis Child.* 1981;135:1063–1064.

168. Holt GR, McManus, Newman RK, Potter JL, Tinsley PP. Computed tomography in the diagnosis of deep-neck infections. *Arch Otolaryngol.* 1982;108:693–696.

169. Rauschkolb EN, Keen SJ, Patel S. High-dose computed tomography in the evaluation of low attenuation lesions in the neck. *J Comput Tomogr.* 1983;7:159–166.

170. Keyes JW, Thrall JH, Carey JE. Technical considerations in in vivo thyroid studies. *Semin Nucl Med.* 1978;8:43–57.

171. O'Connor MK, Freyne PJ, Cullen MJ. Low-dose radioisotope scanning and quantitative analysis in the diagnosis of congenital hypothyroidism. *Arch Dis Child.* 1982;57:490–494.

172. Hayek A, Stanbury JB. The diagnostic use of radionuclides in the thyroid disorders of childhood. *Semin Nucl Med.* 1971;1:334–344.

173. Ghahremani GG, Hoffer PB, Oppenheim BD, Gottschalk A. New normal values for thyroid uptake of radioactive iodine. *JAMA.* 1971;217:337–339.

174. Sty JR, Starshak RJ, Miller JH. Thyroid imaging. In: *Pediatric Nuclear Medicine.* Norwalk, Conn: Appleton-Century-Crofts; 1983:149–158.

175. Dussault JH. An update on screening for congenital hypothyroidism. *Thyroid Today.* 1985;7:1–4.

176. Price DA, Ehrlich RM, Walfish PG. Congenital hypothyroidism. Clinical and laboratory characteristics in infants detected by neonatal screening. *Arch Dis Child.* 1981;56:845–851.

177. Barnes ND. Screening for congenital hypothyroidism: the first decade. *Arch Dis Child.* 1985;60:587–592.

178. Fisher DA, Dussault JH, Foley TP Jr, et al. Screening for congenital hypothyroidism: results of screening one million North American infants. *J Pediatr.* 1979;94:700–705.

179. Arnold MB, Arulananthani K, Bapat V, et al. Characteristics of infantile hypothyroidism discovered on neonatal screening. *J Pediatr.* 1984;104:539–544.

180. Fisher DA. Clinical review 19: management of congenital hypothyroidism. *J Clin Endocrinol Metab.* 1991;72:523–529.

181. Fort P, Lifshitz F, Bellisario R, et al. Abnormalities of thyroid function in infants with Down syndrome. *J Pediatr.* 1984;104:545–549.

182. Fisher DA. Second International Conference on Neonatal Thyroid Screening: progress report. *J Pediatr.* 1983;102:653–654.

183. Fisher DA, Klein AH. Thyroid development and disorders of thyroid function in the newborn. *N Engl J Med.* 1981;304:702–712.

184. Takasu N, Mori T, Koizumi Y, Takeuchi S, Yamada T. Transient neonatal hypothyroidism due to maternal immunoglobulins that inhibit thyrotropin-binding and post-receptor processes. *J Clin Endocrinol Metab.* 1984;59:142–146.

185. Hulse JA, Jackson D, Grant DB, Byfield PGH, Hoffenberg R. Different measurements of thyroid function in hypothyroid infants diagnosed by screening. *Acta Paediatr Scand.* 1979;277(suppl):21–25.

186. Czernichow P, Schlumberger M, Pomarede R, Fragu P. Plasma thyroglobulin measurements help determine the type of thyroid defect in congenital hypothyroidism. *J Clin Endocrinol Metab.* 1983;56:242–245.

187. Wells RG, Sty JR, Duck SC. Technetium-99m pertechnetate thyroid scintigraphy: congenital hypothyroid screening. *Pediatr Radiol.* 1986;16:368–373.

188. Heyman S, Crigler JF Jr, Treves S. Congenital hypothyroidism: 123-I thyroidal uptake and scintigraphy. *J Pediatr.* 1982;101:571–574.

189. Kim EE, Domstad PA, Choy YC, DeLand FH. Avid thyroid uptake of (Tc-99m) sodium pertechnetate in children with goitrous cretinism. *Clin Pediatr.* 1981;20:437–439.

190. Kaplan M, Kauli R, Lubin E, Grunebaum M, Laron Z. Ectopic thyroid glands: a clinical study of 30 children and review. *J Pediatr.* 1978;92:205–209.

191. Davy T, Daneman D, Walfish PG, Ehrlich RM. Congenital hypothyroidism: the effect of stopping treatment at 3-years of age. *Am J Dis Child.* 1985;139:1028–1030.

192. Miller JH. Lingual thyroid gland: sonographic appearance. *Radiology.* 1985;156:83–84.

193. Bachrach LK, Daneman D, Daneman A, Martin DJ. Use of ultrasound in childhood thyroid disorders. *J Pediatr.* 1983;103:547–552.

194. Inoue M, Taketani N, Sato T, Nakajima H. High incidence of chronic lymphocytic thyroiditis in apparently healthy school children: epidemiological and clinical study. *Endocrinol Jpn.* 1975;22:483–488.

195. Rallison ML, Dobyns BM, Keating FR, Rall JE, Tyler FH. Occurrence and natural history of chronic lymphocytic thyroiditis in childhood. *J Pediatr.* 1975;86:675–682.

196. Winter J, Eberlein WR, Bongiovanni AM. The relationship of juvenile hypothyroidism to chronic lymphocytic thyroiditis. *J Pediatr.* 1966;69:709–718.

197. Weetman AP, McGregor AM. Autoimmune thyroid disease: developments in our understanding. *Endocr Rev.* 1984;5:309–355.

198. Maceri DR, Sullivan MJ, McClatchney KD. Autoimmune thyroiditis: pathophysiology and relationship to thyroid cancer. *Laryngoscope.* 1986;96:82–86.

199. Brown J, Solomon DH, Beall GN, et al. Autoimmune thyroid diseases: Graves' and Hashimoto's. *Ann Intern Med.* 1978;88:379–391.

200. Greenberg AH, Czernichow P, Hung W, Shelley W, Winship T, Blizzard RM. Juvenile chronic lymphocytic thyroiditis: clinical, laboratory and histological correlations. *J Clin Endocrinol Metab.* 1970;30:293–301.

201. Ling SM, Kaplan SA, Leitzman JJ, et al. Euthyroid goiters in children: correlation of needle biopsy with other clinical and laboratory findings in chronic lymphocytic thyroiditis and simple goiter. *Pediatrics.* 1969;44:695–708.

202. Sklar CA, Qazi R, David R. Juvenile autoimmune thyroiditis: hormonal status at presentation and after long-term follow-up. *Am J Dis Child.* 1986;140:877–880.

203. Hopwood NJ, Rabin BS, Foley TP, Peake RL. Thyroid antibodies in children and adolescents with thyroid disorders. *J Pediatr.* 1978;93:57–61.

204. Hayashi N, Tamaki N, Konishi J, et al. Sonography of Hashimoto's thyroiditis. *J Clin Ultrasound.* 1986;14:123–126.

205. Poyhonen L, Lenko HL. Ultrasound imaging in diffuse thyroid disorders of children. *Acta Paediatr Scand.* 1986;75:272–278.

206. Lucaya J, Berdon WE, Enriquez G, Regas J, Carreno JC. Congenital pyriform sinus fistula: a cause of acute left-sided suppurative thyroiditis and neck abscess in children. *Pediatr Radiol.* 1990;21:27–29.

207. Abe K, Taguchi R, Okuno A, Matsuura N, Sasaki H. Acute suppurative thyroiditis in children. *J Pediatr.* 1979;94:912–914.

208. Mann CM. Thyroid abscess in a 3½-year-old child. *Arch Otolaryngol.* 1977;103:299–300.

209. Rich EJ, Mendelman PM. Acute suppurative thyroiditis in pediatric patients. *Pediatr Infect Dis J.* 1987;6:936–940.

210. Clair MR, Mandelblatt S, Baim RS, Perkes E, Goodman K. Sonographic features of acute suppurative thyroiditis. *J Clin Ultrasound.* 1983;11:222–224.

211. Bernard PJ, Som PM, Urken ML, Lawson W, Biller HF. The CT findings of acute thyroiditis and acute suppurative thyroiditis. *Otolaryngol Head Neck Surg.* 1988;99:489–493.

212. Greene JN. Subacute thyroiditis. *Am J Med.* 1971;51:97–108.

213. Hamburger JI. The various presentations of thyroiditis. Diagnostic considerations. *Ann Intern Med.* 1986;104:219–224.

214. Bartels PC, Boer RO. Subacute thyroiditis (de Quervain) presenting as a "cold" nodule. *J Nucl Med.* 1987;28:1488–1490.

215. Hamburger JI. The clinical spectrum of thyroiditis. *Thyroid Today.* 1980;3:1–6.

216. Benker G, Olbricht T, Weindeck R, et al. The sonographical and functional sequelae of de Quervain's subacute thyroiditis: long-term follow-up. *Acta Endocrinol (Copenh).* 1988;117:435–441.

217. Tokuda Y, Kasagi K, Iida Y, et al. Sonography of subacute thyroiditis: changes in the findings during the course of the disease. *J Clin Ultrasound.* 1990;18:21–26.

218. Hayek A. Thyroid storm following radioiodine for thyrotoxicosis. *J Pediatr.* 1978;93:978–980.

219. Zakarija M, McKenzie M, Banovac K. Clinical significance of assay of thyroid-stimulating antibody in Graves' disease. *Ann Intern Med.* 1980;93: 28–32.

220. Charkes ND, Maurer AH, Siegel JA, Radecki PD, Malmud LS. MR imaging in thyroid disorders: correlation of signal intensity with Graves disease activity. *Radiology.* 1987;164:491–494.

221. Duck SC, Sty J. Technetium thyroid uptake ratios in pediatric Graves disease. *J Pediatr.* 1985;107:905–909.

222. Studer H, Ramelli F. Simple goiter and its variants: euthyroid and hyperthyroid multinodular goiters. *Endocr Rev.* 1982;3:40–61.

223. Gefter WB, Spritzer CE, Eisenberg B, et al. Thyroid imaging with high–field-strength surface-coil MR. *Radiology.* 1987;164:483–490.

224. Sandler MP, Patton JA. Multimodality imaging of the thyroid and parathyroid glands. *J Nucl Med.* 1987;28:122–129.

225. Silverman PM, Newman GE, Korobkin M, et al. Computed tomography in the evaluation thyroid disease. *AJR.* 1984;142:897–902.

226. Chrousos GP. Endocrine tumors. In: Pizzo PA, Poplack DG, eds. *Principles and Practice of Pediatric Oncology.* Philadelphia: Lippincott; 1989:733–757.

227. De Keyser LF, Van Herle AJ. Differentiated thyroid cancer in children. *Head Neck Surg.* 1985;8:100–114.

228. Scott MD, Crawford JO. Solitary thyroid nodules in childhood: is the incidence of thyroid carcinoma declining? *Pediatrics.* 1978;58:521–525.

229. Jereb B, Lowhagen T. Carcinoma of the thyroid in children and young adults. A review of 32 patients. *Acta Radiol.* 1972;11(suppl): 411–421.

230. Hung W, August GP, Randolph JG, Schisgall RM, Chandra R. Solitary thyroid nodules in children and adolescents. *J Pediatr Surg.* 1982; 17:225–229.

231. Reiter EO, Root AW, Rettig K, Vargas A. Childhood thyromegaly: recent developments. *J Pediatr.* 1981;99:507–518.

232. Abe K, Konno M, Sato T, Matsuura N. Hyperfunctioning thyroid nodules in children. *Am J Dis Child.* 1980;134:961–963.

233. Hopwood NJ, Carroll RG, Kenny FM. Functioning thyroid masses in childhood and adolescence. Clinical, surgical and pathological correlation. *J Pediatr.* 1976;89:710–718.

234. Osburne RC, Goren EN, Bybee DE, Johnsonbaugh RE. Autonomous thyroid nodules in adolescents: clinical characteristics and results of TRH testing. *J Pediatr.* 1982;100:383–386.

235. Ashcraft MW, Van Herle AJ. Management of thyroid nodules. I. History and physical examination, blood tests, x-ray tests, and ultrasonography. *Head Neck Surg.* 1981;3:216–230.

236. Dodd GD. The radiologic features of multiple endocrine neoplasia types IIA and IIB. *Semin Roentgenol.* 1985;20:64–90.

237. Keiser HR, Beaven MA, Doppman J, Wells S Jr, Buja LM. Sipple's syndrome: medullary thyroid carcinoma, pheochromocytoma and parathyroid disease. Studies in a large family. *Ann Intern Med.* 1973;78:561–579.

238. Jones BA, Sisson JC. Early diagnosis and thyroidectomy in multiple endocrine neoplasia type 2b. *J Pediatr.* 1983;102:219–223.

239. Maxon HR, Hertzberg V, Vasavada P, Pu MY, Volarich D. The continuing impact of thyroid scintigraphy in the diagnosis of thyroid enlargement. *Clin Nucl Med.* 1986;11:306–307.

240. Nagai GR, Pitts WC, Basso L, Cisco JA, McDougall IR. Scintigraphic hot nodules and thyroid carcinoma. *Clin Nucl Med.* 1987;12: 123–127.

241. Fisher DA. Thyroid nodules in childhood and their management. *J Pediatr.* 1976;89:866–868.

242. Melnick JC, Stemkowski PE. Thyroid hemiagenesis (hockey stick sign): a review of the world literature and a report of four cases. *J Clin Endocrinol Metab.* 1981;52:247–251.

243. Fawcett HD, Winsett MZ, Yudt WM, Sayle BA. Hyperthyroidism and the single lobe. *Clin Nucl Med.* 1987;12:57–64.

244. Vieras F. Preoperative scintigraphic detection of cervical metastases from thyroid carcinoma with technetium-99m pertechnetate. *Clin Nucl Med.* 1985;10:567–569.

245. Noyek AM, Greyson ND, Steinhardt MI, et al. Thyroid tumor imaging. *Arch Otolaryngol.* 1983;109:205–224.

246. Solbiati L, Volterrani L, Rizzatto G, et al. The thyroid gland with low uptake lesions: evaluation by ultrasound. *Radiology.* 1985;155:187–191.

247. Higgins CB, McNamara MT, Fisher MR, Clark OH. MR imaging of the thyroid. *AJR.* 1986;147:1255–1261.

248. Mountz JM, Glazer GM, Dmuchouski C, Sisson JC. MR imaging of the thyroid: comparison with scintigraphy in the normal and diseased gland. *J Comput Assist Tomogr.* 1987;11:612–619.

249. Stone WM, Van Heerden JA, Zimmerman D. An 8-year-old patient with complicated primary hyperparathyroidism. *J Pediatr Surg.* 1989;24: 1113–1114.

250. Allo M, Thompson NW, Harness JK, Nishiyama RH. Primary hyperparathyroidism in children, adolescents, and young adults. *World J Surg.* 1982;6:771–776.

251. Picard D, D'Amour P, Carrier L, Chartrand R, Poisson R. Localization of abnormal parathyroid gland(s) using thallium-201/iodine-123 subtraction scintigraphy in patients with primary hyperparathyroidism. *Clin Nucl Med.* 1987;12:60–64.

252. Winzelberg GG, Hydovitz JD, O'Hara KR. Parathyroid adenomas evaluated by thallium-201/technetium-99m pertechnetate subtraction scintigraphy and high resolution ultrasonography. *Radiology.* 1985;155: 231–235.

253. Simeone JF, Mueller P, Ferrucci JT. High-resolution real-time sonography of the parathyroid. *Radiology.* 1981;141:745–751.

254. Scheible W, Deutsch AL, Leopold GR. Parathyroid adenoma: accuracy of preoperative localization by high-resolution real-time sonography. *J Clin Ultrasound.* 1981;9:325–330.

255. Gooding GAW, Okerlund MD, Stark DD, Clark OH. Parathyroid imaging: comparison of double-tracer (T1-201, Tc-99m) scintigraphy and high-resolution ultrasound. *Radiology.* 1986;161:57–64.

256. Basarab RM. Parathyroid scintigraphy. In: van Nostrand D, Baum S, eds. *Atlas of Nuclear Medicine.* Philadelphia: Lippincott; 1988:115–143.

257. Peck WW, Higgins CB, Fisher MR, Ling M, Okerlund MD, Clark OH. Hyperparathyroidism: comparison of MR imaging with radionuclide scanning. *Radiology.* 1987;163:415–420.

258. Higgins CB, Auffermann W. MR imaging of thyroid and parathyroid glands: a review of current status. *AJR.* 1988;151:1095–1106.

259. Gardner TW, Zaparackas ZG, Naidich TP. Congenital optic nerve colobomas: CT demonstration. *J Comput Assist Tomogr.* 1984;8:95–102.

260. Pagon RA. Ocular coloboma. *Surv Ophthalmol.* 1981;25:223–236.

261. Weiss A, Greenwald M, Martinez C. Microphthalmos with cyst: clinical presentations and computed tomographic findings. *J Pediatr Ophthalmol Strabismus.* 1985;22:6–12.

262. Traboulsi EI, O'Neill JF. The spectrum in the morphology of the so-called "Morning glory disc anomaly." *J Pediatr Ophthalmol Strabismus.* 1988;25:93–97.

263. Mafee MF, Jampol LM, Langer BG, Tso M. Computed tomography of optic nerve colobomas, morning glory anomaly, and colobomatous cyst. *Radiol Clin North Am.* 1987;25:693–699.

264. Haik BG, St Louis L, Smith ME, Abramson DH, Ellsworth RM. Computed tomography of the nonrhegmatogenous retinal detachment in the pediatric patient. *Ophthalmology.* 1985;92:1133–1142.

265. Hopper KD, Katz NNK, Dorwart RH, Margo CE, Filling-Katz M, Sherman JK. Childhood leukokoria: computed tomographic appearance and differential diagnosis with histopathologic correlation. *RadioGraphics.* 1985; 5:377–394.

266. Sherman JL, McLean IW, Brallier DR. Coats' disease: CT-pathologic correlation in two cases. *Radiology.* 1983;146:77–78.

267. Chang MM, McLean IW, Merritt JC. Coats' disease: a study of 62 histologically confirmed cases. *J Pediatr Ophthalmol Strabismus.* 1984;21:163–168.

268. Haik BG, Saint Louis L, Smith ME, et al. Magnetic resonance imaging in the evaluation of leukocoria. *Ophthalmology.* 1985;92:1143–1152.

269. Mafee MF, Goldberg MF, Greenwald MJ, Schulman J, Malmed A, Flanders AE. Retinoblastoma and simulating lesions: role of CT and MR imaging. *Radiol Clin North Am.* 1987;25:667–682.

270. Wells RG, Miro P, Brummond R. Color-flow Doppler sonography of persistent hyperplastic primary vitreous (PHPV). *J Ultrasound Med.* (In press).

271. Mafee MF, Goldberg MF. Persistent hyperplastic primary vitreous (PHPV): role of computed tomography and magnetic resonance. *Radiol Clin North Am.* 1987;25:683–692.

272. Katz NN, Margo CE, Dorwart RH. Computed tomography with histopathologic correlation in children with leukokoria. *J Pediatr Ophthalmol Strabismus.* 1984;21:50–56.

273. Zimmerman RA, Bilaniuk LT, Metzger RA, Grossman RI, Schut L, Bruce DA. Computed tomography of orbital-facial neurofibromatosis. *Radiology.* 1983;146:113–116.

274. Reed D, Robertson WD, Rootman J, Douglas G. Plexiform neurofibromatosis of the orbit: CT evaluation. *AJNR.* 1986;7:259–263.

275. Wilbur AC, Dobben GD, Linder B. Paraorbital tumors and tumor-like conditions: role of CT and MRI. *Radiol Clin North Am.* 1987; 25:631–646.

276. Naidich TP, Zimmerman RA. Common congenital malformations of brain. In: Brant-Zawadzki MN, Norman D, eds. *Magnetic Resonance Imaging of the Central Nervous System.* New York: Raven Press; 1987:131–150.

277. Singh J, Ghose S, Vashisht S, Goulatia RK. Optic nerve hypoplasia: clinical and ultrasonographic study. *Can J Ophthalmol.* 1985;20:205–210.

278. Acers TE. Optic nerve hypoplasia septo-optic pituitary dysplasia syndrome. *Trans Am Ophthalmol Soc.* 1981;79:425–457.

279. Skarf B, Hoyt CS. Optic nerve hypoplasia in children. Association with anomalies of the endocrine and CNS. *Arch Ophthalmol.* 1984;102:62–67.

280. Zeki SM, Dutton GN. Optic nerve hypoplasia in children. *Br J Ophthalmol.* 1990;74:300–304.

281. Manelfe C, Rochiccioli P. CT of septo-optic dysplasia. *AJR.* 1979; 133:1157–1160.

282. O'Dwyer JA, Newton TH, Hoyt WF. Radiologic features of septo-optic dysplasia: de Morsier syndrome. *AJNR.* 1980;1:443.

283. Chandler JR, Langenbrunner DJ, Stevens ER. The pathogenesis of orbital complications in acute sinusitis. *Laryngoscope* 1970;80:1414–1428.

284. Hornblass A, Herschorn BT, Stern K, Grimes C. Orbital abscess. *Surv Ophthalmol.* 1984;29:169–178.

285. Shapiro ED, Wald ER, Brozanski BA. Periorbital cellulitis and paranasal sinusitis: a reappraisal. *Pediatr Infect Dis.* 1982;1:91–94.

286. Gellady AM, Shulman ST, Ayoub EM. Periorbital and orbital cellulitis in children. *Pediatrics.* 1978;61:272–277.

287. Powell KR, Kaplan SB, Hall CB, Nasello MA Jr, Roghmann KJ. Periorbital cellulitis. Clinical and laboratory findings in 146 episodes, including tear countercurrent immunoelectrophoresis in 89 episodes. *Am J Dis Child.* 1988;142:853–857.

288. Handler LC, Davey IC, Hill JC, Lauryssen C. The acute orbit: differentiation of orbital cellulitis from subperiosteal abscess by computerized tomography. *Neuroradiology.* 1991;33:15–18.

289. Hirsch M, Lifshitz T. Computerized tomography in the diagnosis and treatment of orbital cellulitis. *Pediatr Radiol.* 1988;18:302–305.

290. Eustis HS, Armstrong DC, Buncic JR, Morin JD. Staging of orbital cellulitis in children: computerized tomography characteristics and treatment guidelines. *J Pediatr Ophthalmol Strabismus.* 1986;23:246–251.

291. Rubin SE, Rubin LG, Zito J, Goldstein MN, Eng C. Medical management of orbital subperiosteal abscess in children. *J Pediatr Ophthalmol Strabismus.* 1989;26:21–26.

292. Harr DL, Quencer RM, Abrams GW. Computed tomography and ultrasound in the evaluation of orbital infection and pseudotumor. *Radiology.* 1982;142:395–401.

293. Dillon WP, Som PM, Fullerton GD. Hypointense MR signal in chronically inspissated sinonasal secretions. *Radiology.* 1990;174:73–78.

294. Puliafito CA, Baker AS, Haaf J, Foster CS. Infectious endophthalmitis: review of 36 cases. *Ophthalmology.* 1982;89:921–929.

295. Zinkhan WH. Visceral larva migrans. A review and reassessment indicating two forms of clinical expression: visceral and ocular. *Am J Dis Child.* 1978;132:627–633.

296. Margo CE, Katz NN, Wertz FD, Dorwart RH. Sclerosing endophthalmitis in children: computed tomography with histopathologic correlation. *J Pediatr Ophthalmol Strabismus.* 1983;20:180–184.

297. Char DH, Unsold R. Ocular and orbital pathology. Clinical Aspects and Newton Sobel DF, Salvolini U, Newton TH. Ocular and orbital pathology. Radiological aspects. In: Newton TH, Hasso AN, Dillon WP, eds. *Computed Tomography of the Head and Neck: Modern Neuroradiology.* New York: Raven Press; 1988;3:9.1–9.64.

298. Bishop JO. Retinoblastoma. *Pediatr Ann.* 1979;8:12–33.

299. Nicholson DH, Green WR. Tumors of the eye, lids, and orbit in children. In: Harley RD, ed. *Pediatric Ophthalmology.* Philadelphia: Saunders; 1983:1223–1271.

300. Zimmerman LE, Burns RP, Wankum G, Tully R, Esterly JA. Trilateral retinoblastoma: ectopic intracranial retinoblastoma associated with bilateral retinoblastoma. *J Pediatr Ophthalmol Strabismus.* 1982;19:320–325.

301. Knudson AG Jr, Hethcote HW, Brown BW. Mutation and childhood cancer: a probabilistic model for the incidence of retinoblastoma. *Proc Natl Acad Sci USA.* 1975;72:5116–5120.

302. Shields JA, Bakewell B, Augsburger JJ, Donoso LA, Bernardino V. Space-occupying orbital masses in children. A review of 250 consecutive biopsies. *Ophthalmology.* 1986;93:379–384.

303. Pagani JJ, Bassett LW, Winter J, Gold RH, Brawer M. Osteogenic sarcoma after retinoblastoma radiotherapy. *AJR.* 1979;133:699–702.

304. Meadows AT, D'Angio GJ, Mike V, et al. Patterns of second malignant neoplasms in children. *Cancer.* 1977;40(suppl 4):1903–1911.

305. Francois J. Retinoblastoma and osteogenic sarcoma. *Ophthalmologica.* 1977;175:185–191.

306. Abramson DH, Ellsworth RM, Kitchin FD, et al. Second nonocular tumors in retinoblastoma survivors: are they radiation induced? *Ophthalmology.* 1984;91:1351–1355.

307. White L, Miller JH. Retinoblastoma. In: Miller JH, White L, eds. *Imaging in Pediatric Oncology.* Baltimore: Williams & Wilkins; 1985:95–100.

308. Stannard C, Lipper S, Sealy R, Sevel D. Retinoblastoma: correlation of invasion of the optic nerve and choroid with prognosis and metastases. *Br J Ophthalmol.* 1979;63:560–570.

309. Reed MH, Culham JAG. Skeletal metastases from retinoblastoma. *J Can Assoc Radiol*. 1975;26:249–254.

310. Ellsworth RM. The practical management of retinoblastoma. *Trans Am Ophthalmol Soc*. 1969;67:462–534.

311. Arrigg PG, Hedges TR III, Char DH. Computed tomography in the diagnosis of retinoblastoma. *Br J Ophthalmol*. 1983;67:588–591.

312. Danziger A, Price HI. CT findings in retinoblastoma. *AJR*. 1979; 133:695–697.

313. Schulman JA, Peyman GA, Mafee MF, et al. The use of magnetic resonance imaging in the evaluation of retinoblastoma. *J Pediatr Ophthalmol Strabismus*. 1986;23:144–147.

314. Hoover DL, Robb RM, Petersen RA. Optic disc drusen in children. *J Pediatr Ophthalmol Strabismus*. 1988;25:191–195.

315. Broughton WL, Zimmerman LE. A clinicopathologic study of 56 cases of intraocular medulloepitheliomas. *Am J Ophthalmol*. 1978;85: 407–418.

316. Mafee MF, Peyman GA, McKusick MA. Malignant uveal melanoma and similar lesions studied by computed tomography. *Radiology*. 1985;156: 403–408.

317. Lagos JC, Gomez MR. Tuberous sclerosis: reappraisal of a clinical entity. *Mayo Clin Proc*. 1967;42:26.

318. Harris GJ, Williams AL, Reeser FH, Abrams GW. Intraocular evaluation by computed tomography. *Int Ophthalmol Clin*. 1982;22:197–217.

319. Youssefi B. Orbital tumors in children. A clinical study of 62 cases. *J Pediatr Ophthalmol*. 1969;6:177–185.

320. Pfeiffer RL, Nicholl RJ. Dermoid and epidermoid tumours of the orbit. *Arch Ophthalmol*. 1948;40:639–664.

321. Haye C, Haut J, Romain M. A propos des kystes dermoides de l'orbite. *Arch Ophthalmol (Paris)*. 1966;26:471–480.

322. Sherman RP, Rootman J, Lapointe JS. Orbital dermoids: clinical presentation and management. *Br J Ophthalmol*. 1984;68:642–652.

323. Baum JL, Feingold M. Ocular aspects of Goldenhar's syndrome. *Am J Ophthalmol*. 1973;75:250–257.

324. Mafee MF, Putterman A, Valvassori GE, Campos M, Capek V. Orbital space-occupying lesions: role of computed tomography and magnetic resonance imaging. An analysis of 145 cases. *Radiol Clin North Am*. 1987;25:529–559.

325. Blei L, Chambers JT, Liotta LA, DiChiro G. Orbital dermoid diagnosed by computer tomographic scanning. *Am J Ophthalmol*. 1978;85:58–61.

326. Sullivan JA, Harms SE. Surface-coil MR imaging of orbital neoplasms. *AJNR*. 1986;7:29–34.

327. Kincaid MC, Green WR. Diagnostic methods in orbital diseases. *Ophthalmology*. 1984;91:719–725.

328. Ide CH, Davis WE, Black SP. Orbital teratoma. *Arch Ophthalmol*. 1978;96:2093–2096.

329. Weiss AH, Greenwald MJ, Margo CE, Myers W. Primary and secondary orbital teratomas. *J Pediatr Ophthalmol Strabismus*. 1989; 26:44–49.

330. Hoyt WF, Joe S. Congenital teratoid cyst of the orbit. *Arch Ophthalmol*. 1962;68:196–201.

331. Plonsky L, Virapongse C, Markowitz RI. Congenital orbital teratoma. *J Comput Assist Tomogr*. 1983;7:367–369.

332. Haik BG, Jakobiec FA, Ellsworth RM, Jones IS. Capillary hemangioma of the lids and orbit: an analysis of the clinical features and therapeutic results in 101 cases. *Ophthalmology*. 1979;86:760–792.

333. Flanagan JC. Vascular problems of the orbit. *Ophthalmology (Rochester)*. 1979;86:896–913.

334. Forbes GS, Earnest F IV, Waller R. Computed tomography of orbital tumors, including late-generation scanning techniques. *Radiology*. 1982; 142:387–394.

335. Davis KR, Hesselink JR, Dallow RL, Grove AS Jr. CT and ultrasound in the diagnosis of cavernous hemangioma and lymphangioma of the orbit. *J Comput Tomogr*. 1980;4:98–104.

336. Jones IS. Lymphangiomas of the ocular adnexa: an analysis of 62 cases. *Trans Am Ophthalmol Soc*. 1959;57:602–665.

337. Iliff WJ, Green WR. Orbital lymphangiomas. *Ophthalmology*. 1979;86:914–929.

338. Lallemand DP, Brasch RC, Char DH, Norman D. Orbital tumors in children: characterization by computed tomography. *Radiology*. 1984; 151:85–88.

339. Mafee MF, Schatz CJ. The orbit. In: Som PM, Bergeron RT, eds. *Head and Neck Imaging*. 2nd ed. St. Louis: Mosby; 1991:693–828.

340. Porterfield JF. Orbital tumors in children: a report on 214 cases. *Int Ophthalmol Clin*. 1962;2:319–335.

341. McKeen EA, Bodurtha J, Meadows AT, Douglass EC, Mulvihill JJ. Rhabdomyosarcoma complicating multiple neurofibromatosis. *J Pediatr*. 1978;93:992–993.

342. Schuster SA, Ferguson EC III, Marshall RB. Alveolar rhabdomyosarcoma of the eyelid. Diagnosis by electron microscopy. *Arch Ophthalmol*. 1972;87:646–651.

343. Porterfield JF, Zimmerman LE. Rhabdomyosarcoma of the orbit: a clinicopathologic study of 55 cases. *Virchows Arch A*. 1962;335:329–344.

344. Scotti G, Harwood-Nash DC. Computed tomography of rhabdomyosarcomas of the skull base in children. *J Comput Assist Tomogr*. 1982;6:33–39.

345. Rootman J, Goldberg C, Robertson W. Primary orbital schwannomas. *Br J Ophthalmol*. 1982;66:194–204.

346. Jacoby CG, Go RT, Beren RA. Cranial CT of neurofibromatosis. *AJR*. 1980;135:553–557.

347. Woog JJ, Albert DM, Solt LC, Hu DN, Wang WJ. Neurofibromatosis of the eyelid and orbit. *Int Ophthalmol Clin*. 1982;22: 157–187.

348. Miller NR, Iliff WJ, Green WR. Evaluation and management of gliomas of the anterior visual pathways. *Brain*. 1974;97:743–754.

349. Jakobiec FA, Yeo JH, Trokel SL, et al. Combined clinical and computed tomographic diagnosis of primary lacrimal fossa lesions. *Am J Ophthalmol*. 1982;94:785–807.

350. Byrd SE, Harwood-Nash DC, Fitz CR, Barry JF, Rogovitz DM. Computed tomography of intraorbital optic nerve gliomas in children. *Radiology*. 1978;129:73–78.

351. Duffner PK, Cohen ME. Isolated optic nerve gliomas in children with and without neurofibromatosis. *Neurofibromatosis*. 1988;1:201–211.

352. DeSousa AL, Kalsbeck JE, Mealey J Jr, Ellis FD, Muller J. Optic chiasmatic glioma in children. *Am J Ophthalmol*. 1979;87:376–381.

353. Listernick R, Charrow J, Greenwald MJ, Esterly NB. Optic gliomas in children with neurofibromatosis type 1. *J Pediatr*. 1989;114:788–792.

354. Obringer AC, Meadows AT, Zackai EH. The diagnosis of neurofibromatosis-1 in the child under the age of 6-years. *Am J Dis Child*. 1989;143:717–719.

355. Stern J, DiGiacinto GV, Housepian EM. Neurofibromatosis and optic glioma: clinical and morphological correlations. *Neurosurgery*. 1979; 4:524–528.

356. Azar-Kia B, Naheedy MH, Elias DA, Mafee MF, Fine M. Optic nerve tumors: role of magnetic resonance imaging and computed tomography. *Radiol Clin North Am*. 1987;25:561–581.

357. Lourie GL, Osborne DR, Kirks DR. Involvement of posterior visual pathways by optic nerve gliomas. *Pediatr Radiol*. 1986;16:271–274.

358. Pomeranz SJ, Shelton JJ, Tobias J, Soila K, Altman D, Viamonte M. MR of visual pathways in patients with neurofibromatosis. *AJNR*. 1987;8:831–836.

359. Jakobiec FA, Depot MJ, Kennerdell JS, et al. Combined clinical and computed tomographic diagnosis of orbital glioma and meningioma. *Ophthalmology.* 1984;91:137–155.

360. Stern J, Jakobiec FA, Housepian EM. The architecture of optic nerve gliomas with and without neurofibromatosis. *Arch Ophthalmol.* 1980; 98:505–511.

361. Savoiardo M, Harwood-Nash DC, Tadmor R, Scotti G, Musgrave MA. Gliomas of the intracranial anterior optic pathways in children. The role of computed tomography, angiography, pneumoencephalography, and radionuclide brain scanning. *Radiology.* 1981;138:601–610.

362. Fletcher WA, Imes RK, Hoyt WF. Chiasmatic gliomas: appearance and longterm changes demonstrated by computed tomography. *J Neurosurg.* 1986;65:154–159.

363. Albert A, Lee BC, Saint-Louis L, Deck MDF. MRI of optic chiasm and optic pathways. *AJNR.* 1986;7:255–258.

364. Walsh FB. Meningiomas primary within the orbit and optic canal. In: Glaser JS, Smith JL, eds. *Neuro-Ophthalmology Symposium of the University of Miami and the Bascom Palmer Eye Institute.* St Louis: Mosby; 1975; 8:166–190.

365. Wilson WB. Meningiomas of the anterior visual system. *Surv Ophthalmol.* 1981;26:109–127.

366. Sarkies NJC. Optic nerve sheath meningioma: diagnostic features and therapeutic alternatives. *Eye.* 1987;1:597–602.

367. Daniels DL, Williams AL, Syvertsen A, Gager WE, Harriis GJ. CT recognition of optic nerve sheath meningioma: abnormal sheath visualization. *AJNR.* 1982;3:181–183.

368. Castillo M, Davis PC, Ross WK, Hoffman JC Jr. Case report. Meningioma of the chiasm and optic nerves: CT and MR findings. *J Comput Assist Tomogr.* 1989;13:679–681.

369. Albert DM, Rubenstein RA, Scheie HG. Tumor metastasis to the eye. II. Clinical study in infants and children. *Am J Ophthalmol.* 1967; 63:727–732.

370. Gallet BL, Egelhoff-JC. Unusual CNS and orbital metastases of neuroblastoma. *Pediatr Radiol.* 1989;19:287–289.

371. Nicholson DH, Green WR. Tumors of the eye, lids, and orbit in children. In: Harley RD, ed. *Pediatric Ophthalmology.* Philadelphia: Saunders; 1983:1223–1271.

372. Zimmerman LE, Font RL. Ophthalmologic manifestations of granulocytic sarcoma (myeloid sarcoma or chloroma). *Am J Ophthalmol.* 1975;80:975.

373. Hesselink JR, Weber AL. Pathways of orbital extension of extraorbital neoplasms. *J Comput Assist Tomogr.* 1982;6:593–597.

374. Johnson LN, Krohel GB, Yeon EB, Parnes SM. Sinus tumors invading the orbit. *Ophthalmology.* 1984;91:209–217.

375. Zollars L, Beers J, Carter A. Orbital infiltration in Letterer-Siwe disease. *J Comput Assist Tomogr.* 1984;8:137–138.

376. Hesselink JR, Davis KR, Dallow RL, Roberson GH, Taveras JM. Computed tomography of masses in the lacrimal gland region. *Radiology.* 1979;131:143–147.

377. Balchunas WR, Quencer RM, Byrne SF. Lacrimal gland and fossa masses: evaluation by computed tomography and a-mode echography. *Radiology.* 1983;149:751–758.

378. Mottow LS, Jakobiec FA. Idiopathic inflammatory orbital pseudotumor in childhood. I. Clinical characteristics. *Arch Ophthalmol.* 1978;96:1410–1417.

379. Nugent RA, Rootman J, Robertson WD, Lapointe JS, Harrison PB. Acute orbital pseudotumors: classification and CT features. *AJR.* 1981;137:957–962.

380. Khan JA, Hoover DL, Giangiacomo J, Singsen BH. Orbital and childhood sarcoidosis. *J Pediatr Ophthalmol Strabismus.* 1986;23:190–194.

381. Parelhoff ES, Chavis RM, Friendly DS. Wegener's granulomatosis presenting as orbital pseudotumor in children. *J Pediatr Ophthalmol Strabismus.* 1985;22:100–104.

382. Dresner SC, Rothfus WE, Slamovits TL, Kennerdell JS, Curtin HD. Computed tomography of orbital myositis. *AJR.* 1984;143:671–674.

383. Atlas SW, Grossman RI, Savino PJ, et al. Surface-coil MR of orbital pseudotumor. *AJNR.* 1987;8:141–146.

384. Enzmann DR, Donaldson SS, Kriss JP. Appearance of Graves' disease on orbital computed tomography. *J Comput Assist Tomogr.* 1979;3:815–819.

385. Howard CW, Osher RH, Tomsak RL. Computed tomographic features in optic neuritis. *Am J Ophthalmol.* 1980;89:699–702.

386. Edwards MK, Gilmor RL, Franco JM. Computed tomography of chiasmal optic neuritis. *AJNR.* 1983;4:816–818.

387. McCrary JA III, Demer JL, Friedman DI, Mawad MM. Computed tomography and magnetic resonance imaging in the diagnosis of inflammatory disease of the optic nerve. *Surv Ophthalmol.* 1987;31:352–355.

388. Tolly TL, Wells RG, Sty JR. Case report: MR features of fleeting CNS lesions associated with Epstein-Barr virus infection. *J Comput Assist Tomogr.* 1989;13:665–668.

389. Cabanis EA, Salvolini U, Rodallec A, Menichelli F, Pasquini C, Bonnin P. Computed tomography of the optic nerve: part II. Size and shape modifications in papilledema. *J Comput Assist Tomogr.* 1978;2:150–155.

390. Blank JP, Gill FM. Orbital infarction in sickle cell disease. *Pediatrics.* 1981;67:879–881.

391. Wolff MH, Sty JR. Orbital infarction in sickle cell disease. *Pediatr Radiol.* 1985;15:50–52.

392. Al-Rashid R. Orbital apex syndrome secondary to sickle cell anemia. *J Pediatr.* 1979;95:426.

393. National Society for the Prevention of Blindness. *Data Analysis: Vision Problems in the US.* New York: National Society for the Prevention of Blindness; 1978;24–33.

394. Gallagher SS, Stock L, Bromberg J, Mierzwa K. Childhood and adolescent eye injuries: an overlooked problem. SCIPP Reports (Boston, MA, Statewide Childhood Injury Prevention Program, Massachusetts Department of Public Health). Fall, 1984, 1–3.

395. DeRespinis PA, Caputo AR, Fiore PM, Wagner RS. A survey of severe eye injuries in children. *Am J Dis Child.* 1989;143:711–716.

396. Ball JB. Direct oblique sagittal CT of orbital wall fractures. *AJNR.* 1987;8:147–154.

397. Peyman GA, Mafee H, Schulman J. Computed tomography in choroidal detachment. *Ophthalmology.* 1984;91:156–162.

398. Whyte AM, Byrne JV. A comparison of computed tomography and ultrasound in the assessment of parotid masses. *Clin Radiol.* 1987; 38:339–343.

399. Mandelblatt SM, Braun IF, Davis PC, et al. Parotid masses: MR imaging. *Radiology.* 1987;163:411–414.

400. Rand PK, Ball WS Jr, Kulwin DR. Congenital nasolacrimal mucoceles: CT evaluation. *Radiology.* 1989;173:691–694.

401. Berkowitz RG, Grundfast KM, Fitz C. Nasal obstruction of the newborn revisited: clinical and subclinical manifestations of congenital nasolacrimal duct obstruction presenting as a nasal mass. *Otolaryngol Head Neck Surg.* 1990;103:468–471.

402. Delvert JP, Lafon J. Embryology of the temporal bone. In: Vignaud J, Jardin C, Rosen L, eds. *The Ear. Diagnostic Imaging. CT Scanner, Tomography, and Magnetic Resonance.* New York: Masson; 1986:1–7.

403. Vignaud J, Laval-Jeantet M. Anatomy of the temporal bone and the ear. In: Vignaud J, Jardin C, Rosen L, eds. *The Ear. Diagnostic Imaging. CT Scanner, Tomography, and Magnetic Resonance.* New York: Masson; 1986:8–26.

404. Altman F. Congenital atresia of the ear in man and animals. *Am J Otol Rhinol Laryngol.* 1955;64:824–857.

405. Nager GT, Levin LF. Congenital aural atresia: embryology, pathology, genetics classification and surgical management. In: Paparella

MM, Shumrick DA, eds. *Otolaryngology*. Philadelphia: Saunders, 1980;2:1303–1344.

406. Swartz JD, Wolfson RJ, Marlow FI, et al. External auditory canal dysplasia: CT evaluation. *Laryngoscope*. 1985;95:841–845.

407. Swartz JD, Glazer AU, Faerber EN, et al. Congenital middle ear deafness: CT study. *Radiology*. 1986;159:187–190.

408. Hough JVD. Congenital malformations of the middle ear. *Acta Otolaryngol*. 1963;78:335–343.

409. Sakai M, Miyake H, Shinkawa A, Komatsu N. Klippel-Feil syndrome with conductive deafness and histological findings of removed stapes. *Ann Otol Rhinol Laryngol*. 1983;92(2 pt 1):202–206.

410. Cremers CJ, Hoogland GA, Kuyperss W. Hearing loss in the cervico-oculo-acoustic (Wildervanck) syndrome. *Arch Otolaryngol*. 1984; 110:54–57.

411. Schild JA, Mafee MF, Miller MF. Wildervanck syndrome—the external appearance and radiologic findings. *Int J Pediatr Otorhinolaryngol*. 1984;7:305–310.

412. Harwood-Nash DC. Fractures of the petrous and tympanic parts of the temporal bone in children: a tomographic study of 35 cases. *Am J Roentgenol Radium Ther Nucl Med*. 1970;110:598–607.

413. Schaffer KA, Haughton VM, Wilson CR. High-resolution computed tomography of the temporal bone. *Radiology*. 1980;134:409–414.

Index

Note: Italic page numbers refer to non-text material.

C